Biopsy of Bone
in Internal Medicine

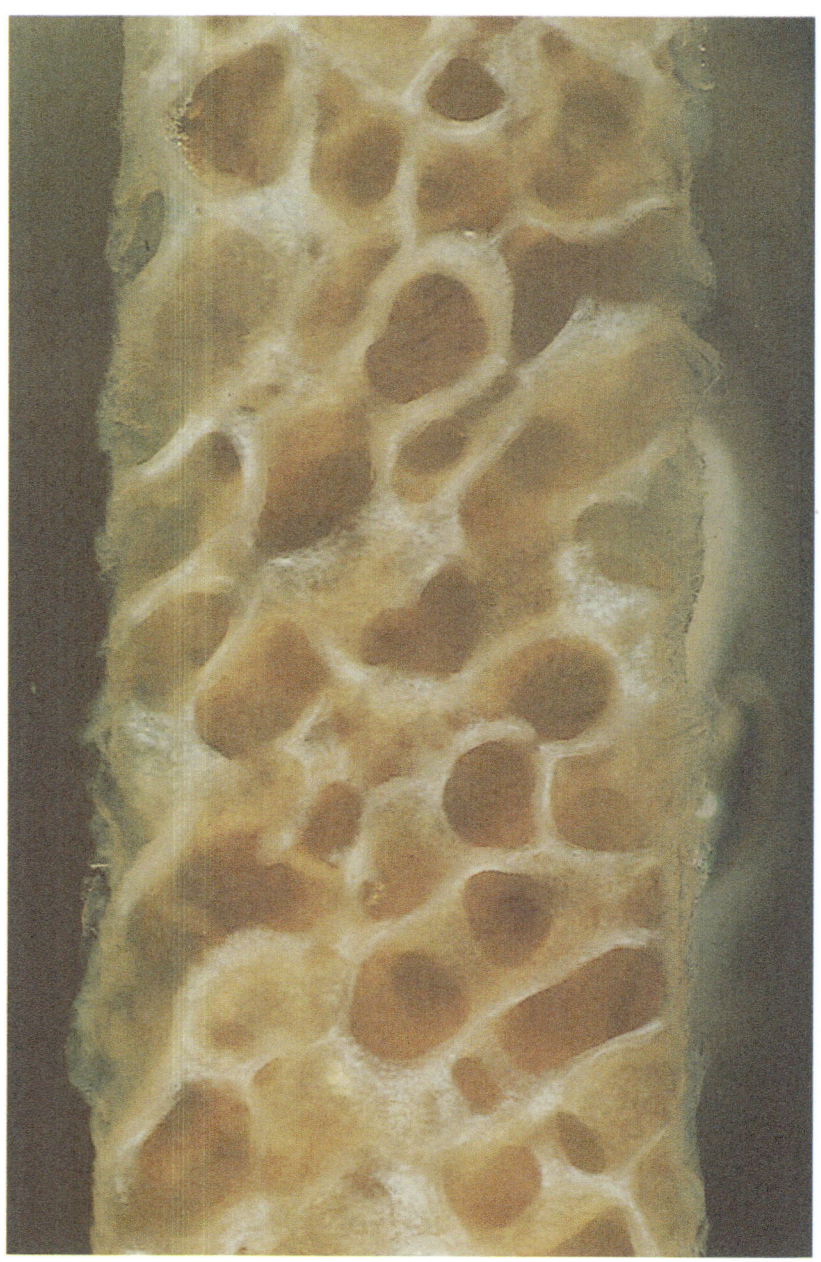

Overview of an iliac crest biopsy (diameter of 4 mm, surface of a trimmed plastic block) showing a normal trabecular structure

Current Histopathology

Consultant Editor
Professor G. Austin Gresham, TD, ScD, MD, FRCPath.
Professor of Morbid Anatomy and Histology, University of Cambridge

Volume Twenty-one

BIOPSY OF BONE IN INTERNAL MEDICINE
AN ATLAS AND SOURCEBOOK

BY
R. BARTL
Unit for Bone and Bone Marrow Diagnosis
Department of Internal Medicine III
Klinikum Großhadern,
University of Munich,
Germany

and

B. FRISCH
Department of Hematology,
Chaim Sheba Medical Center,
Tel-Hashomer
and
Sackler School of Medicine
Tel-Aviv University
Israel

Most X-rays and computed tomographs kindly supplied by Dr B. Mayr, Department of Radiology, Klinikum Großhadern, University of Munich, Germany.

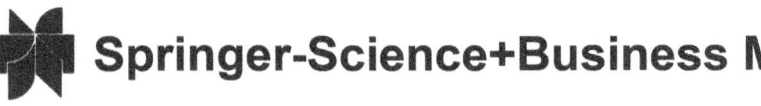

Springer-Science+Business Media, B.V.

A catalogue record for this book is available
from the British Library.

ISBN 978-0-7923-8802-9   ISBN 978-94-011-2222-1 (eBook)
DOI 10.1007/ 978-94-011-2222-1

Copyright

Contents

Current Histopathology Series

Consultant Editor's Note

At the present time books on morbid anatomy and histopathology can be divided into two broad groups: extensive textbooks often written primarily for students and monographs on research topics.

This takes no account of the fact that the vast majority of pathologists are involved in an essentially practical field of general diagnostic pathology providing an important service to their clinical colleagues. Many of these pathologists are expected to cover a broad range of disciplines and even those who remain solely within the field of histopathology usually have single and sole responsibility within the hospital for all this work. They may often have no colleagues in the same department. In the field of histopathology, no less than in other medical fields, there have been extensive and recent advances, not only in new histochemical techniques but also in the type of specimen provided by new surgical procedures.

There is a great need for the provision of appropriate information for this group. This need has been defined in the following terms:

1. It should be aimed at the general clinical pathologist or histopathologist with existing practical training, but should have value for the trainee pathologist.

2. It should concentrate on the practical aspects of histopathology taking account of the new techniques which should be within the compass of the worker in a unit with reasonable facilities.

3. New types of material, e.g. those derived from endoscopic biopsy should be covered fully.

4. There should be an adequate number of illustrations on each subject to demonstrate the variation in appearance that is encountered.

5. Colour illustrations should be used wherever they aid recognition.

Bone biopsy is an increasing part of the work of the histopathologist. Correct interpretation is achieved by cooperation between clinician, haematologist, oncologist and histopathologist. This book is therefore aimed at workers in several aspects of medicine. It will be a valuable addition to the bench manuals of the general histopathologist.

G. A. Gresham

Introduction and aims

Over the past two decades there has been increasing awareness of skeletal participation in numerous disorders in the field of internal medicine as well as in haematology and oncology in which disciplines involvement of the bones has long been appreciated.

The elucidation of the role of osseous tissues in electrolyte balance and associated homeostatic mechanisms, and the demonstration of the sensitivity and reactivity of bone cells to numerous local stimuli and systemic factors (some identified, others still putative), have completely eradicated the concept of bone as a more or less static organ. Thus, bone and its disorders are now studied from the points of view of the anatomist, physiologist, biochemist, cellular and molecular biologist, immunologist, pathologist, physician and surgeon.

Consequently, results of observations and investigations on bone and its cells are widely dispersed in journals relating to these disciplines, in addition to those in journals devoted to calcified tissues. However, a single relatively comprehensive text based on a survey of the literature is not yet available.

Another important aspect is the inter-relationship between bone and marrow. The bones form the framework of the body and protect vital organs such as brain, heart, lungs and bone marrow. But whereas other organs are distinct and separate entities, the bone marrow constitutes an integral part of bone, with which it has a common blood supply. Marrow is required for the maintenance and repair of bone, it provides precursors for the renewal of bone cells, as well as hormones, growth factors and cytokines for its resorption and formation in numerous disorders in internal medicine.

In this volume we have attempted

1. to survey as much as possible the information available in the literature on metabolic and metastatic bone disease, including where possible review articles, and updates on the present state of knowledge;
2. to summarize the data already derived from numerous studies on iliac crest biopsies;
3. to estimate the value of the iliac crest biopsy itself in relation to the diseases in which it is employed as a diagnostic tool; and

4. to present the results of our own experience with approximately 70 000 biopsies of patients with internal medical, haematological and oncological disorders in which the skeleton is involved.

This text deals with osseous disorders most frequently encountered in internal medicine, as well as some that might be considered in the differential diagnosis of various systemic diseases. References to the enormous amount of work done *in vitro* and on animals cannot be included in this book; though sometimes an article which made a point of particular interest to the subject under discussion is referred to.

We hope that this volume will be of use to physicians in internal medicine, haematology and oncology, as well as to pathologists dealing with the interpretation of the bone biopsies.

As in our previous Atlas of the same series *Atlas of Bone Marrow Pathology*, the magnifications of most of the illustrations have been omitted. The magnifications most frequently used are indicated in Fig. 2.S7. In addition, not every detail specifically indicated in a figure or its legend is necessarily mentioned in the text and often a range of observations is illustrated and in these cases the legends are self-explanatory.

ACKNOWLEDGEMENTS

The authors wish to thank all doctors who referred patients or sent biopsies, as well as the technical staff of the laboratories.

We would like to express our appreciation and gratitude to the editor, Mr Phil Johnstone, for his help and advice at every step in the process of producing this volume.

The design and production of the coloured sketches were kindly supported by Boehringer Mannheim®.

We would like to express our appreciation to Professor W. Wilmanns, Director of the Department of Internal Medicine III, University of Munich, for his support and encouragement.

THE SKELETON

Bone, as other connective tissues, consists of cells, fibres and ground substance. But unlike the others, the major part of its extracellular compartment is calcified thus converting it into an extremely hard, rigid structure, ideally suited for its supportive, locomotive and protective *functions*. The skeleton maintains the shape of the body while protecting soft vital organs in the cranial and thoracic cavities. The skeleton also protects and constitutes the framework and part of the microenvironment for the haematopoietic tissue – the blood-forming elements of the bone marrow. It provides facilities for the attachment of the tendons and muscles required for locomotion. In addition to these mechanical functions, the skeleton is the body's major depot for minerals and the regulator of their homeostasis: over 99% of the total body calcium is stored in the skeleton[1,4,12,17,54,134,137,150].

The *axial skeleton* – the trunk – is distinguished from the *appendicular skeleton* – the extremities – by differences in weight-bearing and other functions. Metabolic and inflammatory manifestations as well as metastatic tumour invasion affect various skeletal sites in different ways[63,127,138]. Comprehensive reviews of skeletal structure and function are given in refs 1,12,54,86,94,120,125, 137,138,140,150.

STRUCTURE OF BONES (Plates 1.A–O)

Macroscopically the long bones of the extremities, the flat bones (skull and pelvis), and the short irregular bones (vertebral and carpal bones) consist of an outer shell (cortex) of compact, *cortical bone* and an interior composed of a network of ossicles, trabecular, spongy, *cancellous bone* (Fig. 1.S1)[54,96,104,134]. The normal variations in width and porosity of the cortical bone in the iliac crest are illustrated in Plates 1.G–J and those of the trabecular network in Fig. 1.S2 and Plates 1.A–F. About 80% of the total bone volume is compact, consisting of over 90% matrix with a soft-tissue content of 10% or less. The remaining 20% of bone is cancellous in the form of a three-dimensional lattice of branching bony spicules delimiting a labyrinthine system of intercommunicating spaces[136,139]. This trabecular network encloses either haematopoietic or fatty bone marrow (Fig. 1.S3) and is an important supporting structure for the outer cortices in virtually all bones, except the mid-shaft of the long bones. The spongy structure gives mechanical strength without the disadvantage of undue weight, and the thickest trabeculae are arranged in the direction subjected to the greatest mechanical forces, the trajectorial lines. The cancellous bone with its extensive surface area (about 10 m²!), its lining cells and adjacent sinusoids and its close relationship to the bone marrow, is the site where pathological changes frequently occur and are most readily recognized.

Long bones are divided into three main regions[125,134]: the cylindrical central shaft, or *diaphysis*, and the two

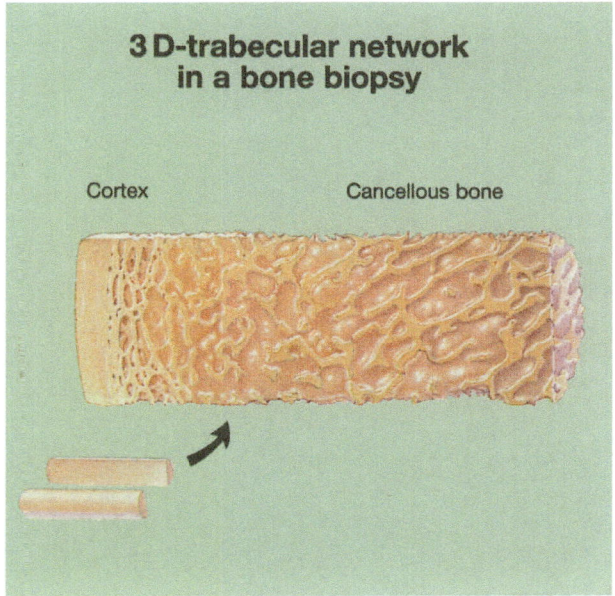

Fig. 1.S1 Three-dimensional sketch of longitudinally cut iliac crest biopsy

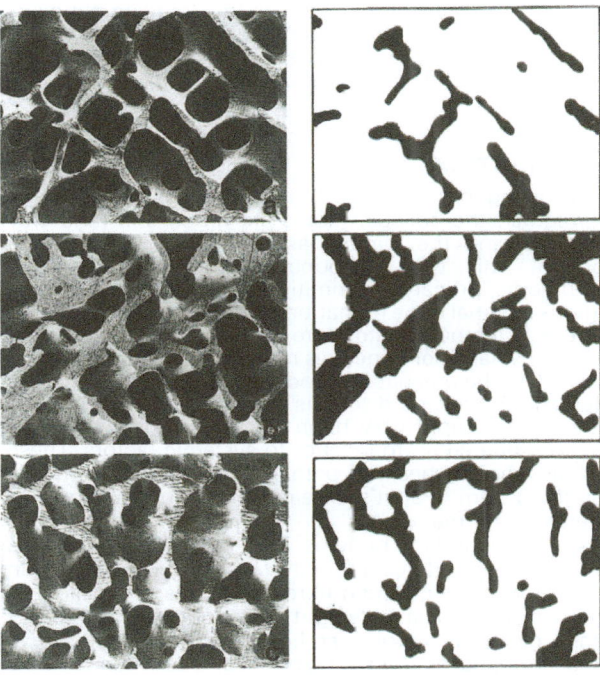

Fig. 1.S2 Scanning electron microscope view of cut and polished surface of trabecular bone of iliac crest of young adult, illustrating variability in trabecular network: **(a)** cancellous bone consisting of fine rods anastomosing to form a meshwork, and showing narrow trabecular plates and moderate anisotropy of pattern. **(b)** Uneven bone architecture with variable bone volumes, trabecular widths and anisotropy, and **(c)** dense trabecular structure consisting of plates and some rods to form a nearly isotropic meshwork. (Reproduced and modified with permission from W. J. Whitehouse (1977). Cancellous bone in the anterior part of the iliac crest. *Calcif. Tissue Res.*, **26**, 67). Diagrams of the corresponding cut surfaces at right

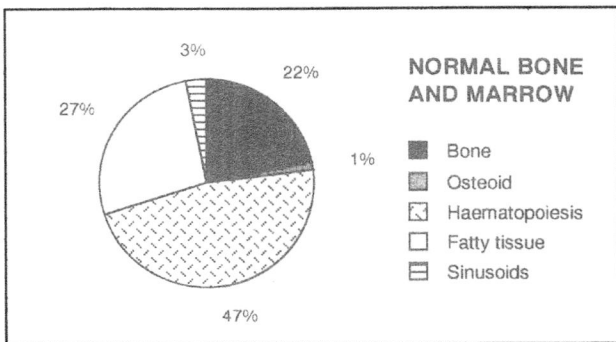

Fig. 1.S3 Histomorphometry of normal bone and marrow components in posterior iliac crest, young to middle-aged individuals

expanded ends, the *epiphyses*. Connecting the diaphysis with each epiphysis is a cone-shaped region, the *metaphysis*. In the child the epiphysis is separated from the metaphysis by a plate of hyaline cartilage known as the *growth plate* (Plate 1.K)[125,150]. On completion of growth this plate is replaced by trabecular bone.

The outer surfaces of the skeleton are covered by a specialized connective tissue, the *periosteum*, which also has osteogenic potential during growth and fracture healing. The cavities of the cancellous and compact bone, i.e. the trabecular and Haversian surfaces, are lined by a layer of thin cells, the *endosteum* (= subcortical and trabecular surfaces) (Plates 1.M–O). It should be pointed out that this endosteal surface constitutes an extremely large area for interchange between the fluid compartment of bone and the systemic circulation. In addition, it is at this endosteal surface that most of the bone remodelling, i.e. resorption and formation, occurs.

BONE MATRIX

In the histogenesis of bone, the first osseous tissue formed is irregular; the collagen fibres are broad and randomly arranged, and the matrix has a relatively low mineral content. This type of bone is called *woven bone* (embryonic, primary, or primitive bone); it is produced in regions of initial bone formation in the embryo[112]. Primitive bone is a temporary structure that is either replaced by secondary, lamellar bone or is removed to mould the bone cavities. In the postnatal period it develops only at special sites and in specific disorders. In adults, woven bone is indicative of rapid new bone formation and high bone turnover due either to local or to systemic factors. These include fracture healing, primary and secondary hyperparathyroidism, Paget's disease of bone, osteomyelosclerosis, and metastases.

Adult, secondary bone is laid down in layers, the *lamellar bone* (Plates 1.D–F,I) (Figs 1EM.1–6). Within each lamella the collagen fibres are thin and parallel but oriented at approximately right angles to those in adjacent lamellae[124]; thus in polarized light microscopy successive lamellae appear as alternating bright and dark bands[80]. The lamellae differ in appearance and in diameter according to their mineralization age. At the outer and inner cortical surfaces, and in the trabeculae, the lamellae are parallel to the surface (the circumference or surface lamellae). In the intermediate areas the lamellae form cylinders (*osteons*) surrounding a central cavity (*Haversian canal*) which contains blood vessels and soft connective tissue elements. The numbers of concentric lamellae vary from a few to 20. The Haversian canals are 30–70 μm in

[continued on p. 27]

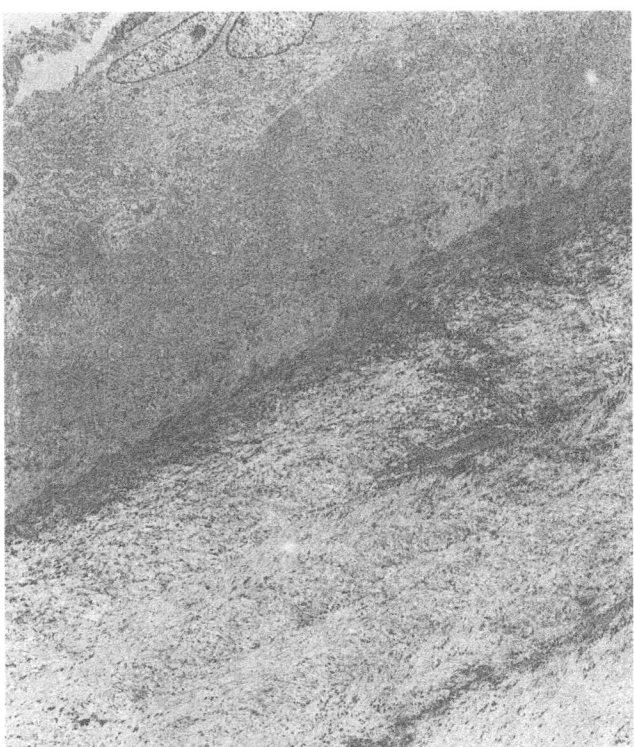

Figs. 1.EM1–EM4 Fine structure of trabecular surface and bone matrix

Fig. 1.EM1 Part of trabecular surface showing osteoblasts (upper left), osteoid and calcification front (centre), and lamellae containing one osteocyte. EM × 1640

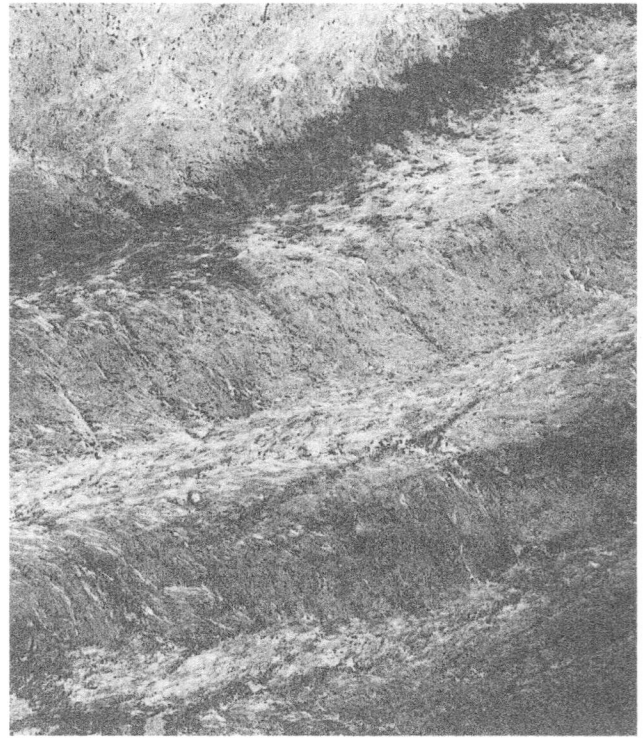

Fig. 1.EM2 Fine structure of bone matrix illustrating the alternating arrangement of collagen fibrils in the lamellae. EM × 4920

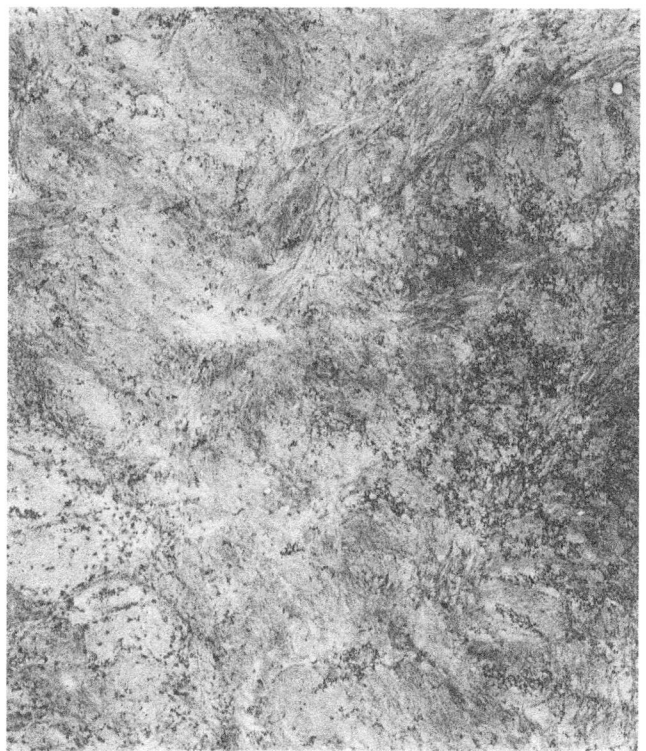

Fig. 1EM3 Collagen fibrils showing lack of lamellar organization with numerous ossification vesicles. EM × 6560

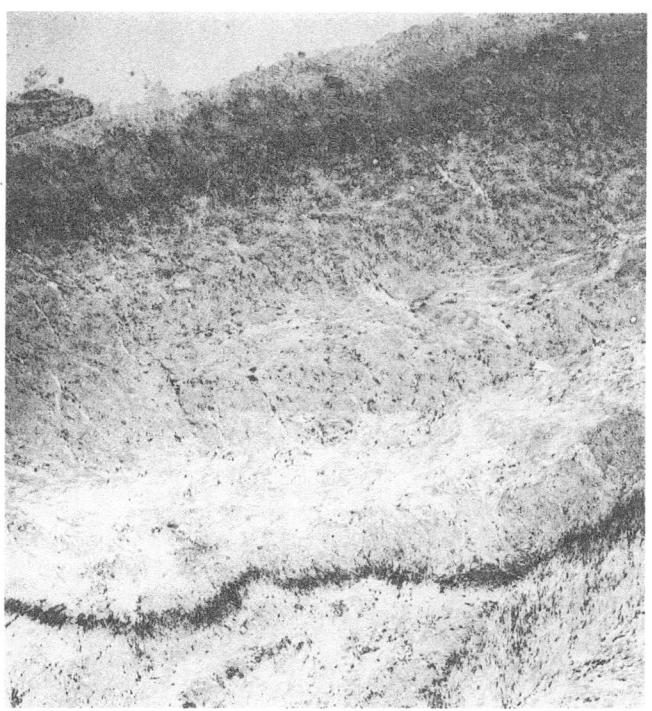

Fig. 1.EM5 Trabecular surface showing part of endosteal cell (above), partially mineralized bone matrix and cement line (below). EM × 1600

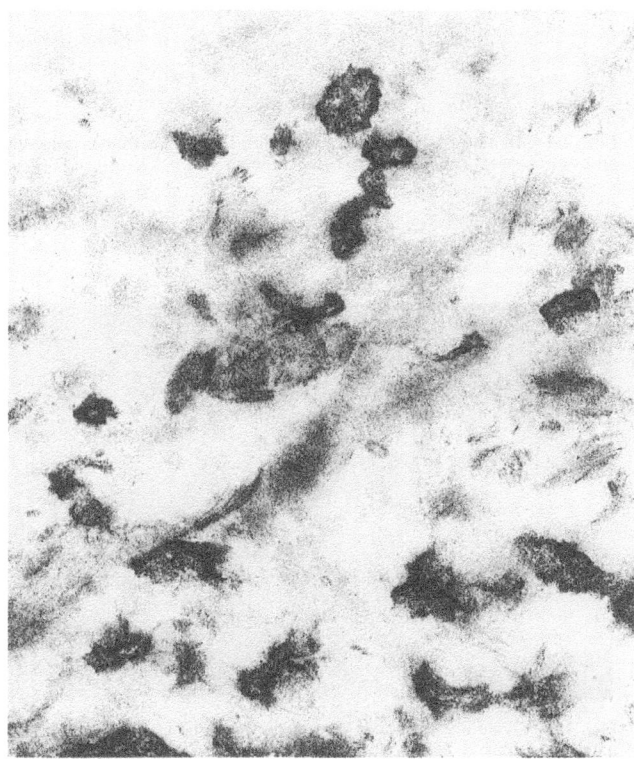

Fig. 1.EM4 Higher magnification of calcification vesicles. EM × 41000

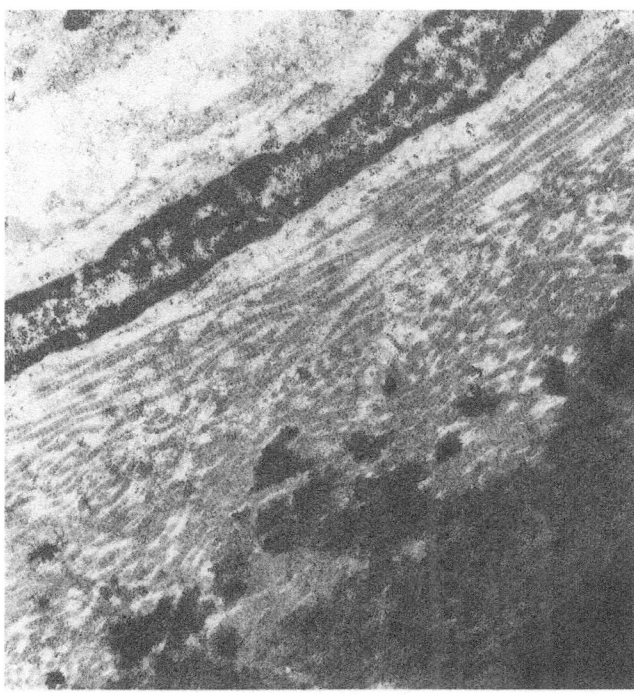

Fig. 1.EM6 Fine structure of bone matrix. Note banded collagen fibrils below the endosteal lining cell and calcifying bone matrix (bottom centre and right). EM × 16400

Plate 1.A

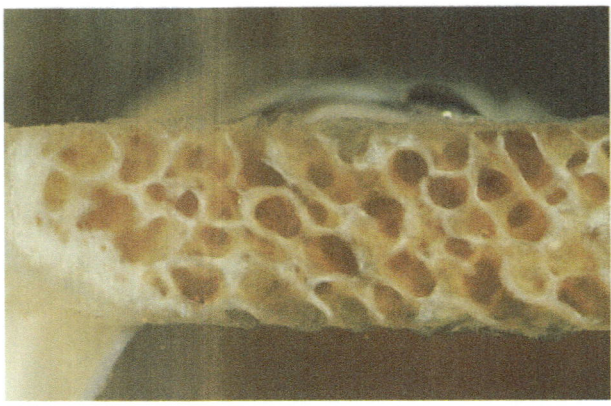

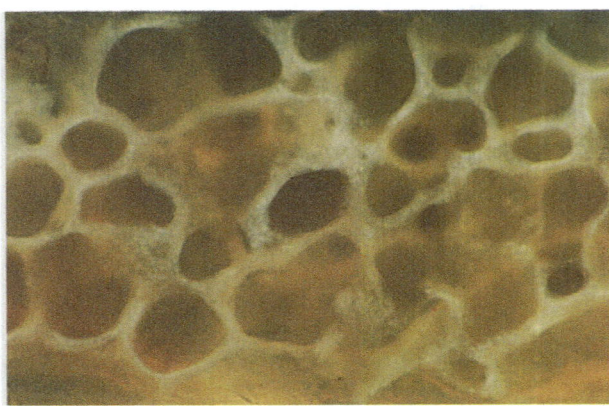

Figs. 1.1–1.6 Aspects of trabecular structure in iliac crest biopsy I

Fig. 1.1 Overview of an iliac crest biopsy (diameter 4 mm, surface of a trimmed plastic block) showing a normal cortex, a fairly uniform trabecular structure, but a moderate anisotropy of pattern

Fig. 1.2 Surface of a trimmed plastic block showing a fairly uniform trabecular network

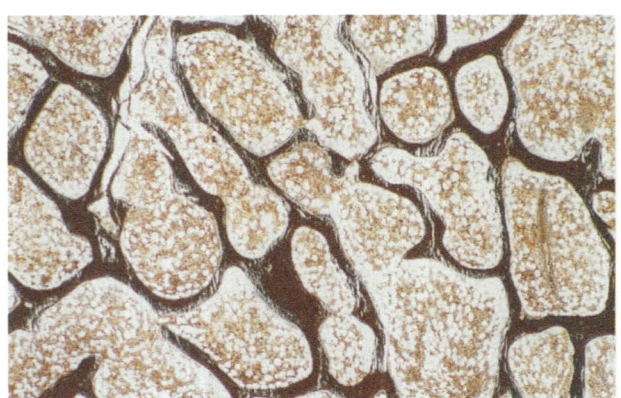

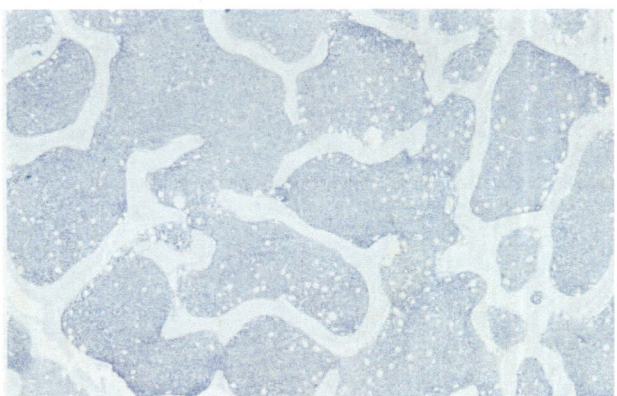

Fig. 1.3 Section of biopsy shown in Fig. 1.1. Gomori

Fig. 1.4 Section of iliac crest biopsy with normal trabecular network and with few fat cells in the marrow. Giemsa

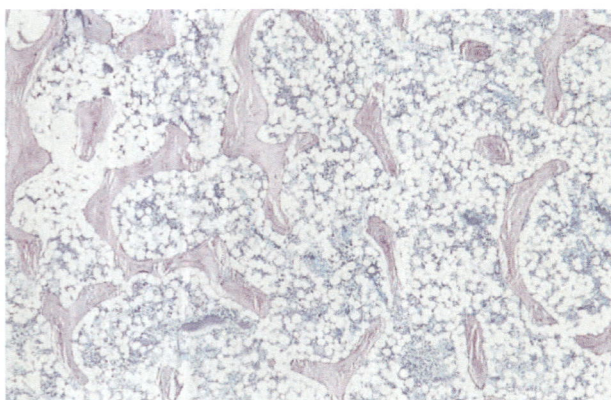

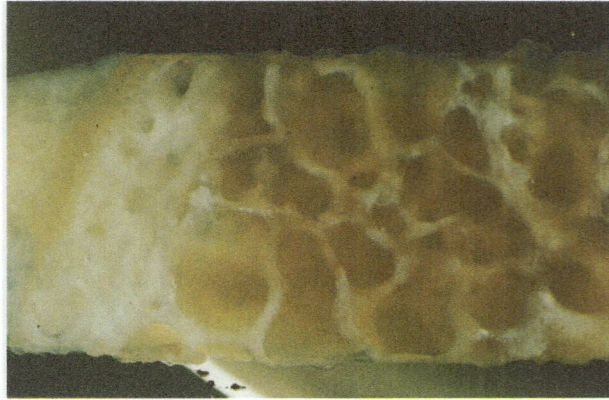

Fig. 1.5 Section of iliac crest biopsy with incipient reduction in trabecular bone, decrease of connected trabeculae and increase in fat cells in the marrow. Haematoxylin and eosin (H&E)

Fig. 1.6 Overview of an iliac crest biopsy (diameter 4 mm, surface of a trimmed plastic block) composed of periosteum (left), broad and spongiosa-like cortex, and uniform trabecular structure with wide marrow spaces

Plate 1.B

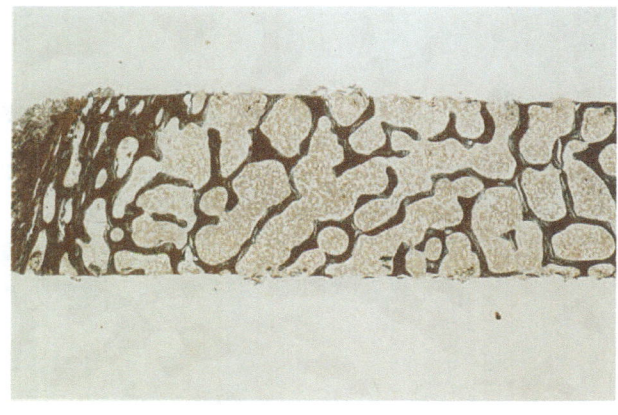

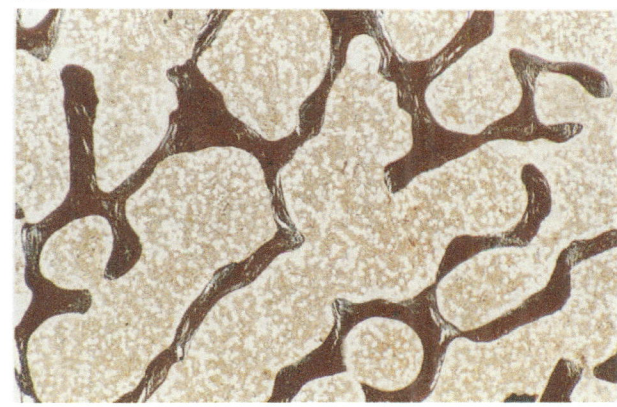

Figs. 1.7–1.12 Aspects of trabecular structure in iliac crest biopsy II

Fig. 1.7 Overview of section of bone biopsy of middle-aged man showing wide cortex and uniform, connected trabecular plates. Gomori

Fig. 1.8 Higher magnification of part of Fig. 1.7. Gomori

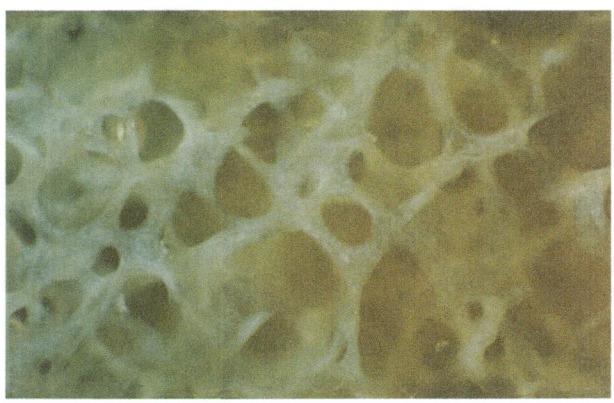

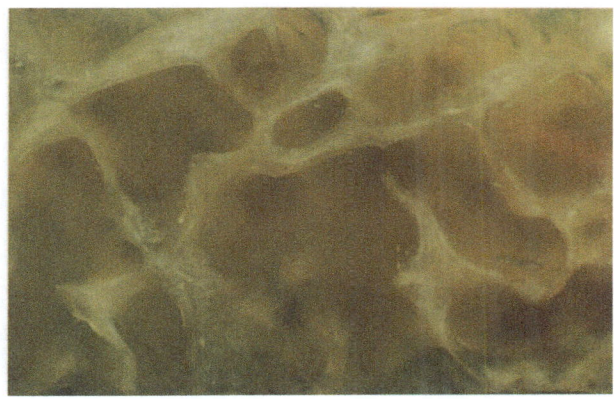

Figs. 1.9 and 1.10 Surfaces of trimmed plastic blocks

Fig. 1.9 Dense trabecular network with small marrow cavities (left)

Fig. 1.10 Widely spaced trabeculae with large marrow spaces

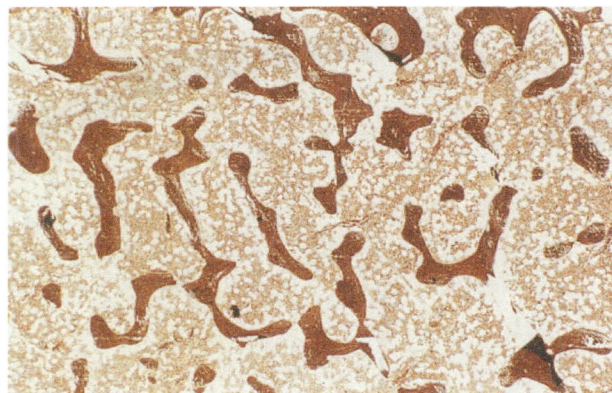

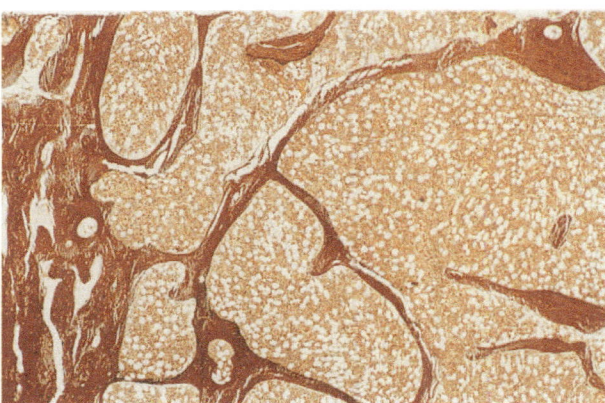

Fig. 1.11 Bone biopsy of young man, section with normal trabecular volume but partial 'discontinuity' of trabecular network. Gomori

Fig. 1.12 Bone biopsy of older man, section showing attenuated but mainly connected trabecular network, with decreased trabecular bone volume on histomorphometry. Gomori

Plate 1.C

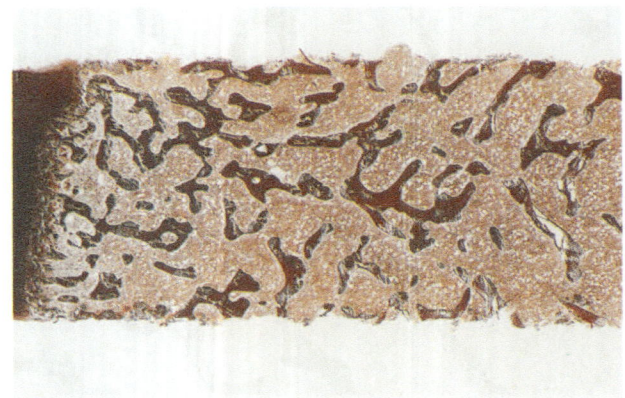

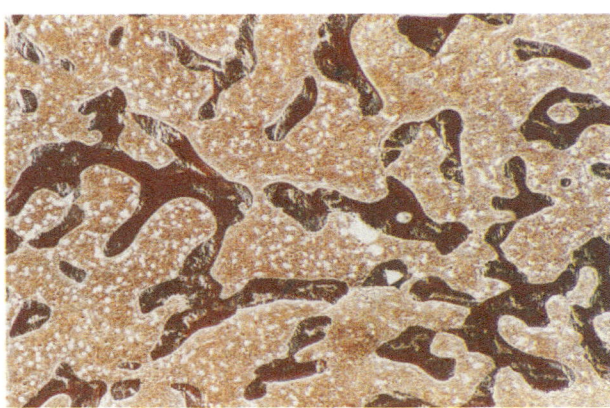

Figs 1.13–1.18 Aspects of trabecular structure in bone biopsy III

Fig. 1.13 Bone biopsy of a 12-year-old child showing growth plate (left), dense but occasionally 'discontinuous' trabeculaer network in subcortical area and more widely separated trabeculae in the 'deeper' part of the biopsy. Gomori

Fig. 1.14 Higher magnification of part of subcortical area shown in Fig. 1.13. Gomori

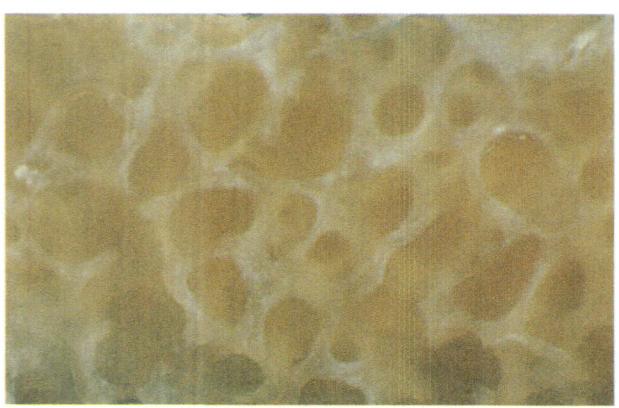

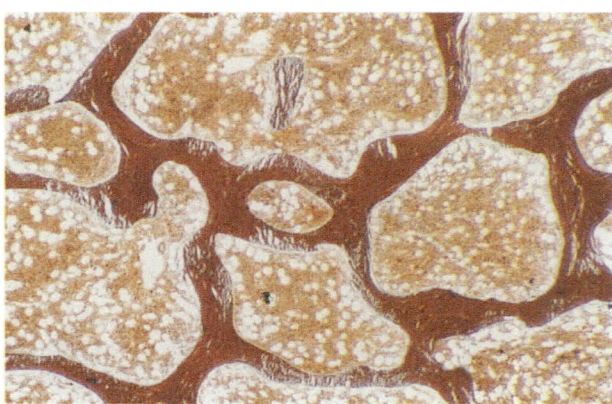

Figs. 1.15 and **1.16** Biopsy of athlete illustrating stout trabecular network

Fig. 1.15 Surface of trimmed plastic block

Fig. 1.16 Section of the same biopsy. Gomori

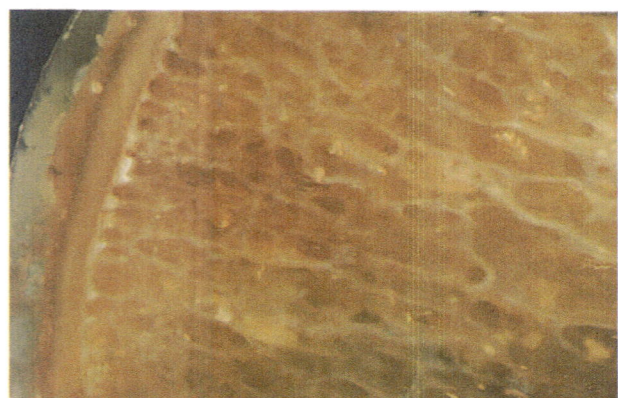

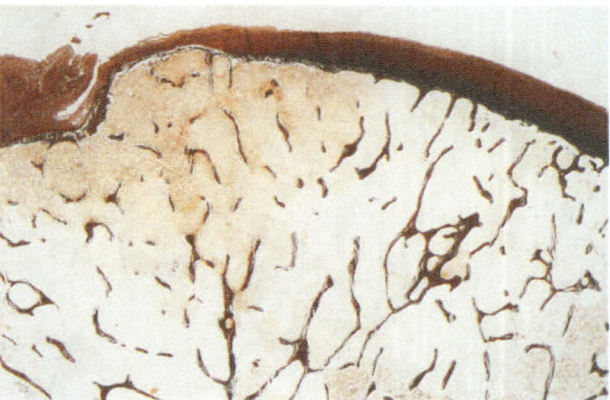

Figs. 1.17 and **1.18** Surgical biopsy of the femoral head of an older patient

Fig. 1.17 Surface of trimmed plastic block

Fig. 1.18 Biopsy section showing variability but no decrease in cortical width and greatly attenuated trabecular network. Note haematopoietic marrow largely replaced by fat cells. Gomori

Plate 1.D

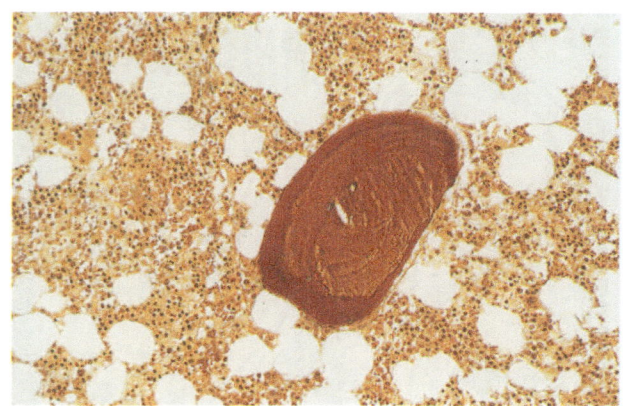

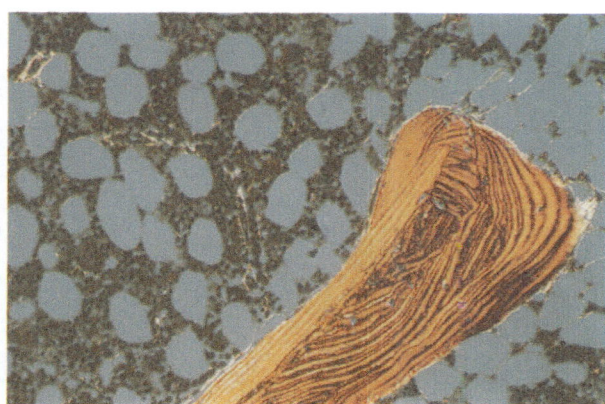

Figs 1.19–1.24 Lamellar structure of cancellous bone in iliac crest biopsy

Fig. 1.19 Transverse section of ossicle with concentric lamellae and osteoid seam. Gomori

Fig. 1.20 Longitudinally cut ossicle with mainly parallel arrangement of lamellae. Note blood vessel (upper left). Gomori, polarized light (polar.)

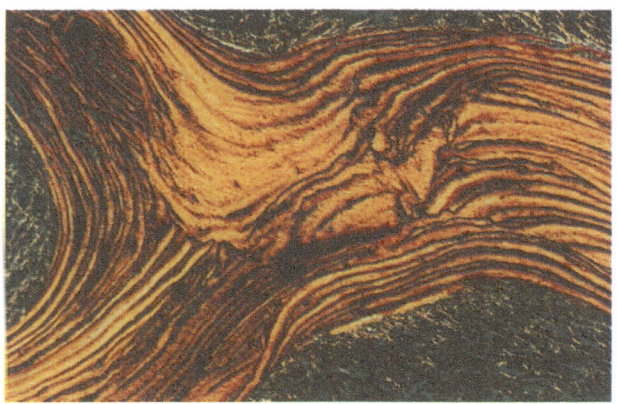

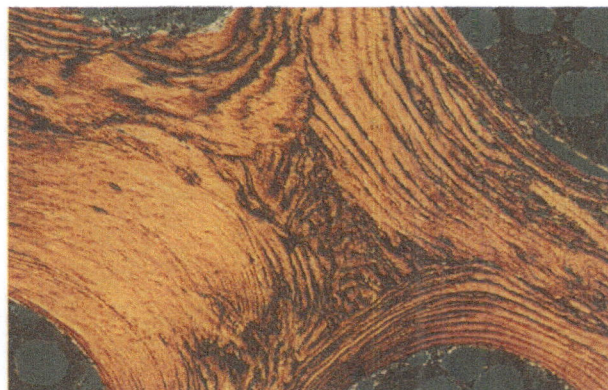

Fig. 1.21 Junction between three trabeculae showing parallel, continuous lamellar orientation. Gomori, polar.

Fig. 1.22 Broad trabecular intersection (packet) without Haversian system. Gomori, polar.

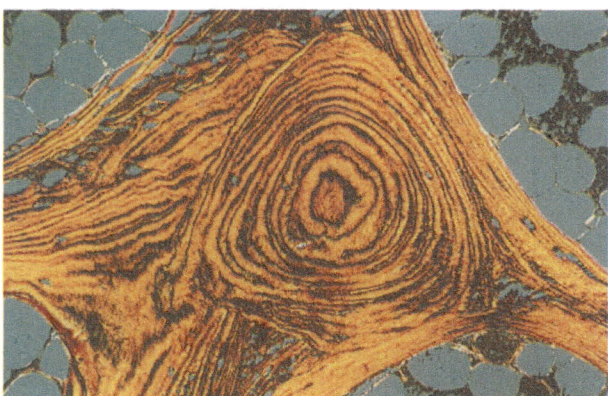

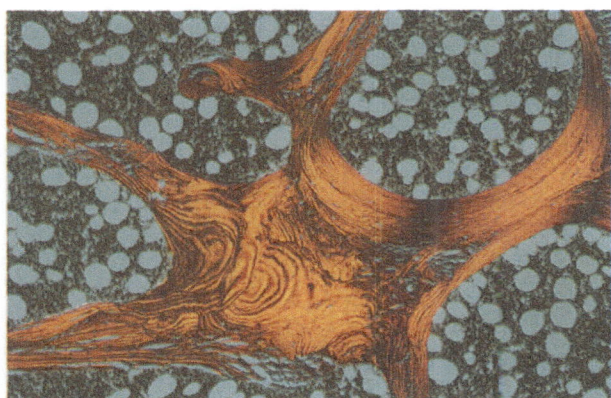

Fig. 1.23 Intersection of four trabeculae showing osteon with concentric lamellae. Gomori, polar.

Fig. 1.24 Intersection of five trabeculae showing osteon with concentric lamellae. Gomori, polar.

Plate 1.E

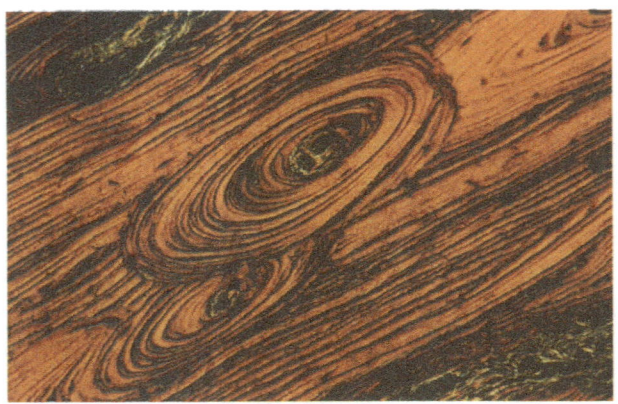

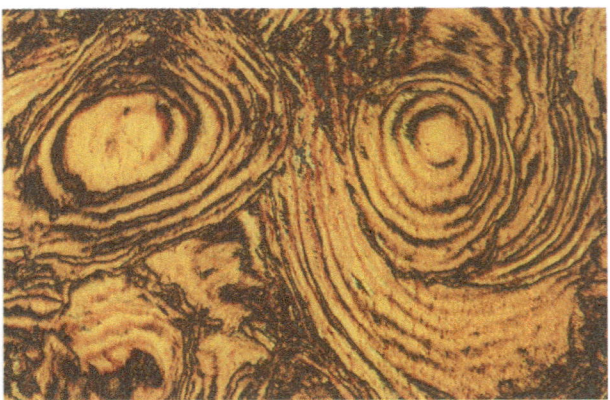

Figs 1.25–1.30 Aspects of lamellar organization and cement lines in cancellous bone

Fig. 1.26 Intersection showing two connected osteons with concentric lamellae. Gomori, polar.

Fig. 1.25 Broad trabeculae with longitudinal and concentric lamellae. Gomori, polar.

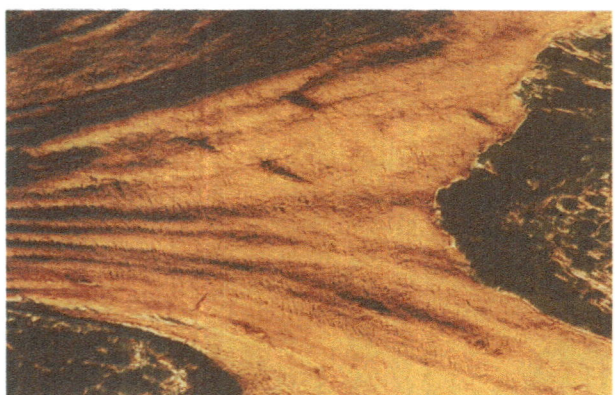

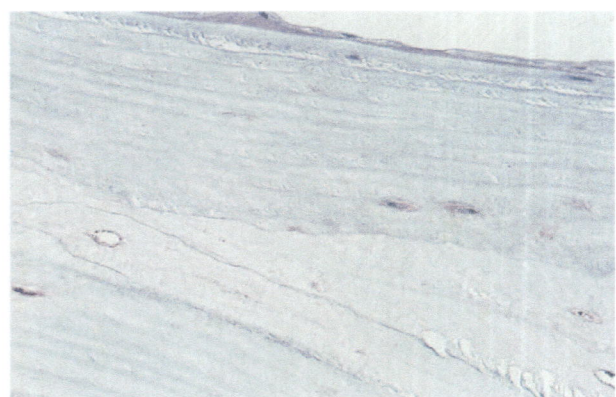

Fig. 1.27 Part of trabecula showing parallel but divergent lamellae. Gomori, polar.

Fig. 1.28 Trabecula showing central zone of 'old' mineralized lamellar bone to which layers of lamellar bone have been added (above and below) and separated by cement lines. Giemsa

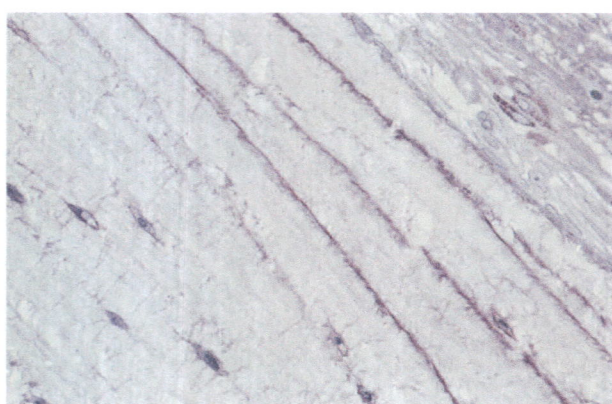

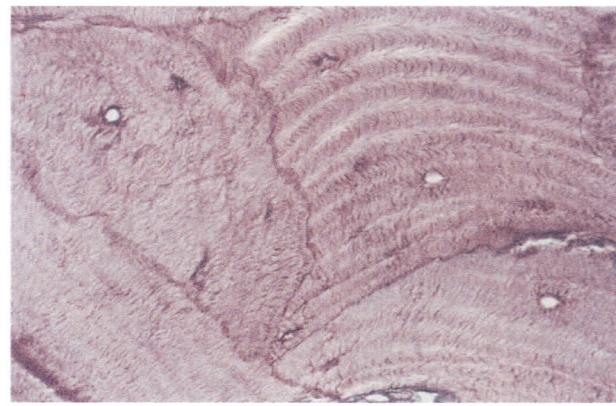

Fig. 1.29 Part of trabecula with multiple, distinct and parallel cement lines. Giemsa

Fig. 1.30 Broad ossicle with multiple, irregular cement lines partly resembling the 'mosaic structure' characteristic for Paget's disease of bone. H&E

Plate 1.F

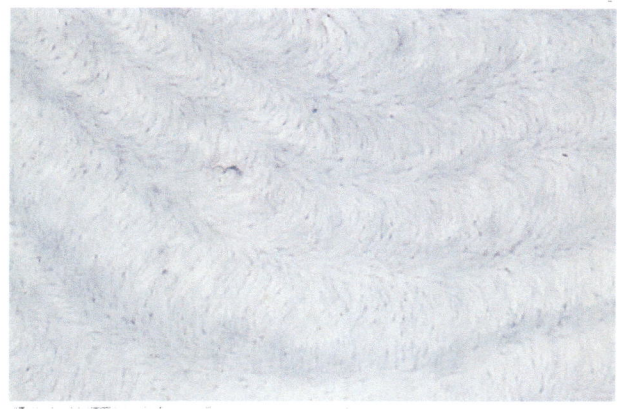

Fig. 1.31 High magnification of parallel lamellae illustrating the variable arrangement of collagen fibres. Giemsa

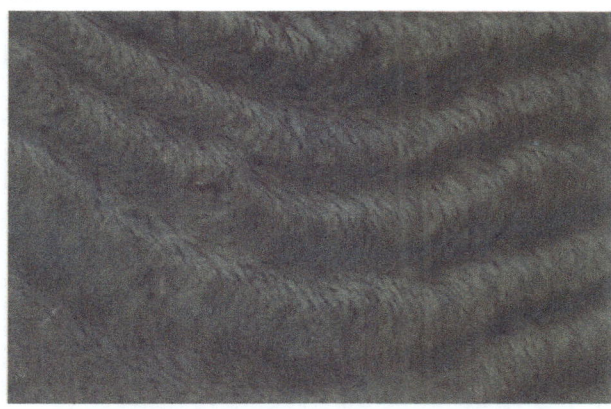

Fig. 1.32 Alternating light and dark 'undulating' lamellae due to arrangement of the collagen fibrils. Fig. 1.31 under po arized light

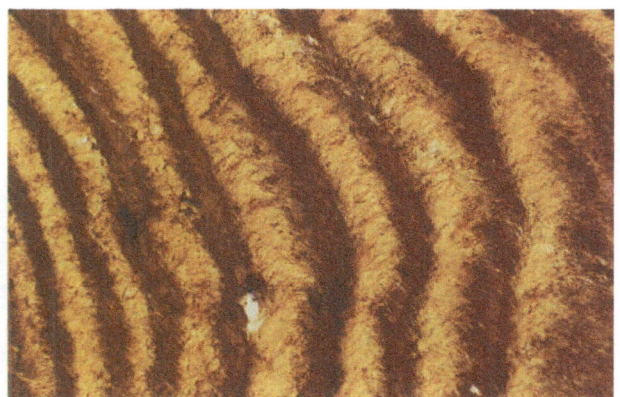

Fig. 1.33 Alternating light and dark 'undulating' lamellae due to arrangement of the collagen fibres. The small white hole represents a transversely cut osteocytic canaliculus. Gomori, polar.

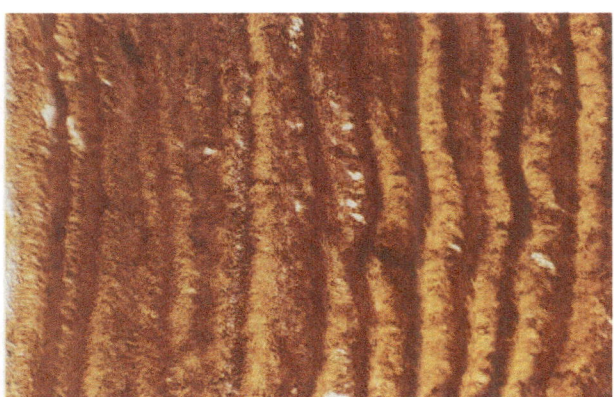

Fig. 1.34 Zones of lamellar maturation ranging from endosteal surface (left) to the mature, sharply delineated lamellae in deeper regions of the ossicle (right). Gomori, polar.

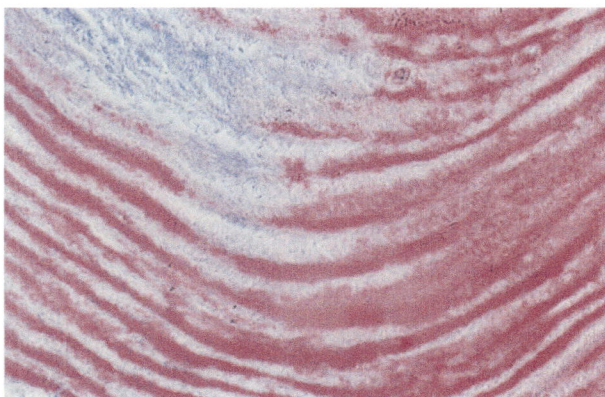

Fig. 1.35 Unmineralized lamellae (red) and patch of mineralized bone (blue). Ladewig

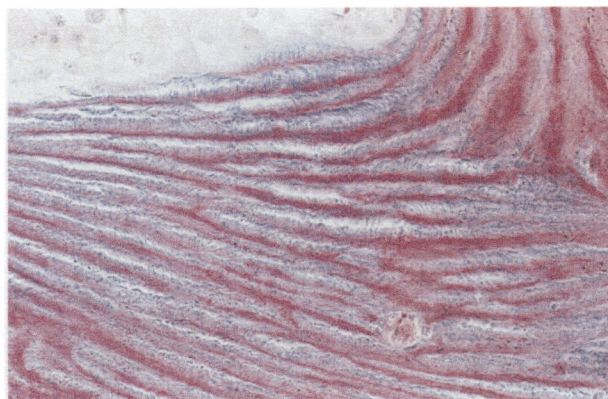

Fig. 1.36 Layers of alternating unmineralized (red) and mineralized (blue) lamellae. Ladewig

Plate 1.G

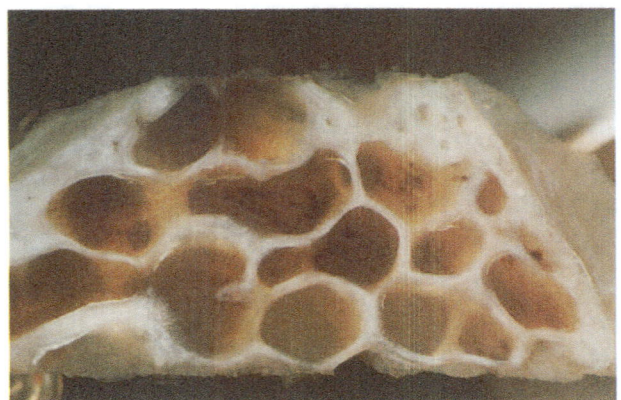

Figs 1.37–1.42 Aspects of cortical bone in iliac crest biopsy I

Fig. 1.37 Plastic-embedded iliac crest biopsy, view of surface of trimmed block ready for sectioning. Note variability of cortical width, and of size of intertrabecular spaces

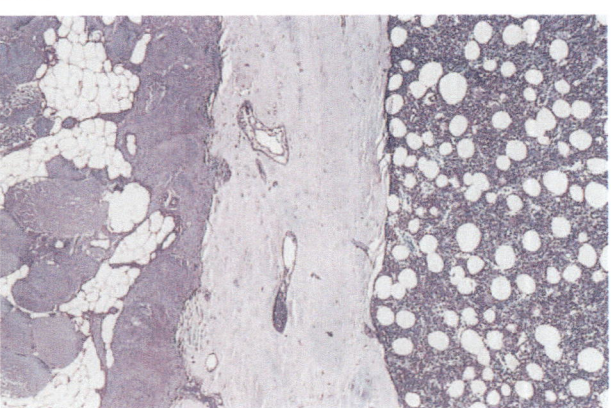

Fig. 1.38 Section showing periosteal tissues (left), solid cortex and normocellular bone marrow. Giemsa

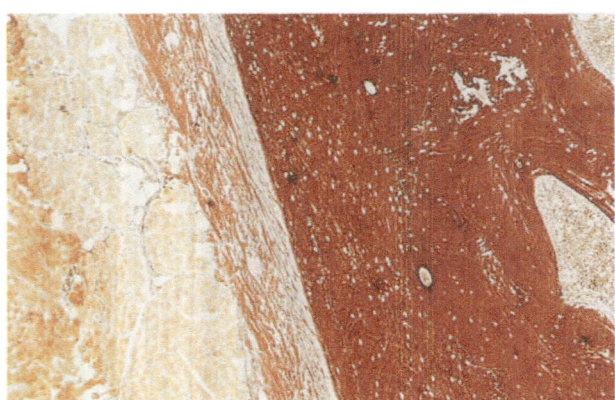

Fig. 1.39 Section showing muscle, periosteal tissues and solid cortex with part of ossicle. Gomori

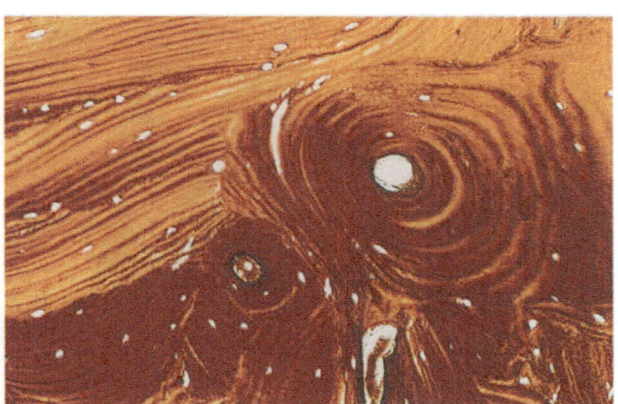

Fig. 1.40 Higher magnification of cortex of Fig. 1.39 showing longitudinal (upper left) and concentric arrangement of lamellae around a Haversian canal. The small white 'spots' are osteocytic lacunae. Gomori, polar.

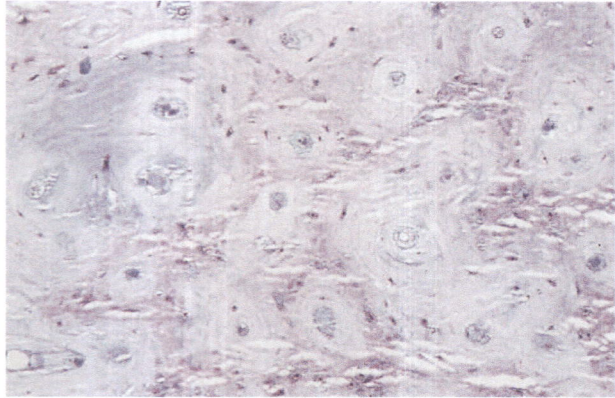

Fig. 1.41 Part of cortex, punctuated by many small canals. Giemsa

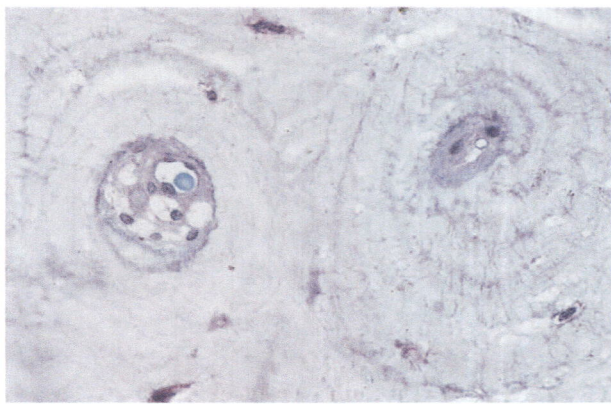

Fig. 1.42 Higher magnification of part of Fig. 1.41 showing one wide and one narrow canal. Giemsa

Plate 1.H

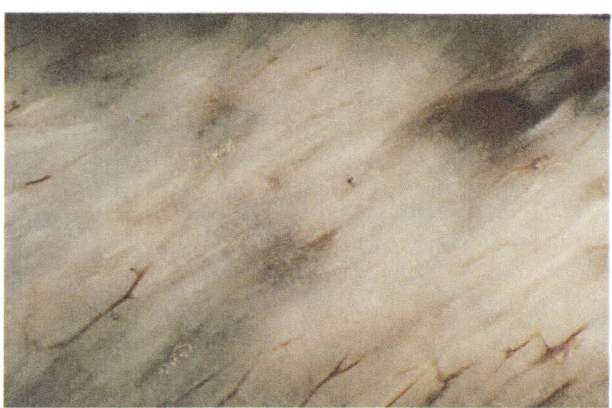

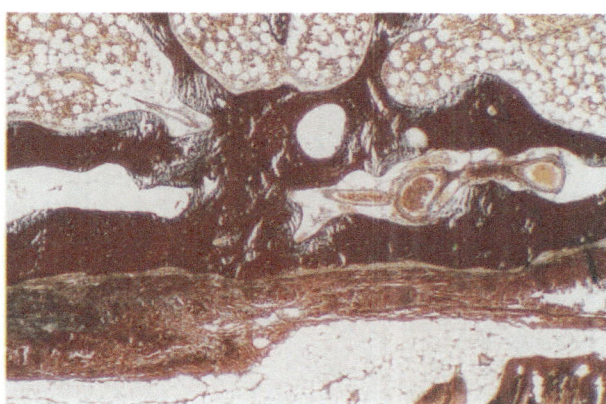

Figs. 1.43–1.48 Aspects of cortical bone in iliac crest biopsy II

Fig. 1.43 High-power view of surface of trimmed plastic block showing blood vessels (thin, slanting reddish-brown lines (lower right) traversing the cortex)

Fig. 1.44 Cortex showing perforating nutrient artery (centre), with subcortical region (upper part) and periosteum, fatty tissue and muscle (lower part). Gomori

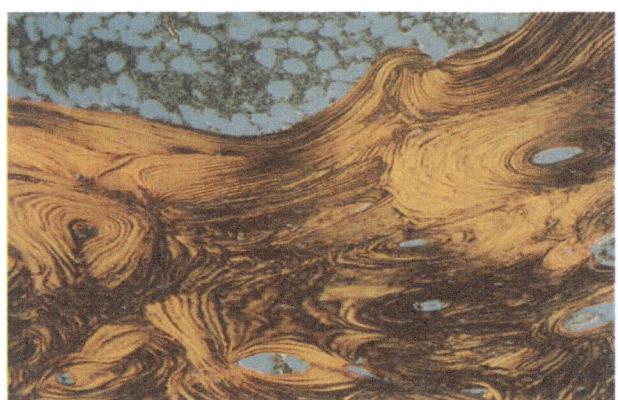

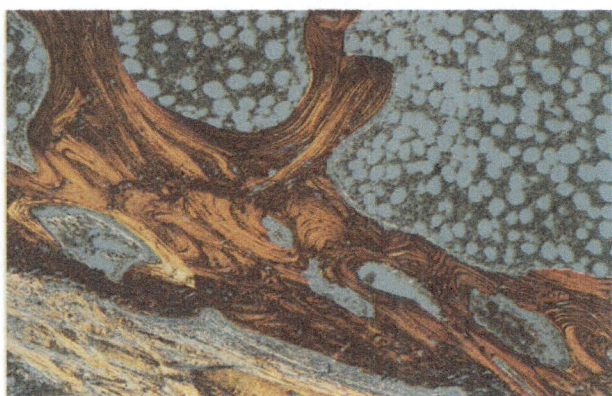

Fig. 1.45 Wide cortex with variably sized Haversian systems. Gomori, polar.

Fig. 1.46 Different cortical area from section shown in Fig. 1.45, smaller, porous cortex with parts of ossicles. Gomori, polar.

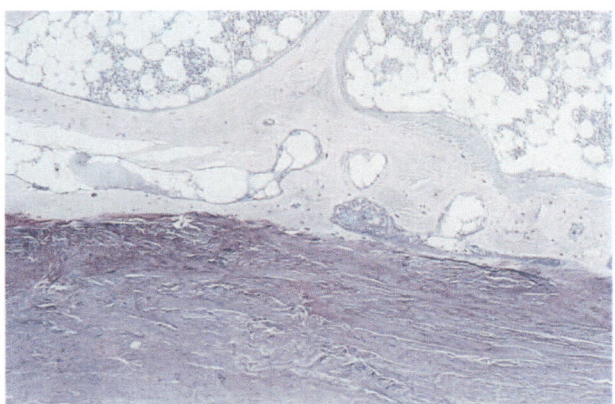

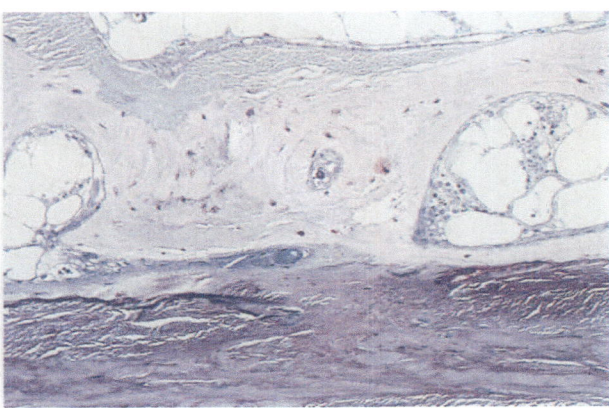

Fig. 1.47 Narrow cortex porous mainly on the periosteal side. Giemsa

Fig. 1.48 Different area from section shown in Fig. 1.47. Note marrow within the cortex and remodelling on the subcortical endosteal surface. Giemsa.

Plate 1.I

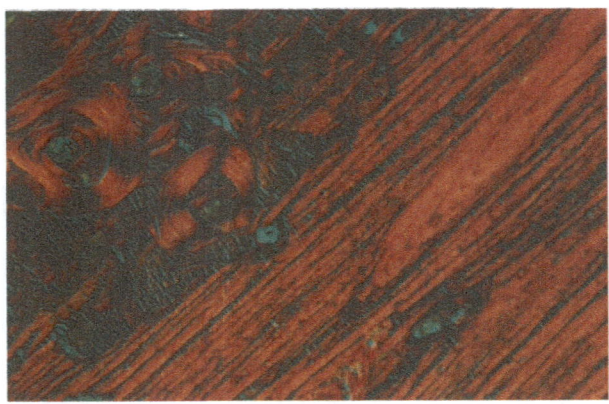

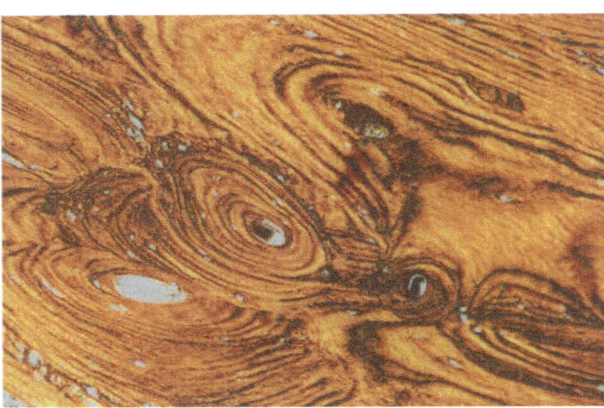

Figs. 1.49–1.54 Aspects of lamellar organization in cortical bone

Fig. 1.49 Longitudinal and concentric arrangement of lamellae of a broad cortex. Gomori, polar.

Fig. 1.50 Cortex predominantly consisting of parallel lamellae, and some variably sized Haversian systems (lower left). Gomori, polar.

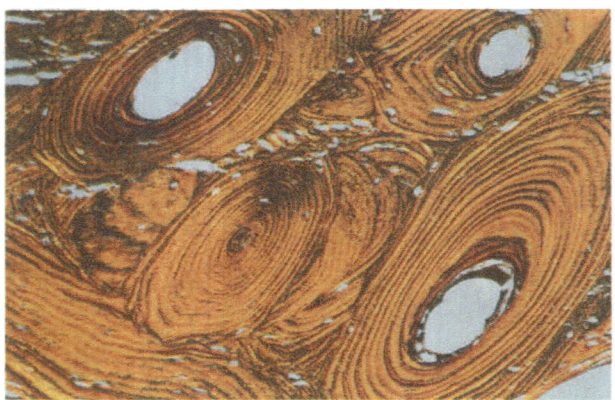

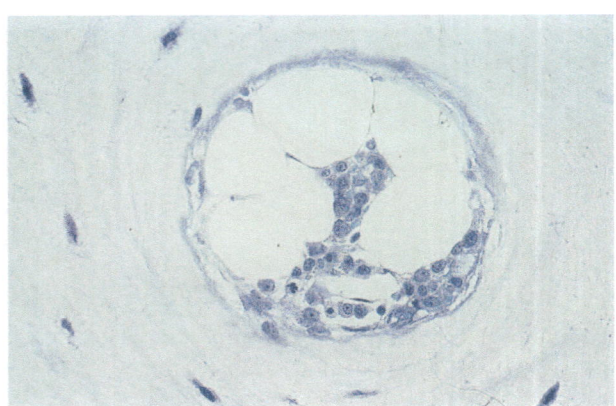

Fig. 1.51 Cortex predominantly consisting of large, sharply delineated Haversian systems. Gomori, polar.

Fig. 1.52 Osteon with concentric lamellae, osteocytes, some fat cells and haematopoietic precursors in the central canal. Giemsa

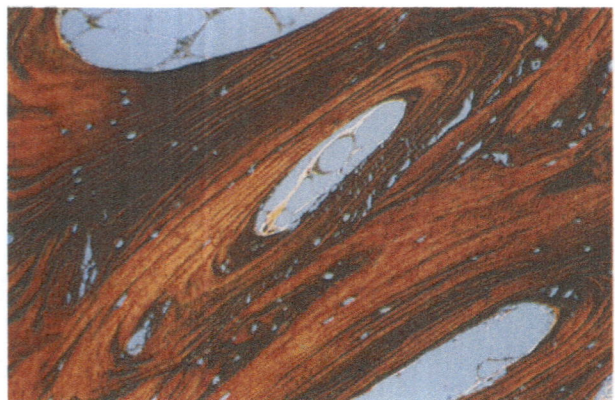

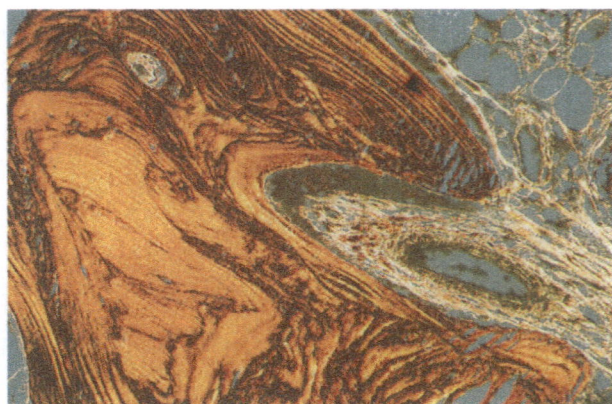

Fig. 1.53 Osteon-like lamellar organization in the subcortical region, with three small marrow cavities. Gomori, polar.

Fig. 1.54 Cortex with subcortical surface showing perforating nutrient artery within fine fibre network. Gomori, polar.

Plate 1.J

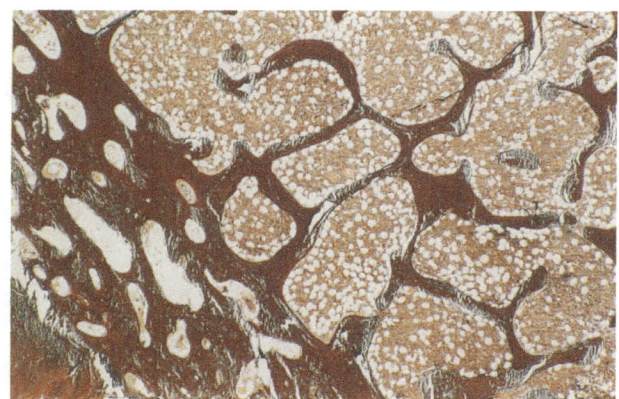

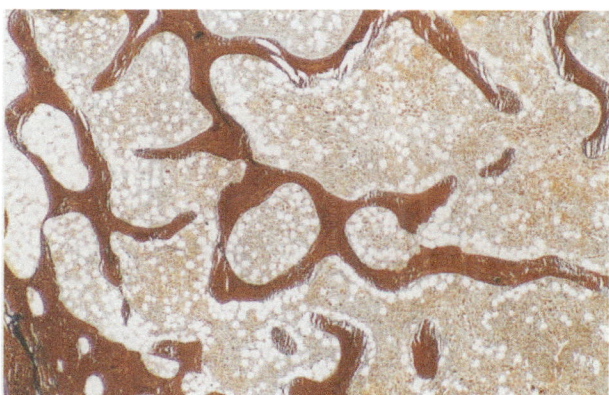

Figs. 1.55–1.60 Variations in cortical structure

Fig. 1.55 Porous compacta, normal trabecular network and normocellular bone marrow. Gomori

Fig. 1.56 Part of porous compacta (lower left), normal trabecular network in the subcortical zone and thin ossicles in the central area. Gomori

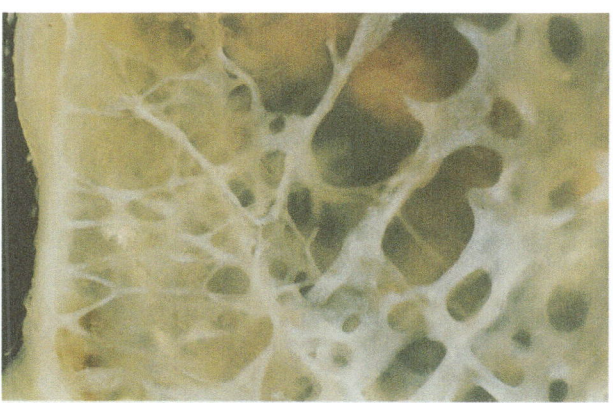

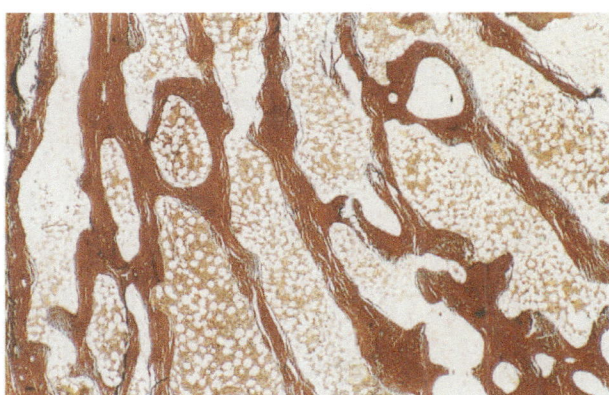

Fig. 1.57 Surface of trimmed plastic block. Note thin, narrow cortex (left) and variability of trabecular network: almost thread-like in subcortical area, to stout broad ossicles on right

Fig. 1.58 Section of biopsy in which the compacta is replaced by series of closely spaced longitudinal trabeculae. Gomori

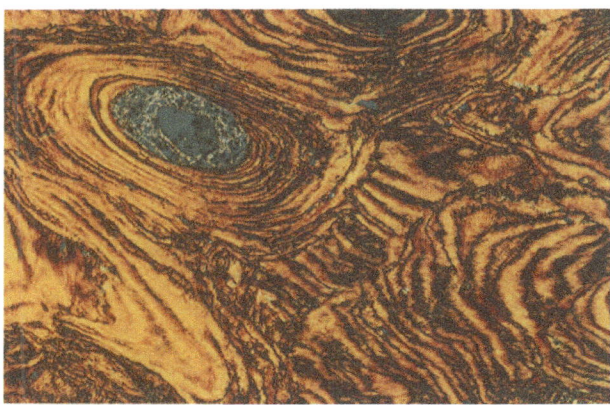

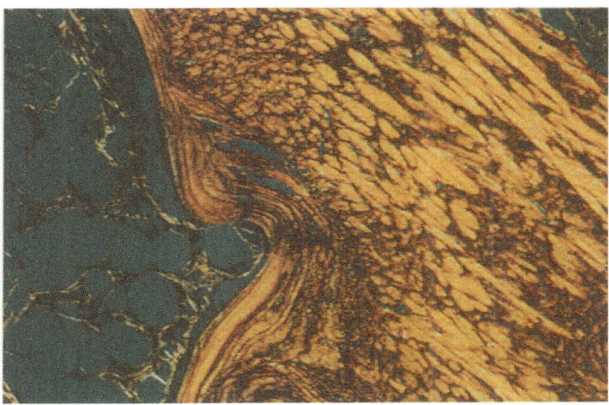

Fig. 1.59 Compacta of older individual showing incipient disorganization of lamellar structure (left). Gomori, polar.

Fig. 1.60 Compacta of 75-year-old patient: instead of parallel layers, the lamellae show a lattice-like arrangement. Gomori, polar.

Plate 1.K

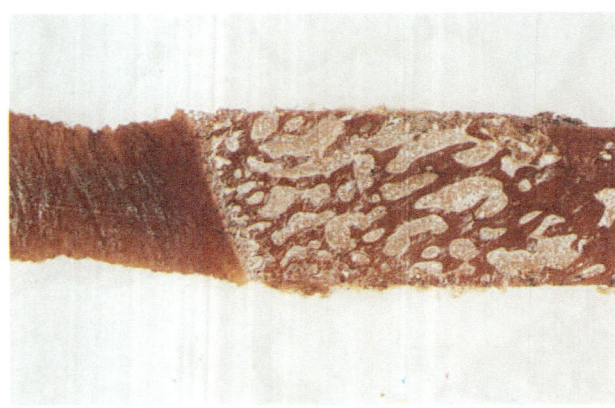

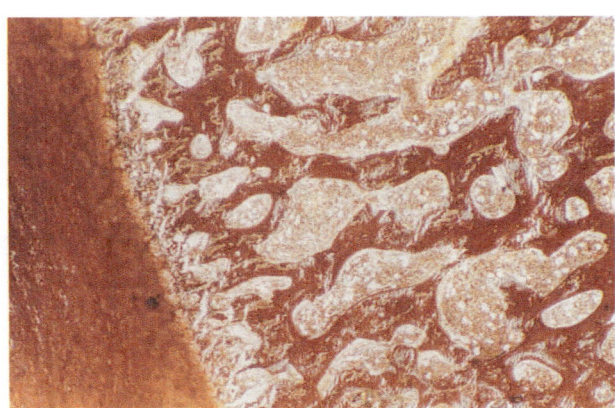

Figs. 1.61–1.66 Growth plate and residual cartilage in iliac crest biopsies of children

Figs. 1.61 and **1.62** Low and higher magnification of iliac crest biopsy of 6-year-old child

Fig. 1.61 Broad layer of cartilage growth plate (left). Gomori, polar.

Fig. 1.62 Dense trabecular network adjacent to growth plate (left). Gomori, polar.

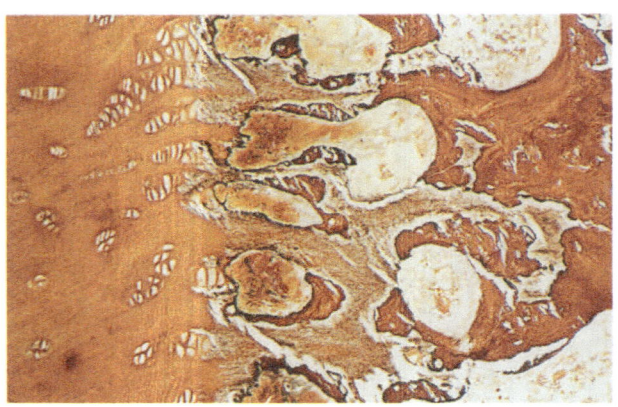

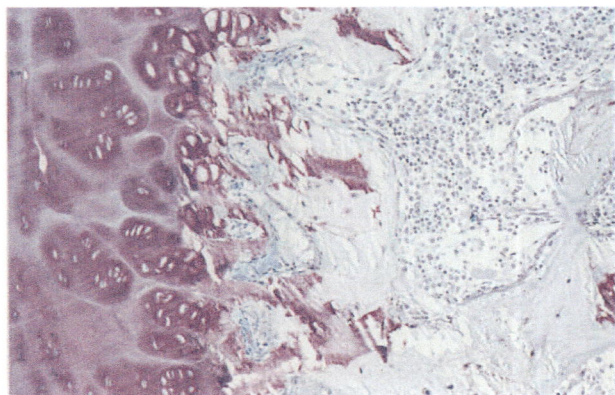

Figs. 1.63 and **1.64** Zones of the cartilaginous and bony components of the growth plate

Fig. 1.63 Large blood vessels between cartilage and bone. Gomori

Fig. 164 Note columns of chondroblasts extending to zone of ossification. Giemsa

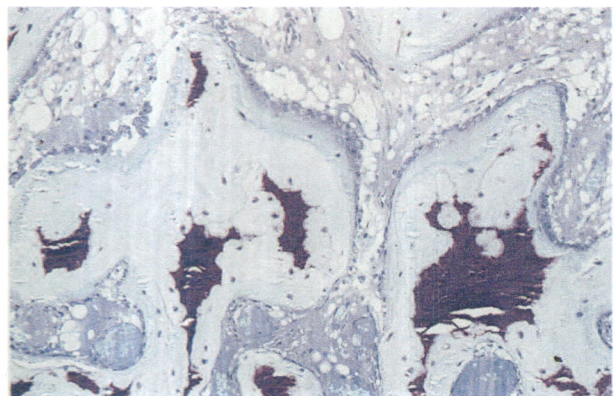

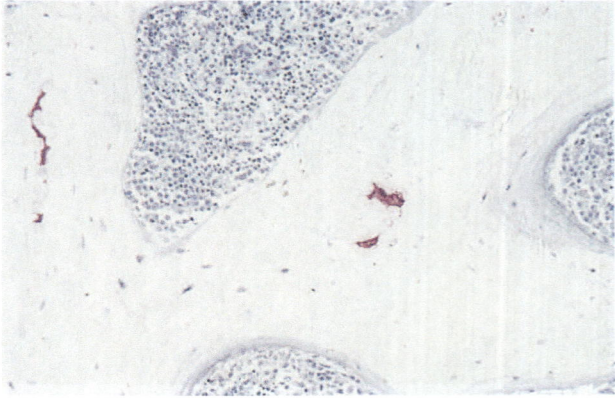

Fig. 1.65 Primary spongiosa with islands of residual cartilage. Note layer of osteoblasts on seams of osteoid (upper centre). Giemsa

Fig. 1.66 Biopsy of older child showing thick trabeculae with lamellar structure and minimal residues of cartilage. Giemsa

Plate 1.L

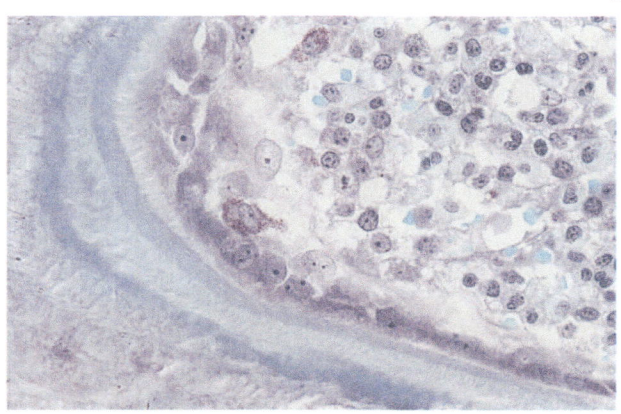

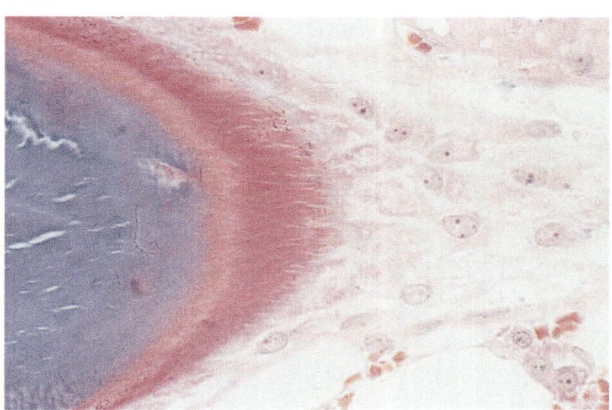

Figs 1.67–1.72 Bone formation and mineralization

Fig. 1.67 Cuboidal, active osteoblasts on lamellae of newly deposited osteoid, separated by calcification front from the mineralized bone. Giemsa

Fig. 1.68 Osteoblasts and layers of newly formed osteoid (red and orange) on mineralized bone. Ladewig

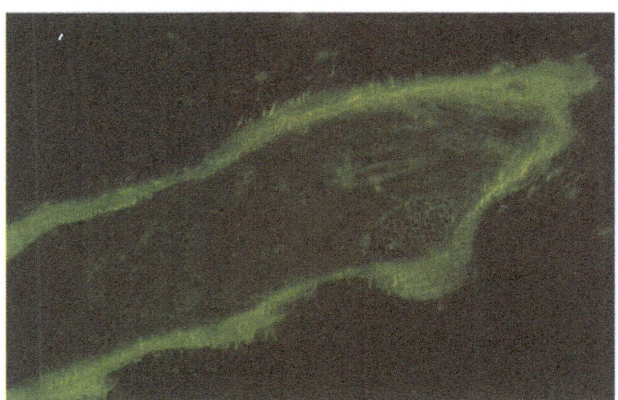

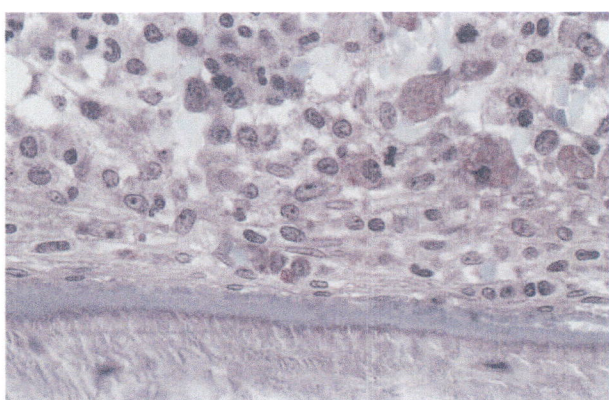

Fig. 1.69 Tetracycline fluorescence in mineralizing osteoid seam at trabecular circumference. Unstained section

Fig. 1.70 Sharp calcification front (dark violet) between osteoid and calcified bone. Giemsa

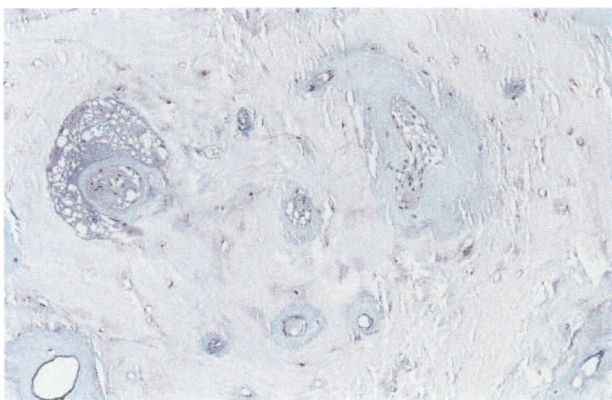

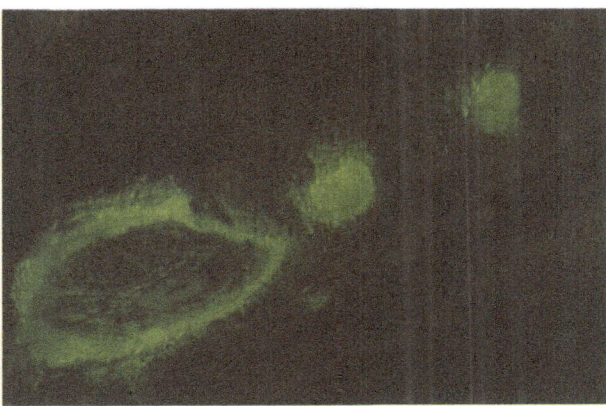

Fig. 1.71 Cortical bone with variably sized osteons containing osteoid seams. Giemsa

Fig. 1.72 Tetracycline fluorescence of the inner layers of Haversian systems. Unstained section

Plate 1.M

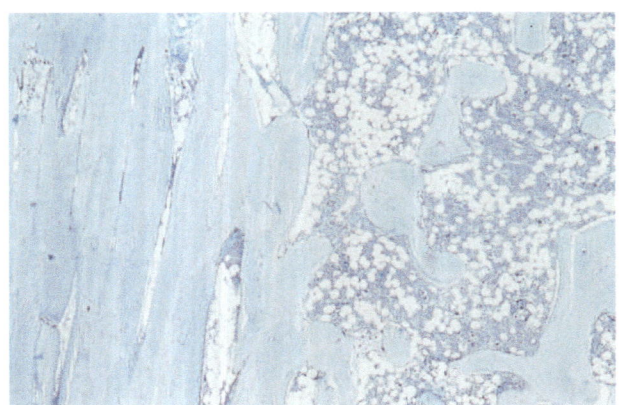

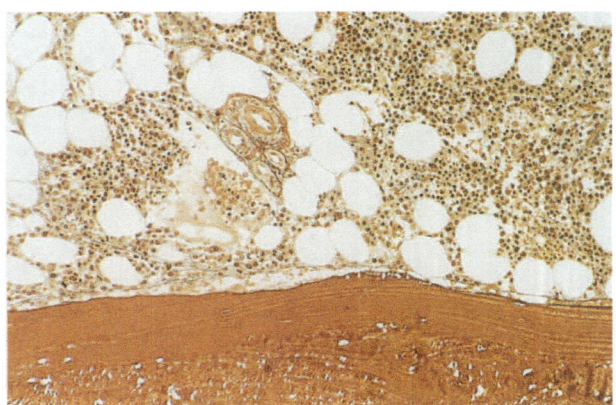

Figs 1.73–1.78 Aspects of subcortical endosteum I

Fig. 1.73 Porous cortical bone at transition between cortex and trabeculae with high endosteal surface area. Giemsa

Fig. 1.74 Flat, inactive cortical surface and normocellular marrow. Gomori

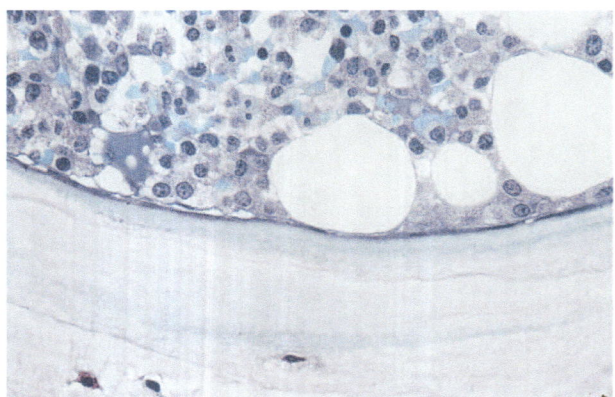

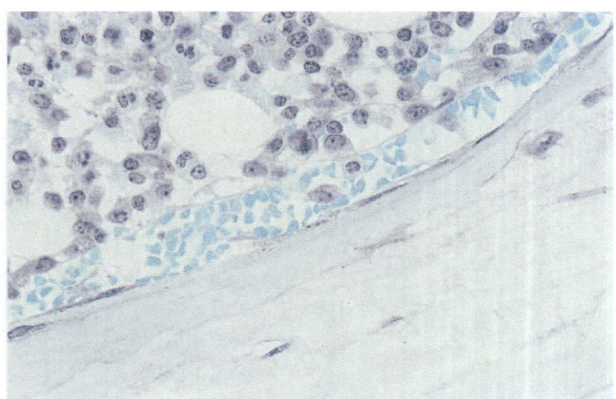

Figs. 1.75 and 1.76 Quiescent subcortical surface

Fig. 1.75 Thin, flat endosteal lining cells. Giemsa

Fig. 1.76 Ditto with paratrabecular sinusoid. Giemsa

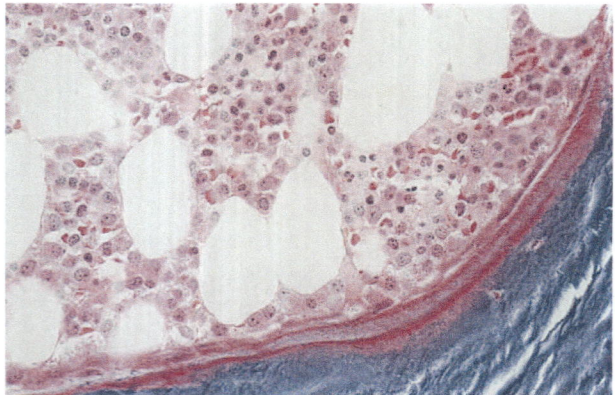

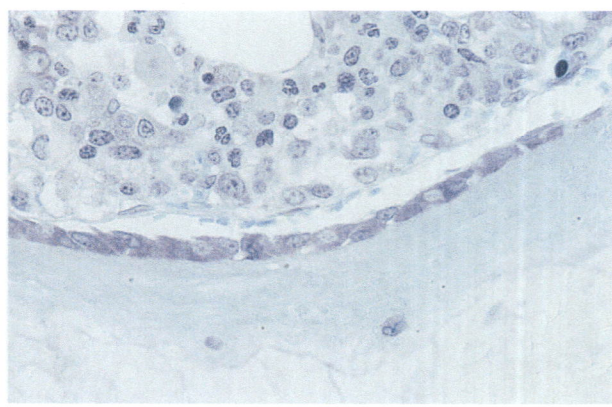

Fig. 1.77 Large extent of subcortical surface lined by layers of osteoid. Ladewig

Fig. 1.78 Broad osteoid seam lined by cuboidal osteoblasts. Note osteocytes in previous resorption cavities above cement line. Giemsa

Plate 1.N

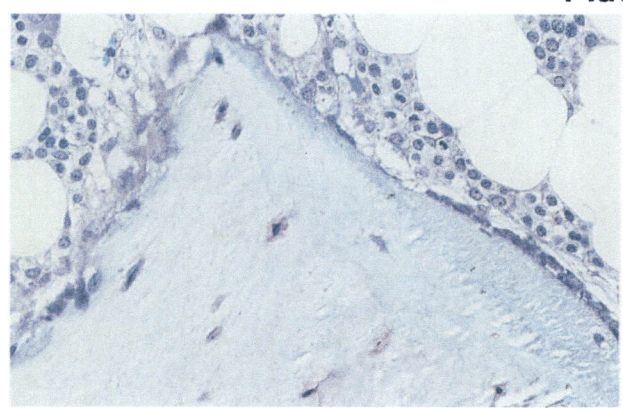

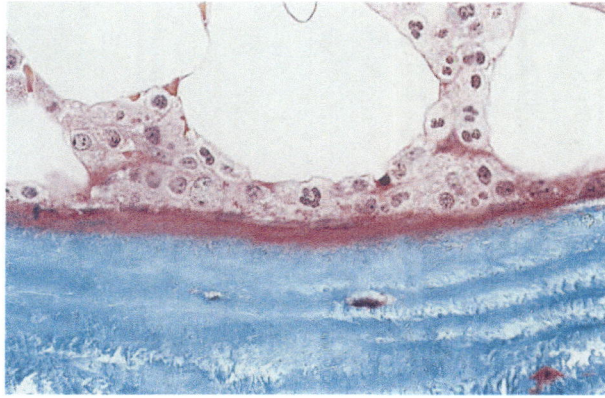

Figs 1.79–1.84 Aspects of subcortical endosteum II

Fig. 1.79 Both osteoclastic (left) and osteoblastic (right) remodelling on subcortical surface. Giemsa

Fig. 1.80 Unmineralized osteoid seam (red) lined by flat endosteal lining cells. Ladewig

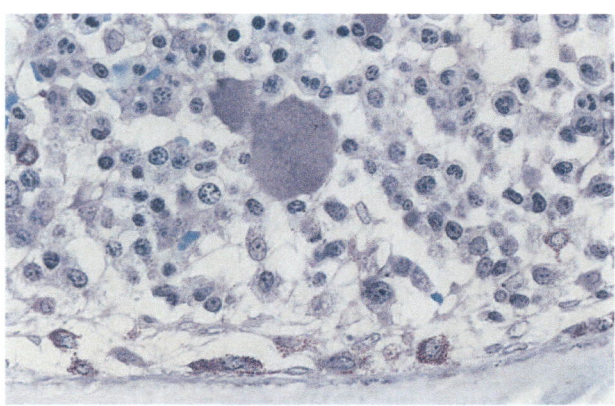

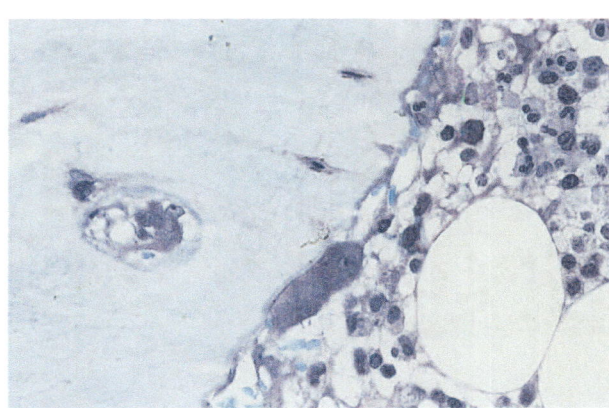

Fig. 1.81 Mast cells in cross and longitudinal sections in close apposition to endosteal lining cells. Giemsa

Fig. 1.82 Osteoclasts in Haversian canal and on endosteal subcortical surface. Giemsa

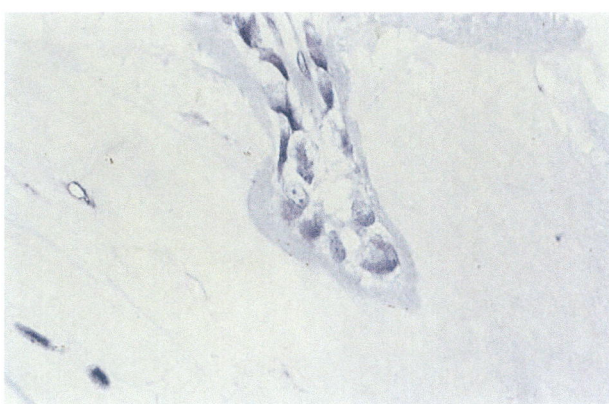

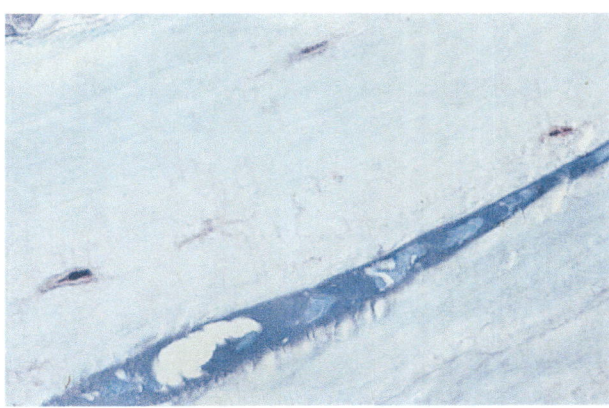

Fig. 1.83 Osteoblastic new bone formation in tunnelling resorption cavity. Giemsa

Fig. 1.84 Volkmann's canal penetrating broad subcortical layer. Giemsa

Plate 1.O

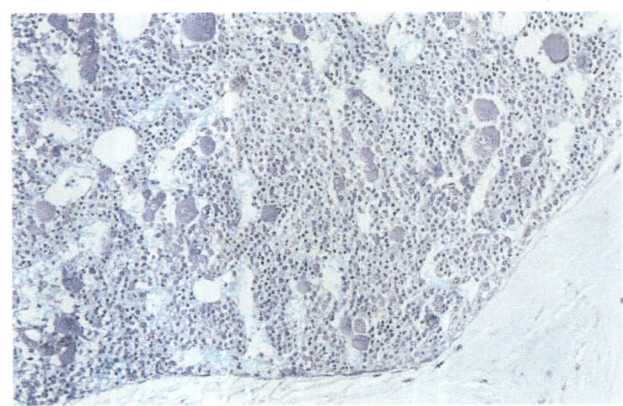

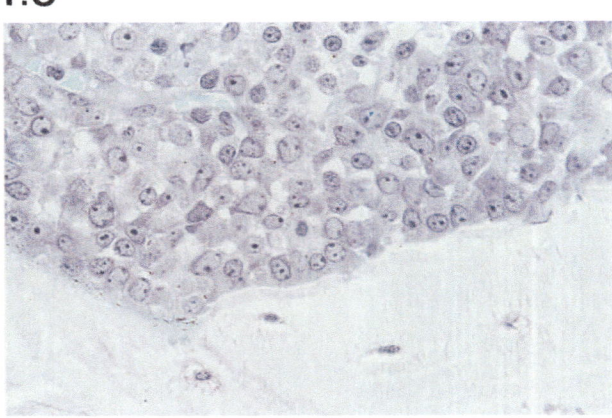

Figs 1.85–1.90 Aspects of trabecular surface in bone biopsies containing marrows with variable cellularity

Fig. 1.86 Broad seam of immature myeloid cells apparently in direct apposition to trabecular surface. Giemsa

Fig. 1.85 Hypercellular bone marrow with quiescent trabecular surface. Giemsa

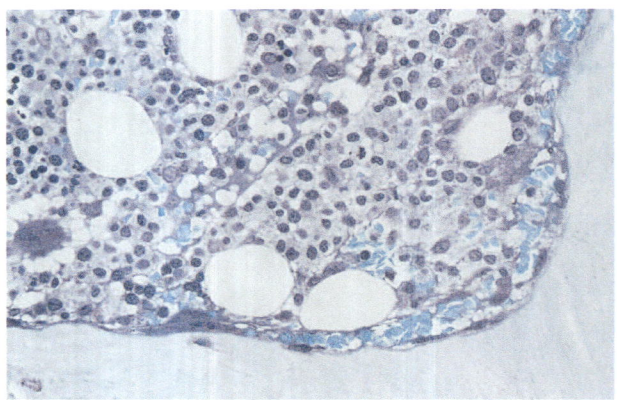

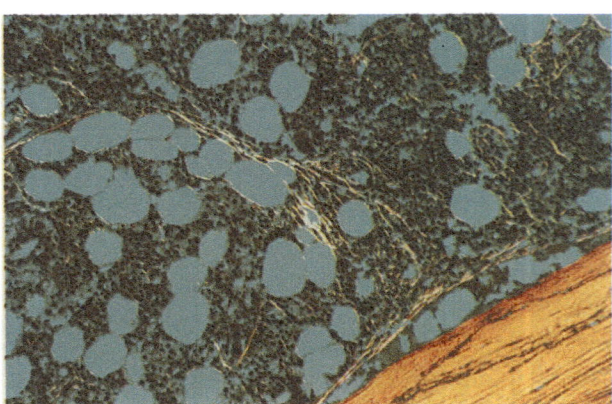

Fig. 1.87 Moderate osteoclastic remodelling in region of paratrabecular sinusoid. Giemsa

Fig. 1.88 Broad endosteal sinusoid on the upper surface of an ossicle, surrounded by normocellular marrow and fine fibrosis. Gomori, polar

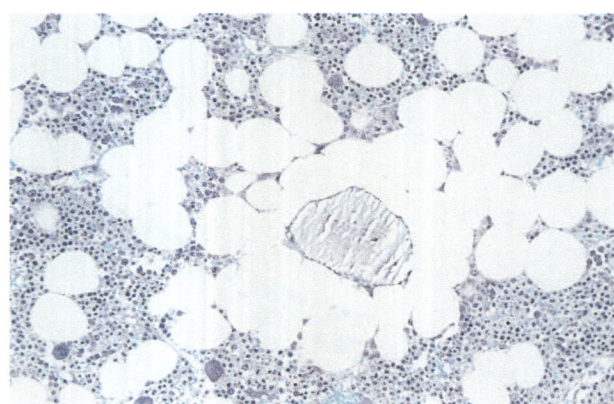

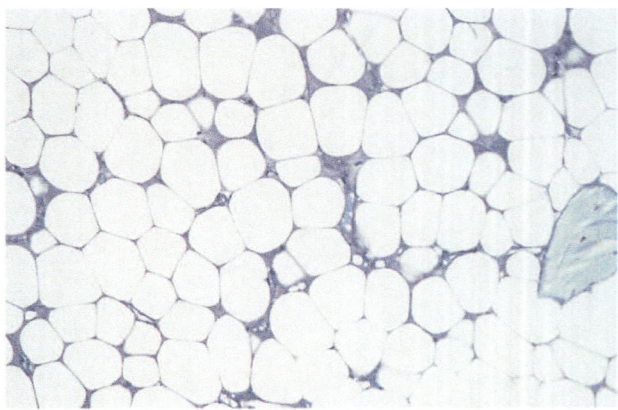

Fig. 1.89 Trabecular bone in cellular bone marrow, nevertheless surrounded by a rim of fat cells. Giemsa

Fig. 1.90 'Button' phenomenon in biopsy of patient with aplastic marrow, exclusively composed of fatty tissue and oedema. Giemsa

diameter; they communicate with the periosteum, the bone marrow and with each other through transverse channels called *Volkmann's canals*. The outer boundary of each osteon is marked by a *cement line*, a 1 μm thick layer of mineralized matrix (Fig. 1.EM5). These lines are poor in collagen, stain differently from other layers of matrix and are not traversed by osteocyte canaliculi. Cement lines are formed wherever resorption is followed by new bone formation[150]. Irregular and scalloped cement lines indicating an unbalanced osseous remodelling are characteristic of Paget's disease of bone.

Most *trabeculae* (ossicles) are less than 0.2 mm thick and do not contain blood vessels. Each trabecula is composed of a mosaic of angular segments, which are formed by parallel sheets of lamellae. A segment is called a *trabecular packet* and is functionally analogous to an osteon, the structural unit of compact bone. A typical trabecular packet is shaped like a shallow crescent with a radius of 600 μm and is about 50 μm thick and 1 mm long. As with compact bone, cement lines hold the trabecular packets together. A few trabeculae are thicker than 0.2 mm and their central portions generally contain an osteon-like structure, with circular rings of lamellae surrounding a blood vessel.

Bone matrix consists predominantly of type I collagen (85–90%) and contains no other interstitial collagens (i.e. types II, III, and IV)[98,116]. Important differences between fibrils in soft tissues and in bone have also been noted in the packing arrangement of their collagen molecules. The region of the fibril containing both holes and overlapped molecules is referred to as the *hole zone*, and the region consisting only of overlapped molecules as the *overlap zone*[125]. Katz and Li also noted the presence of spaces within the fibrils described as 'pores'[76]. The gaps between adjacent molecules in a bone collagen fibril are greater than those in other collagen fibrils, so that the rate of diffusion of ions into the interstices of the fibril is correspondingly greater in bone collagen fibrils. Indeed 90–95% of the mineral present in normal lamellar bone is located in the collagen fibres and only 5–10% in the remaining matrix. Nevertheless the uniqueness of the organic matrix lies in these non-collagenous constituents: the amorphous *ground substance*. Several proteins and proteoglycans are presently known to be specific for bone: osteocalcin, thrombospodin[128], bone sialoprotein I and II and a bone-specific proteoglycan. These components all participate in mineralization. They are highly acidic and have strong aggregation tendencies and calcium-binding properties. Bone morphogenic proteins (BMPs) such as osteogenin can be extracted from demineralized bone matrix, and presumably these proteins stimulate local mesenchymal cells to differentiate into osteoblasts[46]. Osteocalcin, produced by osteoblasts and present in blood, is used as a specific bone marker in many metabolic bone disorders.

Normal bone consists of approximately 65% *mineral*, mainly hydroxyapatite, which is present as needles or thin plates containing many other ions in addition to calcium and phosphate[114]. Trace amounts of fluoride, iron, zinc, copper, aluminium, lead and other metals have also been reported. The hydroxyapatite crystals are distributed evenly along the length of the collagen fibres. Ground substance surrounds and stabilizes these crystals. The interaction of hydroxyapatite with collagen fibres and amorphous ground substance results in the hardness and rigidity of bone. The remainder is amorphous calcium phosphate, has a lower calcium-to-phosphate ratio and occurs in young, active bone.

Approximately 10% of the trabecular surface is covered by osteoid, and about half of the osteoid seams exhibit a zone called mineralization or *calcification front* (Plate 1.L) (Fig. 1.EM7). The precise mechanism of *mineralization*

of bone remains to be clarified[2]. There are two main hypotheses: the extracellular fluid is supersaturated with calcium and phosphate, and only a nucleation site is required to initiate mineralization. This nucleus could be provided by osteonectin or proteoglycans. It is probable that mineralization does not occur normally in other collagenous tissues because of the presence of macro-molecular inhibitors of calcification, and their removal would be necessary to trigger mineralization. The second theory ascribes a central role to alkaline phosphatase in association with matrix vesicles. Calcification starts at the base of the resorption bay along the cement line, dark blue in toluidine blue-stained sections, i.e. at the interface between calcified bone and osteoid (called the mineralization front).

Fig. 1.S4 summarizes the different systems of bone structures – from organ to molecular level.

BONE CELLS (Plates 1.P–T)

The processes of bone formation and resorption are carried out by two major bone cells, the osteoblasts and osteoclasts (Fig. 1.S5). These two lines of specialized bone cells have entirely different embryological origins, and each will be considered separately. It should be noted that there has been an explosion of interest, work and publications on all aspects of bone cells in recent years; some of these studies are summarized in refs. 90–92.

Osteoblasts, osteocytes and lining cells

Osteoblasts synthesize osteoid, the organic bone matrix, and are responsible for its subsequent mineralization (Plates 1.P and Q) (Fig. 1.EM7). In general, active

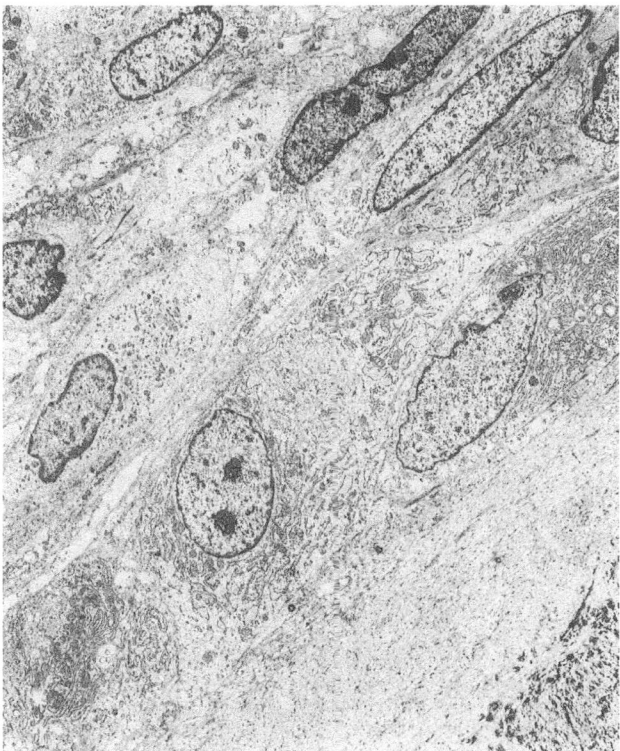

Fig. 1.EM7 From bottom right upwards: small area of mineralized bone matrix, layer of osteoid, parts of two osteoblasts, one with nucleolated nucleus, and endothelial cells. EM × 4200

From macro – to microstructure of bone

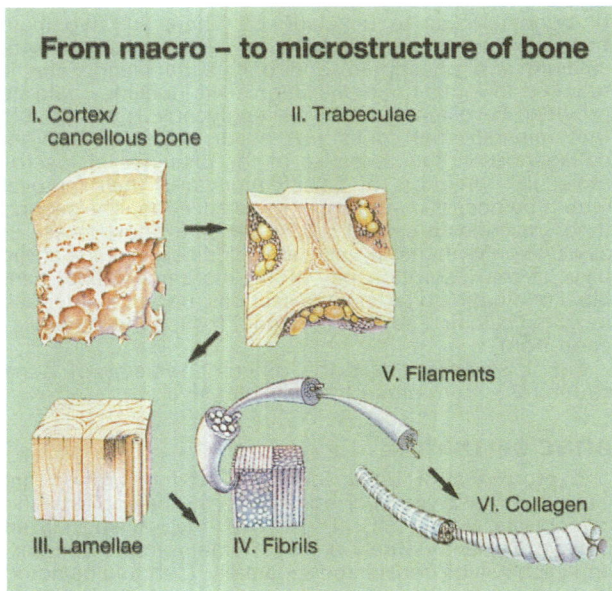

Fig. 1.S4 Diagram of bone architecture – from organ to molecular level

Bone cells

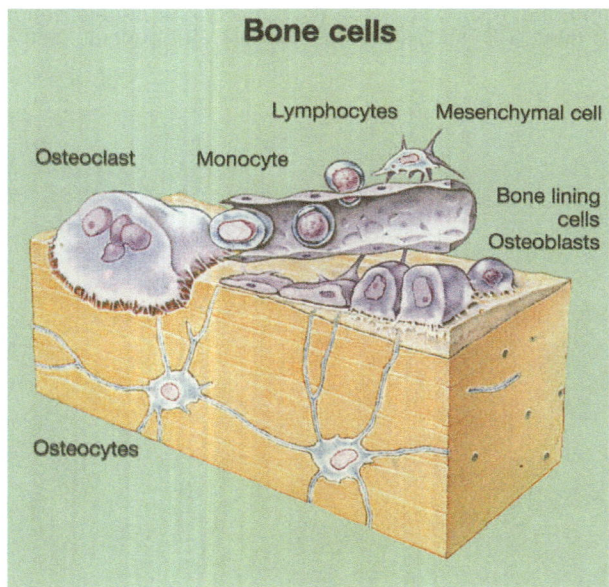

Fig. 1.S5 Sketch of bone cells and accessory cells participating in the remodelling process

osteoblasts are cuboidal, polar, basophilic secretory cells[106]. Mitotic figures are rarely seen. The osteoid is secreted at one end of the cell and in humans is mineralized after approximately 15 days. The osteoblasts apparently regulate the flux of calcium and phosphate in and out of bone[147]. They are target cells and possess receptors for parathyroid hormone and 1,25(OH)$_2$ vitamin D$_3$[11,51–53,69,87,123]. There may be distinct subpopulations of osteo-

blasts, implying that bone cell effectors could have differential effects on each subgroup and even in different areas of the skeleton[43,93]. Other hormones acting on osteoblasts are glucocorticoids, growth factors, insulin and prostaglandins[68,79,95,153]. Osteoblasts also respond to factors and cytokines released by resorbing osteoclasts, and themselves secrete factors for their own stimulation (autocrine pathway), which results in increased production of collagen, osteonectin, alkaline phosphatase and osteocalcin[52,74,119,129,132,142]. It has recently been shown that oestrogen maintains trabecular bone volume not only by suppression of bone resorption but also by stimulation of bone formation[34]. Osteoblast activity also depends on cobalamin, as shown in cobalamin-deficient patients who had significantly lower osteocalcin levels than the control subjects[28]. Osteoblasts also secrete collagenase, which participates in bone resorption, as well as playing a major role in the activation and regulation of osteoclast activity, see below[30,47].

Osteoblasts representing different functional stages can be distinguished: the active secretory cuboidal cell (described above), flatter cells called intermediate osteoblasts and still thinner cells called inactive osteoblasts. The latter are indistinguishable from the *endosteal lining cells* which cover quiescent bone, i.e. about 80% of the trabecular and 95% of the intracortical bone surfaces (Figs. 1.EM8 and 9)[41,70,97]. The lining cells are connected by gap junctions[44]. It seems likely that at least some of the active osteoblasts become lining cells when their matrix-producing phase terminates. Often the lining cells are covered by a layer of flat endothelial cells of endosteal sinusoids. The role of the lining cells is unclear. Are they a source of osteoblasts? Are they an entirely different cell population, separating the marrow and the osseous compartments? Do they play a role in directing the activity of osteoclasts[73]? These are some of the questions currently being addressed[75].

Osteoblasts become *osteocytes* when they lose polarity and form osteoid around themselves (Plate 1.R) (Figs. 1.EM10–18). It is not known how many originally active cuboidal osteoblasts become osteocytes or lining cells. However, the number of osteocytes per volume of bone is relatively constant, which implies that this parameter is regulated. The osteocytes are located in lacunae and are connected with each other and with the surface lining cells by means of cytoplasmic extensions (processes) that run through narrow channels (*canaliculi*) in the bone matrix. These cellular processes are connected via gap junctions, which explains how the osteocytes survive in such an isolated environment. Young osteocytes occupy round lacunae near the surface; subsequently both cells and lacunae become oval or flat. Active osteoblasts on the surface correlate with large, round and basophilic osteocytes in the underlying bone matrix. The size and density of osteocytes is greater in woven than in lamellar bone. Currently, osteocytic osteolysis, i.e. resorption of lacunar walls, is not accepted by most investigators. The function of the osteocytes most probably includes metabolic exchange with the surrounding matrix essential for the maintenance of the structural integrity of bone. When osteocytes die, the involved bone cannot be maintained and becomes a 'sequestrum'.

Osteoclasts (Plates 1.S and T)

Osteoclasts are multinucleated giant cells responsible for bone resorption[31,106,113,133,143,146,149]. The cells range from 20 to over 100 μm in diameter and contain from two to several hundred nuclei. They form by cell fusion. When active the osteoclast rests directly on the surface of the bone were resorption is to take place. Specific changes in the cytoskeletal organization of the osteoclast charac-

[continued on p. 34]

Plate 1.P

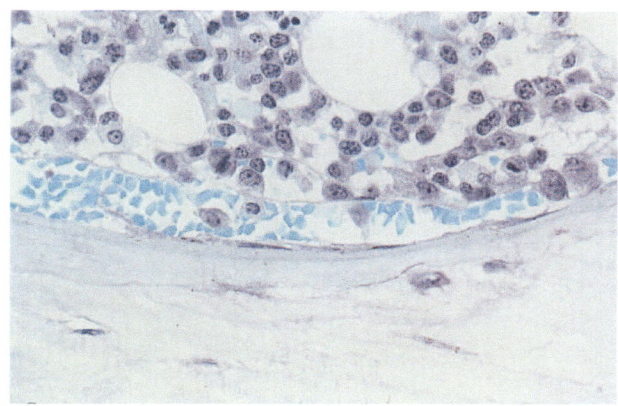

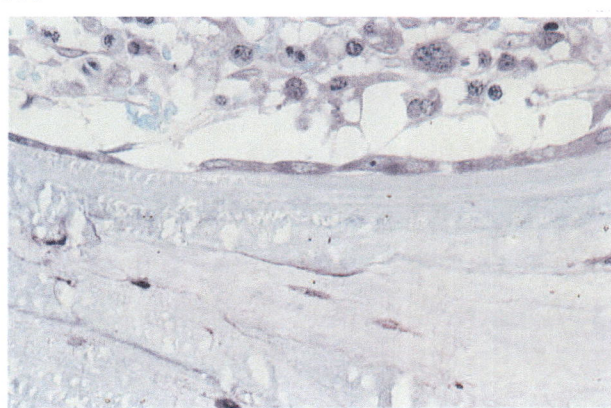

Figs 1.91–1.96 Different degrees of osteoblastic activity

Fig. 1.91 Flat endosteal lining cells and paratrabecular sinusoid. Giemsa

Fig. 1.92 Somewhat plumper endosteal lining cells (already osteoblasts?) on trabecular bone surface. Giemsa

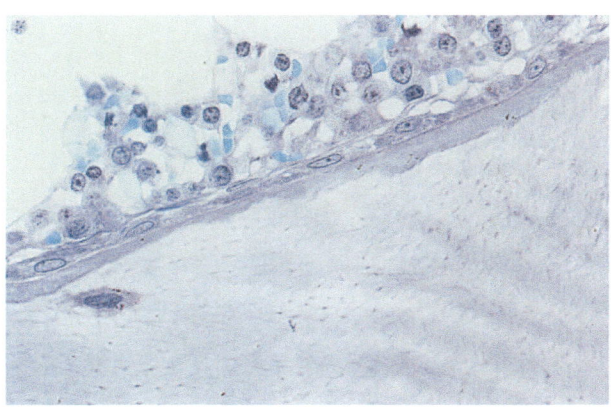

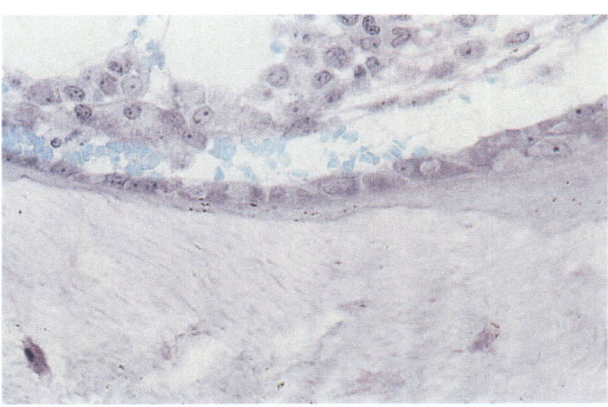

Fig. 1.93 Plumper endosteal lining cells (osteoblasts?) on layer of osteoid. The scalloped surface of the mineralized bone underlying the osteoid appears to be determined by the oblique direction of the lamellae. Giemsa

Fig. 1.94 Active (left) to cuboidal (right) osteoblasts on osteoid seam of variable width and paratrabecular sinusoid. Giemsa

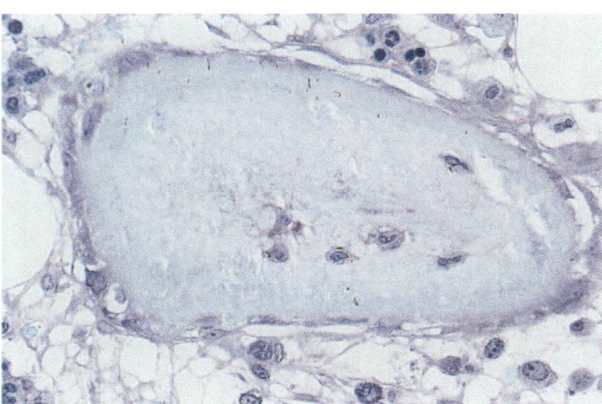

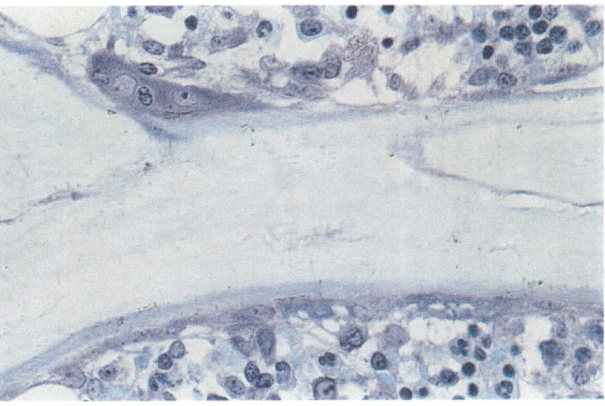

Fig. 1.95 Transverse section of ossicle surrounded by a broad seam of osteoid and a layer of flat to cuboidal osteoblasts. Note osteocytes in the centre of the ossicle. Giemsa

Fig. 1.96 Longitudinally cut ossicle with a broad seam of osteoid covered by osteoblasts (lower surface), and an active osteoclast on the opposite side of the trabecula ('coupled remodelling'). Giemsa

Plate 1.Q

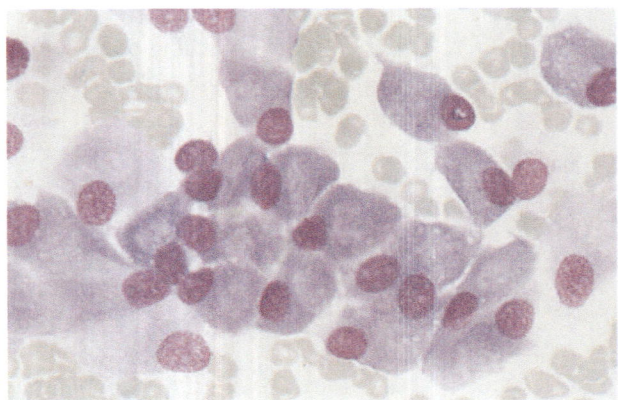

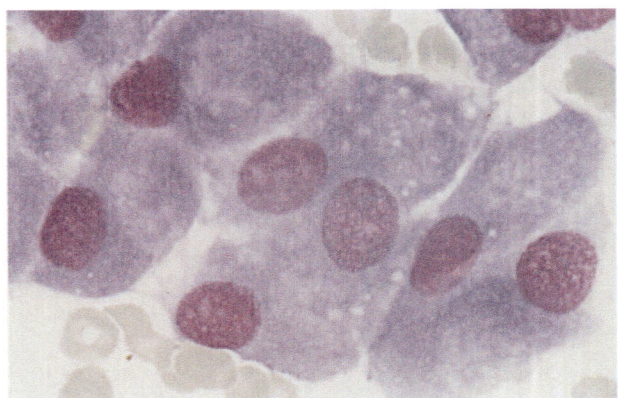

Figs 1.97–1.102 Active osteoblasts

Fig. 1.97 Cluster of osteoblasts as seen in bone marrow aspirates. Pappenheim

Fig. 1.98 Higher magnification of osteoblasts from Fig. 1.97. Pappenheim

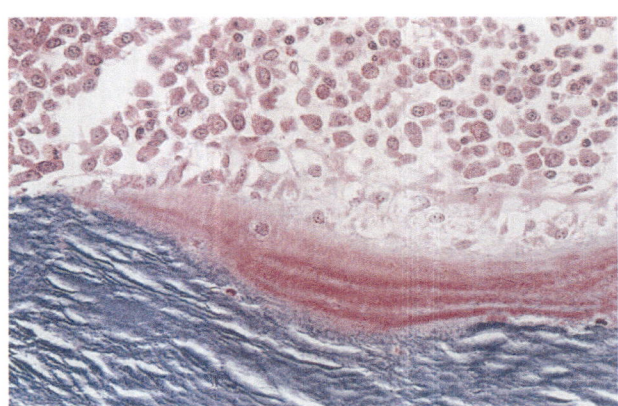

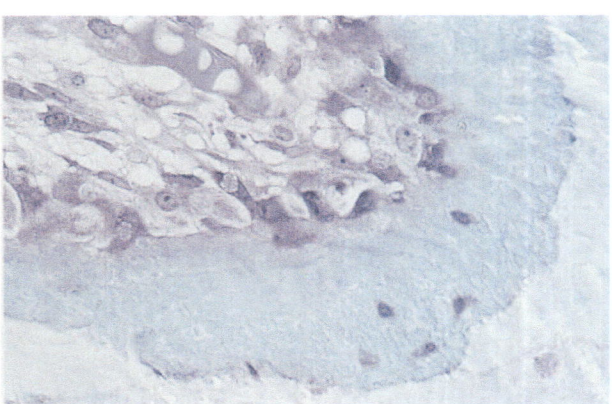

Fig. 1.99 Cuboidal osteoblasts on broad seam of osteoid. Note a single 'young' osteocyte embedded in the osteoid seam. Ladewig

Fig. 1.100 Cuboidal osteoblasts on broad osteoid seam and marked cement line (lower right); several 'young' osteocytes within the osteoid. Giemsa

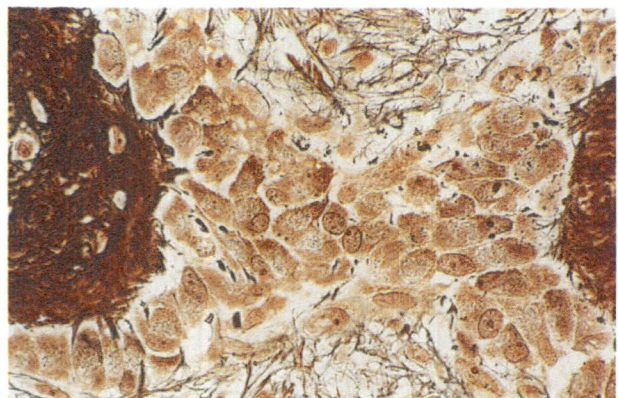

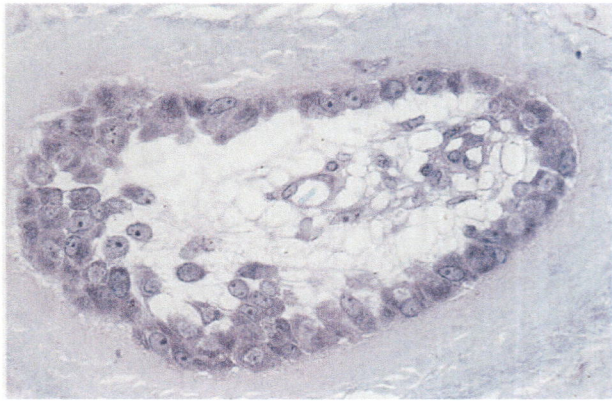

Fig. 1.101 Tangentially cut ossicle with apparent discontinuity and multilayered osteoblasts due to the cutting plane. Gomori

Fig. 1.102 Active cuboidal osteoblasts on layer of osteoid lining Haversian canal. Giemsa

Plate 1.R

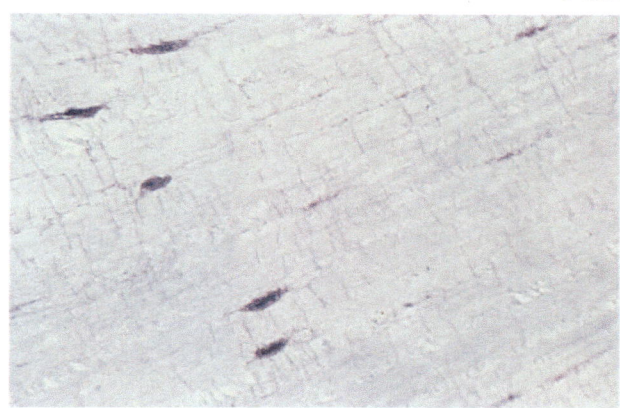

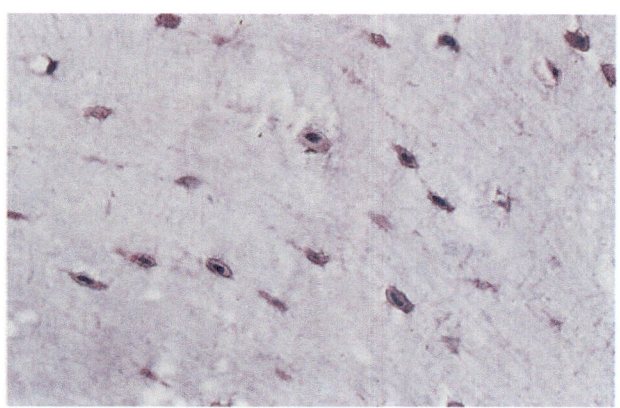

Figs 1.103–1.108 Range of osteocytes in mineralized bone

Fig. 1.103 Flat osteocytes in trabecular bone. Note canaliculi oriented at right angle to the lamellae. Giemsa

Fig. 1.104 Section of trabecular bone illustrating higher density of osteocytes. Giemsa

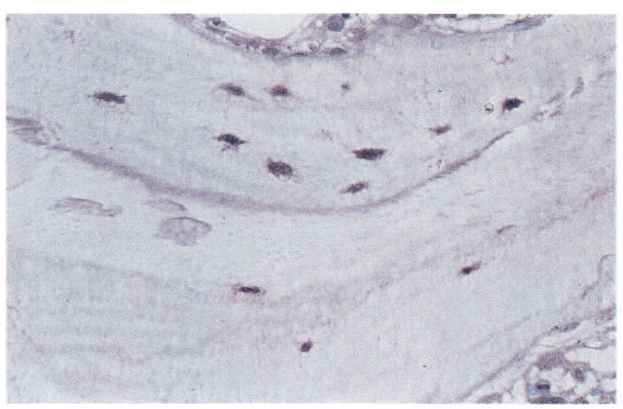

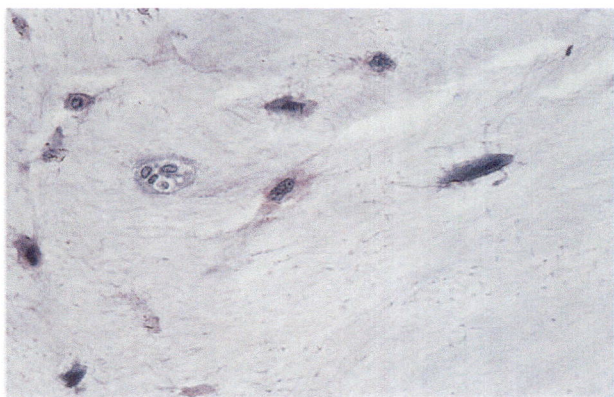

Fig. 1.105 Ossicle with cement lines between 'older' and more recently formed bone which contains apparently larger and more numerous osteocytes (upper centre). Giemsa

Fig. 1.106 Osteocytes cut at different angles in trabecular bone. Note a narrow trabecular canal containing a blood vessel. Giemsa

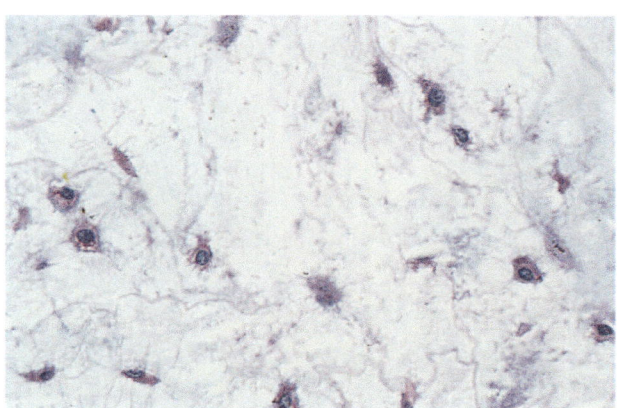

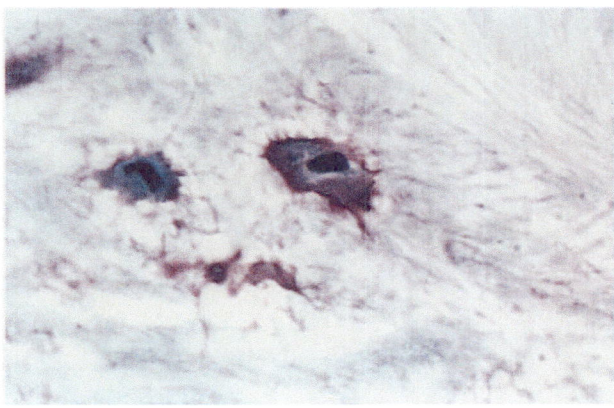

Fig. 1.107 Relatively large osteocytes with round to oval nuclei in an area of newly mineralized bone. Giemsa

Fig. 1.108 Higher magnification of different area of Fig. 1.107 with network of canaliculi. Giemsa

Plate 1.S

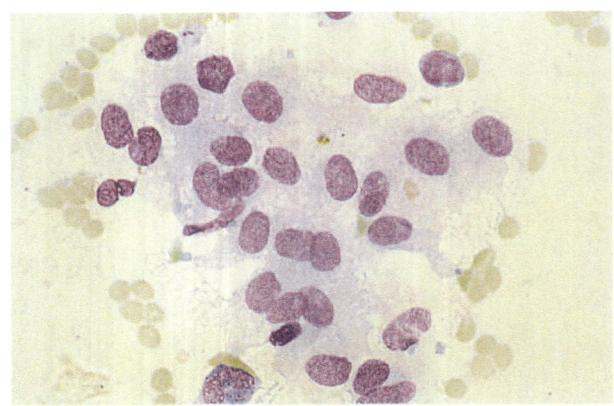

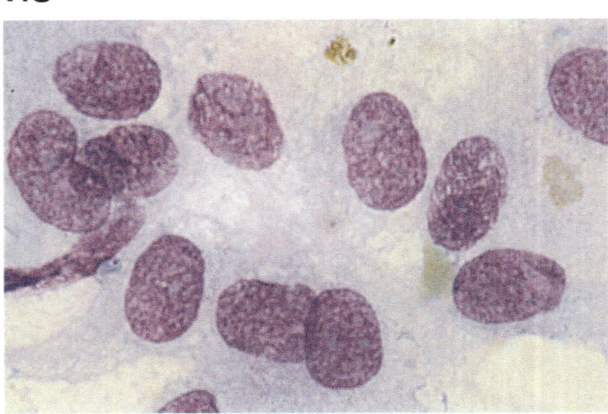

Figs 1.109–1.114 Aspects of osteoclasts I: range in morphology: size, number of nuclei and staining characteristics

Fig. 1.109 Cluster of multinucleated osteoclasts as seen in bone marrow aspirates. Pappenheim

Fig. 1.110 Higher magnification of osteoclasts from Fig. 1.109. Pappenheim

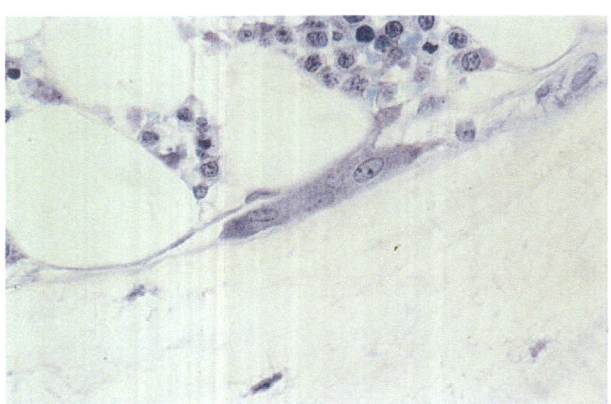

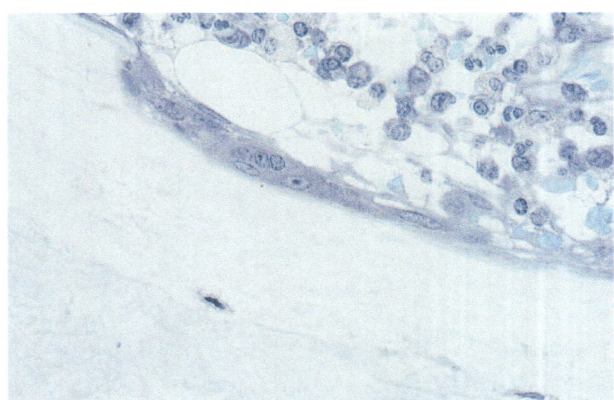

Fig. 1.111 Flat, elongated osteoclast apparently inactive. Giemsa

Fig. 1.112 Flat but multinucleated and active osteoclast within shallow resorption cavity. Giemsa

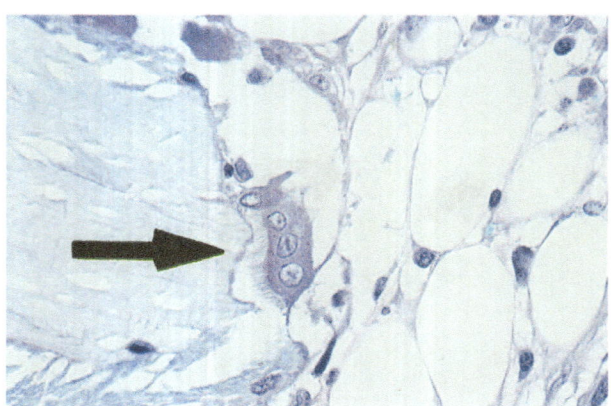

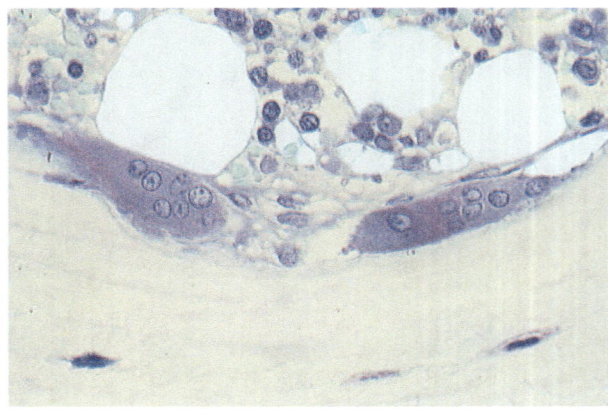

Fig. 1.113 Active osteoclast with ruffled border (arrow) in lacuna associated with paratrabecular sinusoid. Giemsa

Fig. 1.114 Active osteoclasts in wide resorption bay; note pink-stained cytoplasmic areas corresponding to regions containing numerous organelles in electron microscopy (see Fig. 1.EM21). Giemsa

Plate 1.T

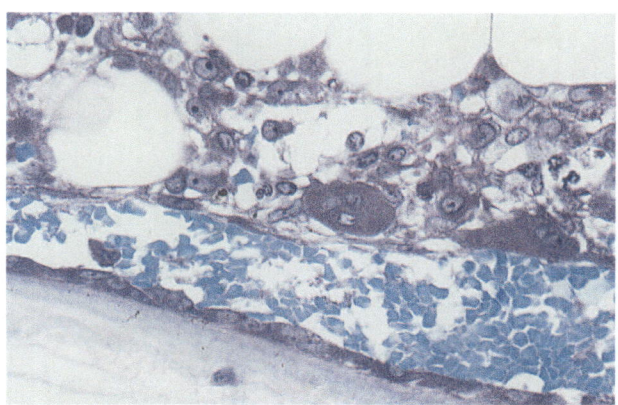

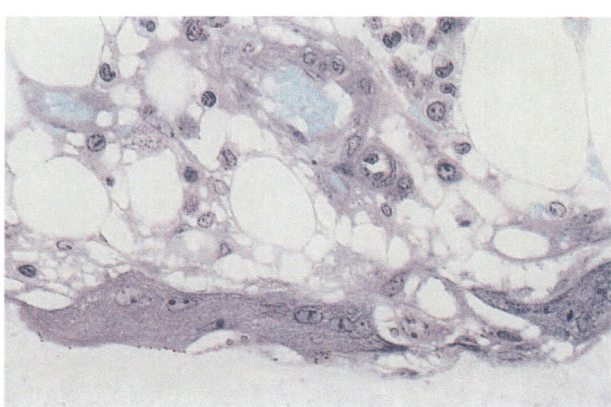

Figs 1.115–1.120 Aspects of osteoclasts II: morphology and activity

Fig. 1.115 Osteoclasts (centre) separated from the trabecular surface by a broad endosteal sinusoid and a seam of endosteal lining cells. Giemsa

Fig. 1.116 Trabecular surface with Howship's lacunae, active osteoclasts and bordered by mesenchymal tissue. Ladewig

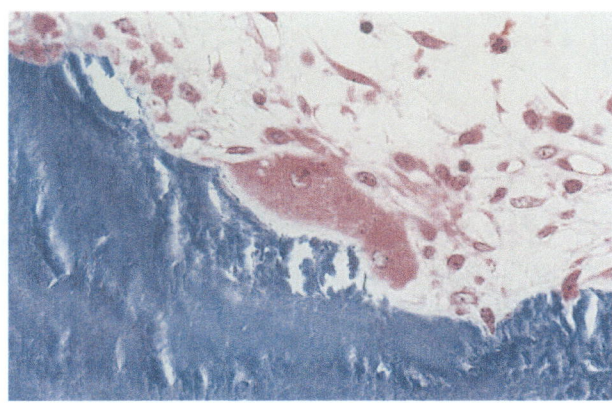

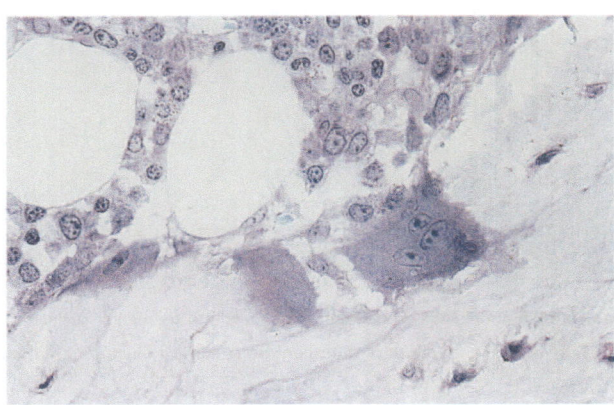

Fig. 1.117 Surface erosion by large multinucleated osteoclast; loose connective tissue with lymphoid and plasma cells. Note absence of osteoid in the Howship's lacuna. Ladewig

Fig. 1.118 Osteoclasts in deep resorption bay: 'tunnelling osteoclastosis'. Note nucleolated osteoclast nuclei. Giemsa

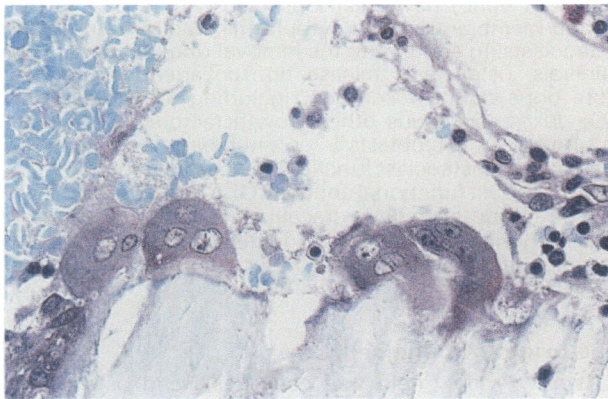

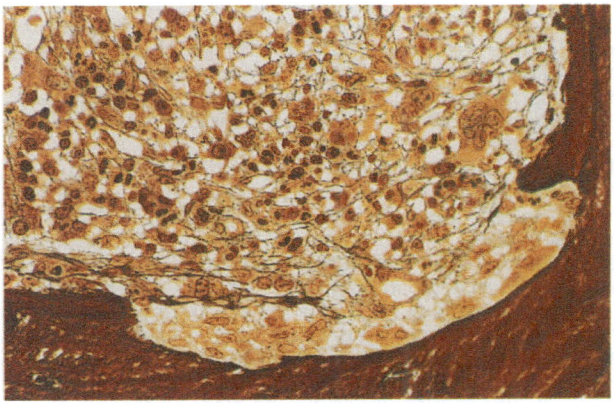

Fig. 1.119 Row of active osteoclasts on trabecular bone surface bordered by an ectatic endosteal sinusoid. Giemsa

Fig. 1.120 Large resorption bay, the lateral edges of which have been undermined by tunnelling osteoclasts. Gomori

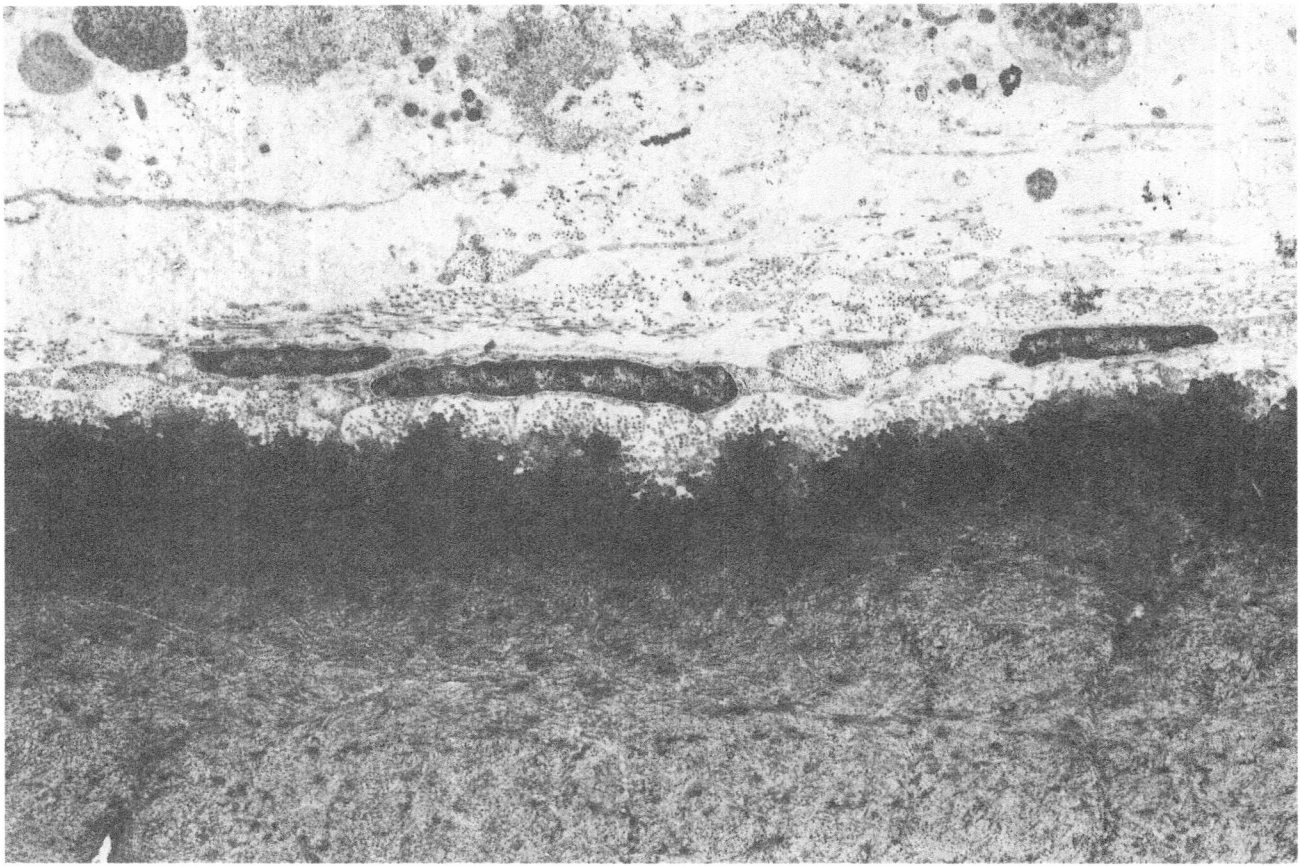

Figs. 1.EM8 and **EM9**   Endosteal lining cells and trabecular surface

Fig. 1.EM8   Fine structure of quiescent bone surface illustrating flat endosteal lining cells. EM × 4500

terize the 'attachment zone', mediated by integrin-type receptors[107,145]. Bone resorption takes place inside the attachment zone. As a result of its activity, a shallow bay, called *Howship's lacuna* or resorption bay, is formed in the bone directly under the osteoclast[40]. However, many questions still remain open: What determines sites on bone surfaces to which osteoclasts are attracted (other than damage)? What determines the size–length–width–depth of the resorption cavities? Which signals switch the osteoclasts 'on' and 'off'? How exactly does the osteoclast remove bone? It is now thought that osteoclasts secrete *proteinases* at the ruffled border and these remove organic matrix; they produce *hydrogen ions* by means of carbonic anhydrase and proton pumps of vacuolar type ATPase – for dissolution of hydroxyapatite crystals, thereby both matrix and minerals are resorbed[5,13,14,65,145]. In some cases osteoclasts may resorb to a depth of about 60 μm from the surface and then continue to excavate sideways parallel to the surface.

In the light microscope the surface of the osteoclast adjacent to the bone often has a striated appearance; in the electron microscope this corresponds to an area of extensive membrane undulations called the *ruffled border*, which in turn is surrounded by the clear or sealing zone (Figs 1.EM19–22).

Cinematographic studies of osteoclasts have shown that *processes* are continually extended and retracted and change their positions. In the sealed-off extracellular

resorption area between the ruffled border and the bone surface, bone mineral is dissolved presumably by acidification (see above). It is generally believed that osteoclasts do not resorb non-mineralized osteoid, though they may be found on osteoid seams, especially in conditions such as osteomalacia[16]. Fragments of electron-dense material (chips of bone) have been observed within folds of the ruffled membrane and in cytoplasmic vacuoles in active osteoclasts. In addition to the removal of bone matrix and minerals, osteoclasts release non-collagenous proteins from bone during resorption, including factors such as TGF-β[103] and various other growth factors[102,122], which in turn act on osteoblasts[71,151]. A number of receptors for mediators of osteoclast function have been identified[71,121]. The osteoclast functional antigen (OFA), shown to belong to the tissue-specific extracellular matrix receptors – the integrins – and possibly identical to the vitronectin receptor, may have functional importance in the regulation of bone resorption[10,32,38,89].

The origin of bone cells

It is now widely held that osteoclasts and osteoblasts have separate origins[67,90,99,105]. The osteoclastic lineage is thought to derive from a blood-borne source. There is strong evidence that this is a haematopoietic cell, possibly a progenitor belonging to the monocyte–macrophage lineage[19,20,33,66,89,125]: a monoclonal antibody (anti-L-35)

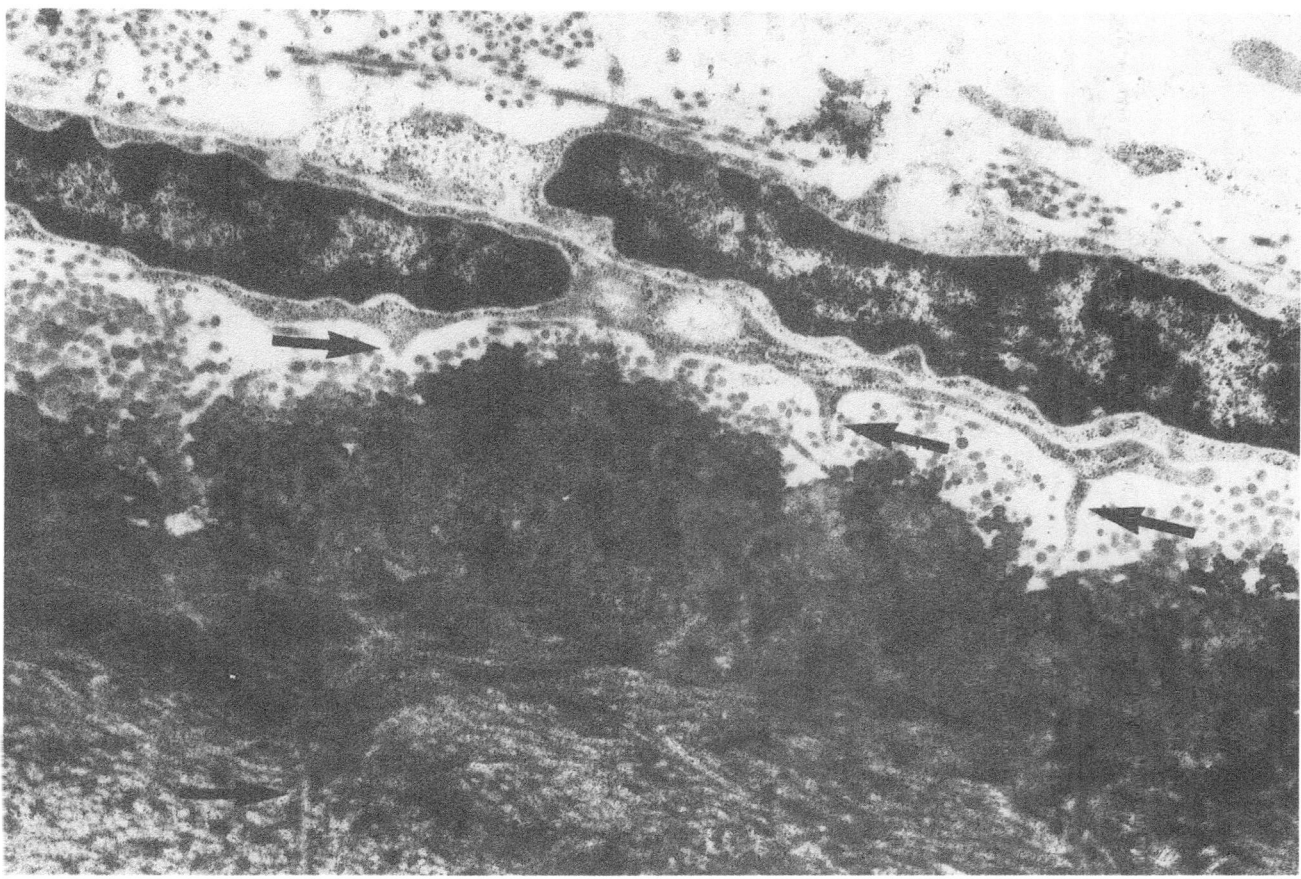

Fig. 1.EM9 At higher magnification, collagen in transverse section under the flat endosteal lining cells, and in longitudinal section in lower part of micrograph. Note processes of endosteal lining cells (arrows) extending between collagen fibres, presumably to connect with processes of osteocytes within the canaliculi. EM × 11300

reacts with both human osteoclasts and cells of the mononuclear phagocyte system[6–9,81,155].

The origin of the osteogenic lineage (osteoblasts, osteocytes, endosteal lining cells) has not been identified, but probably involves cells of the primitive mesenchyme[45,130,131]. Recently Owen proposed a lineage pathway derived from stromal stem cells with the capacity to differentiate into any of several directions – reticular, fibroblastic, adipocytic and osteogenic[108]. However, the mesenchymal origin of osteoblasts in the adult organism has been challenged[152].

OSTEOGENESIS

Embryologically, bone tissue may be detected by 8 weeks in the developing human fetus[3]. As described above, histogenesis of bone proceeds by the initial formation of primary (woven) bone, which is later replaced by secondary (lamellar) bone. This sequence of formation occurs via two pathways: intramembranous and enchondral ossification, which differ by the material on which the woven bone is formed.

Intramembranous ossification takes place within an area of well-vascularized primitive connective tissue[144]. Initially mesenchymal cells differentiate into osteoblasts followed by the secretion of osteoid. Several such foci arise simultaneously at an ossification centre; fusion of the growing spicules then forms the primitive spongiosa (spongy, cancellous or trabecular bone). In early embryos, prior to the appearance of cartilage, the primitive mesen-chymal cells produce type I collagen as the extracellular matrix. In the adult, intramembranous ossification occurs under pathological circumstances accompanied by marked mesenchymal activity, as for example in osseous metastases, osteomyelosclerosis and Paget's disease of bone.

When bone formation develops in pre-existing cartilage it is called enchondral or *intracartilagenous ossification*. The vertebral column, the pelvis and the extremities are formed by this type of ossification. Essentially all increases in length occur at the *epiphyseal growth plate*, where approximately 90% of all trabecular bone is initially generated. Five zones are distinguished within the growth plate: (1) the zone of resting cells, (2) the zone of cell proliferation, (3) the zone of cell maturation, (4) the zone of cell hypertrophy, and (5) the zone of provisional calcification.

THE CONCEPT OF BONE REMODELLING

The process of *bone modelling* is responsible for determining the shape and size of bone and it stops at adulthood. *Remodelling* occurs throughout life and is essential for the maintenance of normal bone structure[88,101]. It involves a balanced sequence of resorption and formation[109]. Approximately 5–10% of all the existing bone is replaced every year, while the turnover of trabecular bone probably reaches 20%. A striking characteristic of bone remodelling is its non-uniformity: it varies from one bone to another, from axial to appendicular skeleton,

[continued on p. 39]

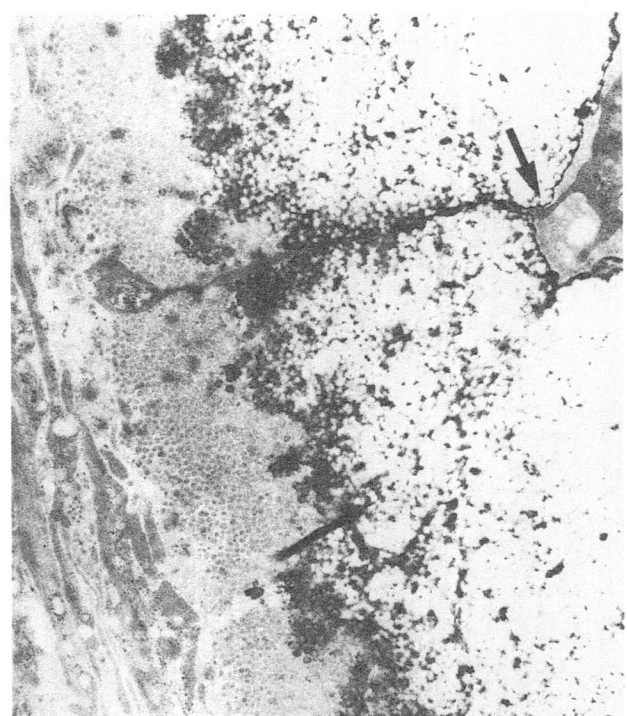

Fig. 1.EM10 Section of trabecular surface illustrating osteocytic canaliculus containing osteocyte process (arrow) and penetrating the bone matrix and osteoid. The layer of osteoid contains transversely sectioned collagen fibrils. EM × 6560

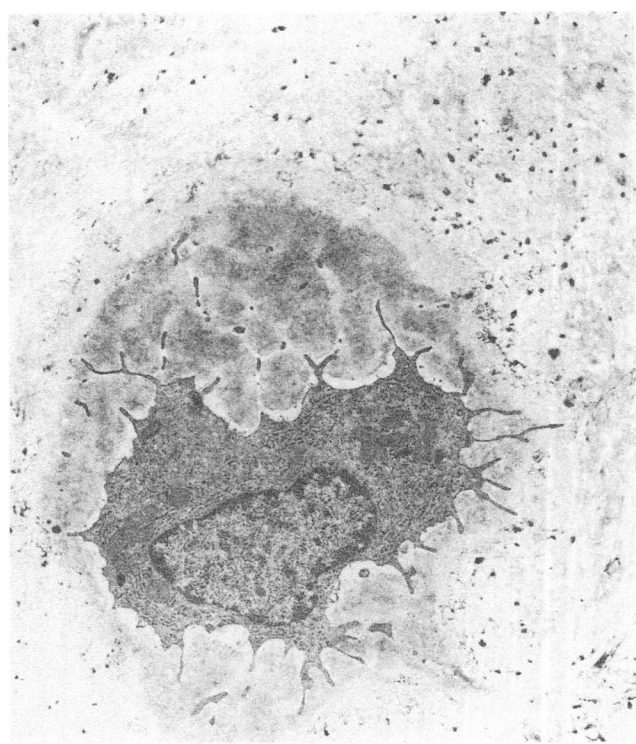

Fig. 1.EM12 Osteocyte nucleus showing mainly euchromatin. Note mitochondria and numerous cytoplasmic extensions. EM × 8000

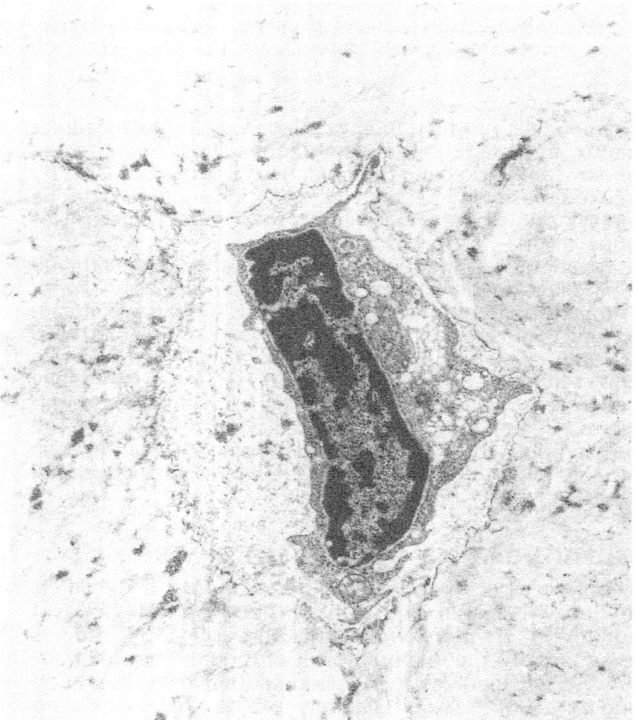

Figs. 1.EM11–EM14 Cytological details of osteocytes

Fig. 1.EM11 Osteocyte nucleus with clumped heterochromatin; numerous cytoplasmic organelles including a centriole. EM × 18 000

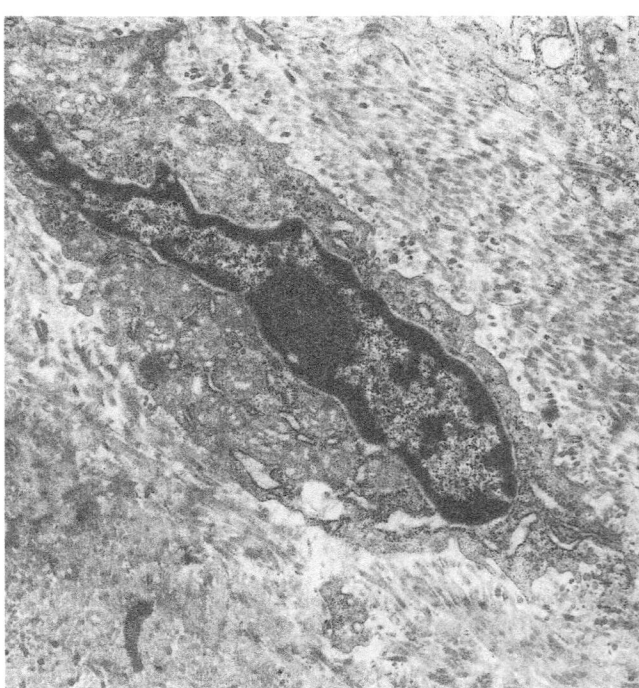

Fig. 1.EM13 Somewhat elongated osteocyte with nucleolated nucleus. Note endoplasmic reticulum, some with dilated cisternae. EM × 9600

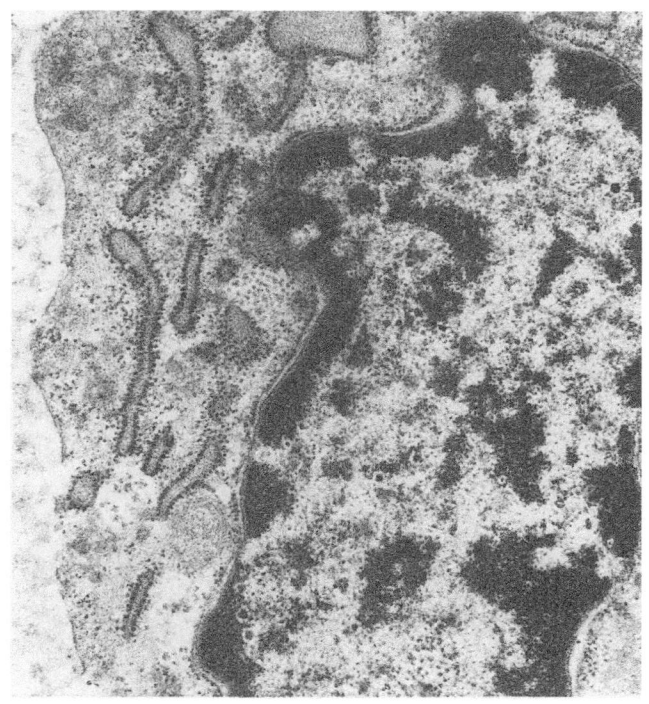

Fig. 1.EM14 Higher magnification illustrating the rough (ribosome studded) endoplasmic reticulum. EM × 41 000

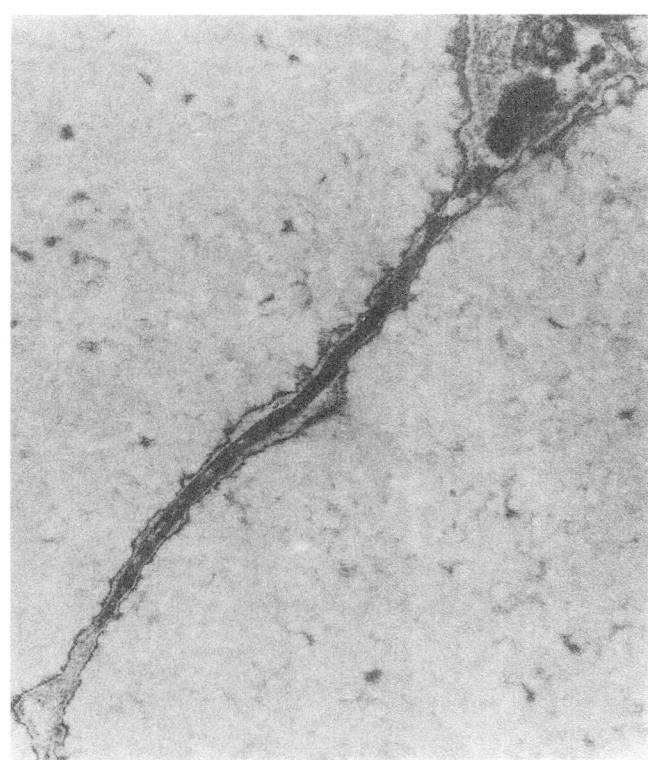

Fig. 1.EM16 Higher magnification of Fig. 1.EM15 showing long filamentous process within a canaliculus. EM × 8800

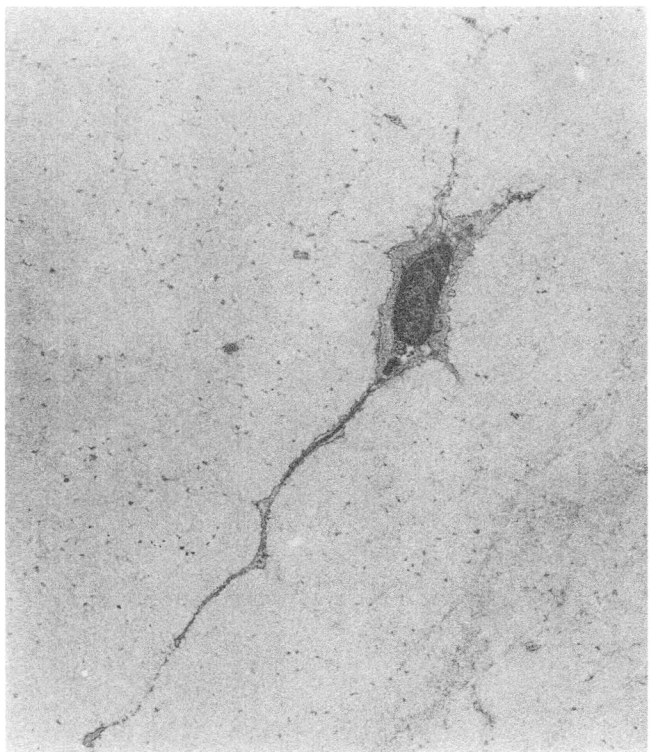

Figs. 1.EM15–EM18 Osteocytes and their processes in canaliculi

Fig. 1.EM15 Osteocyte, osteocytic lacuna and canaliculi. EM × 3200

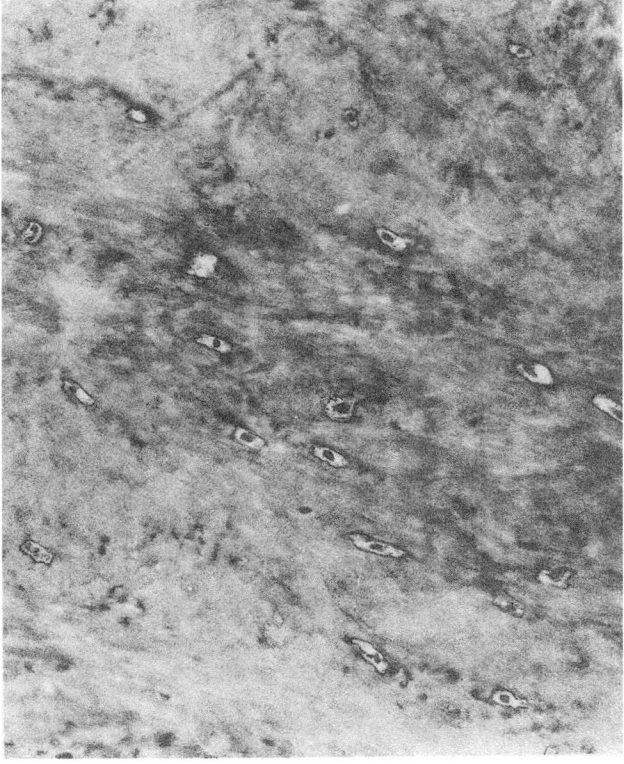

Fig. 1.EM17 Osteocytic canaliculi, many containing cellular processes cut in cross-section. EM × 8200

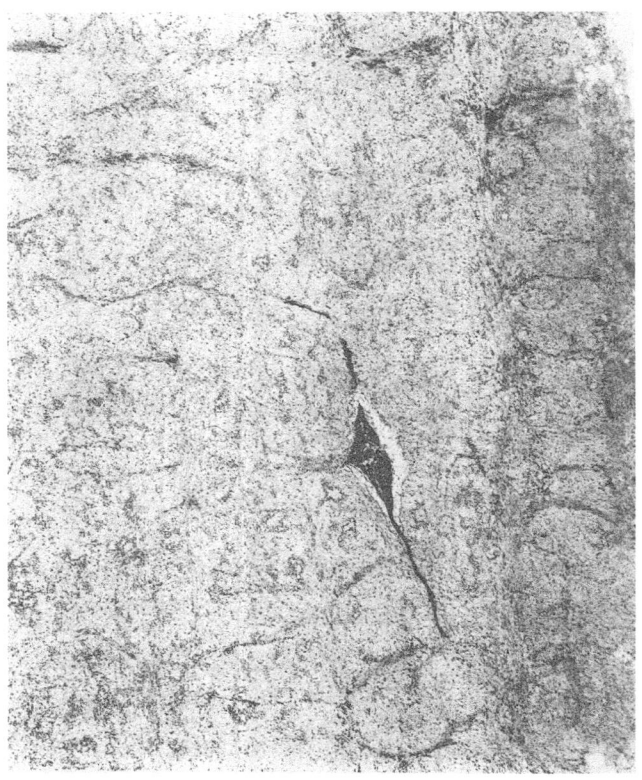

Fig. 1.EM18 Osteocyte at low magnification illustrating extension of nucleus into a canaliculus. This phenomenon was frequently observed in electron micrographs of iliac crest biopsies. EM × 1640

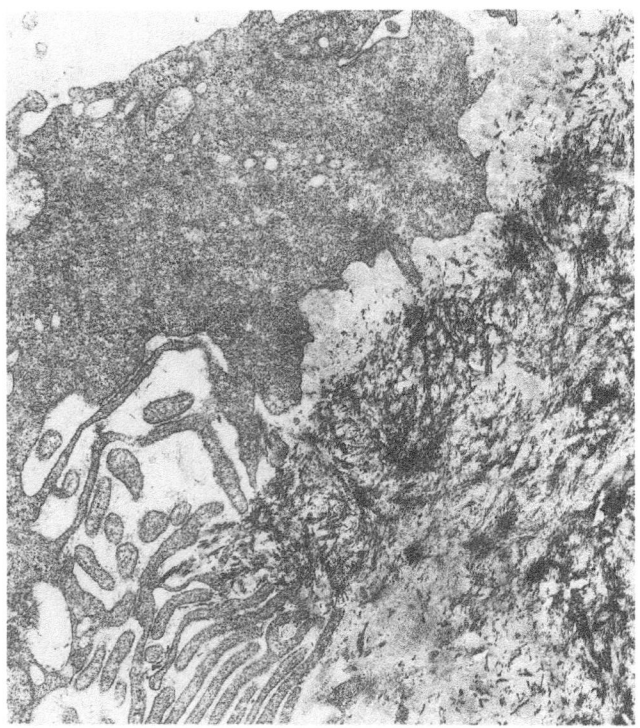

Fig. 1.EM20 Osteoclast attacking mineralized bone matrix. Note cross and longitudinal sectioned villi of ruffled membrane (lower left). EM × 28 500

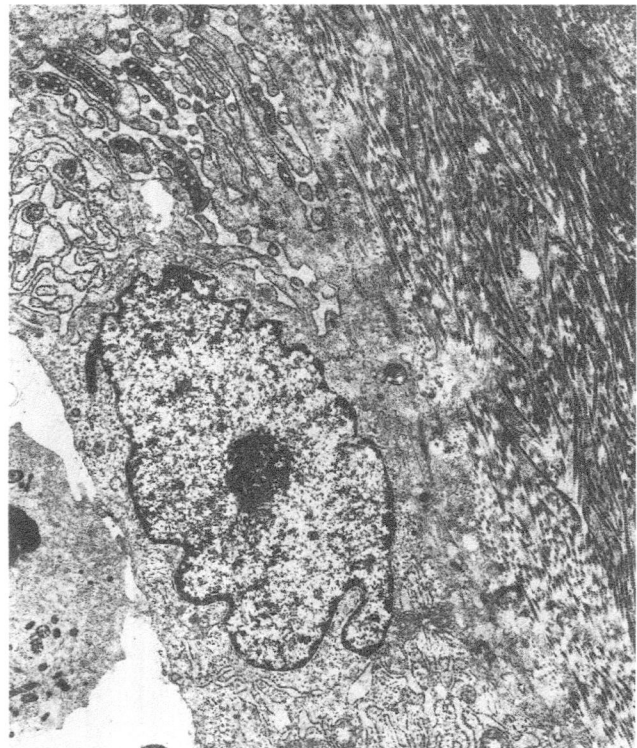

Figs. 1.EM19–EM22 Aspects of osteoclastic resorption

Fig. 1.EM19 Part of osteoclast showing ruffled membrane (upper left and bottom). EM × 17 200

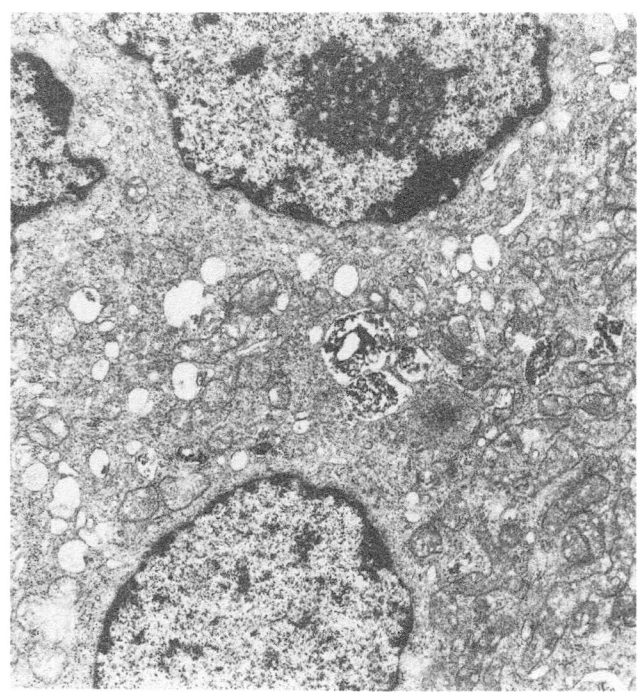

Fig. 1.EM21 Part of multinucleated osteoclast illustrating cytoplasmic vacuoles containing electron-dense material (calcified bone matrix). EM × 27 000

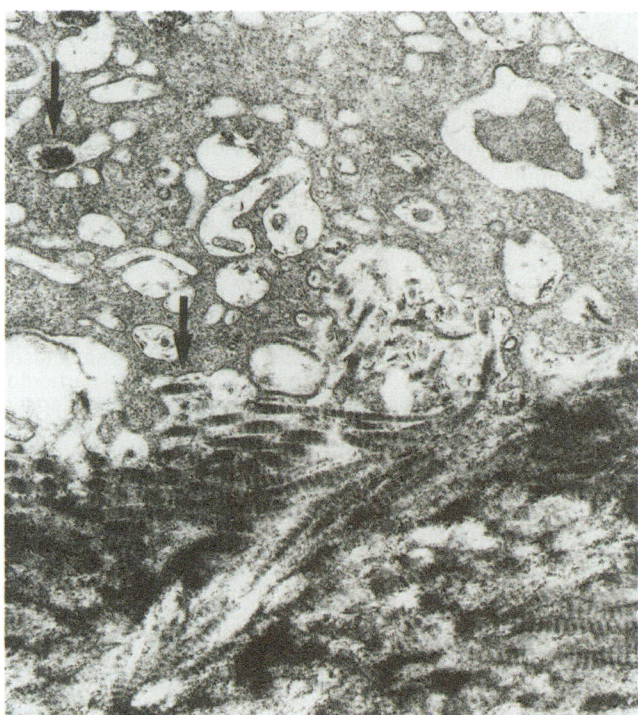

Fig. 1.EM22 Osteoclastic resorption of collagen fibres (centre) and mineralized bone matrix. Note fragments of both in osteoclastic vacuoles (arrows). EM × 40 000

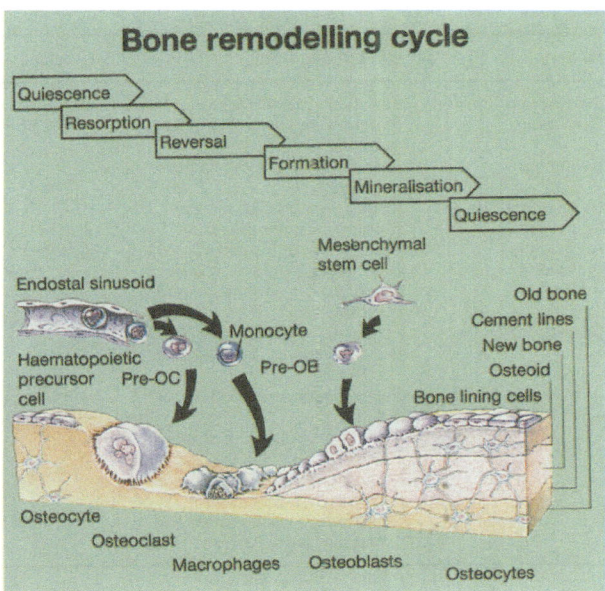

Fig. 1.S6   Diagram of the five phases of bone remodelling

from cortical to trabecular bone and even from one ossicle to another[37].

The concept of bone remodelling was formulated by Frost in 1964 and since then has been elaborated by numerous investigators[59]. Several stages of cellular activity are distinguished: (A) activation of osteoclasts, (R) resorptive phase, (Rev) reversal phase with deposition of a cement line, (F) activation of osteoblasts with formation of osteoid, and (Rest) resting phase after complete mineralization of the osteoid (Fig. 1.S6)[50,117,120].

Trabecular remodelling usually occurs on the surface, whereas in cortical remodelling the osteoclasts tunnel through the bone. Parfitt has proposed two types of trabecular remodelling[110,111]. In the first, resorption is completed before new bone formation begins and in the second new bone formation starts while resorption is still in progress. The complete trabecular bone remodelling cycle takes about 200 days.

The rate of remodelling depends on the number of 'basic multicellular units' (BMU) of bone remodelling operative at any given time. In the normal human skeleton, activation of a unit occurs about every 10 s, and the total number of BMU has been calculated to be about 35 million. It seems likely that the initiation of remodelling is triggered by different stimuli in weight-bearing as opposed to non-weight-bearing bones.

In summary: the formation of functionally competent and adapted bone is the culmination of several closely integrated processes: (1) intramembranous ossification, (2) intracartilagenous ossification, (3) bone growth, (4) the 'modelling' of bone into the required shape and size, and, in the adult skeleton, (5) the constant replacement, 'turnover', of bone by 'remodelling'; and a variety of methods is now available for its measurement[49], though the complete mechanism and pathways of regulation have not yet been unravelled.

INTERACTIONS IN CONTROL OF BONE REMODELLING

The functions of bone cells are regulated by the actions of systemic, circulating *hormones* such as vitamin D, parathyroid hormone and calcitonin, by a variety of locally produced *growth factors*[25,26], by *cytokines*[27,61] and by *cellular connections* between the bone cells themselves and other connective tissue cells in their vicinity such as mast cells (Fig. 1.S7)[102,103,117,145]. Some of these factors have now been identified and characterized (Table 1.1): bone cells synthesize fibroblast growth factors (FGF), platelet-derived growth factor (PDGF), insulin-derived

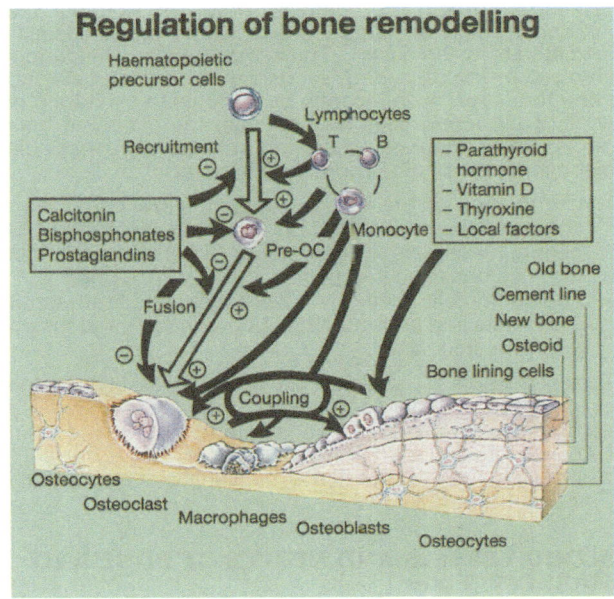

Fig. 1.S7   Sketch of the highly complex regulation of bone remodelling (present state of knowledge)

Table 1.1 Mediators of bone metabolism (present state of knowledge)

Hormones	Growth factors	Cytokines
Parathyroid hormone	Fibroblast growth factors (FGF)	M-CSF
Calcitonin	Platelet-derived growth factors (PDGF)	GM-CSF
Vitamin D	Transforming growth factors (TGF)	IL-1
Glucocorticoids	Insulin-like growth factors (IGF)	IL-6
Oestrogens	Binding proteins (BP)	TNF-α
Androgens	Beta-2-microglobulin (β_2-M)	Interferon
Thyroxine	Osteoinductive factors (OIFs)	
Insulin	Parathyroid hormone-related protein (PTH-rP)	
Growth hormone	Epidermal growth factor (EGF)	
	Oxygen-derived free radicals (ODFR)	
	Plasminogen tissue activator (PTA)	
	Bone morphogenic proteins (BMP)	
	Macrophage-derived growth factor (MDGF)	
	Inhibitors of collagenase and metallo-proteinases	

growth factors (IGF) and transforming growth factor β (TGF-β)[29,115]. Other factors now known to be involved in bone cell metabolism include the bisphosphonates[78], the osteo-inductive factors and various cytokines[64]. Cytokines in particular serve as biological response modifiers[122], and many cells secrete and respond to these mediators, but not all the communication pathways thus established are as yet recognized in bone remodelling as in other biological processes[64]. Consequently a better understanding of activity, synthesis and receptors of the growth factors may result in the therapeutic use of these molecules to enhance growth of bone or repair of fractures[29,35,36]. Additional stimuli are also involved, including electrical[18], magnetic and biomechanical[48,60,72,82,83,135] ones. The concept of interactions between osteoblasts and osteoclasts is an integral component of the 'coupling' theory of bone remodelling first put forward by Frost, 1964[57-59]. However, the idea that cells of the osteoblast lineage can direct osteoclast function is relatively new: for example the inhibitory effect of parathyroid hormone on osteoclasts mediated by osteoblasts[67]. The interactions and mediators involved in the cascading sequence of events leading to bone formation have recently been outlined by Rodan et al.[129]. Bone lining cells may mediate the action of hormones that stimulate resorption through two possible mechanisms, as pointed out by Martin et al.[90]:

1. Contraction of the lining cells may allow osteoclasts access to the mineralized matrix. Once resorption has begun, the release of chemotactic factors would attract more osteoclastic precursors.
2. The lining cells themselves release factors that recruit precursors and promote their differentiation and fusion to form osteoclasts.

These concepts of osteoclast activation are also supported by structural evidence in bone biopsies. A detailed account of current ideas on different factors and their complex interactions has been given by Martin et al.[90]; and for bone cells in particular by Canalis et al.[27] and by Burr and Martin[24].

BLOOD VESSELS AND NERVES OF BONE AND MARROW (Plates 1.U–X)

Bone and marrow are highly vascularized organs which account for about 10% of resting cardiac output. *Nutrient arteries*, the principal source of blood for bones, penetrate the cortex through the nutrient canal. Each nutrient artery is accompanied by nerve fibres, and it branches within the marrow cavities. In long bones it bifurcates into ascending and descending branches from which radial arteries arise, but this does not occur in flat bones like the pelvis. The smaller branches divide into *arterioles* and *capillaries* which either enter the cortex via Volkmann's canals to become cortical capillaries, or lead to a highly branching network of medullary and endosteal *sinusoids* (Fig. 1.S8). These form a spongy network of channels of variable width and length, physiologically characterized by a very low rate of blood flow. A retrograde venous blood flow caused by muscle contractions has been observed in the endosteal sinusoids and this may play an important role in the process of osseous metastases (Batson's vertebral venous plexus)[15]. At any particular time portions of the sinusoidal channels may be collapsed and therefore difficult to identify even in optimal sections. The microvascular system is in a state of constant dynamic change and its expansion and contraction are probably controlled by locally produced factors and by the accompanying *nerve fibres*, which innervate the sphincter mechanisms and specialized thickened endothelial cells present at the bifurcation of smaller arteries[42]. These regulate the blood flow in the different regions of bone and marrow. Within the intertrabecular space central sinusoids are associated with erythrons and megakaryocytes, while endosteal sinusoids of variable number and width accompany the trabeculae. The medullary sinusoids drain into the periosteal venules and veins. Traction of attached muscles may also assist venous drainage. There are close vascular relationships between bone and marrow. For example, changes in haematopoietic activity modify the dynamics of the regional circulation and set up a new equilibrium between bone cells and their environment, resulting in alterations in remodelling and possibly structure, while interference with the blood supply may lead to avascular necrosis of bone. Comprehensive reviews of the bone vasculature are given in refs 22,39,42,55,56,77,126,150,154.

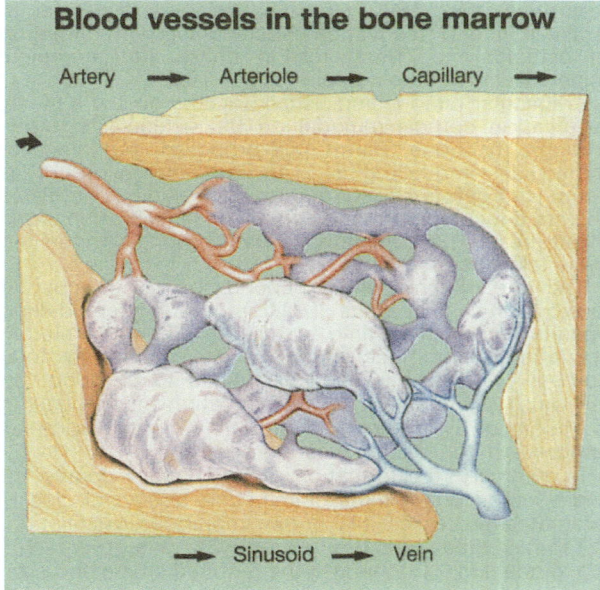

Blood vessels in the bone marrow

Artery → Arteriole → Capillary →

→ Sinusoid → Vein

Fig. 1.S8 Vascular system as seen in a marrow cavity in iliac crest biopsy. The sinusoids may be wide and engorged as illustrated by the two in the foreground, or collapsed and narrow as shown in the background

[continued on p. 45]

Plate 1.U

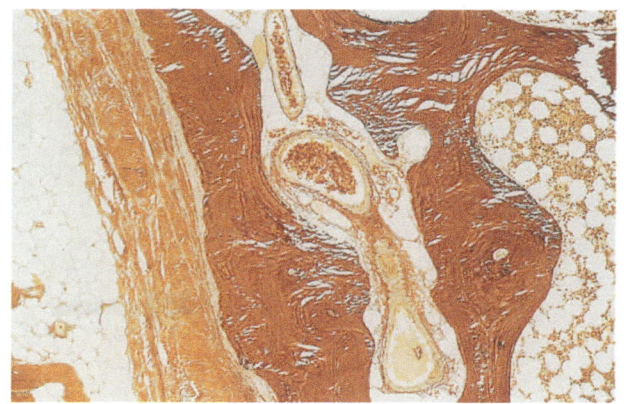

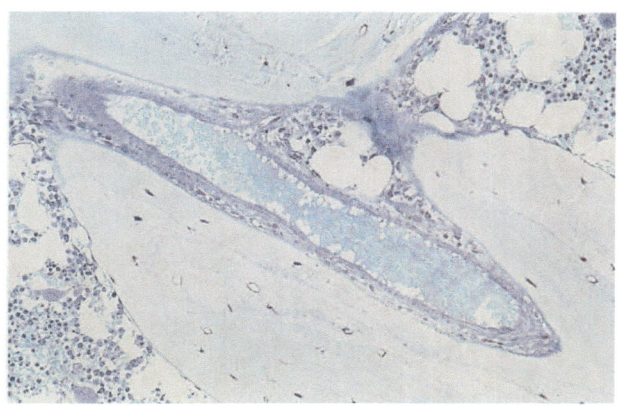

Figs 1.121–1.126 Range of blood vessels in bone and marrow I: larger vessels

Fig. 1.121 Nutrient artery penetrating cortical bone. Gomori

Fig. 1.122 Nutrient artery penetrating subcortical trabecula. Giemsa

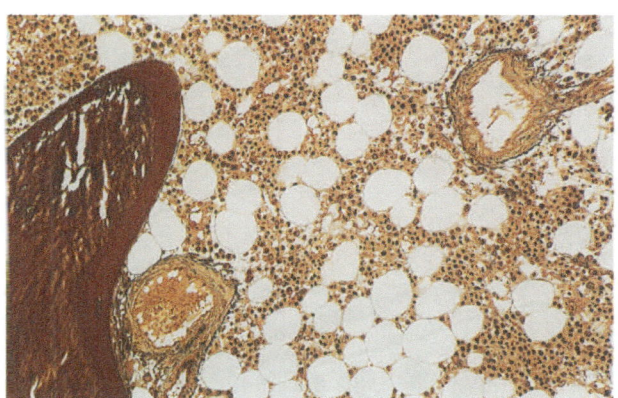

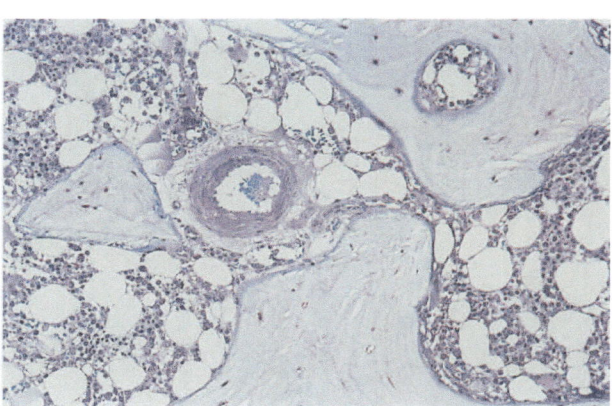

Fig. 1.123 Inter- and paratrabecular arteries. Gomori

Fig. 1.124 Paratrabecular artery within niche formed by erosion of bone, as seen by remodelling on the osseous surface below the artery. Giemsa

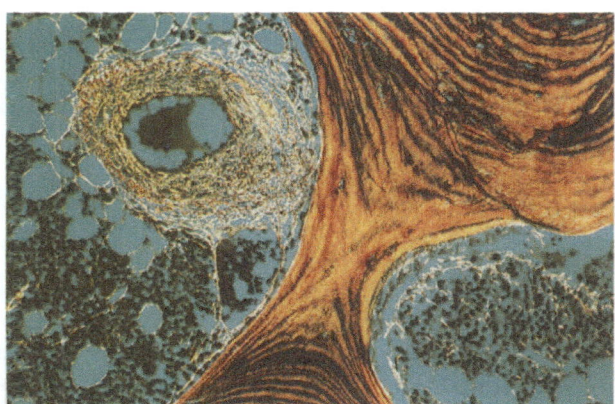

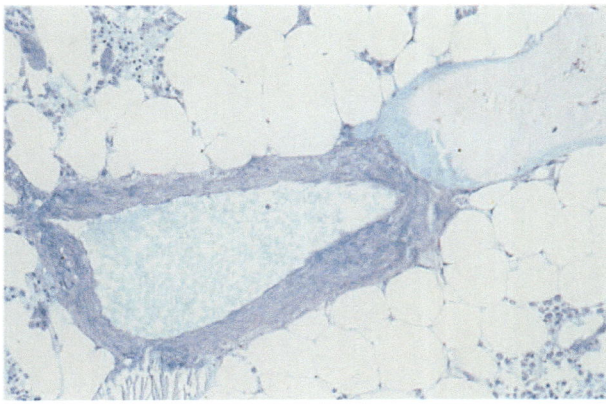

Fig. 1.125 Small artery with more perivascular fibrosis than would be seen in the Giemsa stain. Gomori, polar.

Fig. 1.126 Artery with wide lumen perforating a trabecula. Note osteoid seam adjacent to the vessel wall (upper right). Giemsa

Plate 1.V

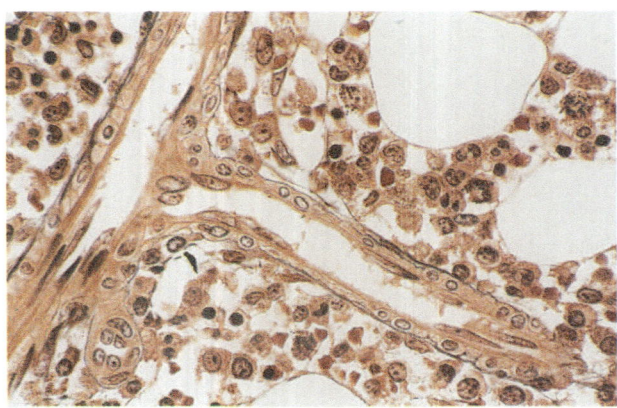

Figs 1.127–1.132 Range of blood vessels in bone and marrow II: smaller vessels

Fig. 1.127 Small artery (left) with branch at right angle. Note endothelial cells (arrow) functioning as sphincter at bifurcation. Gomori

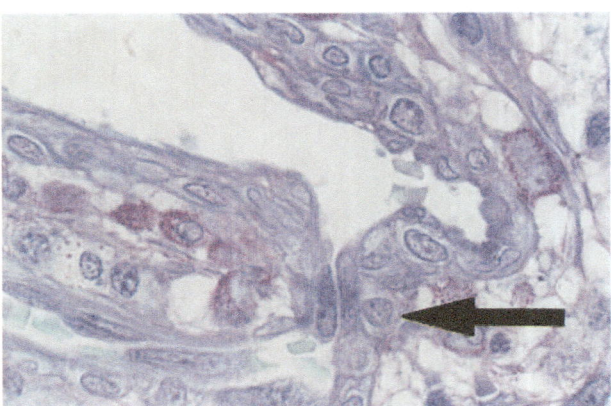

Fig. 1.128 Higher magnification to illustrate sphincter mechanism (arrow) at branching of small artery. Note mast cells and plasma cells adjacent to the vessels. Giemsa

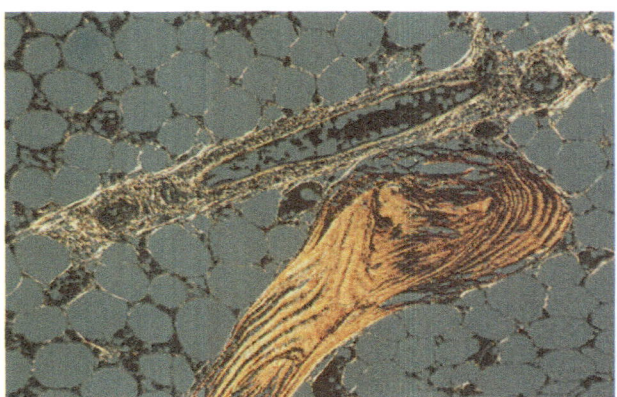

Fig. 1.129 Small artery adjacent to trabecula longitudinally cut, in hypocellular fatty bone marrow. Gomori, polar.

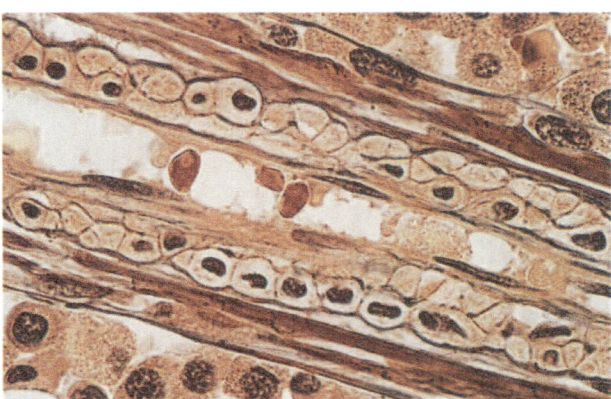

Fig. 1.130 High magnification showing details of the layers of a small artery, from the lumen outwards: flat endothelial cells, row of nuclei of cross-sectioned media, longitudinally cut adventitia and perivascular plasma cells. Gomori

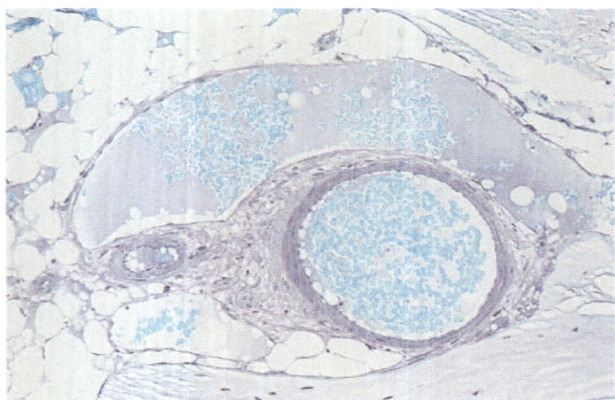

Fig. 1.131 Cross-sections of blood vessels of varying calibres ranging from wide artery to adjacent ectatic sinusoid to small arteries, capillaries and sinusoids (left). Giemsa

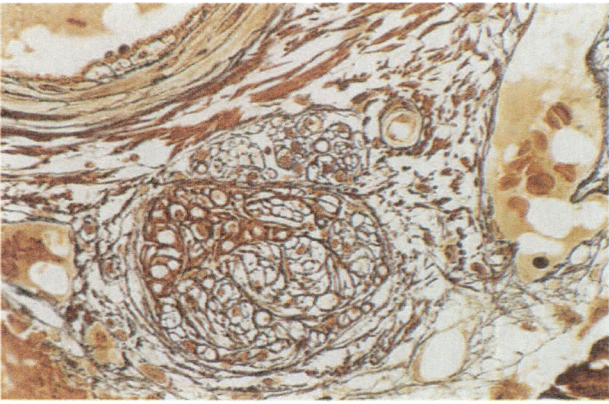

Fig. 1.132 Nerve fibre bundle adjacent to artery (upper left) and sinusoid (upper right) in bone marrow. Gomori

Plate 1.W

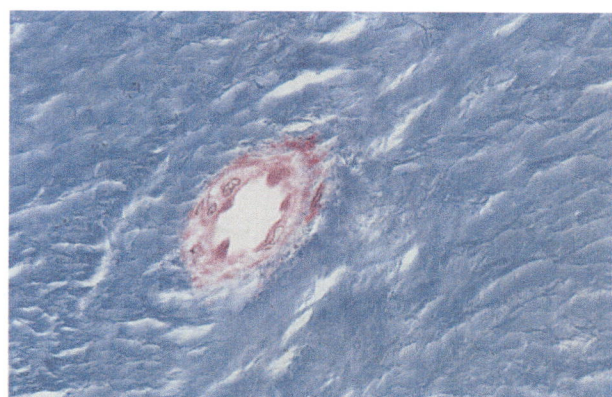

Figs 1.133–1.138 Range of blood vessels in bone and marrow III: small arteries, arterioles and capillaries

Fig. 1.133 Small artery in cortical bone. Ladewig

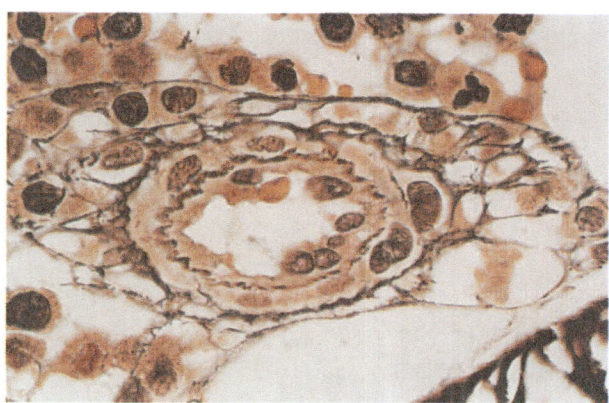

Fig. 1.134 Cross-section of small artery showing endothelial cells, media and adventitia. Gomori

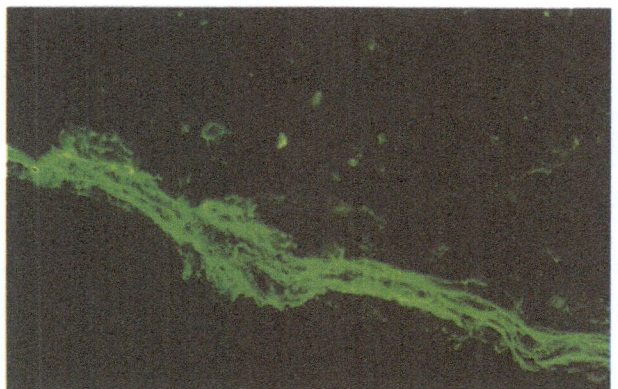

Fig. 1.135 The perivascular fibres consist of collagen type III as shown by immunofluorescent labelling. Cryostat section

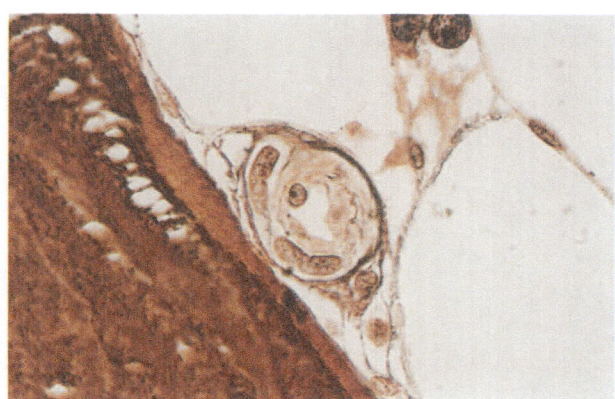

Fig. 1.136 Arteriole on trabecular surface. Gomori

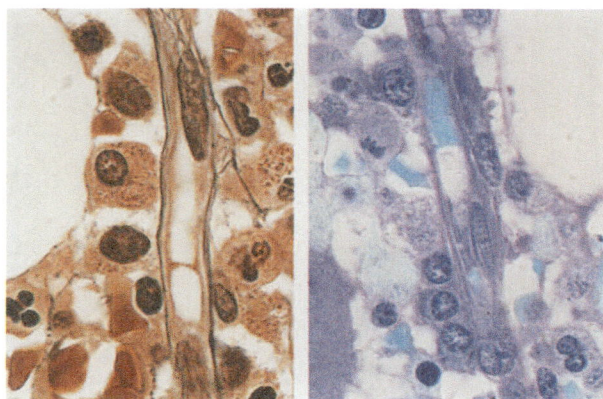

Fig. 1.137 Longitudinal section of capillary with adjacent plasma cells. Gomori and Giemsa

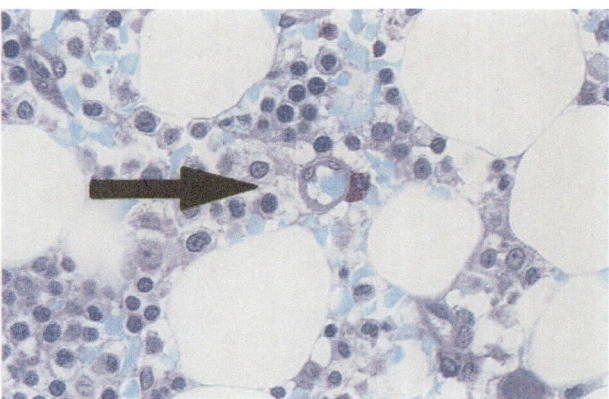

Fig. 1.138 Cross-section of capillary (arrow) in bone marrow. Note mast cell at right of vessel. Giemsa. It is doubtful whether the capillaries illustrated in Fig. 1.137 and 1.138 would be identified in paraffin sections

Plate 1.X

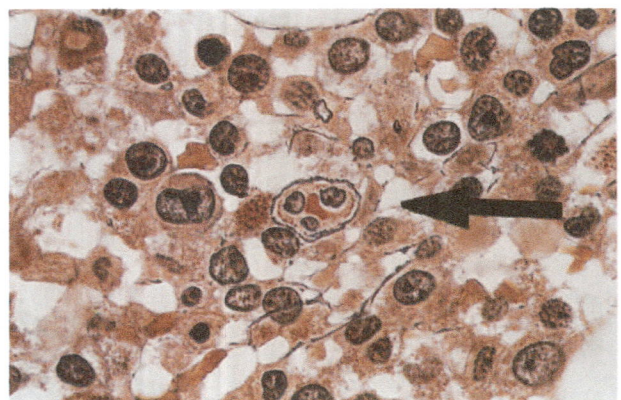

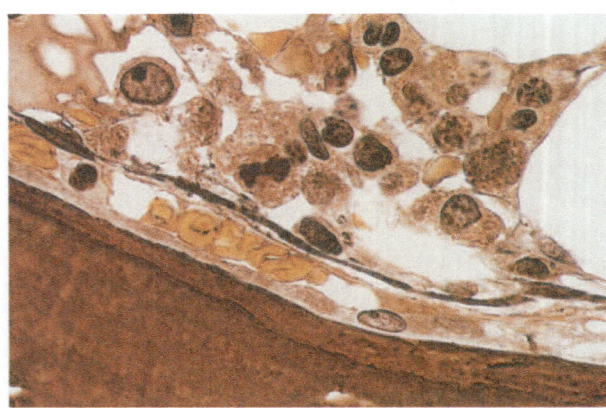

Figs. 1.139–1.144 Range of blood vessels in bone and marrow IV: sinusoids

Fig. 1.140 Narrow endosteal sinusoid filled with erythrocytes (orange). Gomori

Fig. 1.139 Small collapsed sinusoid cut in cross-section at arrow. Gomori

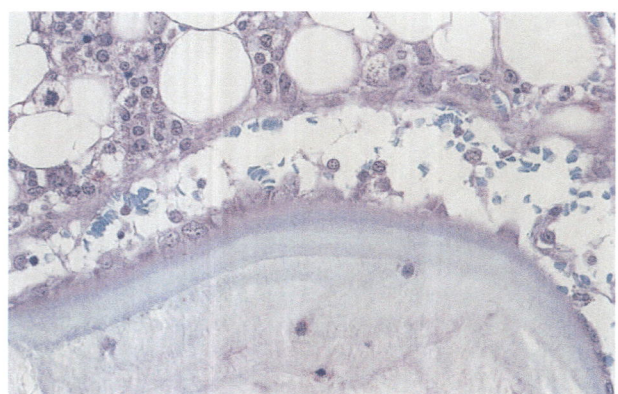

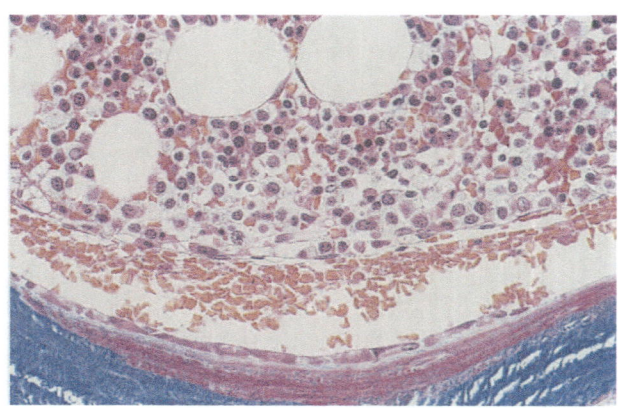

Fig. 1.141 Broad but tapering endosteal sinusoid (centre) with adjacent osteoblastic new bone formation. Giemsa

Fig. 1.142 Broad endosteal sinusoid filled with erythrocytes (centre) with adjacent layers of osteoblasts and osteoid. Ladewig

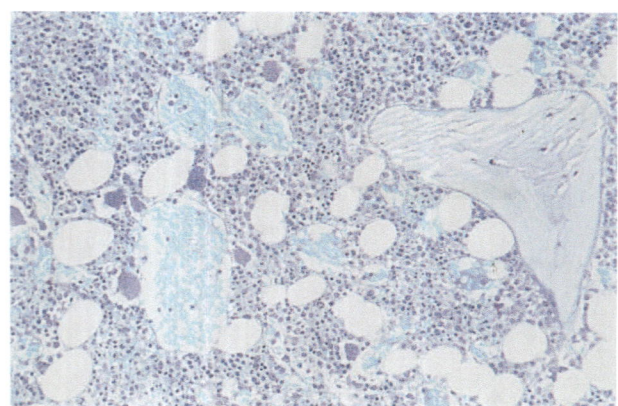

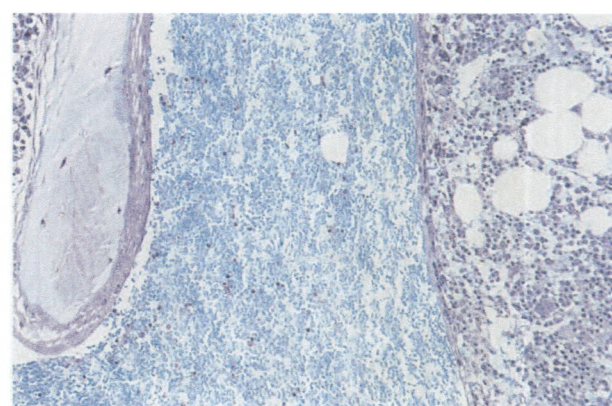

Fig. 1.143 Hyperplastic, engorged intertrabecular sinusoids. Giemsa

Fig. 1.144 Very large, ectatic peritrabecular sinusoid. Giemsa. Such a sinusoid if cut could lead to bleeding during and after taking the biopsy

The *sinusoidal wall* is composed of a thin continuous layer of endothelial cells, a thin interrupted basement membrane and a discontinuous coat of adventitial cells and collagen fibres. The endothelial cells of the sinusoids are actively endocytic and form the interface, the barrier and the control system for substances and particles entering and leaving the haematopoietic and intraosseous spaces. A network of reticular cell cytoplasmic processes and argentophilic fibres extends from one sinusoid to another. Usually the bone lining cells and one layer of endothelial cells of the endosteal sinusoids are closely apposed, sometimes indistinguishable from one another. Mast cells, mesenchymal cells, fibroblasts, macrophages and lymphoid cells are loosely dispersed close to the trabecular surface.

Bone and marrow possess both myelinated and unmyelinated *nerves* which are found in close proximity to the arteries as they enter and branch within the bone marrow. Small unmyelinated nerves have been observed in the Haversian canals near the capillaries. The function of the nerves is probably related to the vascular flow, controlling the expansion and contraction of the vascular system within the rigid bony cage (as described above). Such nerves apparently have free endings.

Lymphatic vessels have not been recognized in bone and marrow.

BONE MARROW

Bone and marrow are closely interrelated organs[55,56,85]: they have one vascular and stromal system, and disorders of the one invariably affect the other to a lesser or greater degree: for example osteoporosis in aplastic and haemolytic anaemias, 'hair on end' skull in thalassaemia, osteolysis in multiple myeloma and bone marrow insufficiency in osteopetrosis[21,22,65,118,148]. Even focal changes in the bone marrow inevitably influence the structure and turnover of the adjacent trabeculae, as has frequently been demonstrated in bone biopsies. Though beyond the scope of this atlas, a brief outline of the main histological features of bone marrow is given below. A detailed description of the marrow is available in the *Atlas of Bone Marrow Pathology* in this series[55].

Haematopoiesis is situated in the extravascular marrow spaces, surrounded and protected by the trabecular network[55,56]. Early *myeloid precursors* occupy the paratrabecular regions close to the endosteal surface, while the more mature granulocytes are found in the central marrow areas. *Erythrons* and *megakaryocytes* are situated close to the sinusoids in the central regions of a marrow space (Fig. 1.S9). *Lymphoid cells* belong to the normal marrow population, and are dispersed among fat cells or form aggregates or nodules. These have been found in 1% to over 40% of bone biopsies, particularly in the older age groups. *Plasma cells* lie in close apposition to capillaries and arterioles. *Mast cells* may be found adjacent to endothelial cells of sinusoids, at the endosteal surface, at the periosteum and around arterial vessels. Bone marrow stroma forms the framework which supports the extravascular haematopoietic compartment and constitutes the *'haematopoietic microenvironment'*[84,141]. It consists of reticular cells, fat cells, fibroblasts and their collagen fibres, mesenchymal cells and the network of small blood vessels. The close association between the mesenchymal elements of bone and marrow – the endothelial cells, the endosteal lining cells, osteoclasts and osteoblasts, macrophages and reticular cells – has induced much speculation and experimental work on their possible origins and capabilities of transformation and differentiation, and the factors and inter-cellular interactions involved in these processes.

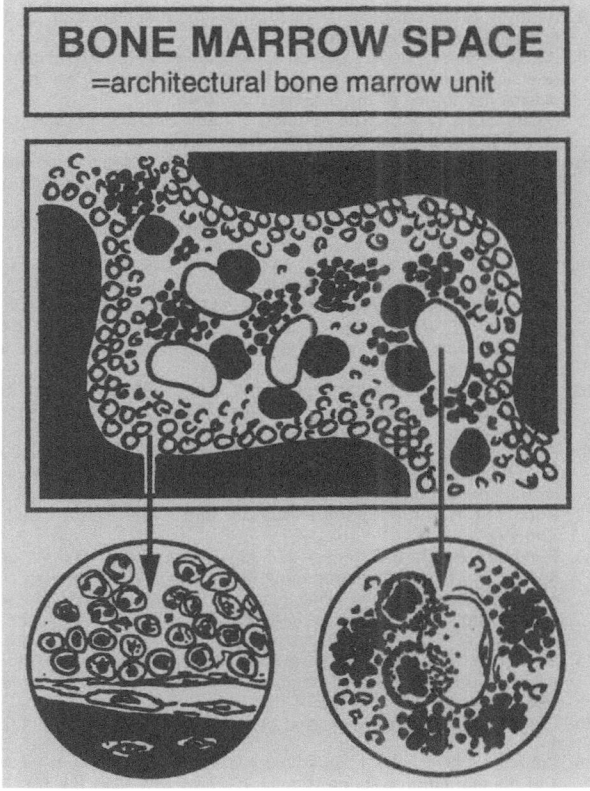

Fig. 1.S9 Normal architecture of the bone marrow, with granulopoietic precursors at endosteal surface (left circle), erythrons and megakaryocytes around the central sinusoids (right circle). This topographic arrangement may be altered when osseous changes are present, such as trabecular osteopenia

References

1. Adler C.-P. (1983). *Knochenkrankheiten*. Stuttgart: Thieme
2. Anderson H. C. (1989). Biology of disease: mechanism of mineral formation. *Lab. Invest.*, **60**, 320
3. Arey L. B. (1965). *Developmental Anatomy: A Textbook and Laboratory Manual of Embryology*. Philadelphia: Saunders
4. Arnaud C. D. (1988). Mineral and bone homeostasis. Wyngaarden J. B. and Smith L. H., *Cecil Textbook of Medicine* (p. 1469). Philadelphia: Saunders
5. Arnett T. R. and Dempster T. W. (1990). Protons and osteoclasts. *J. Bone Miner. Res.*, **5**, 1099
6. Athanasou N. A., Hall D. A., d'Ardenn A. J., Quinn J. and McGee J. O. (1988). A monoclonal antibody (anti-L-35) which reacts with human osteoclasts and cells of the mononuclear phagocyte system. *Brit. J. Exp. Pathol.*, **69**(2), 309
7. Athanasou N. A., Heryet A., Quirn J., Gatter K. C., Mason D. Y. and McGee J. O. (1986). Osteoclasts contain macrophage and megakaryocyte antigens. *J. Pathol.*, **150**, 239
8. Athanasou N. A., Quinn, J. and McGee J. O. (1988). Immunocytochemical analysis of the human osteoclast: phenotypic relationship to other marrow-derived cells. *Bone Miner.*, **3**(4), 317
9. Athanasou N. A., Quinn J. and McGee J. O. (1987). Leucocyte common antigen is present on osteoclast. *J. Pathol.*, **153**, 121
10. Athanasou N. A., Quinn J., Horton M. A. and McGee I. D. (1990). New sites of cellular vitronectin receptor immunoreactivity detected with osteoclast reacting monoclonal antibodies 13C2 and 23C6. *Bone Miner.*, **8**(1), 7
11. Avioli L. V., Hruska K. and Civitelli R. (1990). Activation of the (Ca 2+)i message system by parathyroid-hormone-related protein in osteoblastic cells. *Adv. Second Mess.-Phosphoprotein Res.*, **24**, 529
12. Avioli L. V. and Krane S. M. (1990). *Metabolic Bone Disease*. Philadelphia: Saunders

13. Baron R. (1989). Molecular mechanisms of bone resorption by the osteoclast. *Anat. Rec.*, **224**, 317

14. Baron R., Neft L., Roy C., Boivert A. and Caplan M. (1986). Evidence of a high and specific concentration of (Na + K +)ATPase in the plasma membrane of the osteoclast. *Cell*, **46**, 311

15. Batson O. V. (1940). The function of the vertebral veins and their role in spread of metastases. *Ann. Surg.*, **112**, 138

16. Blair H. C., Kahn A. J. and Crouch E. C. (1986). Isolated osteoclasts resorb the organic and inorganic components of bone. *J. Cell Biol.*, **102**, 1164

17. Bouvier M. (1989). The biology and composition of bone. Cowin St. C., *Bone Mechanics* (p. 1). Boca Raton: CRC Press

18. Brighton C. T. and McCluskey W. P. (1986). Cellular response and mechanisms of action of electrically induced osteogenesis. Peck W. A., *Bone and Mineral Research/4* (p. 213). Amsterdam: Elsevier

19. Burger E. H., VanDerMeer J. W. N. and Nijweide P. J. (1984). Osteoclast formation from mononuclear phagocytes: role of bone-forming cells. *J. Cell Biol.*, **99**, 1901

20. Burger E. H. and VanDerMeer J. W. M. (1984). Precursor cell proliferation during osteoclast formation from bone marrow phago-cytes. *Calcif. Tissue Int.*, **36**, 454

21. Burgio G. R., Arico M., Caselli D., Beluffi G. and Calligaro A. (1987). Bone and bone marrow syndromes: a causal, not only casual connection? *Haematologia*, **72**, 363

22. Burkhardt R. (1971). *Bone Marrow and Bone Tissue*. Berlin: Springer

23. Burkhardt R., Bartl R., Frisch B., Jäger K., Mahl G., Hill W. and Kettner G. (1984). The structural relationship of bone forming and endothelial cells of the bone marrow. Arlet J., Ficat R. P. and Hungerford D. S., *Bone Circulation* (p. 2). Baltimore: Williams & Wilkins

24. Burr D. B. and Martin R. B. (1989). Errors in bone remodelling: toward a unified theory of metabolic bone disease. *Amer. J. Anat.*, **186**, 186

25. Canalis E. (1988). Bone-related growth factors. *Triangle*, **27**(1/2), 11

26. Canalis E., McCarthy T. and Centrella M. (1988). Growth factors and the regulation of bone formation. *Endocrine Rev.*, **83**, 60

27. Canalis E., McCarthy T. L. and Centrella M. (1991). Growth factors and cytokines in bone cell metabolism. *Ann. Rev. Med.*, **42**, 17

28. Carmel R., Lau K.-H. W., Baylink D. J., Saxena S. and Singer F. R. (1988). Cobalamin and osteoblast-specific proteins. *N. Engl. J. Med.*, **319**, 70

29. Centrella M., McCarthy T. and Canalis E. (1991). Current concepts review: transforming growth factor-beta and remodeling of bone. *J. Bone Jt. Surg.*, **73A**, 1418

30. Chambers T. J. (1982). Osteoblasts release osteoclasts from calci-tonin-induced quiescence. *J. Cell Sci.*, **57**, 247

31. Chambers T. J. (1985). The pathobiology of the osteoclast. *J. Clin. Pathol.*, **38**, 241

32. Chambers T. J. and Hall T. J. (1991). Cellular and molecular mechanisms in the regulation and function of osteoclasts. *Vitam.-Horm.*, **46**, 41

33. Chilosi M., Gilioli E., Lestani M., Menestrina F. and Fiore-Donati L. (1988). Immunohistochemical characterization of osteoclasts and osteoclast-like cells with monoclonal antibody MBI on paraffin-embedded tissues. *J. Pathol.*, **156**, 251

34. Chow J., Tobias J. H., Colston K. W. and Chambers T. J. (1992). Estrogen maintains trabecular bone volume in rats not only by suppression of bone resorption but also by stimulation of bone formation. *J. Clin. Invest.*, **89**, 74

35. Colvard D. S., Eriksen E. F., Keeting P. E., Wilson E. M., Lubahn D. B., French F. S., Riggs B. L. and Spelsberg T. C. (1989). Identification of androgen receptors in normal human osteoblast-like cells. *Proc. Natl Acad. Sci.*, **86**, 854

36. Colvard D., Spelsberg T., Eriksen E., Keeting P. and Riggs B. L. (1989). Evidence of steroid receptors on human osteoblast-like cells. *Connect. Tissue Res.*, **20**, 33

37. Davidovitch Z., Hicolay O. F., Hgan P. W. and Shanfield J. L. (1988). Neurotransmitters, cytokines, and the control of alveolar bone remodeling in orthodontics. *Dent. Clin. North Amer.*, **32**(3), 411

38. Davies J., Warwick J., Totty N., Philp R., Helfrich M. and Horton M. (1989). The osteoclast functional antigen, implicated in the regulation of bone resorption, is biochemically related to the vitronectin receptor. *J. Cell Biol.*, **109**, 1817

39. deBruyn P. P. H., Breen P. C. and Thomas T. B. (1970). The microcirculation of the bone marrow. *Anat. Rec.*, **168**, 55

40. Delaisse J. M., Boyde A. and McConnachie E. (1987). The effects of inhibitors of cysteine-proteinases and collagenase on the resorptive activity of isolated osteoclasts. *Bone*, **8**, 305

41. Deldar A., Lewis H. and Weiss L. (1985). Bone lining·cells and hematopoiesis: an electron microscopic study of canine bone marrow. *Anat. Rec.*, **213**, 187

42. Demmler K. (1976). *Das Gefäßsystem des Knochenmarks*. Stuttgart: Ferdinand Enke

43. Dodds R. A., Emery R. J., Klenerman L., Chayen J. and Bitensky L. (1989). Comparative metabolic enzymatic activity in trabecular as against cortical osteoblasts. *Bone*, **10**, 251

44. Doty S. B. (1981). Morphological evidence of gap junctions between bone cells. *Calcif. Tissue Int.*, **33**, 509

45. Editorial. (1990). Fibroblast growth factors: time to take note. *Lancet*, **336**, 777

46. Editorial. (1992). New bone? *Lancet*, **339**, 463

47. Eekhout Y. and Delaisse J. M. (1988). The role of collagenase in bone resorption. An overview. *Pathol. Biol.*, **36**, 1139

48. Einhorn T. A. (1988). Biomechanical properties of bone. *Triangle*, **27**(1/2), 27

49. Epstein S. (1988). Serum and urinary markers of bone remodeling: assessment of bone turnover. *Endocrine Rev.*, **9**(4), 437

50. Eriksen E. F. (1986). Normal and pathological remodeling of human trabecular bone: three dimensional reconstruction of the remodeling sequence in normals and in metabolic bone disease. *Endocrine Rev.*, **7**, 379

51. Evans D. B., Bunning R. A. and Kanis R. G. (1990). The effects of recombinant human interleukin 1 beta on cellular proliferation and the production of prostaglandin E2, plasminogen activator, osteocalcin and alkaline phosphatase by osteoblast-like cells derived from human bone. *Biochem. Biophys. Res. Commun.*, **166**, 208

52. Evans D. B., Russell R. G., Brown B. L. and Dobson P. R. (1989). Agents affecting adenylate cyclase activity modulate the stimulatory action of 1,25-dihydroxy vitamin D3 on the production of osteocal-cin by human bone cells. *Biochem. Biophys. Res. Commun.*, **164**, 1076

53. Evans D. B., Thavarajah M. and Kanis S. A. (1990). Involvement of prostaglandin E2 in the inhibition of osteocalcin synthesis by human osteoblast-like cells in response to cytokines and systemic hormones. *Biochem. Biophys. Res. Commun.*, **167**, 194

54. Fawcett D. W. (1986). *Bloom and Fawcett – a Textbook of Histology*. Philadelphia: Saunders

55. Frisch B. and Bartl R. (1990). *Atlas of Bone Marrow Pathology*. Dordrecht: Kluwer

56. Frisch B., Lewis S. M., Burkhardt R. and Bartl R. (1985). *Biopsy Pathology of Bone and Bone Marrow*. London: Chapman & Hall

57. Frost H. M. (1963). *Bone Remodeling Dynamics*. Springfield: Thomas

58. Frost H. M. (1973). *Bone Remodelling and its Relationship to Metabolic Bone Diseases*. Springfield: Thomas

59. Frost H. M. (1964). Dynamics of bone remodelling. Frost H. M., *Bone Biodynamics* (p. 315). Boston: Little, Brown

60. Frost H. M. (1990). Skeletal structural adaptations to mechanical usage (SATMU): 2. Redefining Wolff's law: the remodeling problem. *Anat. Rec.*, **226**(4), 414

61. Garrett R. I., Durie B. G. M. and Nedwin G. E. (1987). Production of lymphotoxin, a bone-resorbing cytokine, by cultured human myeloma cells. *N. Engl. J. Med.*, **317**, 526

62. Gay C. V., Ito M. B. and Schraer H. (1984). Carbonic anhydrase activity in isolated osteoclasts. *Metab. Bone Dis. Rel. Res.*, **5**, 33

63. Grech P., Martin T. J., Barrington N. A. and Ell P. J. (1985). *Diagnosis of Metabolic Bone Disease*. London: Chapman & Hall

64. Gruber H. E. (1991). Bone and the immune system. *Proc. Soc. Exp. Biol. Med.*, **197**, 219

65. Gulati G. L., Ashton J. K. and Hyuan B. H. (1988). Structure and function of the bone marrow and hematopoiesis. *Hematol./Oncol. Clin. N. Amer.*, **2**(4), 495

66. Hanaoka H., Yabe H. and Bun H. (1989). The origin of the osteoclast. *Clin. Orthop.*, **239**, 286

67. Heersche J. N. M. (1991). Bone cells and bone turnover – the basis for pathogenesis. Tam C. S., Heersche J. N. M. and Murray T. M., *Metabolic Bone Disease: Cellular and Tissue Mechanisms* (p. 1). Boca Raton: CRC Press

68. Holick M. F., Krane S. M. and Potts J. T. (1991). Calcium, phosphorus, and bone metabolism: calcium-regulating hormones. Wilson J. D., *Harrison's Principles of Internal Medicine* (p. 1888). New York: McGraw-Hill

69. Huffer W. E. (1988). Morphology and biochemistry of bone remode-ling: possible control by vitamin D, parathyroid hormone, and other substances. *Lab. Invest.*, **59**, 418

70. Islam A., Glomski C. and Henderson E. S. (1990). Bone lining (endosteal) cells and hematopoiesis: a light microscopic study of

70. normal and pathologic human bone marrow in plastic-embedded sections. *Anat. Rec.*, **227**, 300

71. Jandinski J. J. (1988). Osteoclast activation factor is now interleukin-1 beta: historical perspective and biological implications. *J. Oral Pathol.*, **17**, 145

72. Jaworski Z. F. G. (1987). Does the mechanical usage (MU) inhibit bone 'remodeling'? *Calcif. Tissue Int.*, **41**, 239

73. Jilka R. L. (1986). Are osteoblastic cells required for the control of osteoclastic activity by parathyroid hormone? *Bone Miner.*, **1**, 261

74. Junth G., Berghauser K. H., Termine J. D. and Schulz A. (1987). Osteonectin – a differentiation marker of bone cells. *Cell Tissue Res.*, **248**, 409

75. Kahn A. J. and Partridge N. C. (1987). New concepts in bone remodelling: an expanding role for the osteoblast. *Amer. J. Otolaryngol.*, **8**, 258

76. Katz E. P. and Li S-T. (1973). Structure and function of bone collagen fibrils. *J. Mol. Biol.*, **80**, 1

77. Kelly P. J. and Montgomery R. J. (1990). Circulation in bone. McCollister Evarts C., *Surgery of the Musculoskeletal System*, 2nd edn (p. 71). New York: Churchill Livingstone

78. Khokher M. A. and Dandona P. (1989). Diphosphonates inhibit human osteoblast secretion and proliferation. *Metabolism*, **38**, 184

79. Koshihara Y. and Kawamura M. (1989). Prostaglandin D2 stimulates calcification of human osteoblastic cells. *Biophys. Res. Commun.*, **159**, 1206

80. Kragstrup J., Melsen F. and Mosekilde L. (1983). Thickness of lamellae in normal human iliac trabecular bone. *Metab. Bone Dis. Rel. Res.*, **4**, 291

81. Kukita T. and Roodman G. D. (1989). Development of a monoclonal antibody to osteoclasts formed *in vitro* which recognizes mononuclear osteoclast precursors in the marrow. *Endocrinology*, **125**, 630

82. Lanyon L. E. (1986). Biomechanical factors in adaptation of bone structure. Uhthoff H. K. and Stahl E. *Current Concepts of Bone Fragility* (p. 19). Berlin: Springer

83. Lanyon L. E. (1987). Functional strain in bone tissue as an objective, and controlling stimulus for adaptive bone remodelling. *J. Biochem.*, **20**, 1083

84. Lichtman M. A. (1981). The ultrastructure of the hematopoietic environment of the marrow: a review. *Exp. Hematol.*, **9**(4), 391

85. Lips P., VanGinkel F. C. and Netelenbos J. C. (1985). Bone marrow and bone remodelling. *Bone*, **6**, 343

86. Little K. (1973). *Bone Behaviour*. London: Academic Press

87. Lomri A. and Marie P. J. (1990). Changes in cytoskeletal proteins in response to parathyroid hormone and 1,25-dihydroxy vitamin D in human osteoblastic cells. *Bone Miner.*, **10**(1), 1

88. Marcus R. (1987). Normal and abnormal bone remodeling in man. *Annu. Rev. Med.*, **38**, 129

89. Marks S. C. (1989). Osteoclast biology: lessons from mammalian mutations. *Am. J. Med. Genet.*, **34**(1), 43

90. Martin T. J., Ng K. W. and Suda T. (1989). Bone cell physiology. *Endocrinol. Metab. Clin. N. Amer.*, **18**(4), 833

91. Martin T. J., Ng K. W. and Nicholson G. C. (1988). Cell biology of bone. Martin T. J., *Metabolic Bone Disease* (p. 1). London: Baillière Tindall

92. Martin T. J., Raisz L. G. and Rodan G. (1987). Calcium regulation and bone metabolism. Martin T. J. and Raisz L. G., *Clinical Endocrinology of Calcium Metabolism* (p. 1). New York: Marcel Dekker

93. Matsuyama T., Lau K.-H. and Wergedal J. E. (1990). Monolayer cultures of normal human bone cells contain multiple subpopulations of alkaline phosphatase positive cells. *Calcif. Tissue Int.*, **47**, 276

94. McGuire J. L., Marks S. C. and Drezner M. K. (1989). Metabolic bone disease. Kelley W. N., *Textbook of Internal Medicine* (p. 2232). Philadelphia: Lippincott

95. Melsen F., Mosekilde L., Eriksen E. F., Charles P. and Steinike T. (1989). *In vivo* hormonal effects on trabecular bone remodeling, osteoid mineralisation, and skeletal turnover. Kleerekoper M. and Krane S. M., *Clinical Disorders of Bone and Mineral Metabolism* (p. 25). New York: Liebert

96. Milgram J. W. (1990). *Radiologic and Histologic Pathology of Nontumorous Diseases of Bones and Joints*. South Lane Northbrook: Northbrook Publ. Co.

97. Miller S. C. (1987). The bone lining cell: a distinct phenotype? *Calcif. Tissue Int.*, **41**, 1

98. Miller E. J. and Martin G. R. (1968). The collagen of bone. *Clin. Orthop.*, **59**, 195

99. Minkin C. and Shapiro I. M. (1986). Osteoclasts, mononuclear phagocytes, and physiological bone resorption. *Calcif. Tissue Int.*, **39**, 357

100. Mosekilde L. (1990). Consecuences of the remodelling process for vertebral trabecular bone structure: a scanning electron microscopic study (uncoupling of unloaded structures). *Bone Miner.*, **10**, 13

101. Mundy G. R. (1987). Bone resorption and turnover in health and disease. *Bone*, **8**, Suppl., 9

102. Mundy G. R. (1989). Local factors in bone remodelling. *Rec. Progr. Horm. Res.*, **45**, 507

103. Mundy G. R. and Bonewald L. F. (1990). Role of TGFβ in bone remodeling. *Ann. N.Y. Acad. Sci.*, **593**, 91

104. Murray R. O., Jacobson H. G. and Stocker D. J. (1990). *The Radiology of Skeletal Disorders*. Edinburgh: Churchill Livingstone

105. Nijweide P. J., Burger E. H. and Feyen J. H. M. (1986). Cells of bone: proliferation, differentiation, and hormonal regulation. *Physiol. Rev.*, **66**, 855

106. Nijweide D. J., v.d.Plas A. and Olthof A. A. (1988). Osteoblastic differentiation. *Ciba Foundation Symp.*, **136**, 61

107. Osdoky P., Oursler M. J., Salino-Hugg T. and Krukovsky M. (1988). Osteoclast development: the cell surface and the bone environment. *Ciba Foundation Symp.*, **136**, 108

108. Owen M. (1985). Lineage of osteogenic cells and their relationship to the stromal system. Peck W. A., *Bone and Mineral Research*, vol. 3 (p. 1). Amsterdam: Elsevier

109. Palle S., Chappard D., Vico L., Riffat G. and Alexandre C. (1989). Evaluation of the osteoclastic population in iliac crest biopsies from 36 normal subjects: a histoenzymologic and histomorphometric study. *J. Bone Miner. Res.*, **4**, 501

110. Parfitt A. M. (1983). The physiologic and clinical significance of bone histomorphometric data. Recker R. R., *Bone Histomorphometry: Techniques and Interpretation* (p. 143). Boca Raton: CRC Press)

111. Parfitt A. M. (1987). Trabecular bone architecture in the pathogenesis and prevention of fracture. *Amer. J. Med.*, **82**, 68

112. Patten B. M. and Carlson B. M. (1974). *Foundations of Embryology*. New York: McGraw-Hill

113. Pierce A. N., Lindskog S. and Hammerstrom L. (1991). Osteoclasts: structure and function. *Electron-microsc. Rev.*, **4**, 1

114. Posner A. S. (1985). The mineral of bone. *Clin. Orthop. Rel. Res.*, **200**, 87

115. Price P. A. (1988). New bone markers. *Triangle*, **27**(1/2), 21

116. Prockop D. J., Mivirikko K. I., Tuderman L. and Guzman N. A. (1979). The biosynthesis of collagen and its disorders. *N. Engl. J. Med.*, **301**, 13

117. Raisz L. G. (1988). Bone metabolism and its hormonal regulation. *Triangle*, **27**(1/2), 5

118. Raisz L. G. (1981). What marrow does to bone. *N. Engl. J. Med.*, **304**, 1485

119. Raisz L. G. and Kream B. E. (1983). Regulation of bone formation. *N. Engl. J. Med.*, **83**, 309

120. Rasmussen H. and Bordier P. (1974). *The Physiological and Cellular Basis of Metabolic Bone Disease*. Baltimore: Williams & Wilkins

121. Reddi A. H. (1985). Regulation of bone differentiation by local and systemic factors. Peck W. A., *Bone and Mineral Research*, vol. 3 (p. 27). Amsterdam: Elsevier

122. Rees R. C. (1992). Cytokines as biological response modifiers. *J. Clin. Pathol.*, **45**, 93

123. Reichel H., Koeffler P. and Norman A. W. (1989). The role of the vitamin D endocrine system in health and disease. *N. Engl. J. Med.*, **320**, 980

124. Reid S. A. (1986). A study of lamellar organisation in juvenile and adult human bone. *Anat. Embryol.*, **174**, 329

125. Revell P. A. (1986). *Pathology of Bone*. Berlin: Springer

126. Rhinelander F. W. (1972). Circulation of bone. Bourne G. H., *The Biochemistry and Physiology of Bone*, vol. 2 (p. 1). New York: Academic Press

127. Riggs B. L., Wahner H. W. and Melton L. J. (1986). Rates of bone loss in the appendicular and axial skeletons of women. *J. Clin. Invest.*, **77**, 1487

128. Robey P. J., Young M. F., Fisher L. W. and McClain T. D. (1989). Thrombospodin is an osteoblast-derived component of mineralized extracellular matrix. *J. Cell Biol.*, **108**, 719

129. Rodan G. A. (1991). Autocrine/paracrine regulation of osteoblast growth and differentiation. *Lab. Invest.*, **64**(5), 593

130. Rodan G. A., Heath J. K., Yoon K., Noda M. and Rodan S. B. (1988). Diversity of the osteoblastic phenotype. *Ciba Foundation Symp.*, **136**, 78

131. Rodan S. B., Wesolovsky G., Thomas K. A., Yoon K. and Rodan G. A. (1989). Effects of acidic and basic fibroblast growth factors on osteoblastic cells. *Connect. Tissue Res.*, **20**, 283

132. Romanowski R., Jundt G., Termine J. D., vonderMark K. and Schulz A. (1990). Immunoelectron microscopy of osteonectin and type I collagen in osteoblasts and bone matrix. *Calcif. Tissue Int.*, **46**, 353
133. Roodman G. D. (1991). Osteoclast differentiation. *Crit. Rev. Oral Biol. Med.*, **2**, 389
134. Ross M. H., Reith E. J. and Romrell L. J. (1989). *Histology – A Text and Atlas*. Baltimore: Williams & Wilkins
135. Rubin C. T. and Lanyon L. E. (1987). Osteoregulatory nature of mechanical stimuli: function as a determinant for adaptive remodeling in bone. *J. Orthop. Res.*, **5**, 300
136. Singh I. (1978). The architecture of cancellous bone. *J. Anat.*, **127**(2), 305
137. Smith L. H. and Thier S. O. (1985). *Pathophysiology*. Philadelphia: Saunders
138. Smith R. (1987). Disorders of the skeleton. Weatherall D. J., Ledingham J. G. G. and Warrell D. A., *Oxford Textbook of Medicine* (p. 17.1). Oxford: Oxford University Press
139. Steiniche T., Vesterby A., Eriksen E. F., Mosekilde L. and Melsen F. (1986). A histomorphometric determination of iliac bone structure and remodelling in obese subjects. *Bone*, **7**, 77
140. Tam C. S., Hersche J. N. M. and Murray T. M. (1989). *Metabolic Bone Disease: Cellular and Tissue Mechanisms*. Boca Raton: CRC Press
141. Tavassoli M. and Friedenstein A. (1983). Haematopoietic stromal microenvironment. *Amer. J. Hematol.*, **15**, 195
142. Termine J. D. (1983). Osteonectin and other newly described proteins of developing bone. Peck W. A., *Bone and Mineral Research*, vol. 1 (p. 114). Amsterdam: Elsevier
143. Testa N. G., Allen T. D., Molineux G., Lord B. I. and Onions D. (1988). Haematopoietic growth factors: their relevance in osteoclast formation and function. *Ciba Foundation Symp.*, **136**, 257
144. Trueta J. (1963). The role of vessels in osteogenesis. *J. Bone Jt Surg.*, **45B**, 402
145. Vaananen H. K., Hentunen T., Lakkakorpi P., Parvinen E. K., Sundquist K. and Tuukanen J. (1988). Mechanism of osteoclast mediated bone resorption. *Ann. Chir. Gynaecol.*, **77**, 193
146. Vaes G. (1988). Cellular biology and biochemical mechanism of bone resorption. A review of recent developments on the formation, activation and mode of action of osteoclasts. *Clin. Orthop.*, **231**, 239
147. Vaughan J. (1981). *The Physiology of Bone*. Oxford: Clarendon Press
148. Walker D. G. (1975). Control of bone resorption by hematopoietic tissue; the induction and reversal of congenital osteopetrosis in mice through use of bone marrow and splenic transplants. *J. Exp. Med.*, **142**, 651
149. Wallach S., Carstens J. B. and Avioli L. V. (1990). Caicitonin, osteoclasts and bone turnover. *Calcif. Tissue Int.*, **47**, 388
150. Weiss L. (1988). *Cell and Tissue Biology – A Textbook of Histology*. Baltimore: Urban & Schwarzenberg
151. Wegedal J. E., Mohan S. and Lundy M. (1990). Skeletal growth factor and other growth factors known to be present in bone matrix stimulate proliferation and protein synthesis in human bone cells. *J. Bone Mineral Res.*, **5**, 179
152. Wlodarsky K. H. (1990). Properties and origin of osteoblasts. *Clin. Orthop.*, **252**, 276
153. Yeh C.-K. and Rodan G. A. (1984). Tensile forces enhance prostaglandin E synthesis in osteoblastic cells grown on collagen ribbons. *Calcif. Tissue Int.*, **36**, 567
154. Zamboni L. and Pease D. C. (1961). The vascular bed of red bone marrow. *Ultrastruct. Res.*, **5**, 65
155. Zheng M. H., Nicholson G. C., Warton A. and Papadimitriou J. M. (1991). What's new in osteoclast ontogeny. *Pathol. Res. Pract.*, **187**, 117
156. Coe F. E. and Farus M. J. (1992). *Disorders of Bone and Mineral Metabolism*. New York: Raven Press

The following recent reference reflects the continuing search for non-invasive methods of monitoring bone resorption and the possible clinical applications.

Editorial. (1992). Pyridinium crosslinks as markers of bone resorption. *Lancet*, **340**, 278

Bone biopsy

2

POTENTIAL OF BONE BIOPSY IN CLINICAL PRACTICE

Many clinicians still maintain that clinical history and examination combined with a biochemical profile, radiology and a bone scan provide sufficient information in most cases to make the diagnosis of bone disease. However, the limitations of the radiological examinations in these disorders are well known, particularly the difficulties in recognition of early or minor bone changes. While a bone scan is more sensitive than radiology (for example in detecting metastases) it is also much less specific and a wide variety of osseous disorders including many benign ones produce abnormalities in isotope uptake. A number of non-invasive measurements of bone mass have also been developed, with varying degrees of accuracy and reproducibility[8,13,19,23,25,32,46,47,49,55,60].

More widespread use of these methods has led to the realization that:

1. changes in the bone mass of individuals are site-specific and cannot be extrapolated from one area to another;
2. cortical bone behaves differently from trabecular bone;
3. changes in the axial skeleton do not necessarily relate closely to those in the appendicular skeleton.

To determine bone mass and its changes at any one site with acceptable accuracy one must measure that site. Furthermore, there are many pitfalls in relying exclusively on biochemistry and/or radiology, especially in the interpretation of the findings and the diagnosis of patients with some hyperosteoid and malignant states (e.g. osteomalacia, renal bone disease and metastases in bone). It is therefore reasonable to take a bone biopsy[27]

1. when the diagnosis is in doubt;
2. when confirmation is sought of a specific process (e.g. metastases, multiple myeloma or systemic mastocytosis);
3. when further categorization is required for therapeutic decisions (e.g. low and high turnover variants of osteoporosis, different subtypes of renal osteodystrophy or of multiple myeloma); and
4. when follow-up and monitoring of therapy is necessary as in osteomalacia or malignant lymphomas[7].

Moreover, the unique attraction of a bone biopsy is that it allows *direct visualization of bone and its cells*[32]. Jowsey (1977) stressed that relevant if not always crucial diagnostic and therapeutic information can be obtained only from the observation of tissue itself[39]. By embedding the biopsy in plastic, the histological sections permit reliable identification of both calcified bone and osteoid ('mineralized bone histology')[2,3,9,27,42].

Various morphological *parameters* can be quantified (histomorphometry) in sections of undecalcified biopsies[4,6,20,27,43,44,51]. These measurements reflect the amount and behaviour of bone[5,48,56] and its cells in areas of remodelling[35,52]. Histomorphometric parameters also provide information on the rate of turnover, by quantitation of osteoclastic resorption and osteoblastic formation of bone. Finally the dynamics of formation and calcification can be studied by double-labelling with tetracycline[29,30]. For example, though bone histomorphometry has contributed little to the diagnosis of osteoporosis, it has provided unique information on the heterogeneity of bone cell behaviour in osteoporosis: low-turnover ('inactive') versus high-turnover ('active') states. Analysis at the level of the basic bone remodelling unit, and therefore of the underlying pathophysiology, permits a more critical choice of therapeutic regimens in individual cases.

Following the establishment of bone biopsy as a technique for assessing the structure and turnover of bone, attempts have been made to broaden the use of bone biopsy as a diagnostic and investigative too . For example, in the early 1970s high aluminium concentrations were demonstrated in sections of biopsies taken from renal patients on dialysis[31,42]; since then other techniques have been used on parts of the biopsy core or on individual sections to measure concentrations of other elements (quantitative chemical analysis)[2]. A new development has been the use of biopsies to obtain osteoblasts and osteoclasts for *in vitro* cell cultures[7]. In the future we may well see the more widespread use of bone biopsies for the immunohistochemical localization of osteotropic factors and their receptors on bone cells.

BIOPSY SITES

Four main considerations determine choice of the site selected:

1. the biopsy site should be easily accessible, involving a minimum of trauma and danger to the patient;
2. it should provide representative bone structure and turnover;
3. it should contain cortical and trabecular bone; and
4. repeat biopsies with minimal variability should be possible.

The os ilium comes nearest to fulfilling these criteria, and the *anterior* and *posterior iliac crest* are the preferred sites from which the biopsies are taken (Figs 2.S1 and S2,

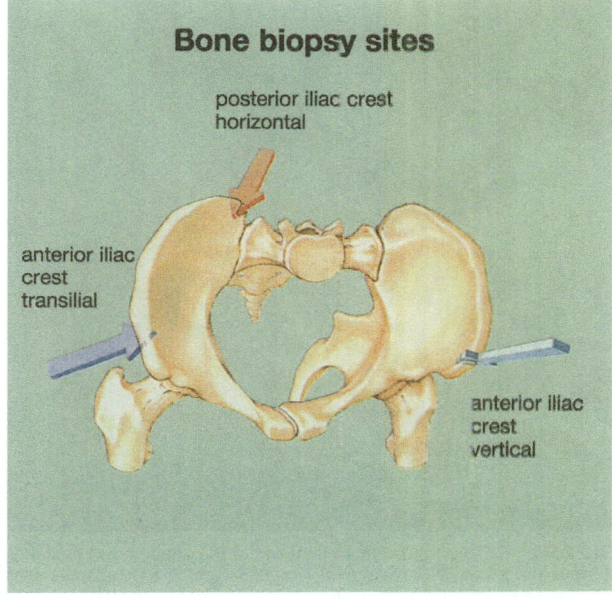

Fig. 2.S1 Sketch illustrating the three sites on the iliac crest from which bone biopsies are generally taken

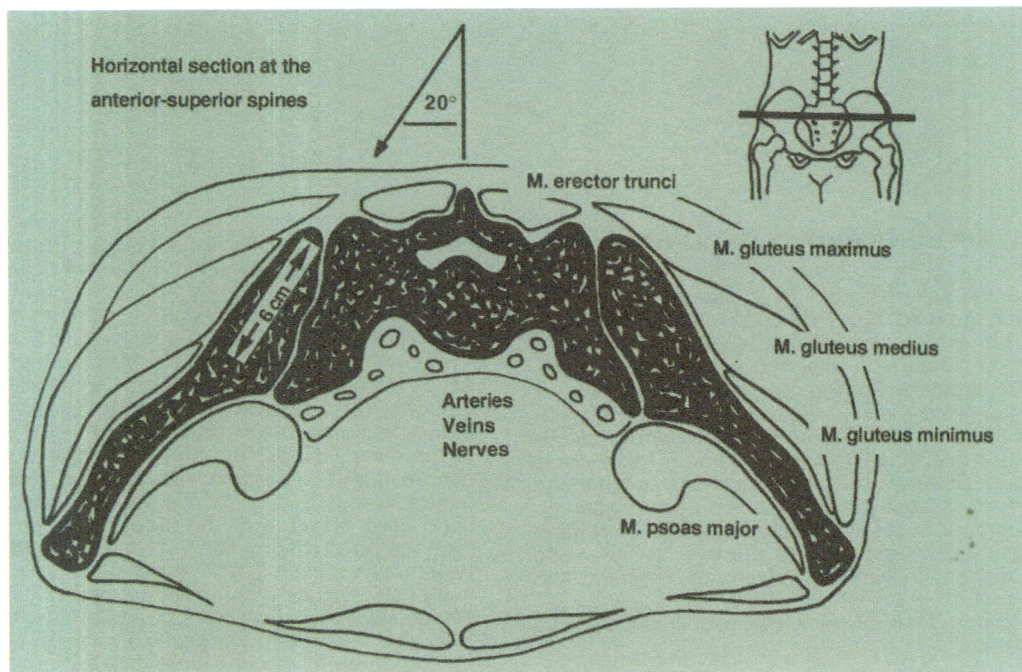

Fig. 2.S2 Sketch of horizontal section at the level of the anterior–superior spinous processes of the ilium (see insert). Note (a) that the posterior ilium is broader than the anterior, and (b) that long biopsies can safely be taken from the posterior ilium. In addition both external and internal surfaces of the ilium are protected by muscles

2.R1 and R2). There are differences in the amounts of cortical and trabecular bone, of bone cells and of marrow in different regions of the ilium, but these have only minor practical significance (Figs 2.S3 and S4). Because follow-up biopsies cannot always be taken from the same region it is essential to know the amount of variation that exists in the iliac crest. Moore and co-workers have shown that

estimates of the percentage of trabecular bone volume deviated systematically, increasing in magnitude from the anterior to the posterior ilium[45]. In contrast, diCarlo *et al.* (1989) doubted whether any region in the anterior ilium was a reliable indicator of cancellous bone volume[16]. Differences have been reported when the biopsies were taken more than 2 cm away from the standard site. Also differences with variations in depth from the iliac crest surface have been published. No striking differences were demonstrable between the right and left iliac crests (important for sequential biopsies!) or between vertical and horizontal iliac crest biopsies, except in the thickness of the cortical bone.

Likewise, histomorphological features of bone and marrow vary in the different parts of the skeleton, as demonstrated in our autopsy study based on 100 cases of accidental death, but there were parallel deviations between the different sites. Nevertheless, there are differences in characteristics of bone taken from different

Fig. 2.R1 CT through pelvis at the level of the anterior and posterior spinous processes. Note width of iliac crest and extent of trabecular bone in the posterior ilium: preferred biopsy site of manual trephine (cm scale at right)

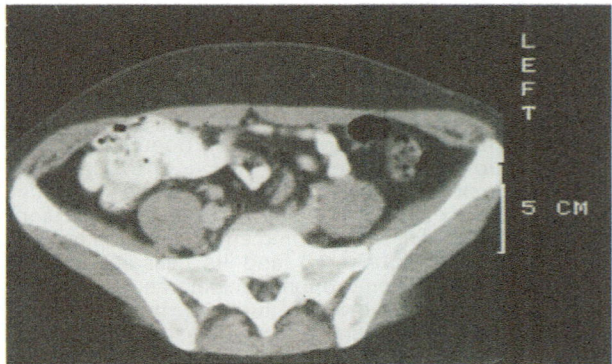

Fig. 2.R2 CT through pelvis showing topography of the anterior and posterior iliac crests, and the protective muscle groups at external and internal surfaces

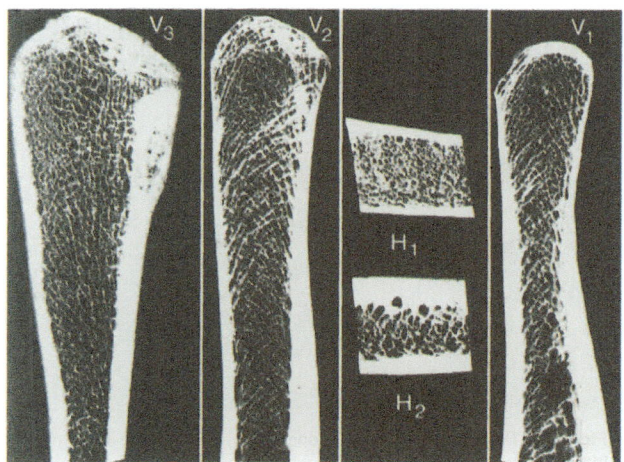

Fig. 2.S3 Vertical sections through the anterior part of the ilium from 25-year-old woman (accidental death) showing the variability in structure and width of the cortical bone, taken at different levels from along the ilium. (Reproduced with permission from W. J. Whitehouse (1977). Cancellous bone in the anterior part of the iliac crest. *Calcif. Tissue Res.*, **26**, 67)

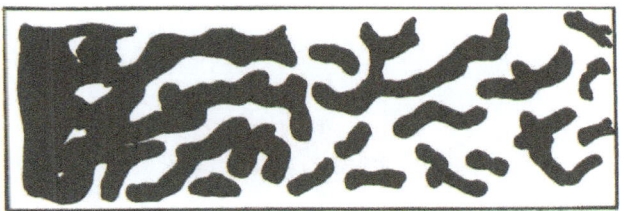

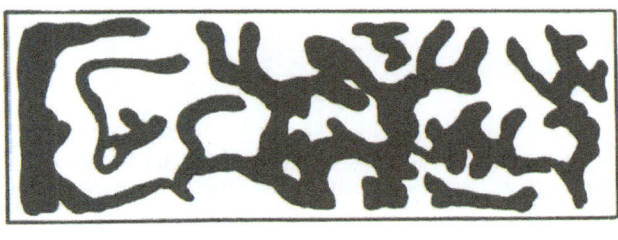

| Cortical region 2 mm | Subcortical region 4 mm | Central region 4–8 mm | "Deeper" region 4 mm |

Fig. 2.S4 Diagram of variations in trabecular bone with increasing depth from the cortex. The four topographic regions and their approximate sizes are indicated on the diagram

skeletal sites which rule out direct extrapolation from one area to another. Biopsies are also taken from other skeletal sites under radiological guidance[40].

BIOPSY INSTRUMENTS (Plates 2.A and B)

There are two main kinds of instruments, namely the *electric drill* and the *manual trephine*[2-4,27,42], various types of which are commercially available. The drill is used for vertical biopsies from the anterior iliac crest[2,9,27], and the wide-bore manual trephine for horizontal transilial biopsies[11,24,26,41,42] – both provide relatively wide cores (4 mm and 8 mm respectively) (Fig. 2.S5). These are recommended when detailed histomorphometric measurements of cortical and trabecular bone are necessary,

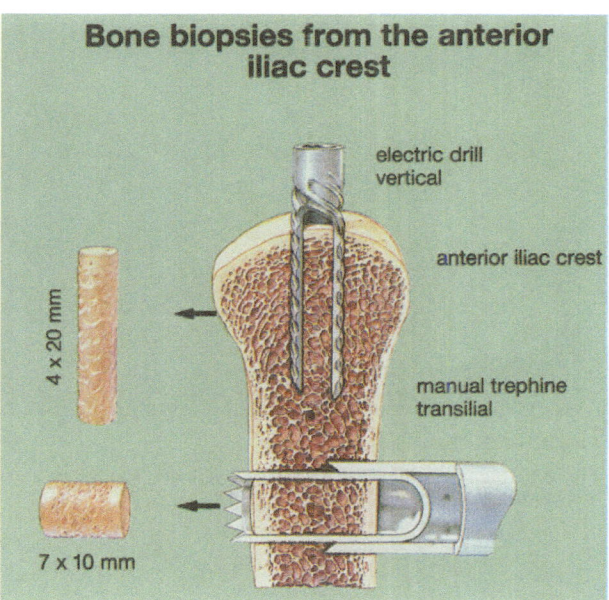

Bone biopsies from the anterior iliac crest

electric drill vertical

anterior iliac crest

4 x 20 mm

manual trephine transilial

7 x 10 mm

Fig. 2.S5 Sketch of electric drill and manual transilial trephine *in situ* in the anterior ilium. Note progressive narrowing of the ilium with distance from the crest

but at the cost of greater invasiveness and rate of complications. It has been shown that biopsy cores of 4 mm diameter and 20 mm length taken vertically from the anterior iliac crest provide excellent sections for qualitative and quantitative evaluation. However, the vast majority of bone biopsies are taken from the posterior iliac crest with an 8-gauge manual trephine (3 mm width)[10,18,21,22,33,36–38,54,57]. Their length varies greatly – up to 70 mm. This needle technique is less invasive, can be performed relatively easily and is particularly suitable for outpatients (Fig. 2.S6)[34]. Though biopsy cores of less

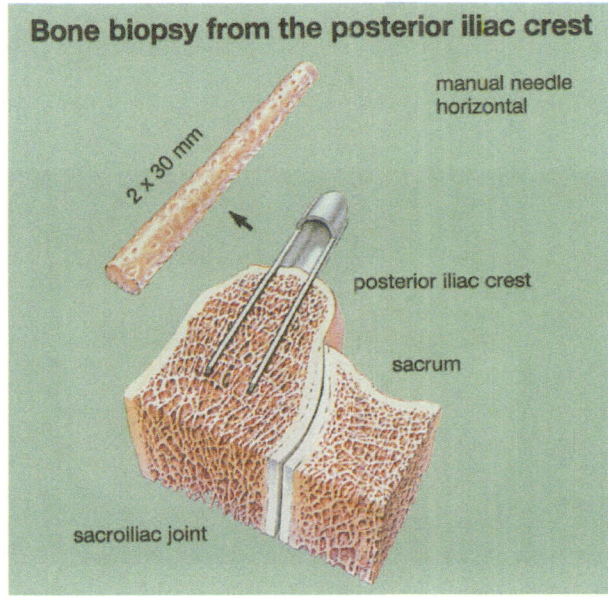

Bone biopsy from the posterior iliac crest

manual needle horizontal

2 x 30 mm

posterior iliac crest

sacrum

sacroiliac joint

Fig. 2.S6 Sketch of manual trephine *in situ* in the posterior ilium. Note width of iliac crest and distance of the needle from the sacroiliac joint

Plate 2.A

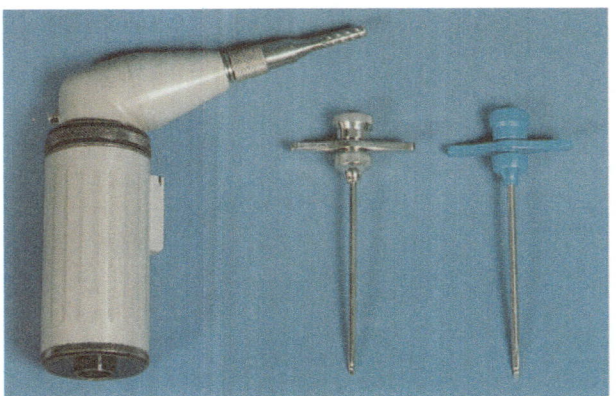

Figs 2.1–2.6   Techniques I

Fig. 2.1   Biopsy instruments used by the authors: manual trephines and electric drill

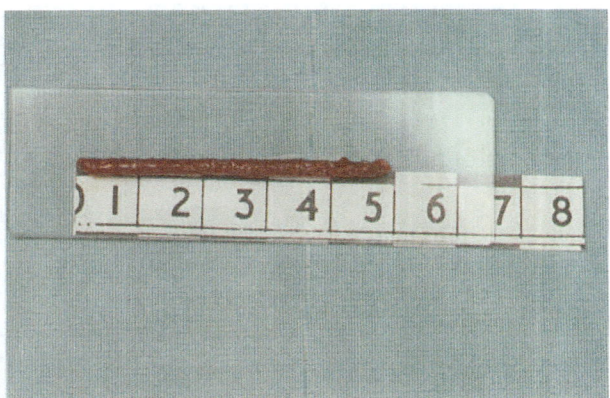

Fig. 2.2   Posterior iliac crest biopsy taken with wide-bore manual trephine

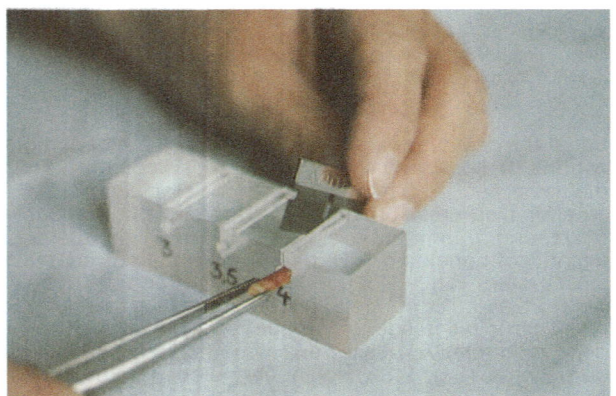

Fig. 2.3   Plastic device for longitudinal halving of the biopsy core

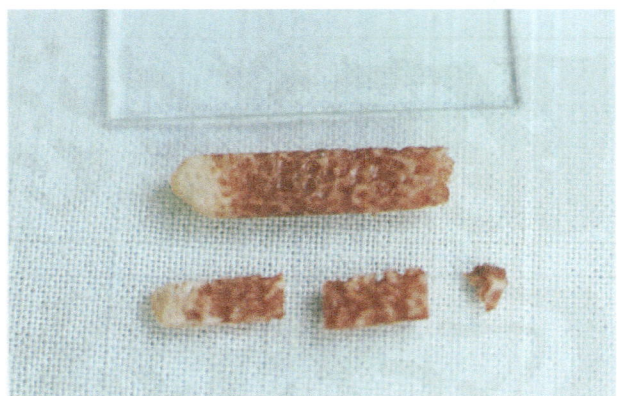

Fig. 2.4   Biopsy longitudinally halved and cut to enable multiparameter studies: plastic histology, cryostat sections, mineral analysis and electron microscopy. Imprints of the cut surface of one biopsy half are also made

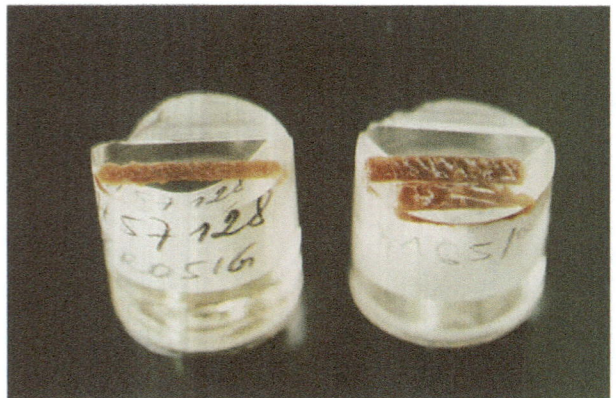

Fig. 2.5   Plastic blocks of iliac crest biopsies taken with the manual needle (left) and the electric drill (right). Note name and biopsy number tag embedded within the plastic, and the top half not containing the biopsy sawn off, and top surface trimmed and ready for cutting

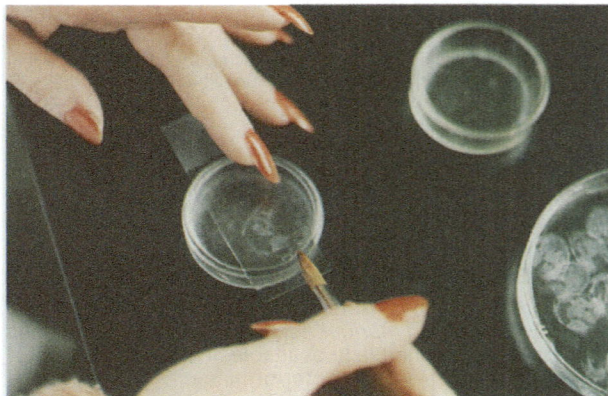

Fig. 2.6.   Mounting of sections. Each section is separately mounted as follows: the section is picked up from the distilled water in a Petri dish (lower right) and placed onto a gelatinized slide, and several drops of 90% alcohol are dropped onto it. After a few seconds the section will soften, and it can be stretched and the folds smoothed out with a soft brush. Alternatively, a roller may be used for rapid mounting of sections

Plate 2.B

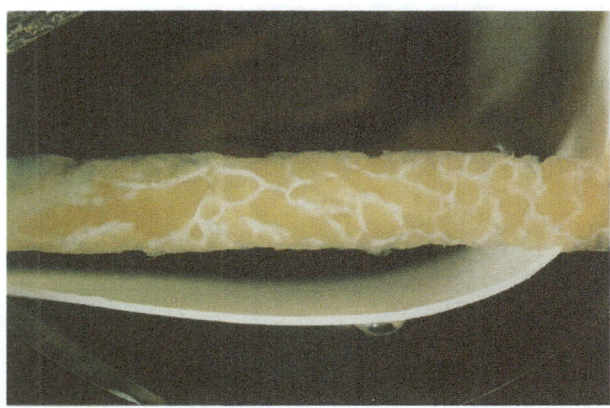

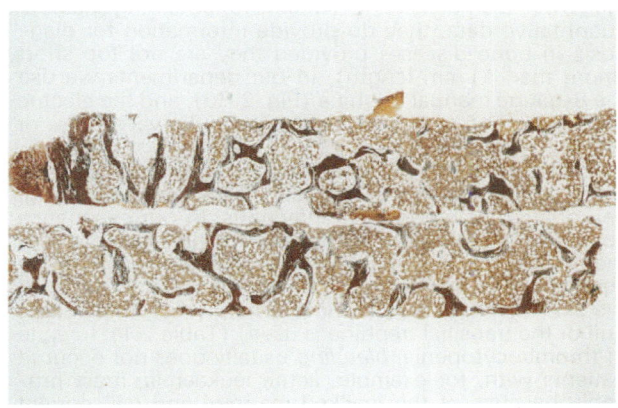

Figs 2.7–2.12 Techniques II

Figs. 2.7 and **2.8** Biopsies taken with narrow-bore manual trephine (2 mm in diameter)

Fig. 2.7 Biopsy in trimmed plastic block

Fig. 2.8 Semithin section showing both halves of long biopsy cut before embedding. Gomori

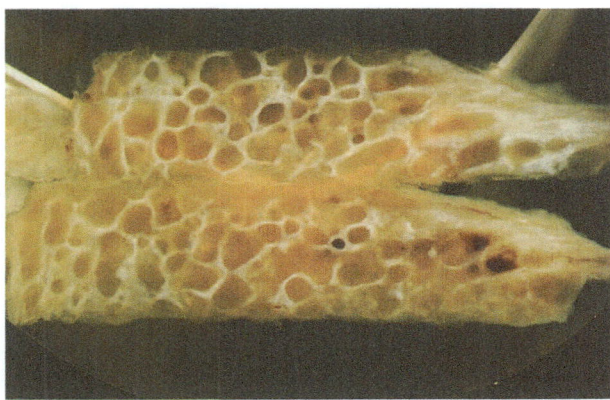

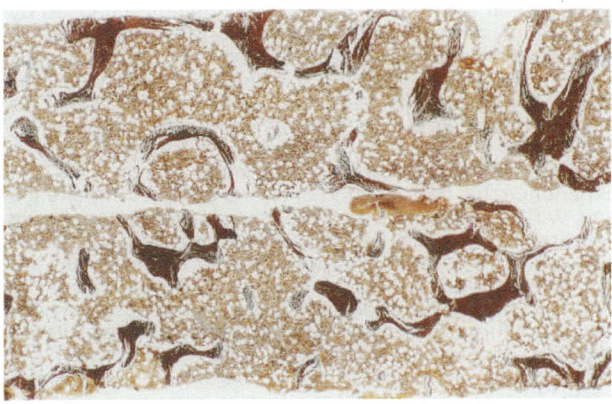

Figs. 2.9 and **2.10** Biopsies taken with wide-bore manual trephine (3 mm in diameter)

Fig. 2.9 Two biopsies taken from the same area, in trimmed plastic block

Fig. 2.10 Semithin section of a wide-bore biopsy taken with manual trephine. Gomori

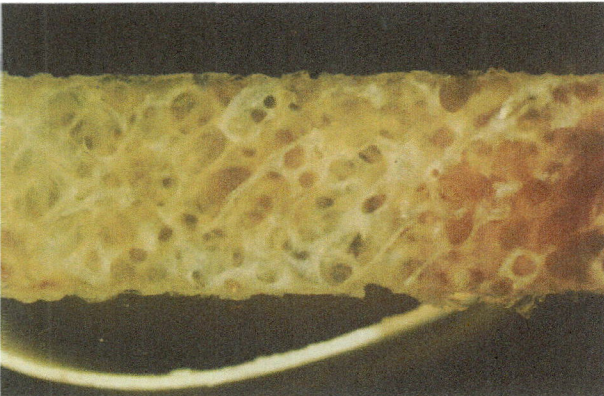

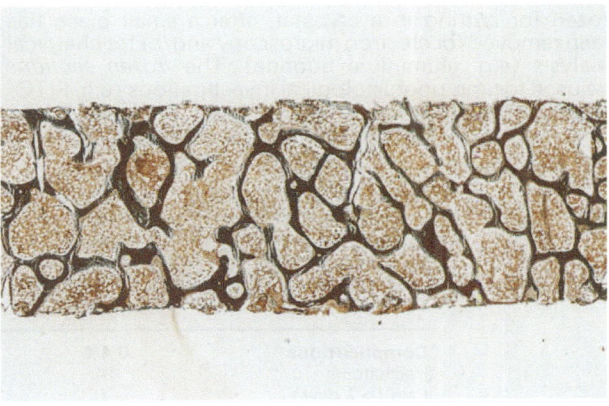

Figs. 2.11 and **2.12** Biopsies taken with electric drill (4 mm in diameter)

Fig. 2.11 Biopsy in trimmed block

Fig. 2.12 Semithin section of a biopsy taken with electric drill. Gomori

than 3 mm diameter are not suitable for obtaining accurate quantitative data, they do provide information for diagnosis in bone diseases provided they are not too short (more than 11 mm length). In our departments we use the 8-gauge manual trephine (Fig. 2.R3), and the electric drill only when the bone is expected to be very dense or soft.

The type and rate of *complications* have been given by Rao[50] and by Duncan *et al.*[17], and they include bleeding, neuropathy, pain and local infections. In our experience complications are very infrequent, in the region of less than 0.5%[27,28]. Generally, manual trephines caused fewer complications, probably owing to a smaller incision in the skin (4 mm versus 10 mm or more when the electric drill or the transilial trephine is used) (Table 2.1). In spite of thrombocytopenia, *bleeding* usually does not occur in patients with, for example, acute leukaemia, most probably because of the 'packed marrow' and consequent compression of the sinusoids. In contrast, bleeding after taking the biopsy may frequently occur in polycythaemia vera; in these cases most probably owing to the increased blood volume and the hyperplastic and engorged sinusoids. Bleeding has also been observed in osteomyelosclerosis, presumably caused by trauma to the ectatic sinusoids with sclerotic and therefore rigid walls, which prevent their collapse or contraction. Bleeding caused by incision of dermal or periosteal blood vessels can be staunched by external pressure for about 2 h. *Pain* radiating into the leg while taking the biopsy occurs occasionally in some patients, but it is transient and causes no motoric disability whatever (at least in our experience).

Recently the question of *secondary tumour deposits in needle biopsy tracks* has again been raised[15]. In our experience this happened in only one patient who already had widespread metastatic disease. However, it should be borne in mind that most patients with carcinomas have circulating tumour cells very early after establishment of the primary tumour. Moreover, should metastases be found in the bone biopsy, the patient obviously already has disseminated disease, so that even should tumour deposits develop in the biopsy track these would not influence the metastatic process, the treatment or prognosis. A completely different situation obtains if a biopsy is taken from a single, encapsulated tumour.

BIOPSY PROCESSING (as carried out in our laboratories) (Plates 2.C and D)

Biopsies with a diameter of 3 mm or more may be longitudinally halved with the aid of a specially designed plastic device[2-4,27]. One half is fixed and the second is frozen for cutting in a cryostat, after a small piece has been removed for electron microscopy and/or for chemical analysis (e.g. aluminium fluoride). The *frozen sections* are used for immunohistological investigations (e.g. FITC-labelled antibodies for collagen types I, II and III) or for rapid diagnosis (e.g. evidence of bone metastases)[2]. The

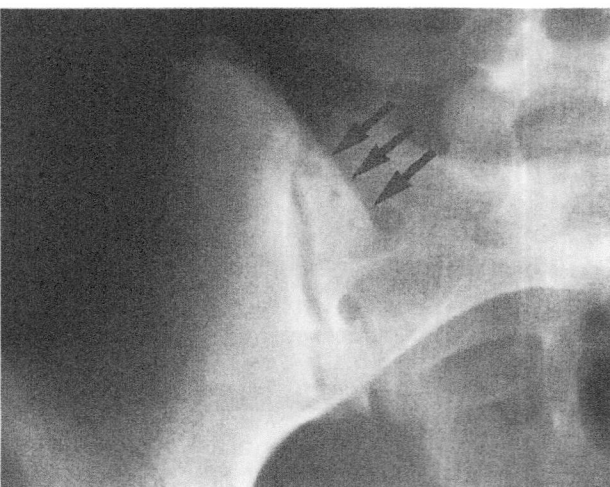

Fig. 2.R3 X-ray of the right posterior iliac crest revealing three small holes at arrows, immediately after taking bone biopsies with a manual trephine, 8 gauge

fixed biopsy halves are dehydrated and embedded in methyl methacrylate without decalcification[1,9,53], and *semithin sections* cut at 2 or 3 μm[9]. The following stains are routinely employed: Gallamin blue–Giemsa for cytological detail, Gomori's stain for bone structure and fibres, PAS stain for glycoprotein and bone cells, Ladewig's and toluidine blue stains for calcified matrix and osteoid, and Berlin blue stain for iron[27]. Details of the methods for processing, cutting and staining are given in Frisch *et al.*[27,28]. However, the method has now been modified[59] and the time required for processing greatly shortened so that the stained sections may be examined and the diagnosis made within 3–4 days after taking the biopsy.

Double *tetracycline labelling* involves the oral administration of two short courses of tetracycline, which is deposited along the calcification front in bone as two distinct lines which can be visualized in bone sections under fluorescent microscopy (Frost, 1969). A typical labelling schedule is[7,29]:

1. 300 mg demethylchlortetracycline twice a day for 2 days,
2. no tetracycline for 10 days,
3. 300 mg demethylchlortetracycline twice a day for 4 days,
4. bone biopsy taken 4–8 days later.

It should be noted that some authors have observed a difference between toluidine-blue-stained and tetracycline-labelled surfaces, especially the calcification front, in iliac crest biopsies[14]. Toluidine blue is thought to stain

[continued on p. 59]

Table 2.1 Complications of three types of bone biopsy instruments

Authors	Rao (ref. 50)		Our series	
Instruments	Manual trephine	Transilial biopsy	Manual trephine	Electric drill
Skeletal sites	Post. iliac crest	Ant. iliac crest	Post. iliac crest	Ant. iliac crest.
Total cases	5780	9131	7361	6529
Complications	**0.4%**	**0.7%**	**0.4%**	**1.1%**
Haematoma	14	22	12	31
Pain (>7 days)	0	17	4	21
Neuropathy, transient	2	11	4	18
Wound infection	4	6	5	16
Osteomyelitis	0	1	0	2
Drug rection	1	0	3	3

Plate 2.C

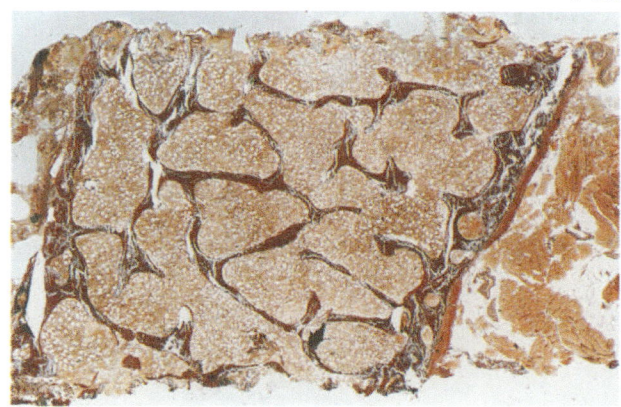

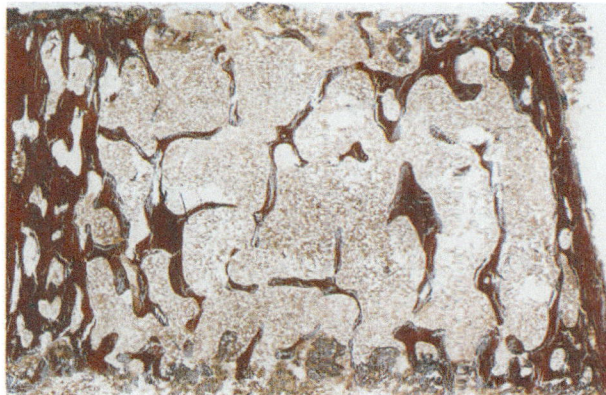

Figs 2.13–2.18 Techniques III

Figs. 2.13 and **2.14** Sections of transiliac biopsies: 7 mm width, cortex to cortex

Fig. 2.13 Trabecular bone and cortices within the normal range both structurally and volumetrically. Gomori

Fig. 2.14 Variable cortical thickness and porosity as well as patchy osteopenia. Gomori

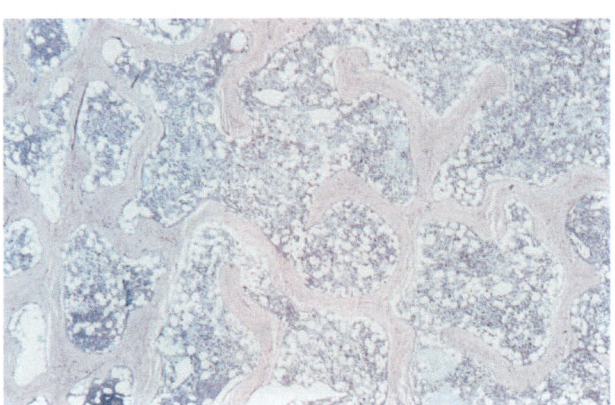

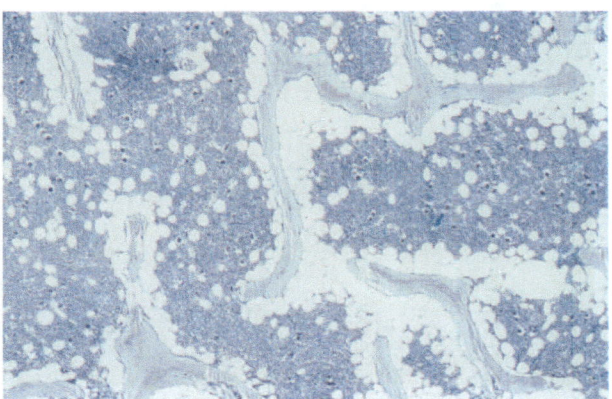

Figs. 2.15–2.18 Sections of plastic-embedded biopsies illustrating the stains commonly used in our laboratories, including Gomori. Not illustrated in this plate, but also useful, are PAS for glycoproteins and Berlin-blue for iron

Fig. 2.15 Haematoxylin and eosin (H&E)

Fig. 2.16 Giemsa for cellular details

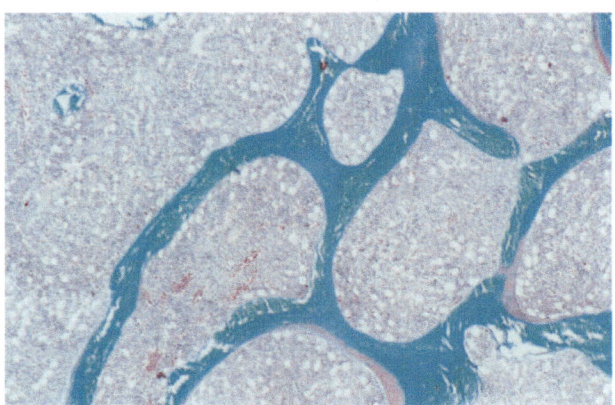

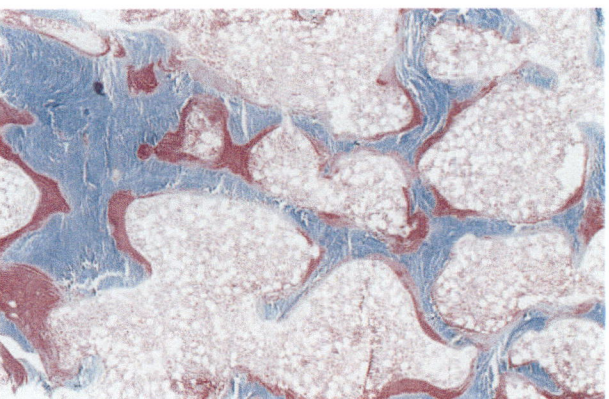

Fig. 2.17 Goldner for osteoid (red) and mineralized bone (green)

Fig. 2.18 Ladewig for osteoid (red) and mineralized bone (blue)

Plate 2.D

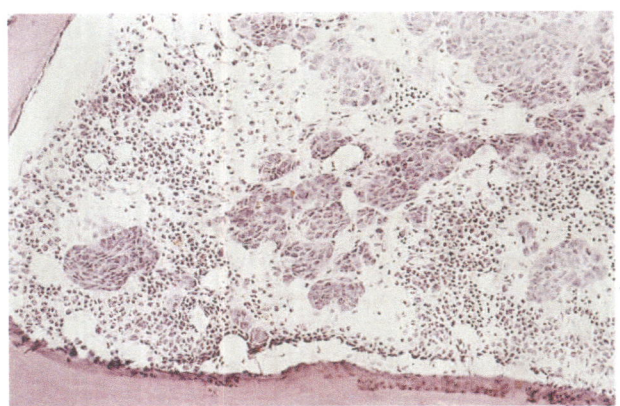

Figs 2.19–2.24 Techniques IV

Fig. 2.19 Cryostat section for rapid diagnosis of metastatic bone disease. Note multiple small metastases in the bone marrow cavity, without any osseous reaction. H&E

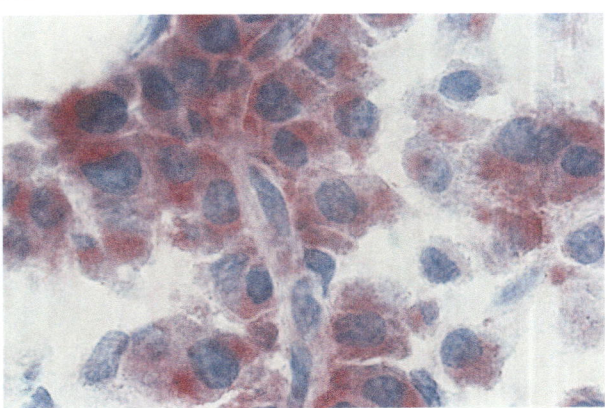

Fig. 2.20 Enzyme histochemistry, e.g. acid phosphatase activity in neoplastic plasma cells in multiple myeloma. Cryostat section

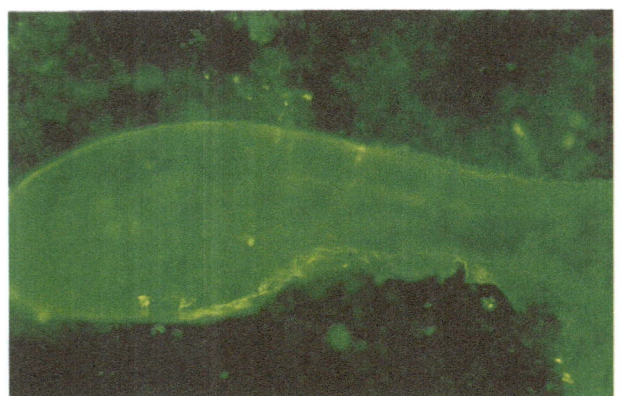

Fig. 2.21 Immunofluorescence demonstrating collagen type I in bone matrix. Cryostat section

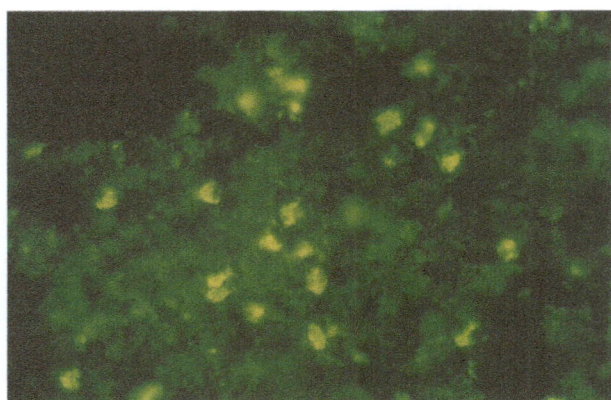

Fig. 2.22 Monoclonal plasma cells in case of early multiple myeloma. Cryostat section

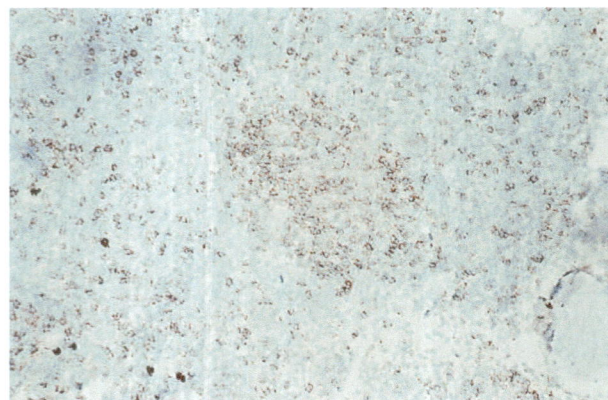

Fig. 2.23 Interstitial and nodular B-lymphocytes in chronic lympho-cytic leukaemia, nodular type. Cryostat section, immunoperoxidase

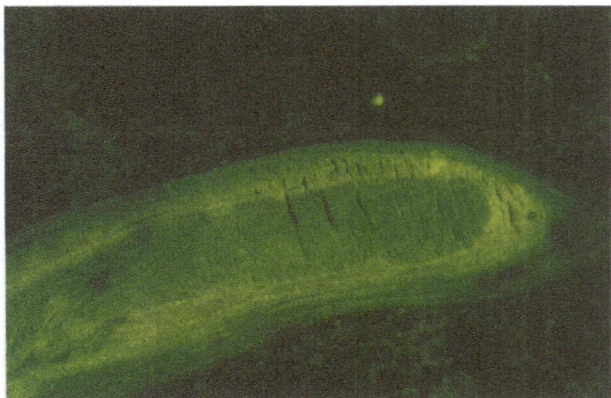

Fig. 2.24 Tetracycline labelling of mineralization in osteoid layer. Plastic section

Plate 2.E

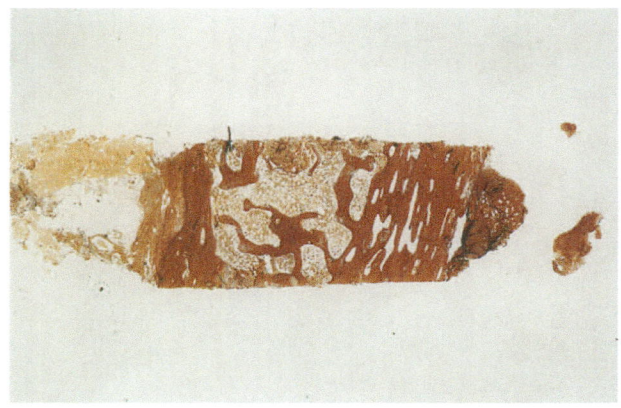

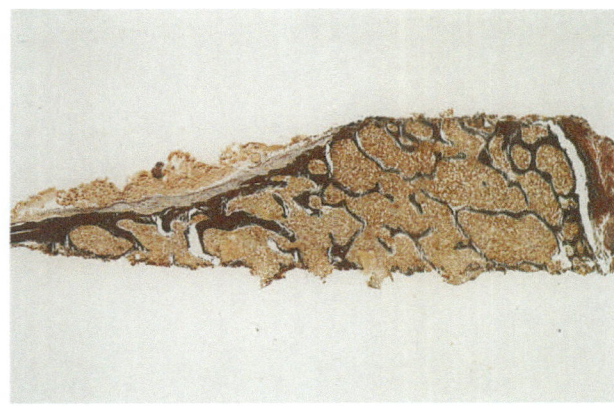

Figs 2.25–2.30 Variations encountered in the biopsy sections due to the direction of the biopsy needle

Fig. 2.25 Short biopsy taken from the edge of the posterior iliac crest, with cortices at both ends and only a few marrow spaces, not appropriate for morphometric evaluation. Gomori

Fig. 2.26 Tangential anterior iliac crest biopsy with cortical bone at both ends. *Gomori*

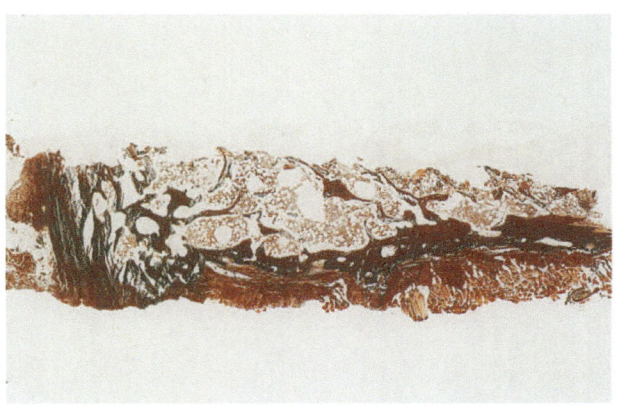

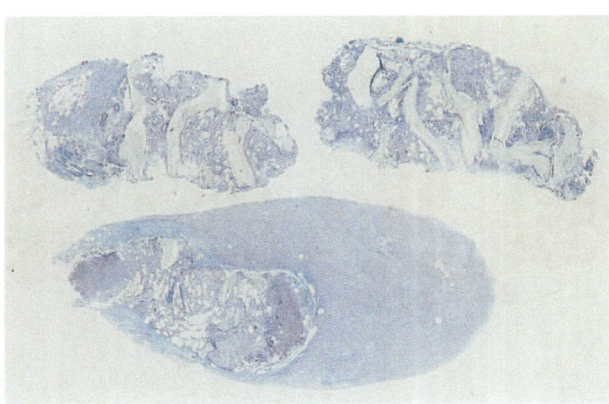

Fig. 2.27 Tangential biopsy showing periosteal tissues, cortical bone and only subcortical trabeculae and marrow. Gomori

Fig. 2.28 Shattered biopsy consisting of fragments and blood clot, not appropriate for morphometric evaluation of bone. Giemsa

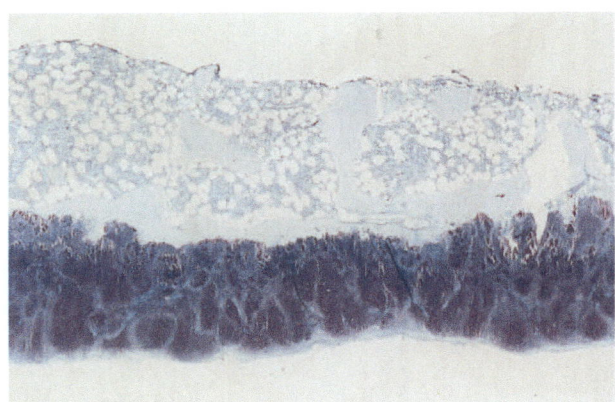

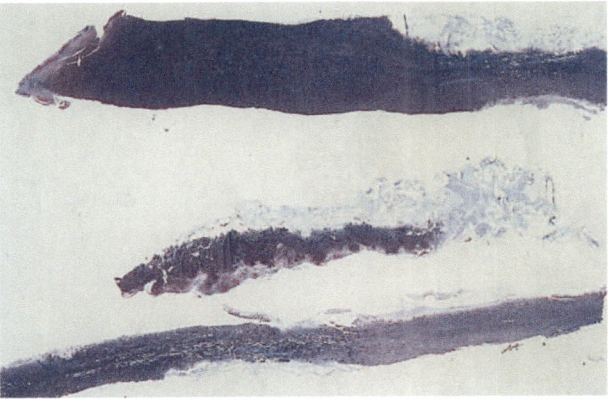

Fig. 2.29 Tangenital biopsy, possibly from region near the sacroiliac joint, showing broad strip of cartilage underlying cortical bone. Giemsa

Fig. 2.30 Tangenital biopsies, almost exclusively consisting of cartilage. Giemsa

Plate 2.F

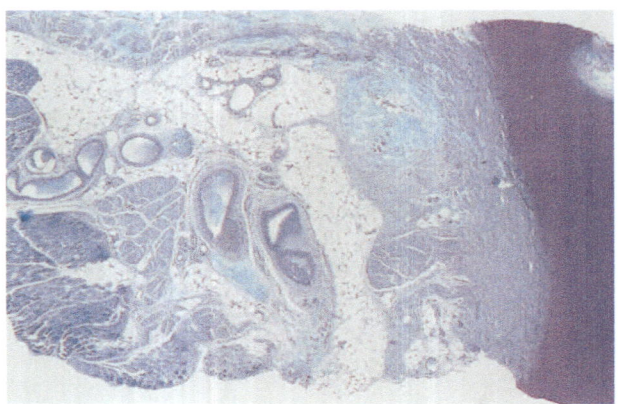

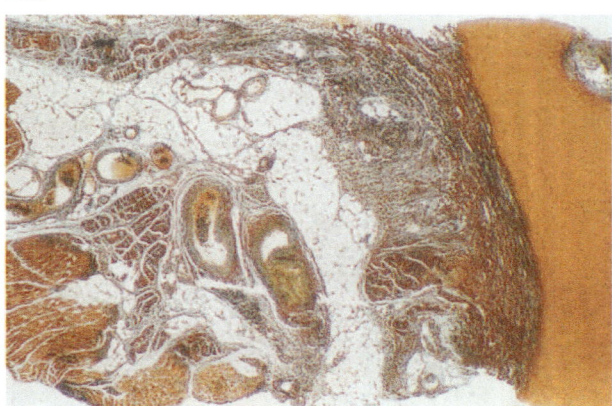

Figs 2.31–2.36 Apparently adequate biopsies but microscopic examination of the sections revealed disproportionate amounts of muscle, vessels, periosteal tissues, cartilage and/or cortical bone

Fig. 2.32 Section of same biopsy stained by Gomori to demonstrate fibrous tissue

Fig. 2.31 Section of biopsy of child showing only muscle, vessels, connective and periosteal tissues, and growth plate. Giemsa

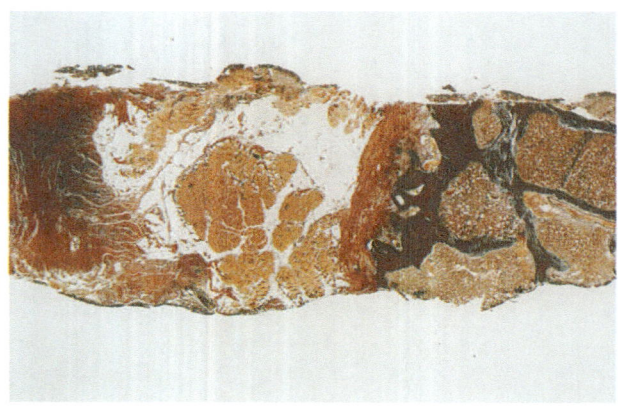

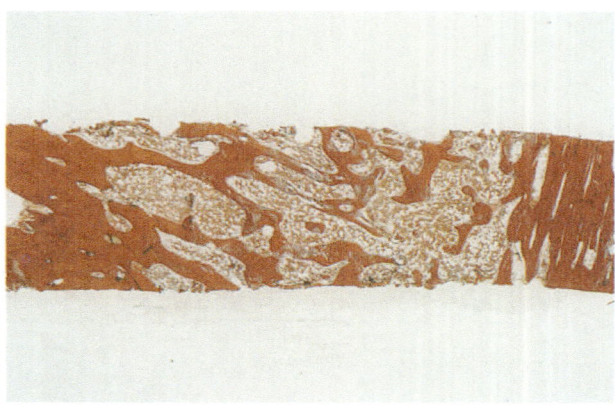

Fig. 2.33 Over half of biopsy consists of extraosseous tissues. Gomori

Fig. 2.34 Section of tangential biopsy with two cortices, with apparently broad cortex at left due to direction of biopsy needle. Gomori

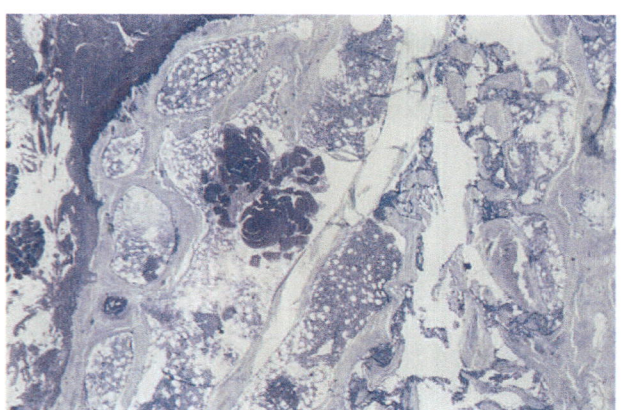

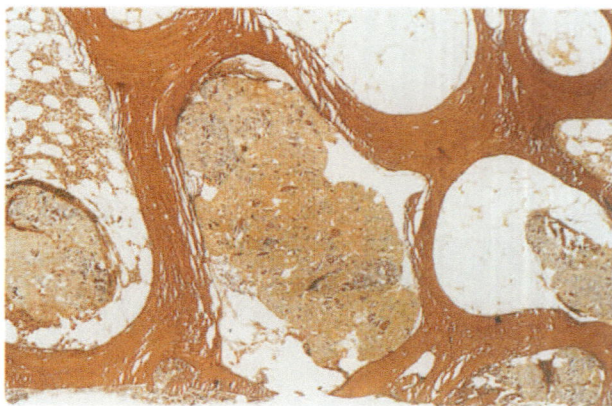

Fig. 2.35 Transilial biopsy with muscle tissue displaced into the subcortical intertrabecular area (centre). Giemsa

Fig. 2.36 Debris due to the electric drill in the marginal marrow spaces. Gomori

the mineralization front, while tetracycline is used for the chelation of calcium deposited on the lamellae during mineralization. The spontaneous fluorescence of tetracycline administered *in vivo* will therefore indicate foci of recent remodelling.

DIAGNOSTIC BIOPSY EVALUATION (Plates 2.E and F)

Sections of biopsies illustrating the range of normal quantitative relationships between cortical and trabecular bone, haematopoietic and adipose tissue are shown in Plates 2.B and C. Part of the anterior and posterior cortex of the iliac crest is porous and of variable thickness[12,58]. Moreover the thickness of the ossicles, as well as the structure of the trabecular network, may be variable even within a single section. Though this text is concerned with bone tissue it is important to consider the bone and marrow together as a single system, because alterations in the one are generally accompanied by changes in the other. It is also important to bear these considerations in mind, especially when histomorphometric measurements, comparative and follow-up studies are made and conclusions for therapy drawn from them. The main *pitfalls*[4] in histological diagnosis are:

1. non-representative tangential biopsies, which are encountered more frequently when biopsies are taken from the narrow anterior iliac crest;
2. presence of misleading artefacts by crushing, distortion, and inclusion of other tissues (dermis, muscles); and
3. histological variations within the same biopsy, with subcortical hypoplasia or alternating fatty and hyperplastic areas in deeper parts of the biopsy, which in turn may affect the bone structure and remodelling.

In our experience 3 mm diameter and 15 mm length, excluding periosteal tissues and cortical bone, proved to be the minimal biopsy size for diagnostic and morphometric evaluation. Nevertheless, in disorders such as osteomalacia, osteitis fibrosa cystica or metastatic bone disease even a single trabecula plus a seam of adjacent marrow may be enough for diagnosis – though not, of course, for histomorphometry.

To complete a *bone and marrow report* (Fig. 2.S7)[4,27] a systematic survey is made beginning with a scan of the whole biopsy section at low power (x 6), to evaluate the periosteum, the cortex, the cancellous bone and the marrow cellularity, and to recognize artefacts (Plates 2.E and F). Then, at intermediate magnifications (x 100 and x 250) lamellar structure, mineralization, bone remodelling, the stroma and the topography of the marrow are studied, ending with examination at high power or oil immersion (x 600 and x 1000), when necessary, of structural and cytological details, especially of the bone cells.

References

1. Baron R., Vignery A., Neff L., Silverglate A. and Santa-Maria A. Processing of undecalcified bone specimens for bone histomorphometry. Recker R. R., *Bone Histomorphometry: Techniques and Interpretations* (p. 13). Boca Raton: CRC Press
2. Bartl R., Buchenrieder B., Sommerfeld, W., Muthmann H., Jäger K., Hoffmann-Fezer G. and Burkhardt R. (1984). Multiparameter studies on 650 bone marrow biopsy cores. Diagnostic value of combined utilisation of imprints cryostat and plastic sections in medical practice. Frisch B. and Bartl R., *Bone Marrow Biopsies Updated. New Prospects for Clinical Diagnostics* (p. 1). Basel: Karger
3. Bartl R., Frisch B. and Burkhardt R. (1984). *Bone Marrow Biopsies Revisited*. Basel: Karger
4. Bartl R., Frisch B. and Burkhardt R. (1991). Bone marrow histology. Catovsky D., *Methods in Hematology: The Leukemic Cell*, vol. 2 (p. 47). Edinburgh: Churchill Livingstone
5. Beck J. S. and Nordin B. E. C. (1960). Histological assessment of osteoporosis by iliac crest biopsy *J. Pathol. Bacteriol.*, **80**, 391
6. Bordier, P., Matrajt H., Miravet H. and Hioco D. (1964). Mesure histologique de la masse et de la résorption des travées osseuses. *Path. Biol.*, **12**, 1238
7. Boyce B. F. (1988). Uses and limitations of bone biopsy in management of metabolic bone disease. Martin T. J., *Metabolic Bone Disease* (p. 31). London: Baillière Tindall
8. Britton J. M. and Davie M. W. J. (1990). Mechanical properties of bone from iliac crest and relationship to the vertebral bone. *Bone*, **11**, 21
9. Burkhardt R. (1971). *Bone Marrow and Bone Tissue. Colour Atlas of Clinical Histopathology*. Berlin: Springer
10. Byers P. and Smith R. (1967). Trephines for full-thickness iliac crest biopsy. *Brit. Med. J.*, **1**, 682
11. Chappard D., Alexandre C., Bousquet G. and Riffat G. (1983). Nouvelles modifications du trocart de Bordier pour la biopsie osseuse quantitative. *Rev. Rheum. Mal. Osteoartic.*, **50**, 307
12. Chavassieux P. M., Arlot M. E. and Meunier P. J. (1985). Intersample variation in bone histomorphometry: comparison between parameter values measured on two contiguous transiliac bone biopsies. *Calcif. Tissue Int.*, **37**, 345
13. Chesnut C. H. (1988). Measurement of bone mass. *Triangle*, **27**(1/2), 37
14. Compston J. E., Vedi S. and Webb A. (1985). Relationship between toluidine blue-stained calcification fronts and tetracycline-labeled surfaces in normal iliac crest biopsies. *Calcif. Tissue*, **37**, 32
15. Denton K. J., Cotton D. W. K., Nakielny R. A. and Goepel J. R. (1990). Secondary tumour deposits in needle biopsy tracks: an underestimated risk? *J. Clin. Pathol.*, **43**, 83
16. DiCarlo E. F., Hoisington S. A. and Bullough P. G. (1989). Site-dependent variation in bone volume and a relative biopsy site on the iliac crest. *Calcif. Tissue*, **44S** (Abstract), S-59 (J9)
17. Duncan H., Rao D. S. and Parfitt A. M. (1980). Complications of bone biopsy. *Metab. Bone Dis. Rel. Res.*, **2**, Suppl., 475
18. Duursma S. A., Visser W. J., Van Zoeren M. and Korver M. F. (1969). A bone biopsy procedure. *Calcif. Tissue Res.*, **4**, 269
19. Edeiken J., Dalinka M. and Karasick D. (1990). *Edeiken's Roentgen Diagnosis of Diseases of Bone*. Baltimore: Williams & Wilkins
20. Ellis H. A. and Peart K. M. (1972). Quantitative observations on mineralised and non-mineralised bone in the iliac crest. *J. Clin. Pathol.*, **25**, 277
21. Ellis L. D., Jensen, W. N. and Westerman M. P. (1964). Needle biopsy of bone marrow. *Arch. Intern. Med.*, **114**, 213
22. Ellis L. D., Jensen W. N. and Westerman, M. P. (1964). Needle

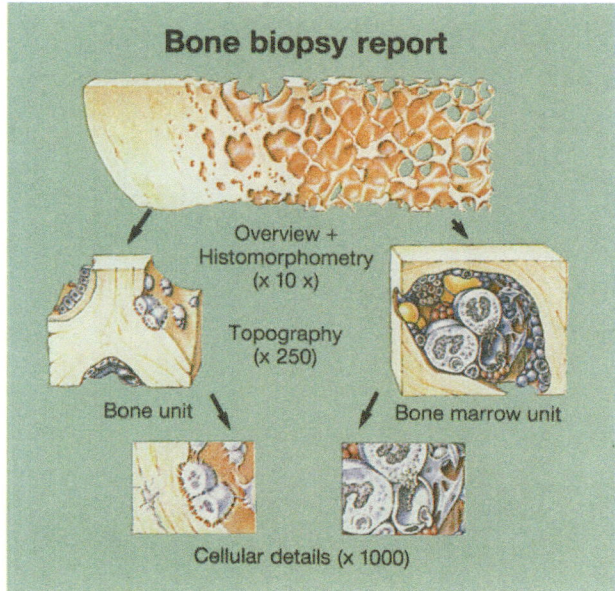

Fig. 2.S7 Sequence of biopsy evaluation

biopsy of bone and marrow. An experience with 1,445 biopsies. *Arch. Intern. Med.*, **114**, 213

23. Epstein S. (1988). Serum and urinary markers of bone remodelling: assessment of bone turnover. *Endocrine Rev.*, **9**(4), 437

24. Faugere M. C. and Malluche H. H. (1983). Comparison of different bone biopsy techniques for qualitative and quantitative diagnosis of metabolic bone diseases. *J. Bone Jt Surg.*, **65**, 1314

25. Fogelman I. (1988). Bone scanning and photon absorptiometry in metabolic bone disease. Martin T. J., *Metabolic Bone Disease* (p. 59). London: Baillière Tindall

26. Fornasier V. L. and Vilaghy M. I. (1973). The results of bone biopsy with a new instrument. *Amer. J. Clin. Pathol.*, **60**, 570

27. Frisch B. and Bartl R. (1990). *Atlas of Bone Marrow Pathology*. Dordrecht: Kluwer

28. Frisch B., Lewis S. M., Burkhardt R. and Bartl R. (1985). *Biopsy Pathology of Bone and Bone Marrow*. London: Chapman & Hall

29. Frost H. M. (1989). Some effects of basic multicellular unit-based remodelling on photon absorptiometry of trabecular bone. *Bone Miner.*, **7**, 47

30. Frost H. M. (1969). Tetracyclin-based histological analysis of bone remodelling. *Calcif. Tissue Res.*, **3**, 211

31. Garner A. and Ball J. (1966). Quantitative observations on mineralised and unmineralised bone in chronic renal azotaemia and intestinal malabsorption syndrome. *J. Pathol. Bacteriol.*, **91**, 545

32. Grech P., Martin T. J., Barrington N. A. and Ell P. J. (1985). *Diagnosis of Metabolic Bone Disease*. London: Chapman & Hall

33. Hocking D. R. (1964). Bone marrow biopsy: a routine including marrow trephine. *Med. J. Aust.*, **2**, 915

34. Hodgson S. F., Johnson K. A. and Muhs J. M. (1986). Outpatient percutaneous biopsy of the iliac crest: methods, morbidity, and patients acceptance. *Mayo Clin. Proc.*, **61**, 28

35. Hufter W. E. (1988). Morphology and biochemistry of bone remodelling: possible control by vitamin D, parathyroid hormone, and other substances. *Lab. Invest.*, **59**(4), 418

36. Islam A. (1982). A new bone biopsy needle with core securing device. *J. Clin. Pathol.*, **356**, 359

37. Jamshidi J. and Swaim R. W. (1971). Bone marrow biopsy with unaltered architecture: a new biopsy device. *J. Lab. Clin. Med.*, **77**, 335

38. Johnson K. A., Kelly P. J. and Jowsey J. (1977). Percutaneous biopsy of the iliac crest. *Clin. Orthop.*, **123**, 34

39. Jowsey J. (1977). The bone biopsy. Avioli L. V., *Topics in Bone and Mineral*. New York: Plenum Medical

40. Kattapuram S. V. and Rosenthal D. I. (1991). Percutaneous biopsy of skeletal lesions. *Amer. J. Radiol.*, **157**, 935

41. Lalor B., Freemont A. and Carlile S. (1986). An improved transiliac crest bone biopsy drill for quantitative histomorphometry. *Bone*, **7**, 273

42. Malluche H. H. and Faugere M.-C. (1986). *Atlas of Mineralized Bone Histology*. Basel: Karger

43. Malluche H. H., Meyer W., Sherman D. and Massry S. G. (1972). Quantitative bone histology in 84 normal American subjects. Micromorphometric analysis and evaluation of variance in iliac bone. *Calcif. Tissue Int.*, **34**, 449

44. Melsen F., Melsen B. and Mosekilde L. (1978). An evaluation of the quantitative parameters applied to bone histology. *Acta Pathol. Microbiol.*, **86**, 63

45. Moore R. J., Durbridge T. C., Woods A. E., and Vernon-Roberts B. (1989). Variation in histomorphometric estimates across different sites of the iliac crest. *J. Clin. Pathol.*, **42**, 814

46. Murray R. O., Jacobson H. G. and Stoker D. J. (1990). *The Radiology of Skeletal Disorders*. Edinburgh: Churchill Livingstone

47. Nielsen H. K., Brixen K., Bouillon R. and Mosekilde L. (1990). Changes in biochemical markers of osteoblastic activity during the menstrual cycle. *J. Clin. Endocrinol. Metab.*, **70**(5), 1431 ·

48. Podenphant J., Gotfredsen A., Nilas L., Norgaard H. and Braendstrup O. (1986). Iliac crest biopsy: representativity for the amount of mineralized bone. *Bone*, **7**, 427

49. Power M. J. and Fottrell P. F. (1991). Osteocalcin: diagnostic methods and clinical applications. *Crit. Rev. Clin. Lab. Sci.*, **28**, 287

50. Rao S. Practical approach to bone biopsy. Recker R. R., *Bone Histomorphometry: Techniques and Interpretation* (p. 3). Boca Raton: CRC Press

51. Rasmussen H. and Bordier P. (1974). *The Physiological and Cellular Basis of Metabolic Bone Disease*. Baltimore: Williams & Wilkins

52. Roberts W. E., Mozsary P. G. and Klingler E. (1982). Nuclear size as a cell-kinetic marker for osteoblast differentiation. *Amer. J. Anat.*, **165**, 373

53. Rowden G., Sacher R. A. and More N. S. (1982). Plastic embedded specimens for evaluation of bone marrow. Roath S., *Topical Reviews in Haematology* (p. 1). Bristol: Wright

54. Stoker D. J., Cobb J. P. and Pringle J. A. S. (1991). Needle biopsy of musculoskeletal lesions. *J. Bone Jt Surg.*, **73-B**, 498

55. Tohme J. F., Seibel M. J., Silverberg S. J., Robins S. P. and Bilezikian J. P. (1991). Biochemical markers of bone metabolism. *Z. Rheumat.*, **50**, 133

56. Visser W. J., Roelofs J. M. M. and Duursma S. A. (1981). Bone density in the iliac crest. *Metab. Bone Dis. Rel. Res.*, **3**, 187

57. Westerman M. P. (1981). Bone marrow needle biopsy: an evaluation and critique. *Sem. Haematol.*, **18**, 293

58. Whitehouse W. J. (1977). Cancellous bone in the anterior part of the iliac crest. *Calcif. Tissue Res.*, **23**, 67

59. Wolf E., Röser K., Hahn M., Welkerling H. and Delling G. (1992). Enzyme and immunohistochemistry on undecalcified bone and bone marrow biopsies after embedding in plastic: a new embedding method for routine application. *Virchows Archiv A. Pathol. Anat.*, **420**, 17

60. Zimmermann M. C., Meunier A., Katz J. L. and Christel P. (1990). The evaluation of cortical bone remodeling with a new ultrasonic technique. *IEEE Trans. Biomed. Eng.*, **37**(5), 433

Histomorphometry

3

Histomorphometry is the method used to quantify histological features of bone (quantitative bone histology)[8,10,15,30–32], in particular static and dynamic parameters of bone structure, formation and resorption. Its main use is in clinical studies in which reproducibility is required[36], especially for the evaluation of the effects of a given treatment on resorptive and formative bone cells[3,4]. In addition it is possible to measure a large number of variables in a biopsy section and from these to derive many more[18,31,34,35]. Thus, some computerized histomorphometric reports can contain so much detail that the recipient may be confused rather than enlightened. The most widely used variables, as well as those assessed in our departments, are given in the following survey. For effective comparison with results of other groups, we have used the unified system of *terminology for bone histomorphometry* of the Nomenclature Committee of the American Society of Bone and Mineral Research (ASBMR), including the three-dimensional description of bone tissue whenever possible (Table 3.1)[26,28].

Table 3.1 Histomorphometric variables used in our laboratories when indicated. TV = tissue volume, BV = bone volume, MV = marrow volume, B.Ar = bone area (2D), M.Ar. = marrow area (2D)

Terminology	Abbreviation	Units	Dimension
Volume			
Bone volume	BV/TV	%	3D
Lamellar bone volume	LBV/TV,		
	LBV/BV	%	3D
Woven bone volume	WBV/TV,		
	WBV/BV	%	3D
Osteoid volume	OV/TV, OV/BV	%	3D
Haematopoiesis volume	HV/TV, HV/MV	%	3D
Fatty tissue volume	FV/TV, FV/MV	%	3D
Sinusoid volume	SV/TV, SV/MV	%	3D
Endosteal sinusoid volume	ESV/TV,		
	ESV/MV	%	3D
Oedema volume	EV/TV, EV/MV	%	3D
Infiltration volume	IV/TV, IV/MV	%	3D
Surface			
Bone surface	BS/BV	mm²/mm³	3D
Osteoid surface	OS/BV	mm²/mm³	3D
Osteoblast surface	Obl.S/BS	%	3D
Osteoclast surface	Ocl.S/BS	%	3D
Eroded surface	ES/BS	%	3D
Thickness			
Trabecular thickness	Tb.Th	μm	3D
Osteoid thickness	O.Th	μm	3D
Cell number			
Osteoclast number	N.Ocl/B.Ar	per mm²	2D
Osteoblast number	N.Obl/B.Ar	per mm²	2D
Lining cell number	N.Lin/B.Ar	per mm²	2D
Osteocyte number	N.Ocy/B.Ar	per mm²	2D
Megakaryocyte number	N.Meg/M.Ar	per mm²	2D
Mast cell number	N.Mas/M.Ar	per mm²	2D
Plasma cell number	N.Pla/M.Ar	per mm²	2D
Vessel number			
Artery number	N.Art/M.Ar	per mm²	2D
Arteriole number	N.Aio/M.Ar	per mm²	2D
Capillary number	N.Cap/M.Ar	per mm²	2D
Sinusoid number	N.Sin/M.Ar	per mm²	2D

All estimates of quantitative histology rely on the use of unbiased sampling methods. Most of our histomorphometry was carried out using the technique of point and line intersect counting with an eyepiece graticule (*grid*)[31,32]. The grid techniques have proved to be precise and, with application of the proper counting statistics, are no more time-consuming than computerized digitizing[10]. We used the Zeiss integration disc II with straight sampling lines (Fig. 3.S1)[1,2]. Initially we also used the cycloid grid with semicircular lines[22,31,33], but there were no differences between results obtained with these grids, at least on sections of iliac crest biopsies. We have also confirmed that the main variance of bone histomorphometry is caused by intra- and interbone variations (Figs. 3.S2 and S3)[5–7,11,12,21,29,37]. Variations also occur when the same

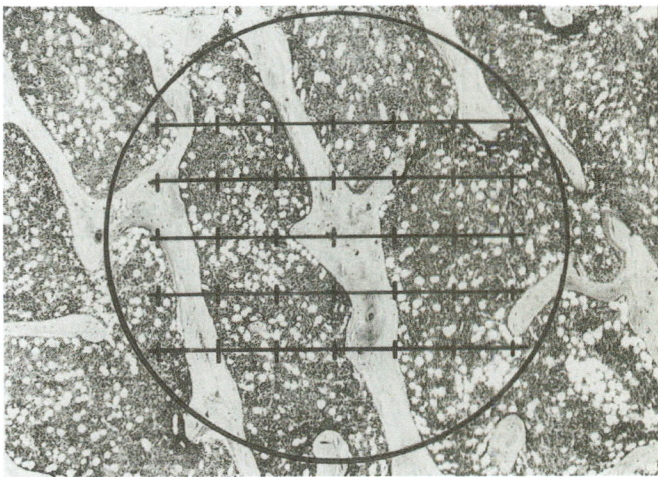

Fig. 3.S1 Grid with straight sampling lines and points superimposed on micrograph of part of bone biopsy section. × 40

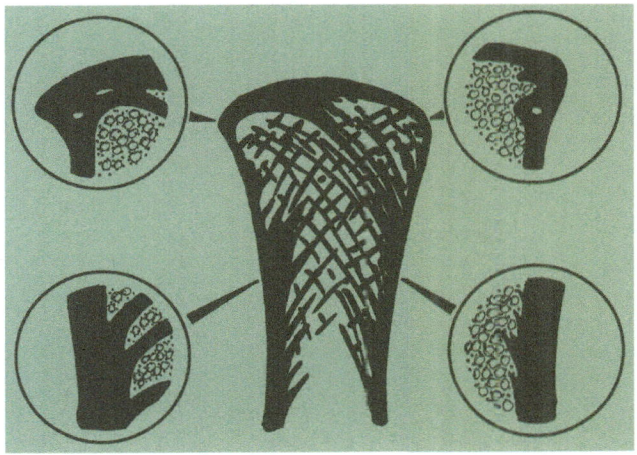

Fig. 3.S2 Diagram of intra-bone variations in longitudinal section of the anterior ilium. Note the variability in width and structure in cortex (in circles), as well as in trabecular network

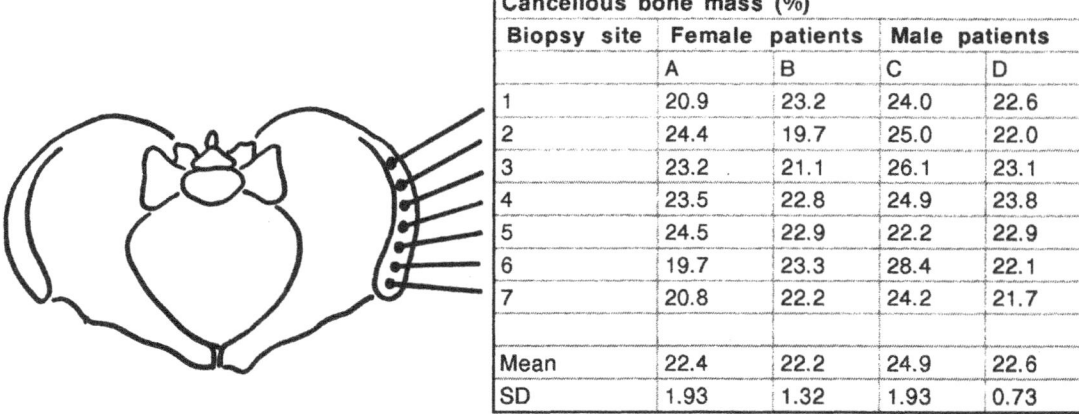

Cancellous bone mass (%)				
Biopsy site	Female patients		Male patients	
	A	B	C	D
1	20.9	23.2	24.0	22.6
2	24.4	19.7	25.0	22.0
3	23.2	21.1	26.1	23.1
4	23.5	22.8	24.9	23.8
5	24.5	22.9	22.2	22.9
6	19.7	23.3	28.4	22.1
7	20.8	22.2	24.2	21.7
Mean	22.4	22.2	24.9	22.6
SD	1.93	1.32	1.93	0.73

Fig. 3.S3 Variations in quantitative measurements of trabecular bone volume (histomorphometry) in biopsies taken from seven different sites along the iliac crest

biopsy sections are evaluated by different observers as well as by different types of grids (Table 3.2)[7]. Therefore we recommend counting the whole trabecular bone area at a relatively low magnification (x100) rather than

Table 3.2 Variations in results of histomorphometry of the same biopsy section between different and the same observers using different grids

			Iliac crest biopsy, volumes, %			
Observer	Grid type	Date	Bone	Osteoid	Haemato-poiesis	Fatty tissue
A	Zeiss	1	20	0.6	45	34
		2	20	0.4	46	34
	Merz	1	22	0.5	47	30
		2	22	1.0	44	33
	Max. deviation		2	0.6	3	4
B	Zeiss	1	23	1.5	46	29
		2	19	1.5	48	31
	Merz	1	21	1.0	50	28
		2	20	1.1	55	24
	Max. deviation		4	0.5	9	7
C	Zeiss	1	19	1.4	55	25
		2	22	1.1	54	23
	Merz	1	22	1.2	56	21
		2	22	0.9	54	23
	Max. deviation		3	0.5	2	4
D	Zeiss	1	20	1.0	56	23
		2	22	1.2	48	29
	Merz	1	19	1.1	56	24
		2	23	0.9	47	29
	Max. deviation		4	0.3	9	6
E	Zeiss	1	21	0.9	46	32
		2	21	1.0	46	32
	Merz	1	21	0.8	43	35
		2	21	0.9	44	34
	Max. deviation		0	0.2	3	3
F	Zeiss	1	20	0.4	49	31
		2	19	0.6	47	34
	Merz	1	20	0.6	46	33
		2	20	0.8	44	35
	Max. deviation		1	0.4	5	4
A–F	Max. deviation		4	0.6	9	7

numerous intersections in smaller and possibly non-representative areas at higher magnifications. Tracing of complete tissue structures with the use of a computerized digitizing device (Videoplan, Kontron) was used for measuring size, structure and volumes of the sinusoidal system. As pointed out by Eriksen, the '*trace method*' (tracing of surface contours with a cursor) demands that complete structures are measured, which is a problem if the section contains artefacts inherent in taking the biopsies and in processing, cutting and staining the sections[10]. Moreover, the act of tracing itself involves a certain inaccuracy because of errors associated with hand movements on the digitizer plate[23]. A difference of only 1.5% was found by Giroux et al. between results based on the use of the Zeiss eyepiece graticule and the Quantimet method[14]. According to Malluche and co-workers, there was no difference in accuracy between point counting and a semi-automatic method with a digitizer tablet[18–20]. We agree with Eriksen's conclusions that the best set-up is probably a programme involving the combination of grid-based sampling methods, digitization of distances and computerized recording of measured data using the unified nomenclature of the ASBMR for comparison[10].

Quantitative histology comprises three main types of primary measurement, expressed in the three-dimensional terminology: *volume*, *surface* and *thickness*[26,27]. *Number*, the fourth type of primary measurement, can only be expressed two-dimensionally, if serial sections are not examined. Other rather sophisticated parameters can be derived from combinations of these primary variables[18,26,31,33].

Bone biopsies are frequently taken to diagnose changes in bone volume, turnover and mineralization, particularly in metabolic bone disease[1–3,16,17,25]. In many cases these parameters can be assessed qualitatively by experienced observers and a descriptive bone report with comments on the degree of abnormalities present is often sufficient for clinical purposes.

The *variables* we use are summarized in Table 3.1. The normal values given for different skeletal sites are derived from post-mortem biopsies taken with the electric drill from 100 normal subjects who died suddenly but had no evidence of bone or marrow disease (Table 3.3 and Figs 3.S4 and S5).

Table 3.3 Normal range of histomorphometric values at different skeletal sites (mean ± SD)

Parameters	Abbreviation	Units	Anterior iliac crest	Posterior iliac crest	Lumbar vertebra	Sternum	Calcaneus	Radius
Bone structure								
Bone volume	BV/TV	%	22 ± 4	22 ± 4	16 ± 4	15 ± 4	20 ± 6	19 ± 5
Bone surface	BS/BV	mm²/mm³	2.8 ± 0.7	2.6 ± 0.8	2.3 ± 0.6	2.7 ± 0.6	3.5 ± 0.8	3.2 ± 1.8
Trabecular thickness	TB.Th	μm	175 ± 42	181 ± 40	178 ± 48	155 ± 42	157 ± 50	161 ± 44
Mineralization								
Osteoid volume	OV/BV	%	2.5 ± 2.2	2.8 ± 2.1	2.3 ± 1.8	1.6 ± 1.8	1.7 ± 1.4	1.3 ± 0.9
Osteoid surface	OS/BV	mm²/mm³	0.6 ± 0.4	0.6 ± 0.4	0.5 ± 0.3	0.4 ± 0.4	0.3 ± 0.2	0.4 ± 0.3
Osteoid thickness	O.Th	μm	4.1 ± 3.4	4.6 ± 3.3	5.4 ± 2.1	4.9 ± 3.5	4.0 ± 3.0	3.5 ± 3.6
Bone cells								
Osteoclasts	N.Ocl/B.Ar	per mm²	1.0 ± 0.9	0.9 ± 0.7	0.9 ± 0.7	1.0 ± 0.8	0.5 ± 0.4	0.4 ± 0.2
Osteoblasts	N.Obl/B.Ar	per mm²	2.5 ± 1.8	3.2 ± 1.1	2.6 ± 1.4	4.1 ± 1.6	2.2 ± 1.7	1.3 ± 0.4
Lining cells	N.Lin/B.Ar	per mm²	2.0 ± 1.3	1.9 ± 1.0	2.0 ± 1.1	1.8 ± 1.0	0.8 ± 0.6	0.9 ± 0.3
Osteocytes	N.Ocy/B.Ar	per mm²	32 ± 6	30 ± 5	24 ± 6	25 ± 6	32 ± 7	28 ± 6
Blood vessels								
Arteries	N.Art/M.Ar	per mm²	0.4 ± 0.4	0.5 ± 0.3	0.6 ± 0.4	0.5 ± 0.5	0.5 ± 0.4	0.4 ± 0.4
Arterioles	N.Aio/M.Ar	per mm²	1.3 ± 0.4	1.4 ± 0.5	1.4 ± 0.6	1.4 ± 0.9	1.4 ± 1.0	1.2 ± 0.9
Capillaries	N.Cap/M.Ar	per mm²	17 ± 5	16 ± 5	16 ± 5	16 ± 5	11 ± 3	11 ± 4
Sinusoids	N.Sin/M.Ar	per mm²	33 ± 7	35 ± 8	36 ± 9	36 ± 8	11 ± 4	11 ± 5
Endosteal sinusoid volume	ESV/TV	%	2.0 ± 1.3	2.1 ± 1.4	2.2 ± 1.4	2.3 ± 1.7	1.8 ± 0.9	1.8 ± 1.0
Stroma								
Fatty tissue volume	FV/MV	%	26 ± 8	25 ± 6	23 ± 7	28 ± 19	96 ± 4	96 ± 5
Mast cells	N.Mas/M.Ar	per mm²	2.3 ± 1.8	2.2 ± 1.9	3.7 ± 3.1	1.9 ± 2.8	0	0
Plasma cells	N.Pla/M.Ar	per mm²	30 ± 12	29 ± 10	31 ± 24	29 ± 14	0	0
Haematopoiesis								
Haematopoiesis volume	HV/MV	%	60 ± 6	62 ± 7	64 ± 7	61 ± 8	0	0
Megakaryocytes	N.Meg/M.Ar	per mm²	14 ± 4	13 ± 4	15 ± 8	16 ± 7	0	0

Terminology, abbreviations and units see Table 3.1. Histomorphometry was performed in collaboration with Dr B. Mallmann

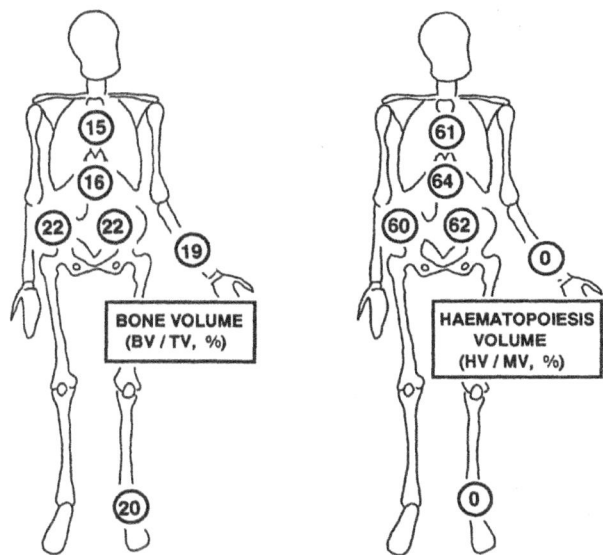

Fig. 3.S4 Cancellous bone mass at different skeletal sites, mean values

Fig. 3.S5 Haematopoietic cellularity at different skeletal sites, mean values

References

1. Bartl R., Frisch B. and Burkhardt R. (1985). *Bone Marrow Biopsies Revisited*. Basel: Karger

2. Bartl R., Frisch B. and Burkhardt R. (1991). Bone marrow histology. Catovsky D., *The Leukemic Cell* (p. 47). Edinburgh: Churchill Livingstone

3. Boyce B. F. (1988). Uses and limitations of bone biopsy in management of metabolic bone disease. Martin T. J., *Metabolic Bone Disease* (p. 31). London: Baillière Tindall

4. Bullough P. G., Bansal M. and D Carlo E. F. (1990). The tissue diagnosis of metabolic bone disease. Role of histomorphometry. *Orthop. Clin. N. Amer.*, **21**(1), 65

5. Chavassieux P. M., Arlot M. E. and Meunier O. J. (1985). Inter-method variation in bone histomorphometry: comparison between manual and computerized methods applied to iliac bone biopsies. *Bone*, **6**, 221

6. Chavassieux P. M., Arlot M. E. and Meunier P. J. (1985). Intersample variation in bone histomorphometry: comparison between parameter values measured on two contiguous transiliac bone biopsies. *Calcif. Tissue Int.*, **37**, 345

7. Compston J. E., Vedi S. and Stellon A. J. (1986) Inter-observer and intra-observer variation in bone histomorphometry. *Calcif. Tissue Int.*, **38**, 67

8. Dunstan C. R. and Evans R. A. (1980). Quantitative bone histology: a new method. *Pathology*, **12**, 255

9. Eriksen E. F., Melsen F. and Mosekilde L. (1984). Reconstruction of the resorptive site in iliac trabecular bone: a kinetic model for bone resorption in 20 normal individuals. *Metab. Bone Dis.*, **5**, 235

10. Eriksen E. F., Steiniche T., Mosekilde L. and Melsen F. (1989). Histomorphometric analysis of bone in metabolic bone disease. *Endocrinol. Metab. Clin. N. Amer.*, **18**(4), 919

11. Eventov I., Frisch B., Cohen Z. and Hammel I. (1991). Osteopenia, hematopoiesis, and bone remodelling in iliac crest and femoral biopsies: a prospective study of 102 cases of femoral neck fractures. *Bone*, **12**, 1

12. Fazzalari N. L., Moore R. J., Manthey B. A. and Vernon-Roberts B. (1989). Comparative study of iliac crest and proximal femur histomorphometry in normal patients. *J. Clin. Pathol.*, **42**, 745

13. Frisch B. and Bartl R. (1990). *Atlas of Bone Marrow Pathology*. Dordrecht: Kluwer

14. Giroux J. M., Courpron P. and Meunier P. (1975). *Histomorphometrie de l'osteopenie physiologique senile*. Lyon: Monographie du Laboratoire de Researches sur l'Histodynamique Osseuse

15. Henning A. (1975). Kritische Betrachtungen zur Volumen- und Oberflächenmessungen in der Mikroskopie. *Zeiss Werkzeitschr.*, **30**, 78

16. Kerndrup G., Pallesen G., Melsen F. and Mosekilde L. (1980). Histomorphometrical determination of bone marrow cellularity in iliac crest biopsies. *Scand. J. Haematol.*, **24**, 110

17. Lauffenburger T., Olah A. J., Dambacher M. A., Guncago J., Lentner C. and Haas H. G. (1977). Bone remodeling and calcium metabolism: a correlated histomorphometric, calcium kinetic, and biochemical study in patients with osteoporosis and Paget's disease. *Metabolism*, **26**(6), 589

18. Malluche H. H. and Faugere M.-C. (1986). *Atlas of Mineralized Bone Histology*. Basel: Karger

19. Malluche H. H. and Faugere M.-C. (1991). Bone biopsies: histology and histomorphometry of bone. Avioli L. V. and Krane S. M., *Metabolic Bone Disease* (p. 283). Philadelphia: Saunders

20. Malluche H. H., Sherman D., Manaka R. and Massey S. G. (1980). Comparison between different histomorphometric methods. *Metab. Bone Dis. Rel. Res.*, **2**(Suppl.), 449

21. Melsen F., Melsen B. and Mosekilde L. (1978). An evaluation of the quantitative analysis of normal bone from the iliac crest. *Acta Pathol. Microbiol. Scand.*, **86**, 63

22. Merz W. A. and Schenk R. K. (1970). Quantitative structural analysis of human cancellous bone. *Acta Anat.*, **75**, 54

23. Meyer P., Schwartz J. and Recker R. R. (1981). Comparison of surface density and volume of human iliac trabecular bone measured directly and by applied stereology. *Calcif. Tissue Int.*, **33**, 561

24. Mosekilde L. (1990). Consequences of the remodelling process for vertebral trabecular bone structure: a scanning electron microscopy study (uncoupling of unloaded structures). *Bone Miner.*, **10**, 13

25. Ott S. M. (1991). Bone density in adolescence. *N. Engl. J. Med.*, **325**, 23

26. Parfitt A. M. (1988). Bone histomorphometry: standardization of nomenclature, symbols and units. Summary of proposed system. *Bone Miner.*, **4**, 1

27. Parfitt A. M. (1983). The stereologic basis of bone histomorphometry. Theory of quantitative microscopy and reconstruction of the third dimension. Recker R. R., *Bone Histomorphometry: Techniques and Interpretations* (p. 53). Boca Raton: CRC Press

28. Parfitt A. M., Drezner M. K., Glorieux F. H., Kanis J. A., Malluche H. H., Meunier P. J., Ott S. M. and Recker R. R. (1987). Bone histomorphometry: standardisation of nomenclature, symbols, and units. *J. Bone Miner. Res.*, **2**(6), 595

29. Podenphant J., Gotfredsen A., Nilas L., Norgaard H. and Braendstrup O. (1986). Iliac crest biopsy: representativity for the amount of mineralized bone. *Bone*, **7**, 427

30. Rasmussen H. and Bordier P. (1974). *The Physiological and Cellular Basis of Metabolic Bone Disease*. Baltimore: Williams & Wilkins

31. Recker R. R. (1983). *Bone Histomorphometry: Techniques and Interpretation*. Boca Raton: CRC Press

32. Revell P. A. (1986). *Pathology of Bone*. Berlin: Springer

33. Schenk R. K. and Olah A. J. (1980). Histomorphometrie. Kuhlencordt F. and Bartelheimer H., *Handbuch der Inneren Medizin: Klinische Osteologie* (p. 437). Berlin: Springer

34. Teitelbaum S. L. and Bates M. (1980). Relationships of static and kinetic histomorphometric features of bone. *Orthop. Rel. Res.*, **146**, 239

35. Vedi S., Compston J. E., Webb A. and Tighe J. R. (1983). Histomorphometric analysis of dynamic parameters of trabecular bone formation in the iliac crest of normal British subjects. *Metab. Bone Dis. Rel. Res.*, **5**, 69

36. Vernejoul M. C., Kuntz D., Miravet L., Goutallier D. and Ryckewaert A. (1981). Bone histomorphometric reproducibility in normal patients. *Calcif. Tissue Int.*, **33**, 369

37. Xipell R. W. and Brown D. J. (1979). Histology of normal bone – a computerized study in the iliac crest. *Pathology*, **11**, 235

Principles of bone biopsy pathology

4

Contrary to the image of the skeleton as an inert structure supporting the rest of the body, bone is a dynamic tissue undergoing constant remodelling throughout life – increasing in size during growth, adapting to physical stresses and repairing structural damage[2,10,15,16,18]. About 2 million bone remodelling units are active at any time in the human skeleton and the removal and replacement rate is about 8% (5–10%) of the total bone per annum. Malfunctioning of this complex cellular system or its regulatory mechanisms, whether due to intrinsic and/or extrinsic factors, will inevitably abolish normal development in childhood and diminish the quantity and/or strength of bone in the adult[2]. Abnormalities of only one type of bone cells or of one regulatory factor may result in seriously disturbed bone turnover with impaired or accelerated bone production or destruction[5,11,14]. The following *four main manifestations* occur in all disorders of bone either singly or in combination, and the manifestations of the major osteopathies are shown in Fig. 4.S1[1,4,7–9,17].

ABNORMALITIES OF BONE MASS (Figs. 4.1–4.4)

Bone mass is a major concern in bone disease. Histomorphometry enables a quantitative measurement of bone mass (volume) usually on sections of bone biopsies[3,12,13,19]. However, it appears that bone mass and changes therein apply only to the measured site and cannot be extrapolated to other sites[6]. Sex- and age-related differences must also be taken into account[2]. *Osteopenia* denotes a decrease in the amount of bone matrix, and this is reflected in morphometric terms as a reduction in trabecular bone volume and in cortical thickness. Osteopenia may be widespread as in involutional osteoporosis or confined to the axial skeleton (osteopenia in young adults), or it may involve the skeleton focally (as in focal inflammatory and neoplastic processes). Therefore normal values of bone volume in an iliac crest biopsy may exclude systemic bone loss, but not the diagnosis of focal disorders or osteoporotic syndromes. *Osteosclerosis* is an expansion of bone volume at the expense of the marrow spaces, i.e. an increase in bone mass[16]. Like osteopenia, the affected areas in the skeleton may be widespread (as in osteopetrosis, fluorosis) or focal as in Paget's disease, in bone tumours or in osteomyelitis; the latter may also be accompanied by osteopenia in the initial phases.

UNDERMINERALIZATION (Figs. 4.5 and 4.6)

This is observed in a variety of bone disorders grouped under the heading of hyperosteoidosis; it denotes an excess of osteoid[19,20]. In these syndromes the amount of osteoid exceeds the normal upper limit, with an increase in the number, extent and thickness of the osteoid seams. There are two main categories of *hyperosteoidosis*: (1) increase of osteoid with defective calcification is known as osteomalacia; rickets is the childhood expression of osteomalacia. The osteoid seams are thick with more than 5 unmineralized lamellae. The extent of the mineralization front is reduced and it is not sharp, but blurred. Calcification defects with broad unmineralized areas spanning the trabeculae are characteristic. The uptake of tetracycline is decreased and there is prolongation of the mineralization lag time. (2) Hyperosteoidosis without defective mineralization is common in high-turnover states such as hyperparathryoidism, Paget's disease of bone and in some cases of metastases of prostatic carcinoma[19]. The calcification front is normal and the mineralization lag time is not increased[3]. Some similar features of bone may be found in conditions of diverse aetiologies.

ABNORMAL BONE ARCHITECTURE

Quantitative morphometry does not provide all the information pertinent to the diagnosis of bone disease. It supplies details of a 'how much?' or a 'how fast?' nature, but gives no information on the presence of qualitative and architectural abnormalities such as woven bone, mosaic structures, alterations of trabecular shape or discontinuities in the trabecular network. These important parameters pertain mainly to bone fragility and are overlooked in measurements of the total trabecular volume. The normal bone lamella of the adult has a low thickness variance between individuals and throughout life. This indicates its importance for the mechanical strength of bone. It would be of interest to estimate lamellar thickness in various metabolic bone diseases, particularly those with qualitative changes in the organization of collagen (e.g. osteogenesis imperfecta or involutional osteoporosis). Woven bone, with its random arrangement of collagen bundles, has a high fragility and is seen in states with rapid bone turnover (e.g. bone tumours, fractures, adjacent to inflammatory or neoplastic processes, some forms of osteogenesis imperfecta).

Bone strength also depends on the architectural arrangement of the trabecular network. Two types are distinguished in osteopenic conditions:

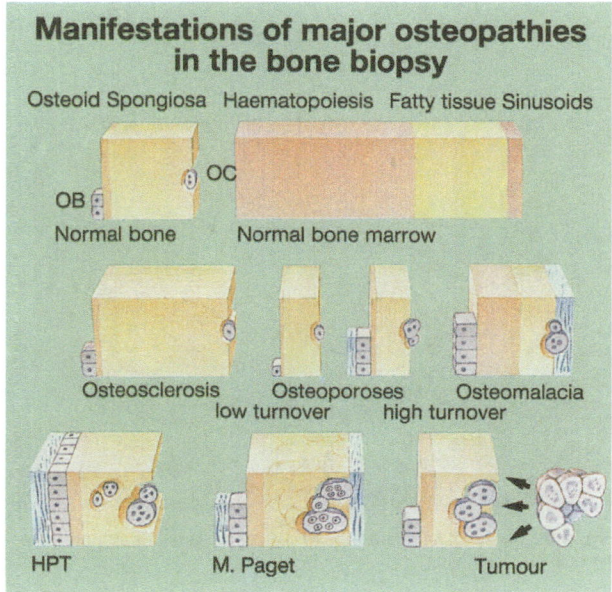

Manifestations of major osteopathies in the bone biopsy

Osteoid Spongiosa Haematopoiesis Fatty tissue Sinusoids

OC
OB
Normal bone   Normal bone marrow

Osteosclerosis   Osteoporoses   Osteomalacia
                  low turnover   high turnover

HPT   M. Paget   Tumour

Fig. 4.S1 Diagram of major osteopathies in iliac crest biopsies

Plate 4.A

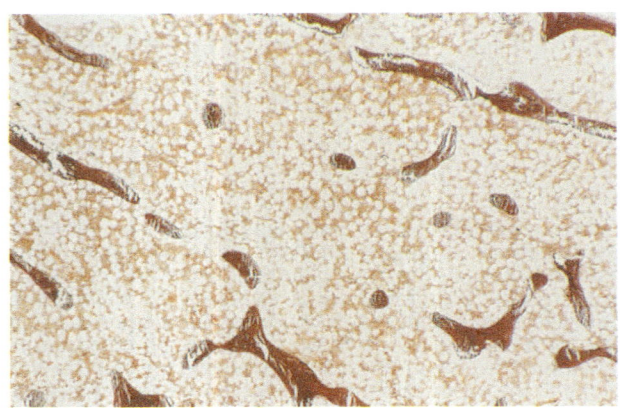

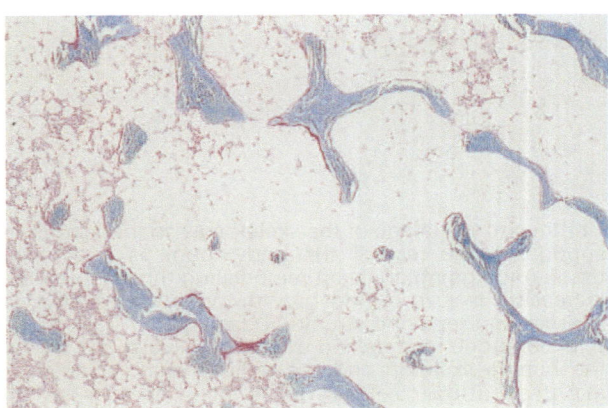

Figs. 4.1–4.6 Main abnormalities of bone volume, structure and mineralization

Fig. 4.1 Marked osteopenia with small islands of bone ('button' phenomenon) and adjacent attenuated trabeculae. Gomori

Fig. 4.2 Patchy osteopenia with 'button' phenomenon (centre) and increased amount of osteoid seams (red): osteoporomalacia. Ladewig

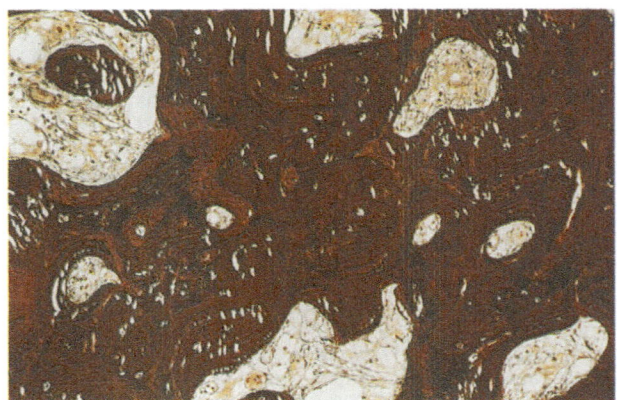

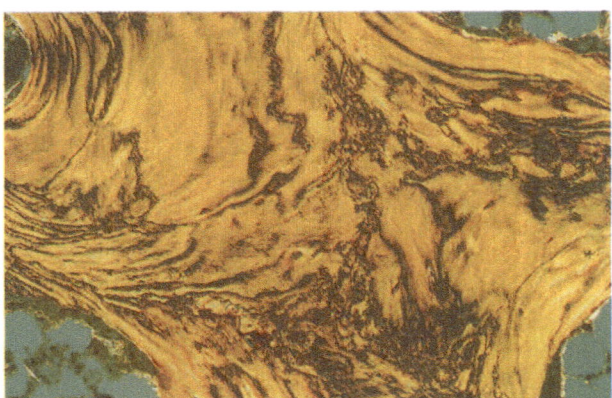

Fig. 4.3 Marked osteosclerosis with narrowing and fibrosis of the marrow cavities (case of 'sclerosing myelitis'). Gomori

Fig. 4.4 Disorganization of lamellae in an old patient with multiple pathologic fractures. Gomori, polar.

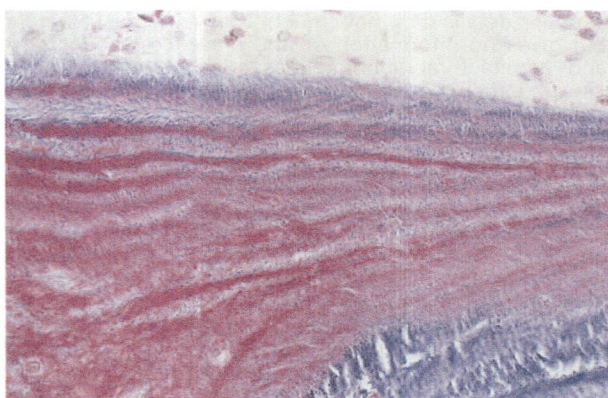

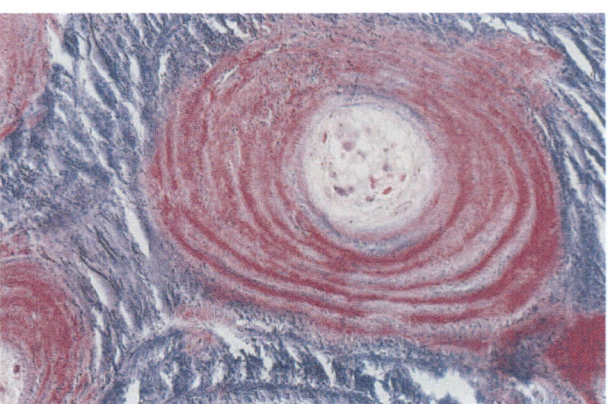

Fig. 4.5 Defect of mineralization (hyperosteoidosis) with broad bands of demineralized parallel lamellae (red). Ladewig

Fig. 4.6 Defect of mineralization of concentric lamellae around Haversian canals. Ladewig

1. osteopenia with attenuated trabeculae, but with preservation of the trabecular connections and network (osteopenia, histological type A); and
2. osteopenia with thick or thin trabeculae, but with disruption of the trabecular network and formation of large marrow spaces (osteopenia, histological type B).

The disposition of the fatty tissue may be of diagnostic value. Sequential biopsies have demonstrated that incipient osteoporosis is characterized by a broad seam of fat cells at the trabecular surface, few and only flat endosteal cells, and a very low bone remodelling activity, indicating an early stage of bone atrophy. In severely osteopenic states biopsy sections show small islands of bone without apparent connections, 'isolated profiles', or the 'button' phenomenon.

ABNORMAL BONE REMODELLING (Plates 4.B–D)

Balanced bone resorption and bone formation (remodelling) maintain skeletal integrity throughout life[14]. A bone biopsy provides the opportunity to examine directly these cellular activities and interactions. The amount of turnover varies with age and sex at different skeletal sites. In general terms, turnover is higher in young, developing individuals and slows down once adulthood is reached. When the skeleton is in balance, the amount of bone formed is equal to the amount of bone resorbed. In 'decoupling', this balance is lost and the normal ratio between resorption and formation is altered. Depending on whether bone resorption is greater than formation or vice versa, 'decoupling' is associated with either osteopenia or osteosclerosis (e.g. osteopenic and osteosclerotic variants in Paget's disease, metastatic disease, and multiple myeloma) (Plates 4.C and D). Deviations from the normal level of bone turnover and 'decoupling' of resorption from formation are two pathophysiologic abnormalities encountered in diseases affecting the bones.

The bone turnover rate is estimated histologically by the population density of the BMU, which is reflected by the density of active osteoblasts and osteoclasts and by the extent of the resorption and formation surfaces[10]. In high and low turnover these values are above or below two standard deviations of the mean. These measurements have clinical relevance and applicability, for example the 'active' and 'inactive' forms of osteoporosis.

Division of the osteoporotic syndrome into high- and low-turnover subtypes has already had consequences for therapy: agents that suppress bone resorption (calcitonin, bisphosphonates) are given in conditions with active remodelling and agents that stimulate formation (vitamin D, fluoride) in inactive states. Characterization of the bone turnover level in other metabolic disorders also gives useful hints for diagnostic and therapeutic decisions.

References

1. Altman R. D. and Gray R. G. (1988). Bone disease. Katz W. A., *Diagnosis and Management of Rheumatic Diseases*, 2nd edn. (p. 620). Philadelpia: Lippincott
2. Alvioli L. and Krane, S. M. (1990). *Metabolic Bone Disease*. Philadelphia: Saunders
3. Boyce B. F. (1988). Uses and limitations of bone biopsy in management of metabolic bone disease. Martin T. J., *Metabolic Bone Disease* (p. 31). London: Baillière Tindall
4. Bullough P. G., Bansal M. and DiCarlo E. F. (1990). The tissue diagnosis of metabolic bone disease. *Orthop. Clin. N. Amer.*, **21**(1), 65
5. Burr D. B. and Martin R. B. (1989). Errors in bone metabolism: toward a unified theory of metabolic bone disease. *Amer. J. Anat.*, **186**(2), 186
6. Chesnut C. H. (1988). Measurement of bone mass. *Triangle*, **27**(1/2), 37
7. Cormier C. (1991). Metabolic bone disease associated with systemic disorders. *Curr. Opin. Rheumatol.*, **3**, 463
8. Frisch B. and Bartl R. (1990). *Atlas of Bone Marrow Pathology*. Dordrecht: Kluwer
9. Frisch B., Lewis S. M., Burkhardt R. and Bartl R. (1985). *Biopsy Pathology of Bone and Bone Marrow*. London: Chapman & Hall
10. Frost H. M. (1973). *Bone Remodeling and its Relationship to Metabolic Bone Diseases*. Springfield: Thomas
11. Little K. (1973). *Bone Behaviour* London: Academic Press
12. Malluche H. H. and Faugere M.-C. (1986). *Atlas of Mineralized Bone Histology*. Basel: Karger
13. Malluche H. H. and Faugere M.-C. (1991). Bone biopsies: histology and histomorphometry of bone. Avioli L. V. and Krane, S. *Metabolic Bone Disease* (p. 283). Philadelphia: Saunders
14. Martin T. J., Ng K. W. and Suda T. (1989). Bone cell physiology. *Endocrinol. Metab. Clin. N. Amer.*, **18**, 833
15. Milgram J. W. (1990). *Radiologic and Histologic Pathology of Nontumorous Diseases of Bones and Joints*. South Lane Northbrook: Northbrook Publ. Co.
16. Revell P. A. (1986). *Pathology of Bone*. Berlin: Springer
17. Rosenberg A. E. (1991). The pathology of metabolic bone disease. *Radiol. Clin. N. Amer.*, **29**(1), 19
18. Smith L. H. and Thier A. O. (1985). *Pathophysiology: Specific Connective Tissues and Mineral Ion Homeostasis*. Philadelphia: Saunders
19. Tam C. S. (1989). The pathogenesis of metabolic bone disease – an overview. Tam C. S., Heersche J. N. M. and Murray T. M., *Metabolic Bone Disease: Cellular and Tissue Mechanisms* (p. 19). Boca Raton: CRC Press
20. Verloog H., DeRoo M., Mortelmans L. and Dequeker J. (1991). Common features of bone in osteomalacia, secondary hyperparathyroidism and renal osteodystrophy. *Clin. Nucl. Med.*, **16**, 372

See also:
Coe F. L. and Favus M. J. (1992). *Disorders of Bone and Mineral Metabolism*. New York: Raven Press

Plate 4.B

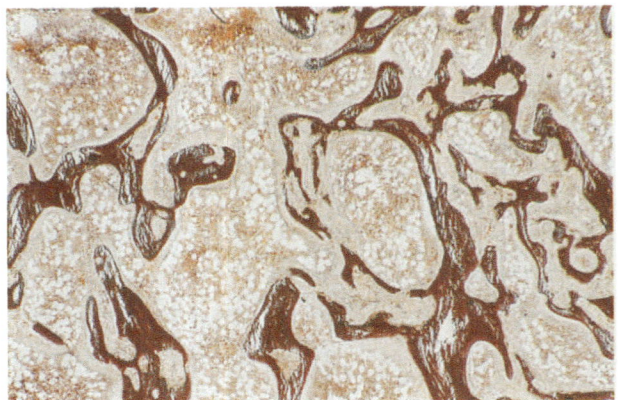

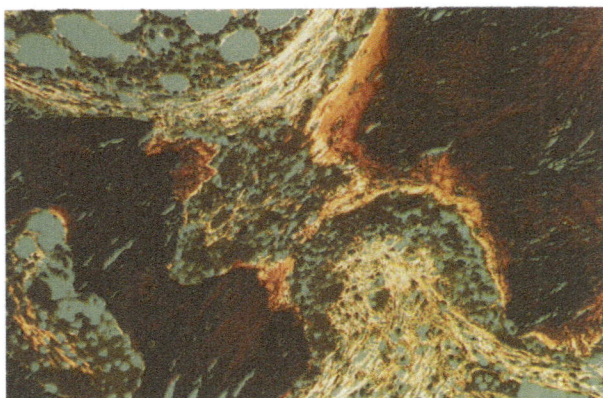

Figs. 4.7–4.12 Main abnormalities in bone cells and remodelling

Fig. 4.7 Substitution of parts of trabecular network by fibrous tissue; case of primary hyperparathyroidism (pHPT). Gomori

Fig. 4.8 Characteristic transecting (centre) and dissecting (left) osteoclastosis in pHPT. Gomori, polar.

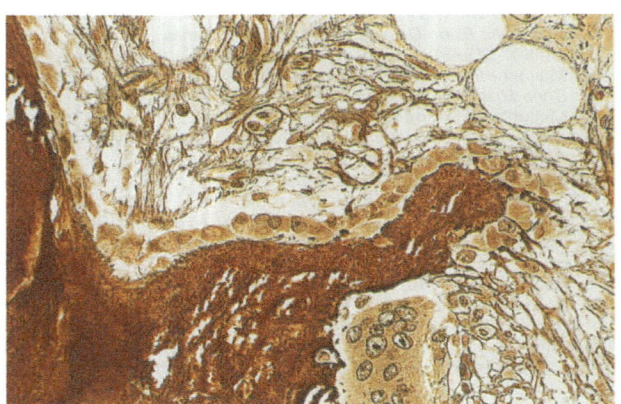

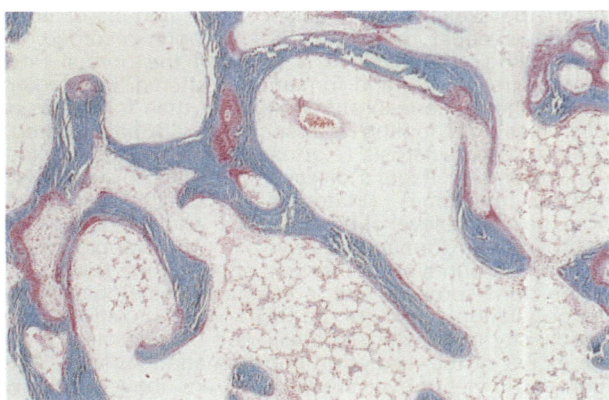

Fig. 4.9 Coupling of osteoclastic bone resorption (lower part) and osteoblastic bone formation (upper part); case of pHPT. Note marked paratrabecular fibrosis (= 'osteodystrophia fibrosa generalisata'). Gomori

Fig. 4.10 Marked dissecting osteoclasia with multiple mineralization defects (red); case of renal osteodystrophy. Ladewig

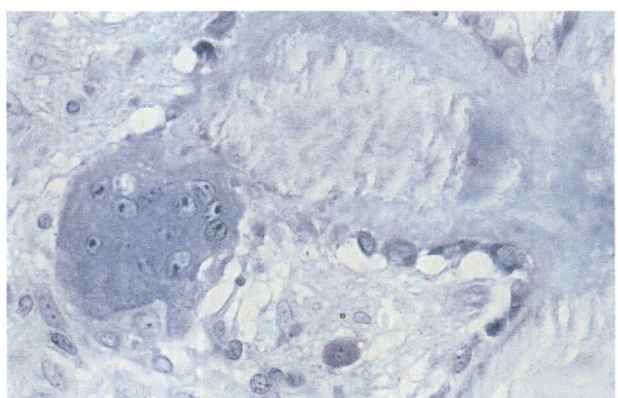

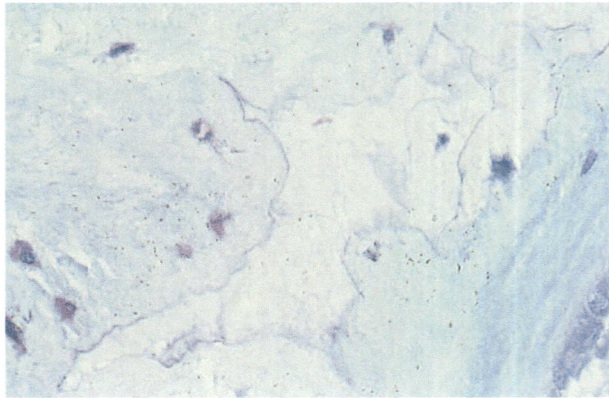

Fig. 4.11 Giant multinucleated and nucleolated osteoclast on bone covered by osteoblasts and osteoid seam; case of Paget's disease of bone. Note marked paratrabecular fibrosis and mast cell (lower centre). Giemsa

Fig. 4.12 Characteristic mosaic structure; case of Paget's disease of bone. Newly formed osteoid seam covered by osteoblasts at lower right. Giemsa

Plate 4.C

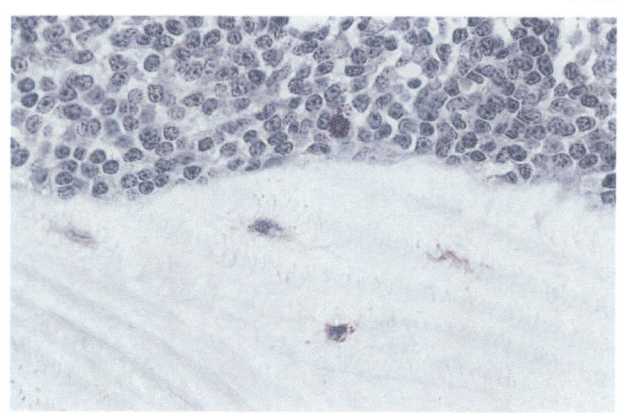

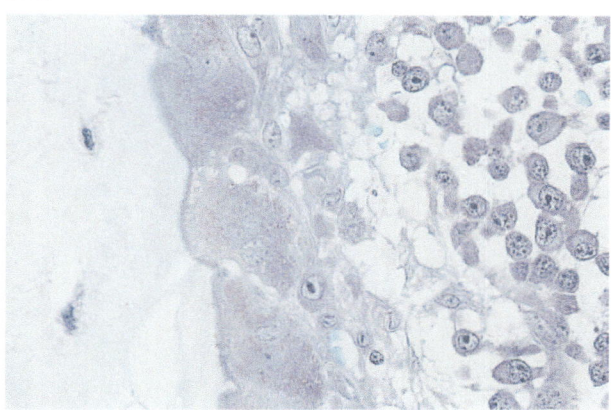

Figs. 4.13–4.18 Aspects of bone resorption in various malignancies

Fig. 4.13 Example of direct trabecular resorption in acute leukaemia, not mediated by osteoclasts. Giemsa

Fig. 4.14 Howship lacunae covered by active osteoclasts and separated from the myeloma cells (secreting osteoclast activating factors) by a band of connective tissue fibres. Giemsa

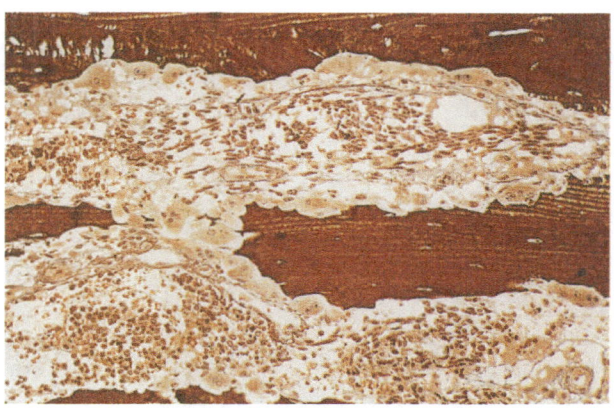

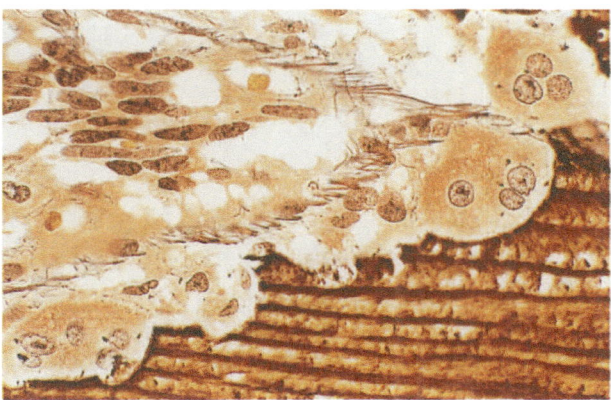

Fig. 4.15 Marked osteoclastic bone resorption in metastatic bone disease (bronchial carcinoma). Gomori

Fig. 4.16 Higher magnification of Fig. 4.15 showing active osteoclasts in deep resorption cavities. Cluster of 'oat cells' upper left. Gomori

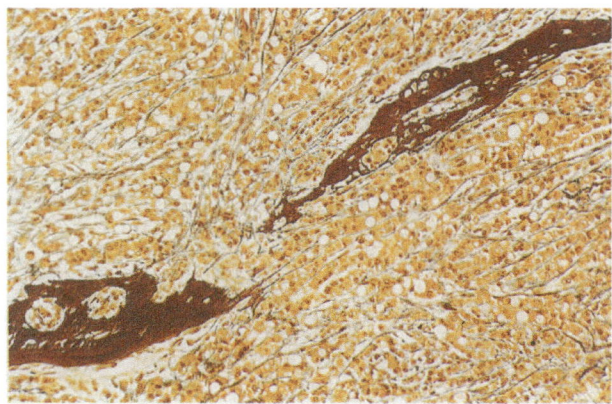

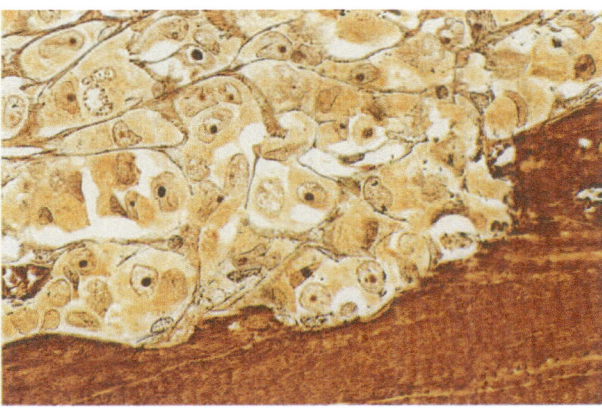

Fig. 4.17 Tumour cells eroding trabecular bone in metastatic bone disease (mammary carcinoma). Gomori

Fig. 4.18 Excavations of trabecular bone surface indicating direct osteolysis by tumour cells. Gomori

Plate 4.D

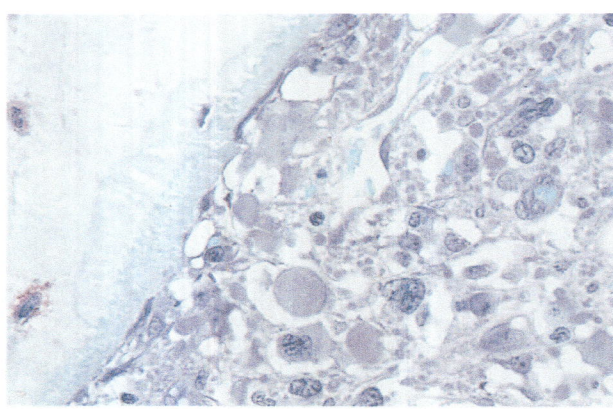

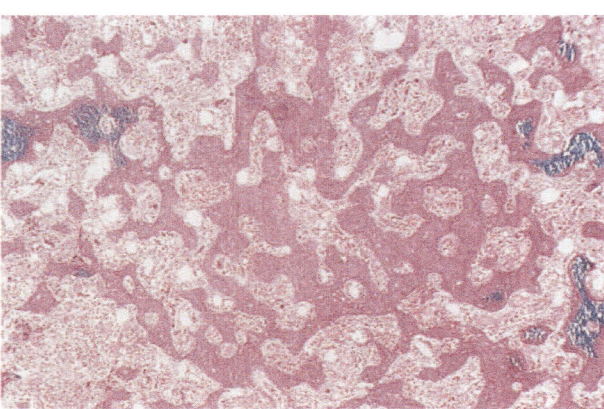

Figs 4.19–4.24 Aspects of bone formation in various malignancies

Fig. 4.19 Loose connective tissue, atypical megakaryocytes and interstitial platelets in OMS, due to a myeloproliferative disorder. The megakaryocytic proliferation and the consequent interstitial platelets are thought to be responsible for the reactive fibrosis and sclerosis. Giemsa

Fig. 4.20 Almost exclusively unmineralized woven bone and lack of lamellar trabecular network in OMS. Skeletal X-ray revealed no osteosclerotic lesions in this case. Ladewig

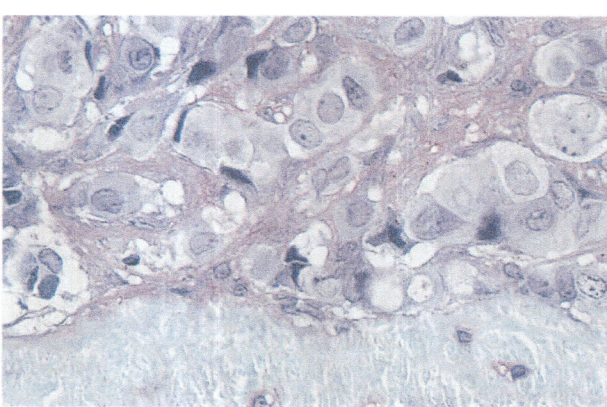

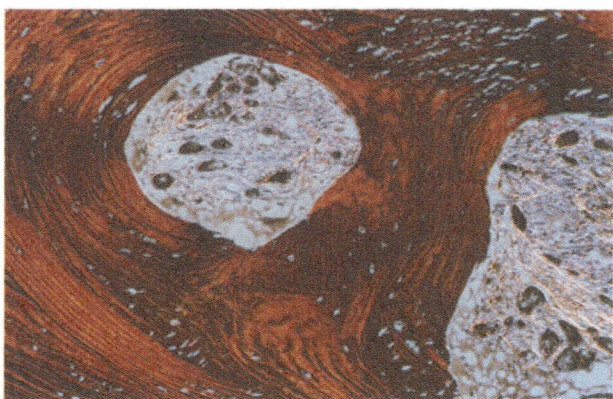

Fig. 4.21 Production of appositional bone and reactive fibrosis close to tumour cells (mammary carcinoma). Giemsa

Fig. 4.22 Narrow marrow spaces filled with carcinomatous tissue and surrounded by broad trabeculae showing lamellar organization (same patient as in Fig. 4.21). Gomori, polar.

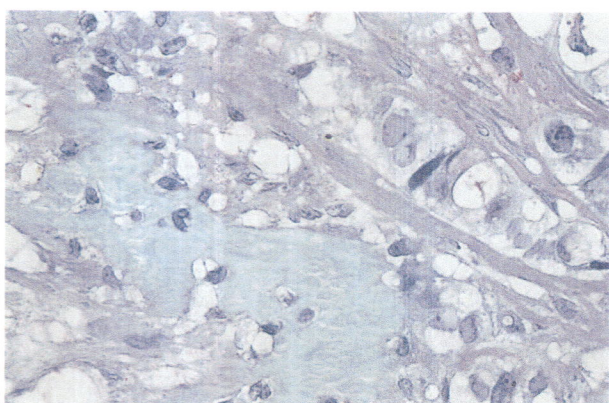

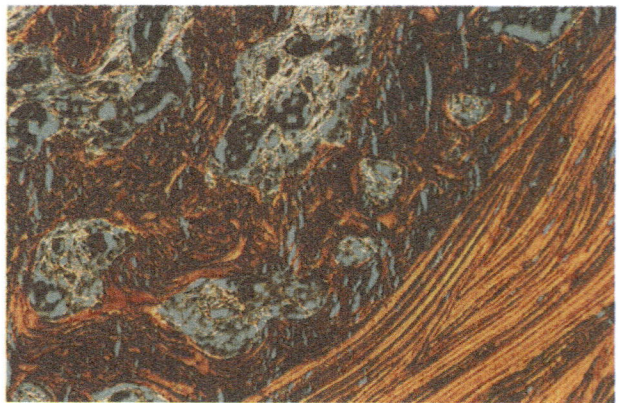

Fig. 4.23 Production of woven bone (lower left) and reactive fibrosis close to tumour cells (prostatic carcinoma). Giemsa

Fig. 4.24 Woven bone, fibrosis and residual tumour cells (upper left) in the marrow cavity surrounded by normal lamellar trabecular bone (lower right) (same patient as in Fig. 4.23). Gomori, polar.

Ageing and bone structure

5

Ageing causes substantial changes in both the structure and the mechanical properties of bone, i.e. quantity and quality[18,31]. Bone loss throughout life has been observed in so many different populations, that it is regarded as a universal feature of ageing, also called 'physiological osteopenia'[6,31,44].

At birth the skeleton weighs approximately 100 g, and doubles during the first year of life. During adolescent growth, bone formation is at its maximum, and bone mineral content increases by about 10% per year[6,24]. By the age of 18 years, however, bone mass is approximately 20% lower in females than in males[6]. *Peak (maximal) bone mass* is achieved at the end of the second decade[22] and is influenced by a number of factors[59], including sex, race[23,50,64,66,68], genetic factors[29,51,56], body weight and lifestyle[60]: thus the skeletal mass is lowest in the 'slim postmenopausal white female'[6]. Other main factors are exercise[35,57], calcium intake and absorption[2,14,57], hormonal status[37,54], pregnancy, cigarette smoking, alcohol consumption[48], use of various drugs, oral contraceptive pills and coexisting diseases.

Bone loss (Figs 5.S1 and S2) begins during or even prior to the third decade, and this onset is likely to be genetically predetermined. Further factors that have been implicated in the phenomenon of age-related bone loss[52,58] include

1. changes in the intestinal absorption and the urinary excretion of calcium[14,20];
2. decrease in the activity of the enzyme 1,25-hydroxylase in the kidney;
3. deficiency of calcitonin in women compared with age-matched men may cause a disruption of the PTH–calcitonin homeostasis, resulting in an accelerated loss of bone[6,63].
4. decline in concentrations of calcium-regulating systemic hormones and local growth factors[6,15,52],
5. thyroid hormone supplementation for the treatment of hypothyroidism in the elderly female or exogenous administration of cortisone may contribute to further imbalance in bone resorption and formation[6].
6. decrease of osteoblastic function leading to impaired bone formation[61];
7. changes in the quality of bone matrix (defects in 'crosslinking' and lamellar arrangement of the collagen molecules) with the consequence of increased bone fragility;
8. alterations in the immune surveillance of bone remodelling[6]; and
9. alterations of bone marrow cellularity and composition[19,25].

Numbers of osteoblasts and osteoclasts in iliac crest biopsies according to age groups are given in Fig. 5.S3, and according to sex in Figs 5.S4 and S5. Contrary to expectations there is a distinct increase in numbers of osteoblasts and osteoclasts in older individuals. Perhaps the increase in numbers represents an attempt to compensate for age-related alterations in function.

Bone mass measurements at a variety of skeletal sites have been used to demonstrate these changes in bone mass with age[5,8,9,27,43,60]. Both men and women reach peak values of bone mass between 20 and 40 years of age[11]. At all adult ages, women have a lower value than men, and this difference widens with advancing age[34]. Over their lifetimes women lose about 35% of their cortical bone and 50% of their trabecular bone, while men lose about three-quarters of these amounts[6,21,22,39,40]. These changes affect all parts of the skeleton, but the *varying patterns of loss* of cortical and trabecular bone at different skeletal sites have not been conclusively defined[3,4,12,13,36,42,53,55,62]. Parfitt *et al.* (1983) have suggested that age-related bone loss is due to removal of entire structural elements of bone, and that the resulting

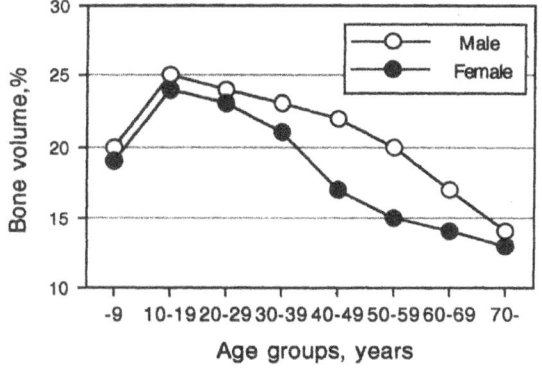

Fig. 5.S1 Peak bone mass and progressive decrease in trabecular bone volume with increasing age in posterior iliac crest biopsies. Note peak in osteoid volume in childhood; another smaller peak occurs in the older age groups

Fig. 5.S2 Trabecular bone volume according to age groups showing differences between males and females

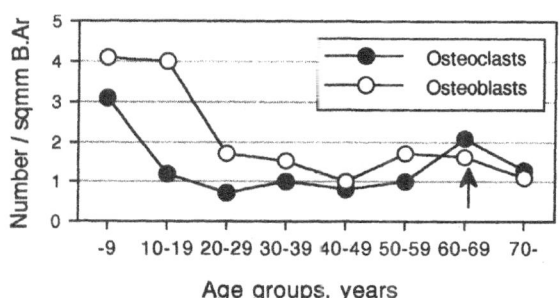

Fig. 5.S3 Number of osteoblasts and osteoclasts according to age groups in posterior iliac crest biopsies

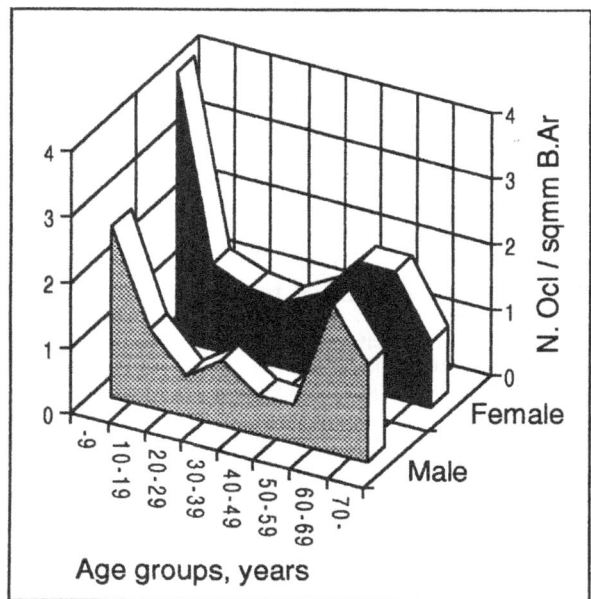

Fig. 5.S4 Osteoclast numbers according to age groups and males and females in posterior iliac crest biopsies

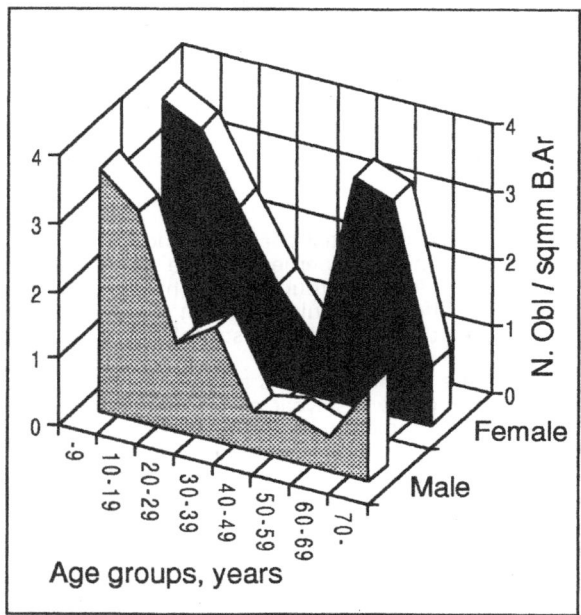

Fig. 5.S5 Osteoblast numbers according to age groups and males and females in posterior iliac crest biopsies

changes are more severe in osteoporotic than in normal subjects[49]. Mosekilde (1990) has studied the whole remodelling process during age-related changes in vertebral trabecular bone by scanning electron microscopy and confirmed the evidence supplied by 'normal' histological studies[45]. We investigated age-related changes in trabecular bone in posterior iliac crest biopsies and at

different skeletal sites; the most important histological parameters are given in Table 5.1 and Fig. 5.S6, respectively.

In summary, bone mass depends on the amount of bone produced during growth and consolidation and its subsequent rate of loss[46,47]. The strength of a bone in compression is related to its density and mineral content[41].

Table 5.1 Histomorphometric parameters measured in posterior iliac crest biopsies according to age groups

Parameters	Abbreviation	Units	Age groups, years							
			−9	10−19	20−29	30−39	40−49	50−59	60−69	70−
Bone structure										
Bone volume	BV/TV	%	20 ± 4	25 ± 5	24 ± 5	22 ± 4	21 ± 5	20 ± 5	17 ± 3	13 ± 1
Bone surface	BS/BV	mm²/mm³	2.9 ± 0.4	2.8 ± 0.6	3.1 ± 0.3	2.9 ± 0.6	3.0 ± 0.6	3.0 ± 0.9	2.6 ± 0.7	2.1 ± 0.5
Trabecular thickness	TB.Th	μm	172 ± 30	222 ± 53	195 ± 44	173 ± 52	179 ± 49	177 ± 39	173 ± 33	171 ± 44
Mineralization										
Osteoid volume	OV/BV	%	7.7 ± 2.4	5.2 ± 4.8	3.4 ± 3.4	2.0 ± 2.4	1.0 ± 1.1	1.9 ± 1.5	2.3 ± 2.3	1.7 ± 2.0
Osteoid surface	OS/BV	mm²/mm³	0.8 ± 0.4	0.9 ± 3.7	0.9 ± 0.5	0.5 ± 0.4	0.3 ± 0.2	0.5 ± 0.5	0.4 ± 0.4	0.5 ± 0.4
Osteoid thickness	O.Th	μm	11 ± 4	6 ± 4	4 ± 3	4 ± 9	4 ± 2	4 ± 5	5 ± 3	3 ± 3
Bone cells										
Osteoclasts	N.Ocl/B.Ar	per mm²	3.1 ± 1.3	1.2 ± 1.0	0.7 ± 0.4	1.0 ± 0.8	0.8 ± 0.5	1.0 ± 0.9	2.1 ± 0.9	1.3 ± 0.9
Osteoblasts	N.Obl/B.Ar	per mm²	3.6 ± 2.9	4.0 ± 2.6	1.7 ± 0.9	1.5 ± 1.3	0.7 ± 0.6	1.7 ± 2.0	1.6 ± 2.1	1.1 ± 1.2
Lining cells	N.Lin/B.Ar	per mm²	5.4 ± 2.8	2.0 ± 1.2	1.9 ± 1.3	1.8 ± 0.9	1.0 ± 0.8	0.9 ± 0.7	1.4 ± 1.0	1.8 ± 1.3
Osteocytes	N.Ocy/B.Ar		24 ± 5	18 ± 5	17 ± 6	20 ± 8	18 ± 8	16 ± 6	18 ± 6	13 ± 3
Blood vessels										
Arteries	N.Art/M.Ar	per mm²	0.3 ± 0.4	0.5 ± 0.6	0.4 ± 0.4	0.4 ± 0.4	0.4 ± 0.4	0.4 ± 0.4	0.5 ± 0.6	0.3 ± 0.4
Arterioles	N.Aio/M.Ar	per mm²	1.3 ± 1.2	1.7 ± 0.9	1.3 ± 0.7	1.3 ± 0.7	1.0 ± 1.0	0.8 ± 0.7	1.2 ± 0.8	1.4 ± 1.2
Capillaries	N.Cap/M.Ar	per mm²	13 ± 4	17 ± 6	18 ± 6	18 ± 6	18 ± 4	20 ± 7	18 ± 8	19 ± 5
Sinusoids	N.Sin/M.Ar	per mm²	37 ± 5	31 ± 8	30 ± 7	34 ± 10	31 ± 7	33 ± 9	39 ± 5	36 ± 7
Endosteal sinusoids	ESV/TV	%	2.5 ± 0.9	2.7 ± 1.0	2.5 ± 1.5	3.0 ± 3.3	1.7 ± 1.7	1.8 ± 0.7	1.7 ± 0.7	1.5 ± 0.5
Stroma										
Fatty tissue	FV/MV	%	12 ± 7	17 ± 5	19 ± 9	26 ± 9	28 ± 11	30 ± 10	31 ± 9	44 ± 14
Mast cells	N.Mas/M.Ar	per mm²	0.4 ± 0.7	0.7 ± 0.8	2.1 ± 1.9	2.2 ± 1.9	2.2 ± 2.4	2.2 ± 1.4	2.6 ± 2.1	3.9 ± 3.8
Plasma cells	N.Pla/M.Ar	per mm²	19 ± 6	32 ± 11	30 ± 9	31 ± 9	29 ± 9	33 ± 9	34 ± 8	30 ± 9
Hematopoiesis										
Haematopoiesis	HV/MV	%	78 ± 13	72 ± 11	70 ± 12	62 ± 11	61 ± 14	59 ± 13	58 ± 11	45 ± 14
Megakaryocytes	N.Meg/M.Ar	per mm²	20 ± 8	16 ± 4	15 ± 6	14 ± 6	15 ± 4	14 ± 5	13 ± 5	10 ± 6

Terminology, abbreviations and units see Table 3.1. Histomorphometry was performed in collaboration with Dr B. Mallmann
Post-mortem biopsies taken with the electric drill from 100 normal subjects, 10 or more cases in each age group

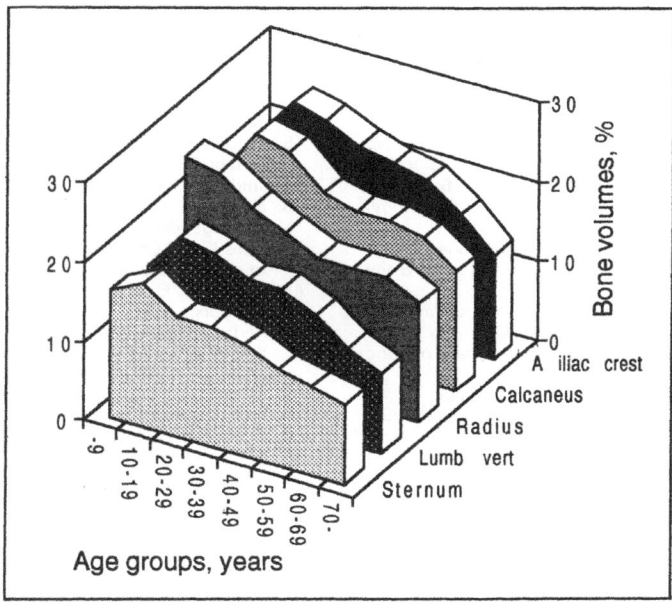

Fig. 5.S6 Trabecular bone volume according to age groups and different skeletal sites

but qualitative aspects of bone structure, as yet imperfectly understood, are also important[28,30]. The tensile strength of bone cannot be predicted from simple measurable indices such as density.

Qualitative defects in ageing bone may take five forms:

1. Bone is a two-component material, and age-related alterations of collagen arrangement and linking and of the hydroxyapatite crystals have a detrimental influence on strength[10,17].
2. Bone tissue possesses a repair mechanism at the microscopic level capable of removing and replacing damaged material. This protective response might become impaired through defective detection of fatigue damage as a result of blunted responsiveness of bone cells (osteocyte/osteoblast) or because of defective and/or unbalanced remodelling.
3. Ineffective architectural arrangement due to reduction in thickness and number of trabeculae as well as decreased connectivity between them increase the fragility of bone[16-18,32,33,67].
4. Osteoid production with a failure of mineralization impairs bone strength (the mixed variant of 'osteoporomalacia' in the elderly).
5. Finally, there may be an overall decrease in bone formation, resulting from the imbalance or uncoupling of the remodelling sequence[26,38].

The role of vitamin D in maintenance of skeletal integrity in the elderly is not yet fully clarified[65].

We conclude that the degree of 'physiological osteopenia' is a consequence of the peak adult skeletal mass attained and the subsequent bone loss (so-called slow and fast bone losers). There may be marked differences of bone loss at different skeletal sites and between trabecular and cortical bone. Bone loss in the elderly has a multifactorial aetiology, which as yet is only partly and poorly understood. This includes alterations in levels and balance of hormones and other factors involving regulation of bone cell activity as well as changes of intestinal and renal functions with subsequent effects on, for example, the parathyroid glands. Furthermore, bone fragility in advanced age is not only a quantitative prob-

lem, but is also influenced by qualitative alterations of bone matrix, mineralization, trabecular architecture and blood supply[6].

References

1. Aaron J. E., Makins N. B. and Sagre ya K. (1987). The microanatomy of trabecular bone loss in normal ageing men and women. *Clin. Orthop.*, **215**, 260
2. Alevizaki C. C., Ikkos D. G. and Singhelakis P. (1973). Progressive decrease of true intestinal calcium absorption with age in normal man. *J. Nucl. Med.*, **14**, 760
3. Arnold J. S. (1970). Focal excess endosteal resorption in aging and senile osteoporosis. Brazel U.S., *Osteoporosis* (p. 80). New York: Grune & Stratton
4. Atkinson P. J. (1965). Changes in resorption spaces in femoral cortical bone with age. *J. Pathol. Bacteriol.*, **89**, 173
5. Atkinson P. J. (1967). Variation in the trabecular structure of vertebrae with age. *Calcif. Tissue Pes.*, **1**, 24
6. Avioli L. V. and Lindsay R. (1990). The female osteoporotic syndrome(s). Avioli L. V. and Krane S. M., *Metabolic Bone Disease* (p. 397). Philadelphia: Saunders
7. Birkenhaeger-Frenkel D. H., Courpron P. and Clermont E. (1986). Trabecular thickness, intertrabecular distance and age related bone loss. *Bone*, **6**, 402
8. Buchanan J. R., Myers C. and Lloyd T. (1988). Early vertebral trabecular bone loss in normal premenopausal women. *J. Bone Miner. Res.*, **3**, 583
9. Chatterji S., Wall J. C. and Jeffrey J. W. (1981). Age-related changes in the orientation and particle size of the mineral phase in human femoral cortical bone. *Calcif. Tissue Int.*, **33**, 567
10. Chatterji S., Wall J. C. and Jeffrey J. W. (1972). Changes in the degree of orientation of bone materials with age in the human femur. *Experimentia*, **28**, 156
11. Delling G. (1974). Age-dependent bone changes. *Klin. Wschr.*, **52**, 317
12. Dequeker J., Remans J., Franssen R. and Waes J. (1971). Ageing patterns of trabecular and cortical bone and their relationship. *Calcif. Tissue Res.*, **7**, 23
13. Dunhill M. S., Anderson J. A. and Whitehead R. (1966). Quantitative histological studies on age changes in bone. *J. Pathol. Bacteriol.*, **94**, 275
14. Eastell R. and Riggs B. L. (1987). Calcium homeostasis and osteoporosis. *Endocrinol. Metab. Clin. N. Amer.*, **16**(4), 829
15. Epstein S., Bryce G. and Hinman J. W. (1986). The influence of age on bone mineral regulating hormones. *Bone*, **7**, 421

16. Eriksen E. F., Mosekilde L. and Melsen F. (1985). Trabecular bone resorption depth increases with age: differences between normal males and females. *Bone*, **6**, 141

17. Ferris B. D., Klenerman L. and Dodds R. A. (1987). Altered organisation of noncollagenous bone matrix in osteoporosis. *Bone*, **8**, 288

18. Foldes J., Parfitt A. M., Shih M. S., Rao D. S. and Kleerekoper M. (1991). Structural and geometric changes in iliac bone: relationship to normal aging and osteoporosis. *J. Bone Miner. Res.*, **6**, 759

19. Frisch B. and Bartl R. (1990). *Atlas of Bone Marrow Pathology*. Dordrecht: Kluwer

20. Gallagher J. C., Goldgar D. and Moy A. (1987). Total bone calcium in normal women: effect of age and menopause status. *J. Bone Miner. Res.*, **2**, 491

21. Garn S. M. (1970). Calcium requirements for bone building and skeletal maintenance. *Amer. J. Clin. Nutr.*, **23**, 1149

22. Garn S. M. (1972). The course of bone gain and the phase of bone loss. *Orthop. Clin. N. Amer.*, **3**, 503

23. Gilsanz V., Roe T. F., Mora S., Costin G. and Goodman W. G. (1991). Changes in vertebral bone density in black girls and white girls during childhood and puberty. *N. Engl. J. Med.*, **325**, 1597

24. Gryfe C. I., Exton-Smith A. W. and Payne P. R. (1971). Pattern of development of bone in childhood and adolescence. *Lancet*, **1**, 523

25. Hartsock R., Smith E. B. and Petty C. S. (1965). Normal variations with aging of the amount of hematopoietic tissue in bone marrow from the anterior iliac crest. *Amer. J. Clin. Pathol.*, **43**(4)

26. Heaney R. P., Recker R. R. and Saville P. D. (1978). Menopausal changes in bone remodeling. *J. Lab. Clin. Med.*, **92**, 964

27. Hedlund L. R. and Gallagher J. C. (1989). The effect of age and menopause on bone mineral density of the proximal femur. *J. Bone Miner. Res.*, **4**, 639

28. Jowsey J. (1960). Age changes in human bone. *Clin. Orthop. Rel. Res.*, **17**, 149

29. Kelly P. J., Eisman J. A. and Sambrook P. N. (1990). Interaction of genetic and environmental influences on peak bone density. *Osteoporosis Int.*, **1**(56),

30. Khairi M. R. A. and Johnston C. C. (1978). What we know – and don't know – about bone loss in the elderly. *Geriatrics*, 67

31. Kiebzak G. M. (1991). Age-related bone changes. *Exp. Gerontol.*, **26**, 171

32. Kragstrup J., Melsen F. and Mosekilde L. (1983). Thickness of lamellae in normal human iliac trabecular bone. *Metab. Bone Dis. Rel. Res.*, **4**, 291

33. Lips P., Courpron P. and Meunier P. J. (1978). Mean wall thickness of trabecular bone packets in the human iliac crest: changes with age. *Calcif. Tissue Res.*, **26**, 13

34. Malluche H. H., Meyer W., Sherman D. and Massry S. G. (1982). Quantitative bone histology in 84 normal American subjects. Micromorphometric analysis and evaluation of variance of iliac crest bone. *Calcif. Tissue Int.*, **34**, 449

35. Marcus R. (1989). Exercise and the regulation of bone mass (Editorial). *Arch. Intern. Med.*, **149**, 2170

36. Marcus R., Kosek J. and Pfefferbaum A. (1983). Age-related loss of trabecular bone in premenopausal women: a biopsy study. *Calcif. Tissue Int.*, **35**, 406

37. Marcus R., Madvig P. and Young G. (1984). Age-related changes in parathyroid hormone and parathyroid hormone action in normal humans. *J. Clin. Endocrinol. Metab.*, **58**, 223

38. Martin R. B., Pickett J. C. and Zinaich S. (1980). Studies of skeletal remodeling in aging man. *Clin. Orthop. Rel. Res.*, **149**, 268

39. Mazess R. B. (1982). On aging bone loss. *Clin. Orthop. Rel. Res.*, **165**, 239

40. Mazess R. B., Barden H. S., Drinka P. J., Bauwens S. F., Orwoll E. S. and Bell N. H. (1990). Influence of age and body weight on spine and femur bone mineral density in U.S. white men. *J. Bone Miner. Res.*, **5**(6), 645

41. McCalden R. W., McGeough J. A., Barker M. B. and Court-Brown C. M. (1991). Mechanical changes in aging cortical bone: the role of changes in porosity, mineralisation and microstructure. *J. Bone Jt Surg.*, **73-B**, 103

42. Meier D. E., Orwoll E. S. and Jones J. M. (1983). Marked disparity between trabecular and cortical bone loss with age in healthy men. *Ann. Intern. Med.*, **101**, 605

43. Melsen F., Melsen B., Mosekilde L. and Bergman S. (1978). Histomorphometric analysis of normal bone from the iliac crest. *Acta Pathol. Microbiol. Scand.*, **86**(70)

44. Meunier P., Courpron P. and Edouard C. (1976). Physiological senile involution and pathological rarefaction of bone. *Clin. Endocrinol. Metab.*, **2**, 239

45. Mosekilde L. (1990). Consequences of the remodelling process for vertebral trabecular bone structure: a scanning electron microscopy study (uncoupling of unloaded structures). *Bone Miner.*, **10**, 13

46. Newton-John H. F. and Morgan D. B. (1970). The loss of bone with age, osteoporosis and fractures. *Clin. Orthop.*, **71**, 229

47. Nilas L. and Christiansen C. (1987). Bone mass and its relationship to age and the menopause. *J. Clin. Endocrinol. Metab.*, **65**, 697

48. Nilsson B. E. and Westlin N. E. (1973). Changes in bone mass in alcoholics. *Clin. Orthop. Rel. Res.*, **90**, 229

49. Parfitt A. M., Matthews C. H. E., Villanueva A. R., Kleerekoper M., Frame B. and Rao D. S. (1983). Relationships between surface, volume and thickness of iliac trabecular bone in ageing and in osteoporosis. Implications for the microanatomic and cellular mechanisms of bone loss. *J. Clin. Invest.*, **72**,1 396

50. Pocock N. A., Eisman, J. A., Mazess R. B., Sambrook P. N., Yeates M. G. and Freund J. (1988). Bone mineral density in Australia compared with the United States. *J. Bone Miner. Res.*, **3**, 601

51. Pocock N. A., Eisman J. A. and Hopper J. L. (1987). Genetic determinants of bone mass in adults. A twin study. *J. Clin. Invest.*, **80**, 706

52. Raisz L. G. (1988). Local and systemic factors in the pathogenesis of osteoporosis. *N. Engl. J. Med.*, **318**, 818

53. Riggs B. L., Wahner H. W., Dunn W. L., Mazess R. B., Offord K. B. and Melton L. J. (1981). Differential changes in bone mineral density of the appendicular and axial skeleton with ageing. *J. Clin. Invest.*, **67**, 328

54. Rigotti N. A., Nussbaum S. R., Herzog D. B. and Neer R. M. (1984). Osteoporosis in women with anorexia nervosa. *N. Engl. J. Med.*, **311**, 1601

55. Rockoff S. D., Sweet E. and Bleustein J. (1969). The relative contribution of trabecular and cortical bone to the strength of human lumbar vertebrae. *Calcif. Tissue Res.*, **3**, 163

56. Smith D. M., Nance W. E. and Kang K. (1973). Genetic factors in determining bone mass. *J. Clin. Invest.*, **52**, 2800

57. Smith E. L. and Gilligan C. (1990). Calcium and exercise in prevention of bone loss in age. *Clin. Nutr.*, **9**, 17

58. Stevenson J. C. (1988). Pathophysiology of osteoporosis. *Triangle*, **27**(1/2), 47

59. Stevenson J. C., Lees B., Devenport M., Cust M. P. and Ganger K. F. (1989). Determinants of bone density in normal women: risk factors for future osteoporosis? *Brit. Med. J.*, **298**, 924

60. Suominen H., Heikkinen E., Vainio P. and Laitinen T. (1984). Mineral density of calcaneus in men at different ages: a population study with special reference to life-style factors. *Age Ageing*, **13**, 273

61. Termine J. D. (1990). Cellular activity, matrix proteins and aging bone. *Exp. Gerontol.*, **25**, 217

62. Thompson D. D. (1980). Age changes in bone mineralisation, cortical thickness, and Haversian canal area. *Calcif. Tissue Int.*, **31**, 5

63. Tonna E. A. (1960). Osteoclasts and the aging skeleton: a cytological, cytochemical and autoradiographic study. *Anat. Rec.*, **37**, 251

64. Trotter M., Broman G. E. and Peterson R. R. (1960). Densities of bones of white and negro skeletons. *J. Bone Jt Surg.*, **42(A)**, 50

65. Tsai K.-S., Wahner H. W., Offord K. P., Melton L. J., Kumar R. and Riggs B. L. (1987). Effect of aging on vitamin D stores and bone density in women. *Calcif. Tissue Int.*, **40**, 241

66. Vedi S., Compston J. E., Webb A. and Tighe J. R. (1982). Histomorphometric analysis of bone biopsies from the iliac crest of normal British subjects. *Bone*, **4**, 231

67. Weinstein R. S. and Hutson M. S. (1987). Decreased trabecular width and increased trabecular spacing contribute to bone loss with aging. *Bone*, **8**, 137

68. Yano K., Wasnich R. D., Vogel J. M. and Heilbrun L. K. (1984). Bone mineral measurements among middle-aged and elderly Japanese residents in Hawaii. *Amer. J. Epidemiol.*, **119**, 751

The term 'osteomyelitis', as used by orthopaedic specialists and surgeons, signifies a local pyogenic infection of bone[43]. This is usually blood-borne and often occurs during bacteraemia. The organisms lodge in the bone marrow, an acute local inflammatory reaction develops, followed by abscess formation and finally necrosis of both marrow and bone. This is sometimes referred as a suppurative destructive necrosis. Osteolytic lesions may result, visible on X-ray usually before the phase of reactive repair during which osteoblastic bone formation may produce a dense sclerosis (Garre's sclerosing osteomyelitis)[43]. Almost any bone may be infected, but the most frequent sites are the lower limbs in children, and the spine in adults[43]. *Staphylococcus aureus* is the commonest organism, although fungal, viral and parasitic infections are also found[19]. Fractures, trauma, operations and intravenous drug abuse provide the main avenues for haematogenous spread of organisms[7,33]. Many of the factors – cytokines and others – which participate in the inflammatory reaction may also be involved in the process of osseous remodelling, in particular osteolysis[35]

Haematologists and osteologists, however, are more frequently confronted with generalized inflammatory conditions of bone and marrow, which occur in the course of systemic disorders of immunological[12,27,29,31,44], infectious[43], haematological[9,18], neoplastic[2,8,47,53] or of unknown origin[24,45,52]: for example, the lytic bone lesions that may occur in acne fulminans[39].

Five main morphological types of inflammatory reactions in the bone marrow have been described[20,22]:

1. *Exudative type* (Plates 6.A–C): this represents an acute inflammation accompanied by dilatation of the sinusoidal lumina, disruption of their walls and extravasation of erythrocytes. There are marked alterations in the stromal compartment with disorganization of the haematopoietic cell lines and oedema. The occurrence of osseous necrosis depends on the degree of the causative noxi: that is, amount of radiation[3,17,28,52], chemotherapy, endotoxins[1] or other agents[16,26]. Marked exudative marrow changes with reactive plasmacytosis are also observed in iliac crest biopsies of patients with active ankylosing spondylitis. This variant of arthritis involves by definition the sacroiliac joints with the adjacent pelvic bones[10]. Therefore bone erosions, lytic lesions with marked osteoclastic activity and later fibrosis, sclerosis and increased bone remodelling are frequent findings in iliac crest biopsies of these patients (Figs 6.R1 and R2, Figs 6.13–16)[15,40].

2. *Atrophic type* (Plate 6.A): this subacute or chronic inflammatory reaction shows large-scale replacement of haematopoiesis by fat cells, oedema and gelatinous material. The affected regions may be almost acellular or infiltrated by lymphocytes, mast cells and plasma cells. Lymphoid nodules may also be found (Plate 6.G). The small vessels often contain PAS-positive deposits in the media, and mast cells in the adventitia. The sinusoids have thickened, sclerotic walls. The trabeculae are lined by osteoblasts and broad seams of osteoid, mainly in regions with conversion of the marrow to gelatinous or serous material. This type of reaction is found in patients after radiation therapy[3,25,28,51], with poor nutrition, chronic infections,

autoimmune disorders[42], drug hypersensitivity, diabetes mellitus and metastatic carcinoma (usually without metastasis in the same biopsy). Gelatinous transformation of the bone marrow occurs as a consequence of inadequate nutrition as in gastric carcinoma and anorexia nervosa; it is completely reversible on resumption of normal nutrition. In 'chronic recurrent multifocal osteomyelitis' microscopic examination of a bone biopsy discloses gelatinous material without

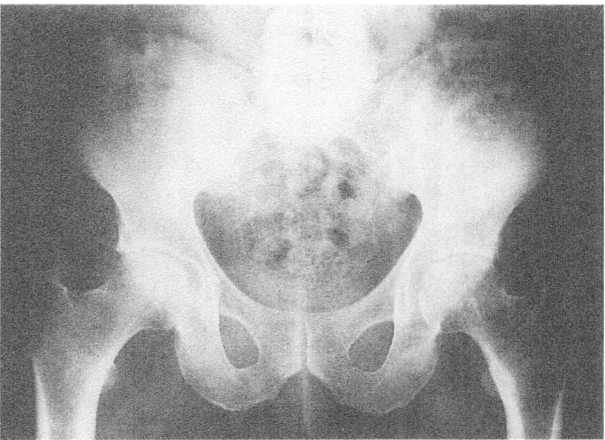

Fig. 6.R1 X-ray of pelvis of the patient with ankylosing spondylitis (as in Figs 6.13–6.16), showing marked sclerosis of spine and ilium

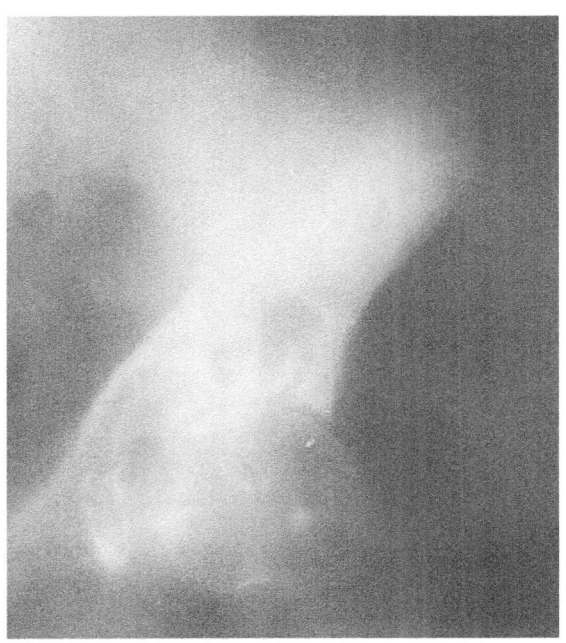

Fig. 6.R2 Tomography of right ilium and hip joint highlighting multiple small subchrondral cysts within sclerotic bone

[continued on p. 79]

Plate 6.A

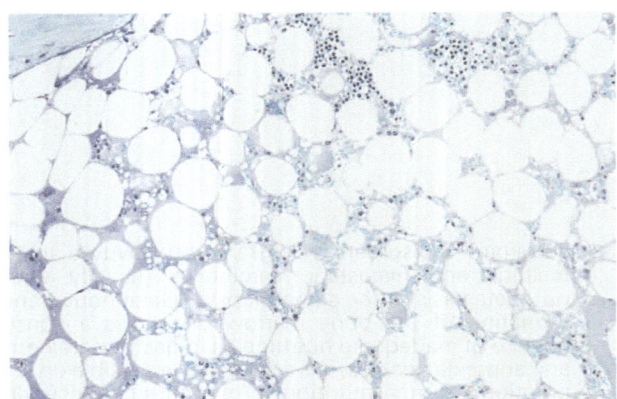

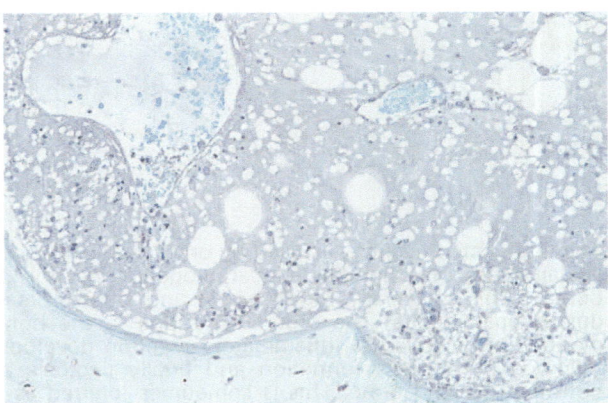

Figs. 6.1–6.6 Examples of exudative and atrophic changes in bone biopsies and their effects on bone

Fig. 6.1 Interstitial oedema between fat cells with some haematopoietic islands (upper centre). Giemsa

Fig. 6.2 Extensive trabecular surface with osteoblastic new bone formation in area of oedematous marrow. Note ectatic sinusoid (upper left) and some osteoclastic bone resorption (lower right). Giemsa

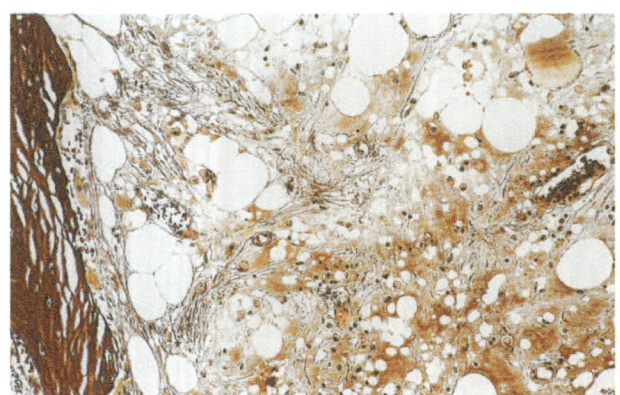

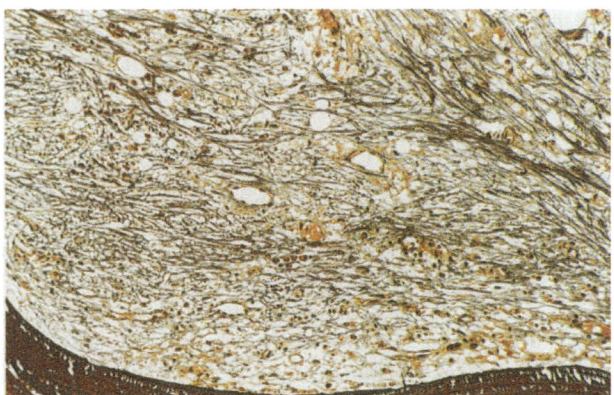

Fig. 6.3 Oedematous intertrabecular cavity showing patchy fibrosis of stroma. Gomori

Fig. 6.4 Later stage of sclerosing myelitis showing complete loss of marrow architecture and replacement by coarse fibrosis. Gomori

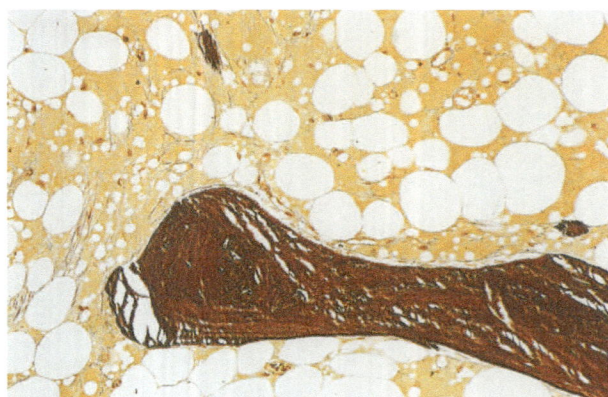

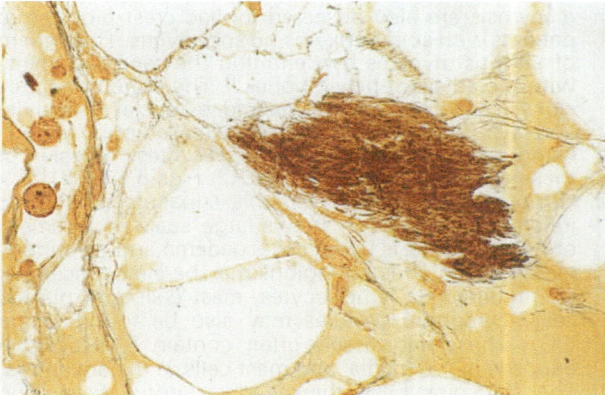

Fig. 6.5 Massive oedematous reaction with complete loss of haematopoiesis and marrow architecture. Note diffuse fine fibrosis and two small islands of newly formed woven bone. Gomori

Fig. 6.6 Higher magnification of different part from Fig. 6.4. Small island of primitive bone from area of exudation. Only a single identifiable osteocyte is present. Gomori

Plate 6.B

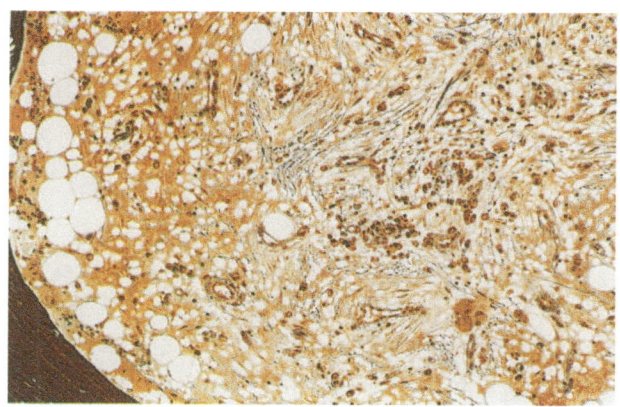

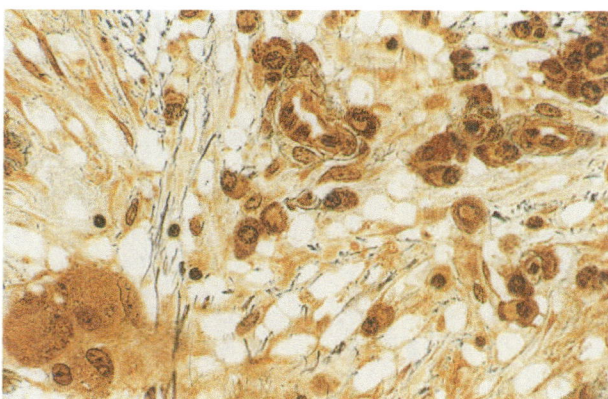

Figs. 6.7–6.11 Varying degree of interstitial and perivascular infiltration by plasma cells in exudative inflammation with osseous reactions

Fig. 6.7 Fibrosis, blood vessels and inflammatory cells in the central area of the marrow space. Gomori

Fig. 6.8 Higher magnification of Fig. 6.7, illustrating perivascular and interstitial plasmacytosis. Gomori

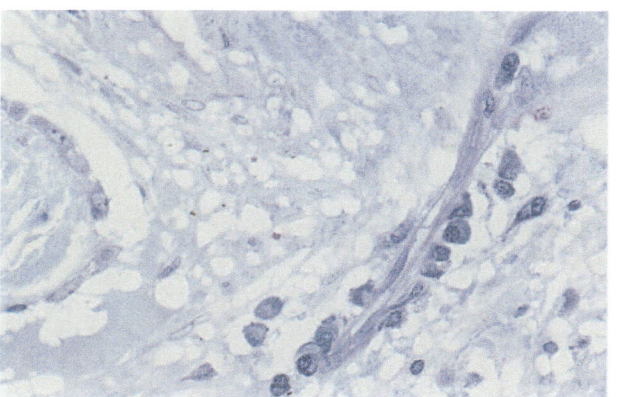

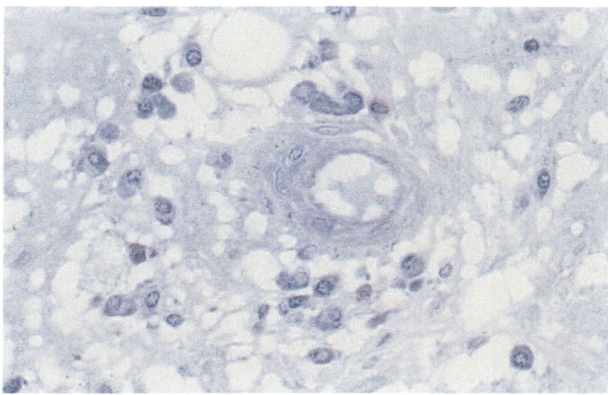

Fig. 6.9 Higher magnification of biopsy from Fig. 6.7. Osteoblasts on trabecular surface at left and capillary traversing oedematous area. Giemsa

Fig. 6.10 Cross-section of small artery with perivascular plasma cells and mast cells. Giemsa

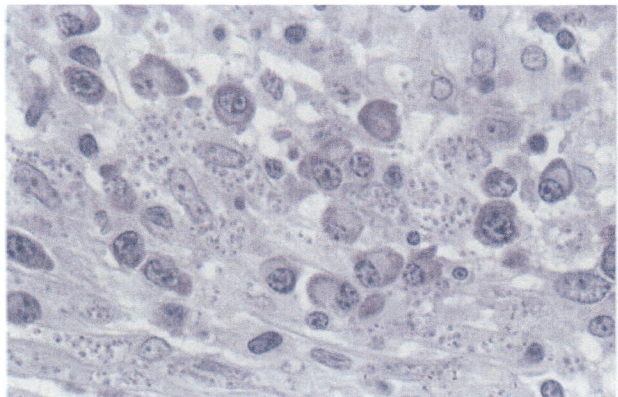

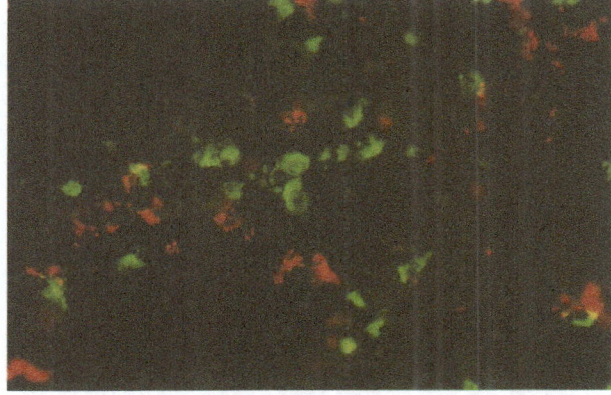

Fig. 6.11 Iliac crest biopsy of a patient with visceral leishmaniasis: demonstration of the parasites in the reticuloendothelial cells of the bone marrow, and concomitant reactive plasmacytosis. Giemsa

Fig. 6.12 Cryostat section incubated with fluorescent conjugated antibodies to immunoglobulins to demonstrate polyclonality of the infiltrating plasma cells. Giemsa

Plate 6.C

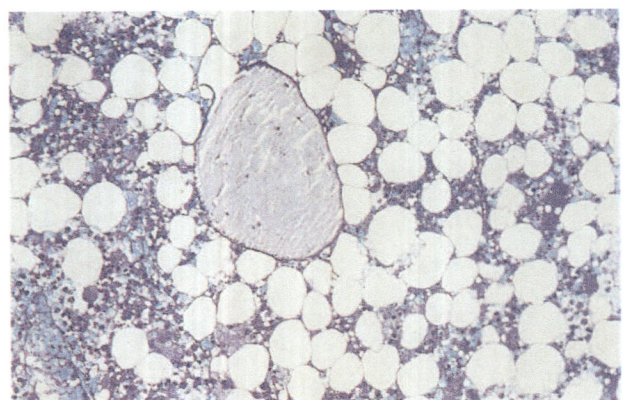

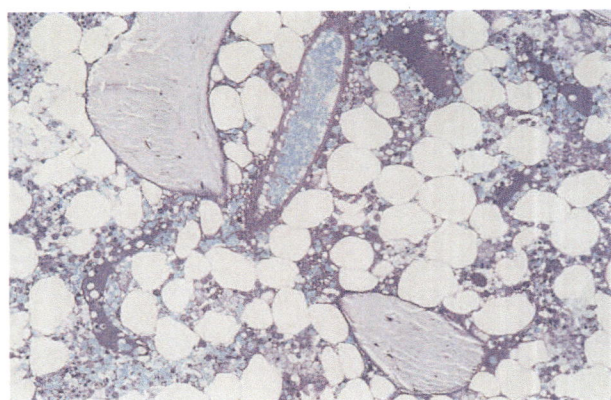

Figs. 6.13–6.16 Characteristics of inflammatory reaction in iliac crest biopsy of a patient with active ankylosing spondylitis

Fig. 6.13 Hypocellular bone marrow with increased fat cells. Giemsa

Fig. 6.14 Section showing disorganization of marrow architecture with large blood vessels, focal interstitial oedema and extravasation of erythrocytes. Giemsa

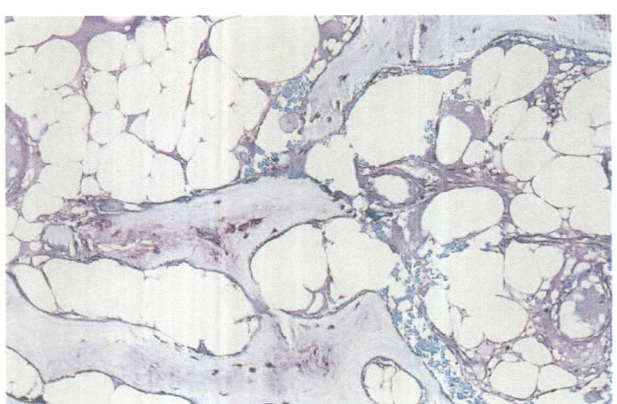

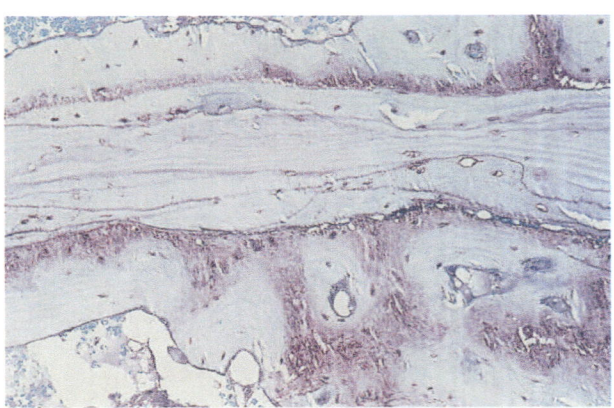

Fig. 6.15 Both reactive appositional and woven new bone formation in empty marrow. Note blood vessels (centre and lower right) with inflammatory changes and fibrosis. Giemsa

Fig. 6.16 Advanced stage documented by sequential biopsy, with osteosclerotic reaction: appositional new bone on both sides of a trabecula. Giemsa

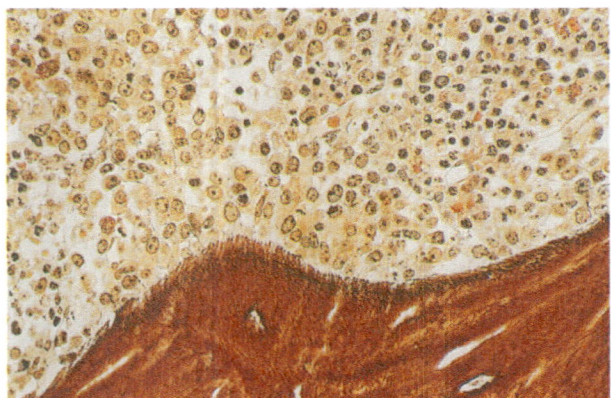

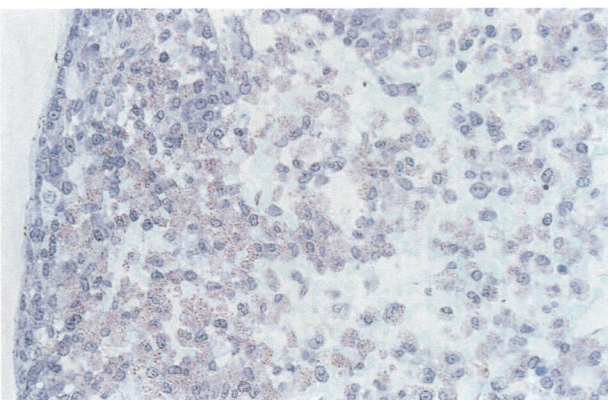

Figs. 6.17–6.18 Inflammatory reaction, proliferative type in bone marrow, with osseous reactions

Fig. 6.17 Proliferative type with primarily neutrophilic hyperplasia. Note endosteal seam of myeloblasts and promyelocytes. Gomori

Fig. 6.18 Proliferative type with primarily eosinophilic hyperplasia. Note dense infiltration in the endosteal zone. Giemsa

obvious evidence of infection. The concomitant inflammatory infiltrate is composed of neutrophils, lymphocytes, eosinophils and histiocyte-like cells; the possibility of eosinophilic granuloma may be considered in the histological differential diagnosis. Fragments of necrotic trabeculae and reactive bone have also been described. In other cases a gelatinous inflammatory reaction in the bone biopsy may terminate in fibrosis or total marrow atrophy with hematopoietic failure, and osteopenia in the affected areas.

3. *Proliferative type*: the hypercellular, sometimes leukaemoid marrow consists mainly of hyperplastic granulopoiesis including eosinophils, together with megakaryocytosis, and increased plasma, mast and lymphoid cells. Bone changes rarely occur. It is a generalized reaction mostly associated with neoplastic (for example Hodgkin's disease) or bacterial processes, and with drug users. In AIDS patients, concomitant myelodysplastic features and mixed inflammatory reactions are frequent findings[21]. Hyperplasia of granulopoiesis with increased numbers of eosinophils, plasma cells and megakaryocytes are often present in autoimmune states, such as rheumatoid arthritis, Felti's syndrome and seronegative arthritides[12,20,45].

4. *Fibrotic type* (Plates 6.D and E), also called 'sclerosing myelitis'[20,45]: there is a generalized coarse fibrosis together with an exudative and inflammatory reaction, replacing most of the haematopoietic and fatty tissues. Infiltrating elements are plasma, mast and lymphoid cells. There is also a high incidence of lymphoid nodules; as well as osteoblastic new bone formation of irregular woven bone. The aetiology of this 'cirrhosis of the bone marrow' or 'myelophthisis' is unknown, but probably chronic immune mechanisms and/or pre-existing myelodysplastic features play an important role in its pathogenesis (Fig. 6.S1)[20,45]. 'Sclerosing myelitis' is also seen in bone biopsies of patients with solid tumours, generally without metastases in the biopsies. In contrast to the myelofibrosis of myeloproliferative disorders, neither atypical, proliferative haematopoiesis nor myeloid metaplasia is found. Transformation to haematological malignancies was observed in about a quarter of the cases with sclerosing myelitis, documented by sequential biopsies; in four cases a primary myelodysplastic syndrome was established as the basic disorder.

5. *Granulomatous type* (Plates 6.F and G): this is defined as the presence of circumscribed nodules within the bone marrow, variably composed of macrophages, epithelioid cells, lymphoid cells, multinucleated giant cells, blood vessels and fibres[4-6]. These granulomas are often surrounded by a cuff of lymphocytes, plasma cells and eosinophils; they are frequently paratrabecular, and a local increase in osteoblastic bone formation was observed in about half of the positive biopsies. Central caseating necrosis (most typical of tuberculosis) is rare in biopsies of the iliac crest; a definite diagnosis of tuberculosis depends on bacterial culture, special stains and serological verification[30]. By combining histological, microbial and serological techniques, an aetiology could be documented in 70% of patients with granulomas in the bone biopsy, and the most frequent diseases associated with bone marrow granulomas are listed in Fig. 6.S2. In our series of 70 000 bone biopsies, granulomas were found in 0.6% of the cases, with increasing numbers in older age groups. In miliary tuberculosis acid-fast bacilli were seen in a third of the positive biopsies, but 'typical' central caseation was infrequent and seen only in confluent granulomatous areas. Slavin and co-workers found that only 22% of autopsied cases having liver granulomas also had them in the bone marrow[48]. In

[continued on p. 84]

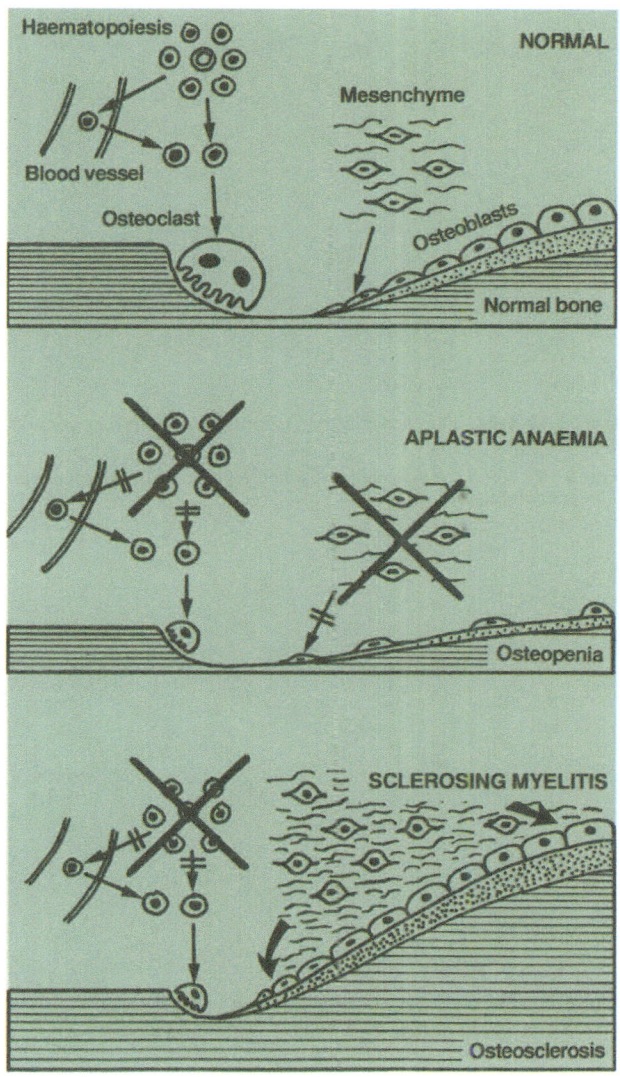

Fig. 6.S1 Hypothetical pathomechanisms of (1) low-turnover osteoporosis in aplastic anaemia (due to failure of haematopoiesis and mesenchyme); and (2) osteosclerosis in sclerosing myelitis (due to failure of haematopoiesis but hyperplasia of stroma)

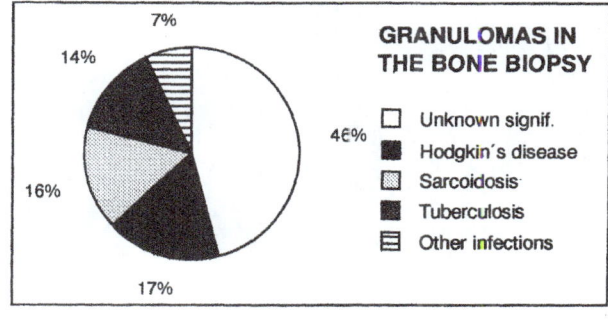

Fig. 6.S2 Underlying clinical conditions in patients with granulomas in iliac crest biopsies

Plate 6.D

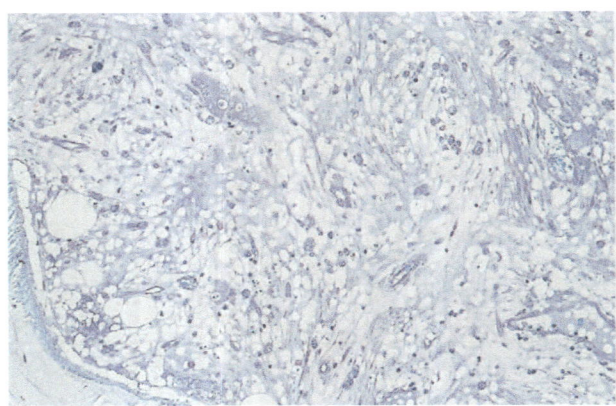

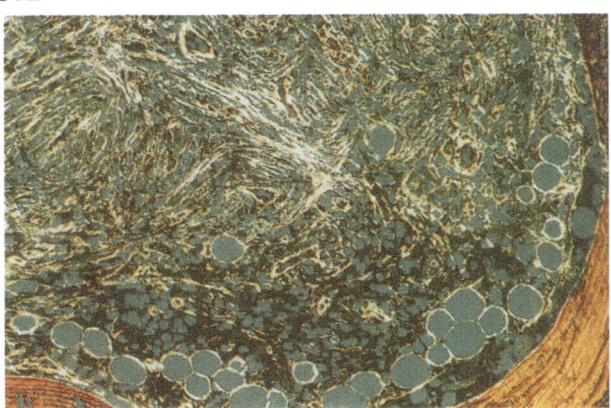

Figs. 6.19–6.24 Fibrotic inflammatory changes in bone biopsies and their effects on bone

Fig. 6.19 Fibrotic inflammatory reaction replacing both haematopoietic and fatty tissues. Gomori

Fig. 6.20 Area of the same biopsy as in Fig. 6.19 demonstrating replacement of haematopoiesis by coarse fibrosis. Note rim of fat cells in the paratrabecular zone, broad endosteal sinusoid (lower right) and smooth trabecular surface. Gomori, polar.

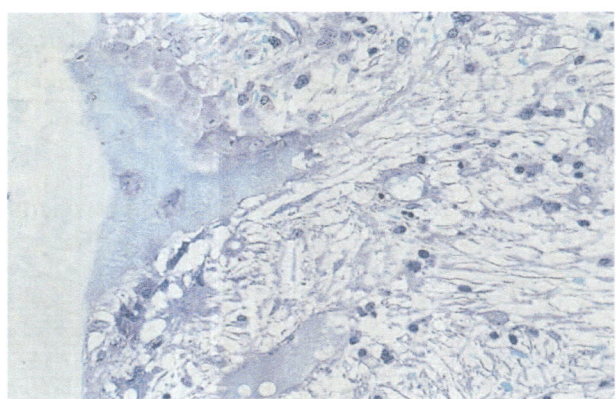

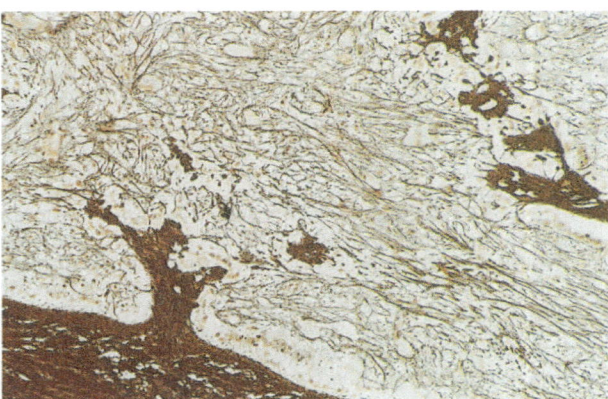

Fig. 6.21 Spicule of woven bone attached to the trabecular surface and surrounded by fibrotic inflammatory reaction. Giemsa

Fig. 6.22 Low-power view from the same biopsy as in Fig. 6.21 illustrating multiple foci of woven bone attached to the ossicle as well as in the fibrous tissue of the marrow cavity. Gomori

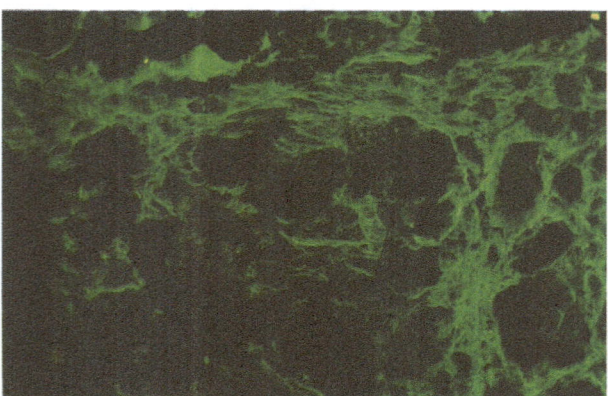

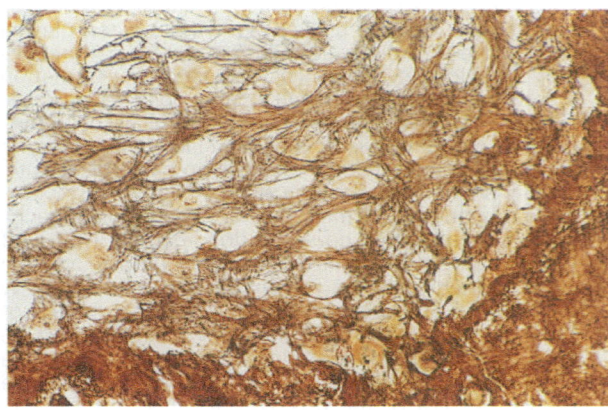

Fig. 6.23 Cryostat section demonstrating collagen type III by immunofluorescent conjugated antibodies in 'sclerosing myelitis'

Fig. 6.24 Osteoblasts on bone surface, and osteoblast-like fibrocytes within coarse fibrosis in case of fibrosing myelitis. Gomori

Plate 6.E

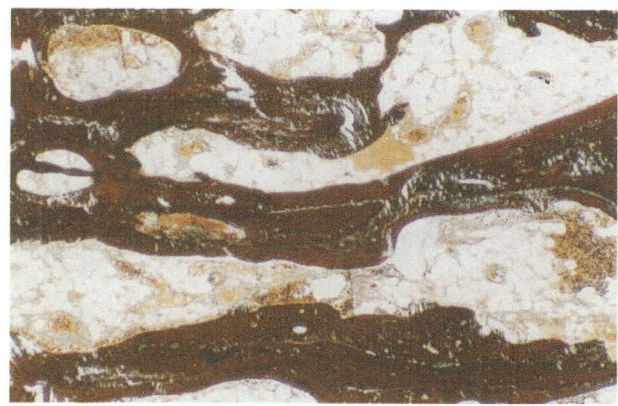

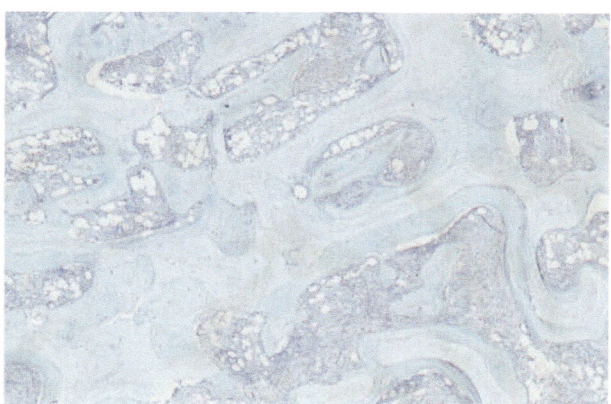

Figs. 6.25–6.30 Sclerosing myelitis with considerably increased trabecular bone volume, all showing reduction in marrow cavities, absence of haematopoiesis and fatty or fibrotic bone marrow

Fig. 6.25 Trabeculae broadened by appositional new bone formation. Gomori

Fig. 6.26 Massive sclerosis of trabecular network and broad osteoid seams. Giemsa

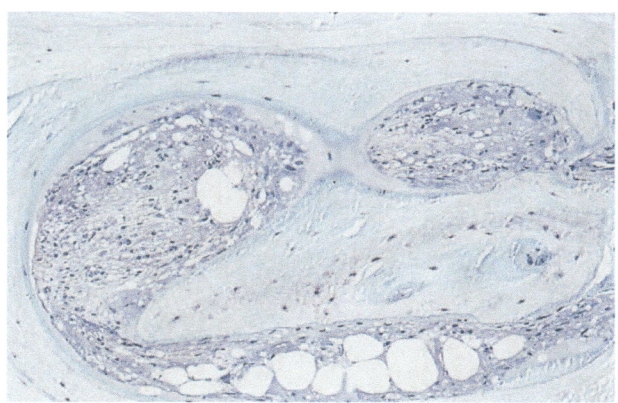

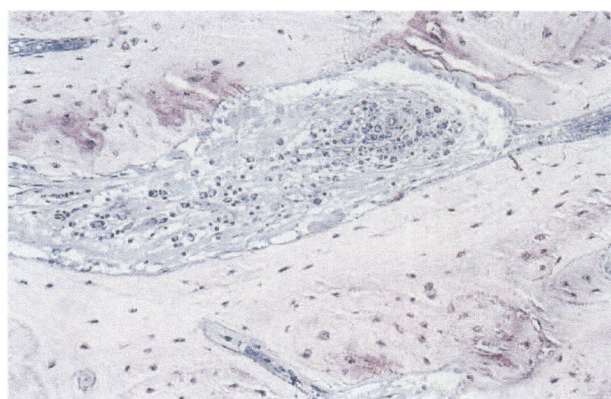

Fig. 6.27 Further encroachment of newly formed bone into a marrow cavity. Giemsa

Fig. 6.28 Newly formed bone containing numerous relatively large osteocytes. Note osteoclasts and osteoblasts as well as inflammatory cells within the fibrotic marrow. Giemsa

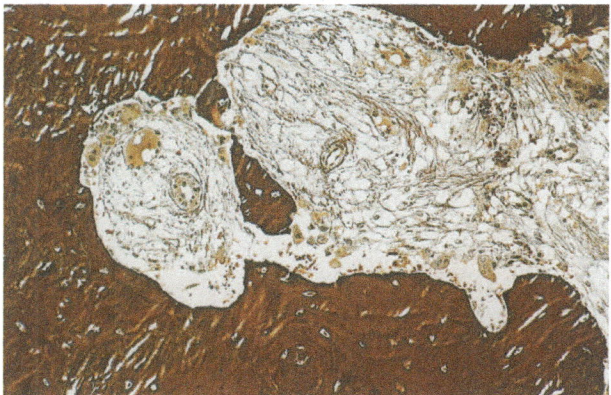

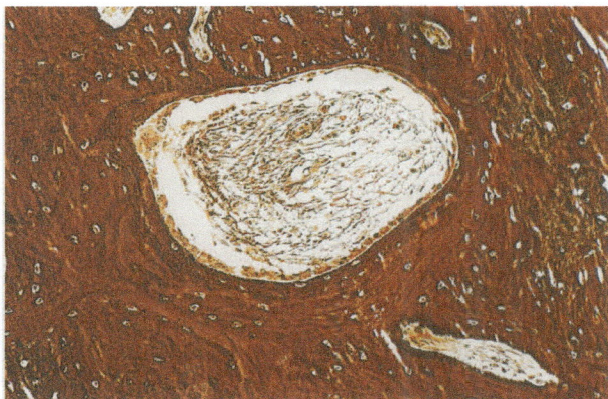

Fig. 6.29 Osteosclerosis and marrow filled with acellular coarse fibrosis and spicules of woven bone. Gomori

Fig. 6.30 Further stage in progressive osteosclerosis based on sclerosing myelitis. Note layer of osteoblasts on bone surrounding the small residual marrow space. Gomori. Striking in all these micrographs is the extreme imbalance of osseous remodelling in favour of bone formation.

Plate 6.F

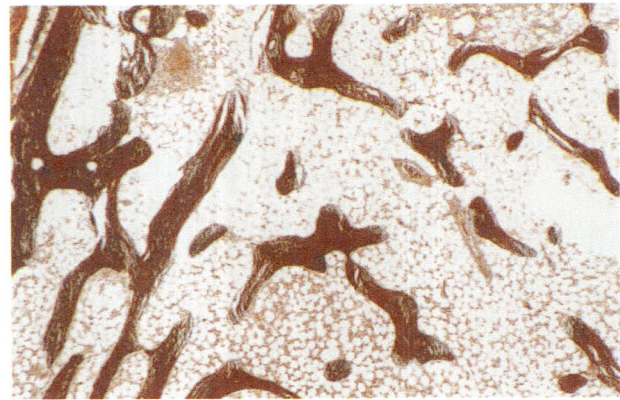

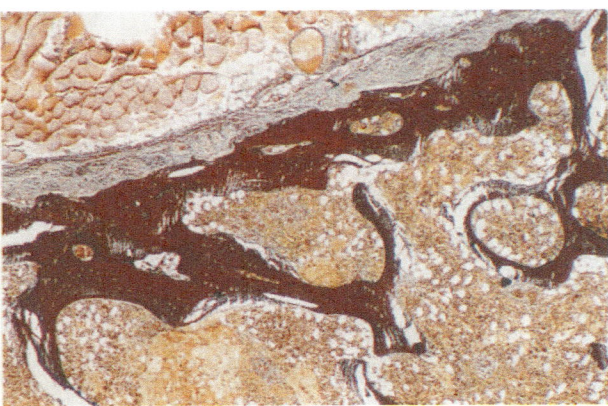

Figs. 6.31–6.36 Sections of bone biopsies with variable granulomatous reactions

Fig. 6.31 Low-power view showing single small granuloma in subcortical region. Gomori

Fig. 6.32 Biopsy section showing small and large granulomas in subcortical region. Gomori

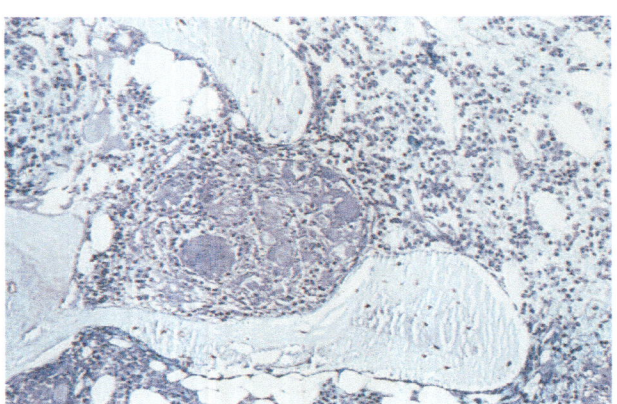

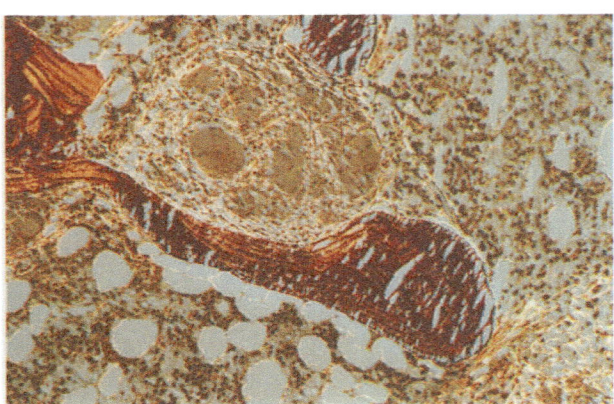

Fig. 6.33 Paratrabecular granuloma showing erosion of bone in normocellular bone marrow. Giemsa

Fig. 6.34 Same section viewed in polarized light to illustrate the fibrosis surrounding the granuloma. Gomori

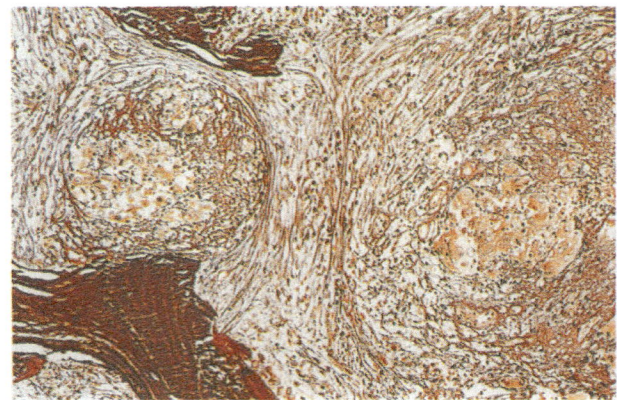

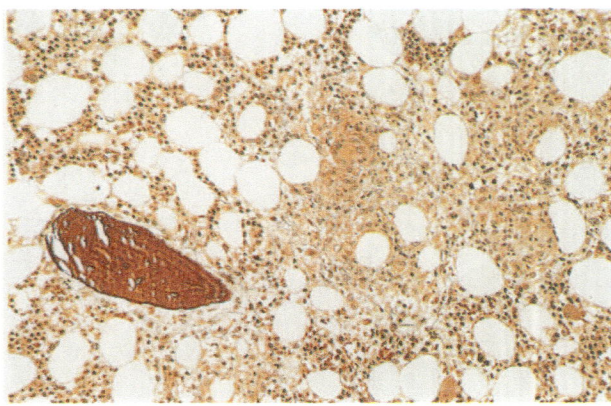

Fig. 6.35 Confluent granulomas in fibrotic bone marrow. Note resorption cavities in trabecular bone (upper and lower left). Gomori

Fig. 6.36 Small epithelioid cell granuloma (centre) in a patient with Hodgkin's disease, indicating a more favourable prognosis. Gomori

Plate 6.G

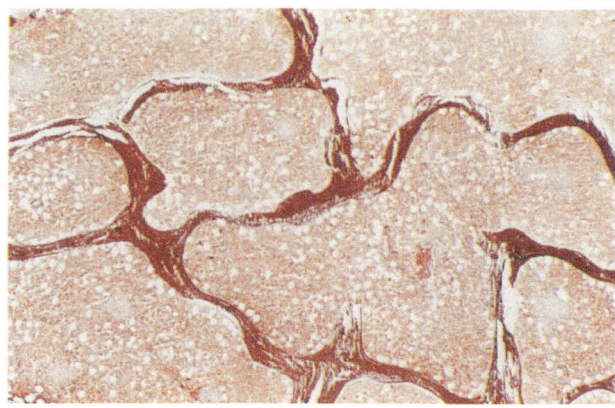

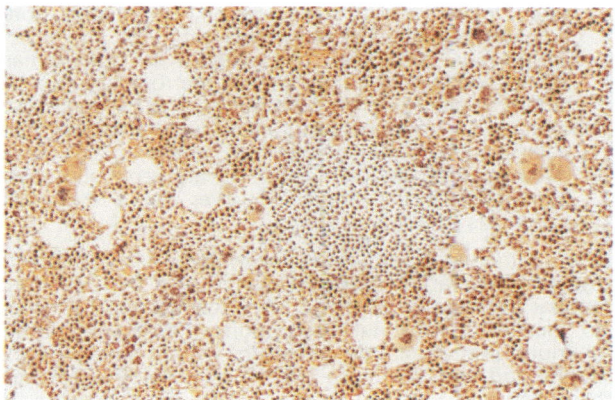

Figs. 6.37–6.42 Sections of bone biopsies with variable lymphoid nodules

Fig. 6.37 Mutiple, but very small lymphoid nodules in the marrow spaces. Gomori

Fig. 6.38 At higher magnification, small lymphoid nodule without sharp delineation from the surroundirg haematopoiesis. Gomori. Such nodules – even large and/or multiple – are often seen in iliac crest biopsies of patients with inflammatory reactions, e.g. rheumatic disorders

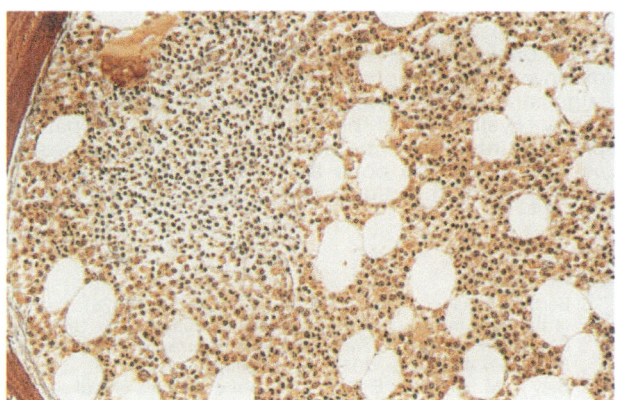

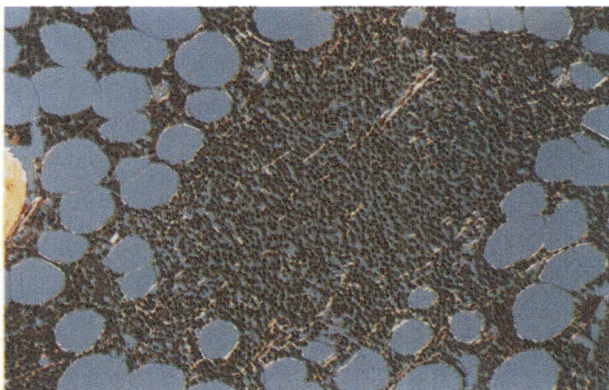

Fig. 6.39 Lymphoid aggregate in the paratrabecular region with rim of fat cells. Gomori

Fig. 6.40 Fine fibrotic network within the lymphoid nodule. Gomori, polar.

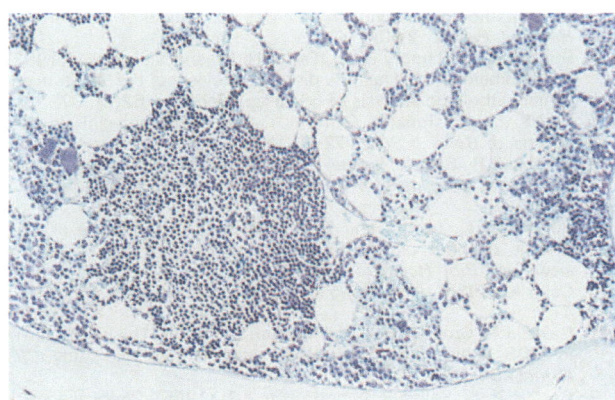

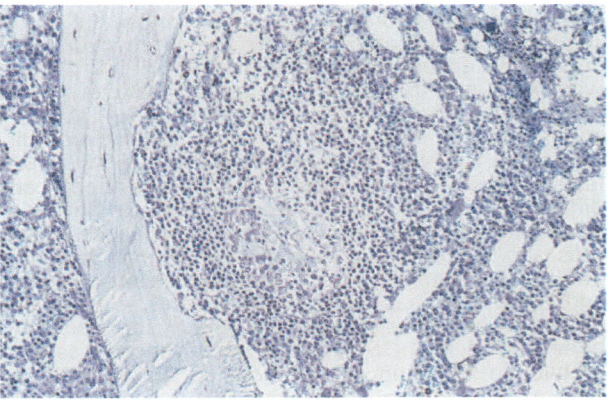

Fig. 6.41 Large lymphoid nodule in hypocellular marrow. Giemsa

Fig. 6.42 Large lymphoid nodule with germinal centre eroding adjacent trabecula. Giemsa

sarcoidosis the reported frequency of positive bone biopsies is higher, ranging between 17% and 50%[4]. Drugs have also been associated with granulomas. The prognosis of patients with marrow granulomas depends mainly on the basic disease. Individuals with multiple or confluent granulomas had a more unfavourable prognosis than those with solitary granulomas. Patients with Hodgkin's disease and epithelioid-cell granulomas in the biopsy, however, had a favourable prognosis in our series.

Granulomatous disorders are known to be associated with *hypercalcaemia*[36,49]. Hypercalcaemia and hypercalciuria appear to reflect accelerated bone resorption in addition to increased intestinal absorption of calcium[34]. Bone changes predominantly affect the small bones of the hands and feet, although lesions of other skeletal sites have also been reported. Pathological fractures may occur. It has been shown that the serum levels of $1,25\text{-}(OH)_2\text{-}D_3$ are elevated in hypercalcaemic patients with sarcoidosis[50]. This vitamin D metabolite is synthesized in the granulomatous tissue[50]. In recent years there has been an upsurge in the incidence of tuberculosis in older people with reduced immunity from whatever cause, and this should be considered in the differential diagnosis of such patients who develop hypercalcaemia. Moreover, extrapulmonary tuberculosis is still a problem in children.

Inflammation has a pivotal role in defence and in healing processes, and thus directly or indirectly contributes to the pathogenesis of many sequelae of these processes, for example the production of granulation tissue and subsequent fibrosis. In liver and kidney the transforming growth factors have been implicated in stimulation of fibroblasts and collagen secretion, and thus as mediators of matrix accumulation in diseases of these organs[13,32,41]. A similar mechanism may well operate in inflammatory processes in the bone marrow, which are then followed by fibrosis and both woven and osteoblastic new bone formation. Under these circumstances bone remodelling is no longer 'coupled', but the balance is tipped in favour of new bone formation without a corresponding increase in resorption.

ACQUIRED IMMUNE DEFICIENCY SYNDROME (AIDS)

Over the past decade reports have appeared in the literature describing bone marrow histopathology in ARC (AIDS-related complex) and AIDS[11,14,21,37,38,46]. The results led to the speculation that the bone marrow is also a target organ in AIDS, and certain constellations of histological features in the bone marrow are highly suggestive, if not pathognomonic of HIV infection[23].

We have investigated bone biopsies of 50 patients with AIDS and the extreme range of bone and marrow manifestations encountered is presented in Table 6.1 and in Plates 6.H and I. Hypo-, normo- and hypercellular marrows, usually together with marked myelodysplastic features, could underlie a cytopénia. Serous atrophy and diffuse fibrosis may contribute to the frequent finding of bone marrow failure. The increase in macrophages, plasma cells and lymphocytes, as well as in benign lymphoid nodules and granulomas, could be ascribed to the additional infections which AIDS patients so frequently undergo. The serous (gelatinous) atrophy reported in the bone marrow in AIDS patients with advanced disease is probably a reflection of their poor condition and inadequate nutrition, as similar changes occur in patients with anorexia nervosa or involuntary starvation.

A normal trabecular structure was found in 76%, and a reduction in the cancellous bone, mostly with moderate osteoblastic and osteoclastic remodelling, in 20%. Two

Table 6.1 Bone and marrow changes in iliac crest biopsies of AIDS patients

	Percentage
Haematopoiesis	
Hypercellular	32
Hypocellular	24
Myelodysplastic	75
Stroma	
Serous atrophy	42
Plasmacytosis	72
Increased iron stores	85
Vasculitis	35
Diffuse fibrosis	25
Lymphoid nodules (follicles)	15
Granulomas	10
Bone	
Osteopenia	20
Osteosclerosis	4
Increased osseous remodelling	20

patients showed increased volumes of bone and osteoid and osteoblast numbers in the biopsy, together with marked inflammatory reactions and diffuse fibrosis in the marrow spaces.

In conclusion, there is a wide spectrum of bone and marrow manifestations in AIDS, but distinctive features suggestive of AIDS were not consistently present in our series. Evaluation of bone biopsies in AIDS patients provides information on the state of the marrow reserve as well as on the bone and marrow reactions to the multitude of infectious and immunological disturbances[20,21].

References

1. Bartl R., Schauer A., Hübner G. and Burkhardt R. (1975). Changes of the bone marrow in endotoxin shock. Urbaschek B., Urbaschek R. and Neter E., *Gram-Negative Bacterial Infections and Mode of Endotoxin Actions* (p. 206). Wien: Springer
2. Baty J. M. and Vogt E. C. (1935). Bone changes of leukaemia in children. *Amer. J. Radiol.*, **34**, 310
3. Beil E., Burkhardt R., Penning W., Bartl R., Kronseder A. and Neumann P. (1976). Histological examination of late changes of bone marrow and bone following local fractionated gamma irradiation in patients with genital carcinoma. *Klin. Wschr.*, **54**, 217
4. Bell N. H. (1990). Sarcoidosis and related disorders. Avioli L. V. and Krane S. M., *Metabolic Bone Disease* (p. 804). Philadelphia: Saunders
5. Bhargava B. A. and Farhi D. C. (1988). Bone marrow granulomas: clinicopathologic findings in 72 cases and review of the literature. *Hematol. Pathol.*, **2**, 43
6. Bodem C. R., Hamory B. H., Taylor H. M. and Kleopfer L. (1983). Granulomatous bone marrow disease. A review of the literature and clinicopathologic analysis of 58 cases. *Medicine*, **62**(6), 372
7. Boll K. L. and Jurik A. G. (1990). Sternal osteomyelitis in drug addicts. *J. Bone Jt Surg.*, **72-B**, 328
8. Burkhardt R., Bartl R., Sandel P. and Binsack T. (1978). Generalized reaction of bone marrow in neoplastic disorders. *Bibl. Haematol.*, **45**, 55
9. Burkhardt R., Zettl K. and Bartl R. (1978). Significance of non-specific changes of the bone marrow tissues: from the bioptic viewpoint. *Bibl. Haematol.*, **45**, 38
10. Calin A. (1985). Ankylosing spondylitis. *Clin. Rheum. Dis.*, **11**(1), 41
11. Castella A., Croxson T. S. and Mildvan D. (1985). The bone marrow in AIDS. A histologic, hematologic and microbiologic study. *Clin. Pathol.*, **84**, 425
12. Castillo B. A., Sallab R. A. and Scott J. T. (1965). Physical activity, cystic erosions and osteoporosis in rheumatoid arthritis. *Ann. Rheum. Dis.*, **24**, 522
13. Creely J. J., Dimari S. J., Howe A. M. and Haralson M. A. (1992). Effects of transforming growth factor β on collagen synthesis by normal rat kidney epithelial cells. *Amer. J. Pathol.*, **140**, 45

Plate 6.H

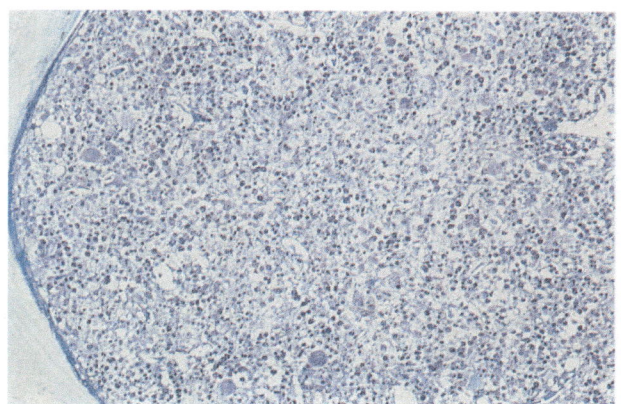

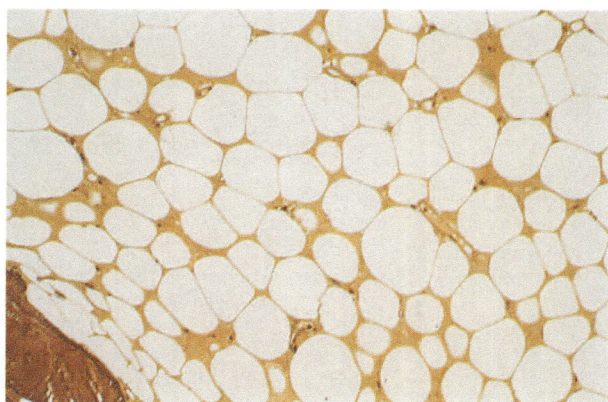

Figs. 6.43–6.48 Bone marrow manifestations in AIDS: cellularity and myelodysplasia

Fig. 6.43 Hypercellularity with topographic disorganization. Giemsa

Fig. 6.44 Aplastic marrow with oedema between the fat cells. Note complete absence of haematopoiesis, in an AIDS patient with severe pancytopenia. Gomori

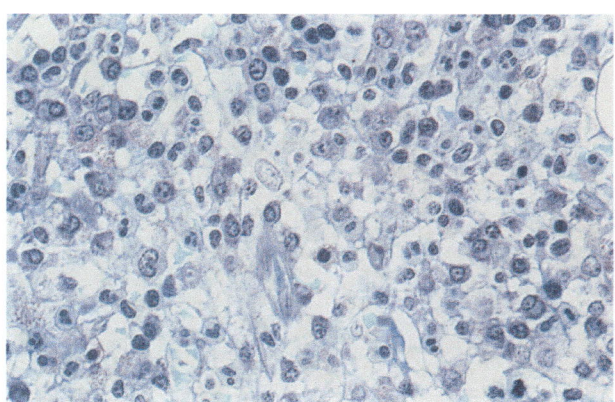

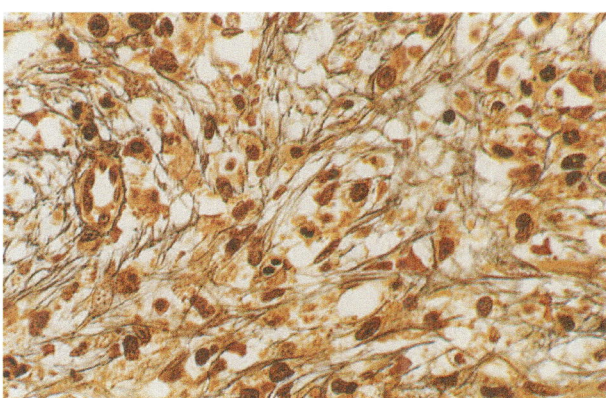

Fig. 6.45 Hypercellular marrow with marked myelodysplastic features (disturbed topographic disorganization and maturation inhibition of all three haematopoietic cell lines). Giemsa

Fig. 6.46 Hypercellular marrow with marked, partly coarse fibrosis (centre). Gomori

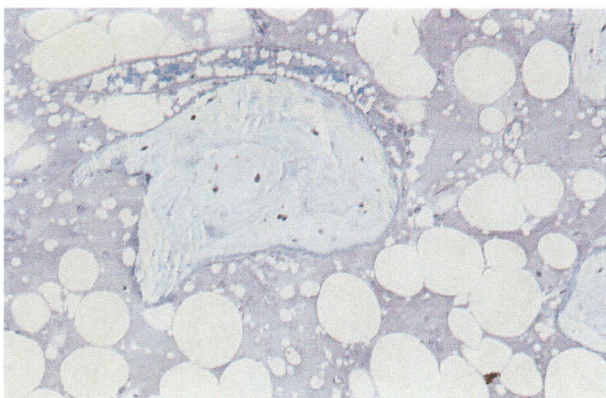

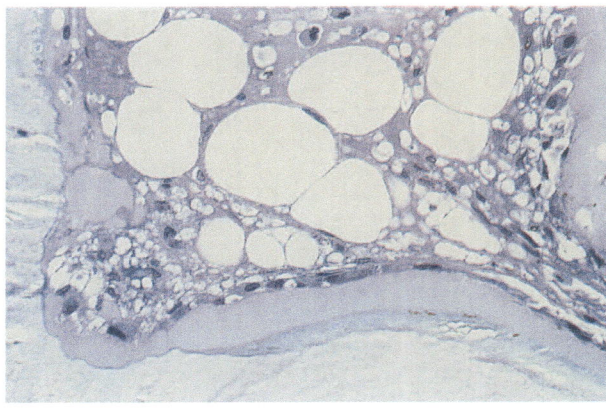

Fig. 6.47 Ossicle surrounded by serous (gelatinous) atrophy of the bone marrow. Giemsa

Fig. 6.48 Marked osteoblastic new bone formation in area of serous atrophy. Giemsa

Plate 6.I

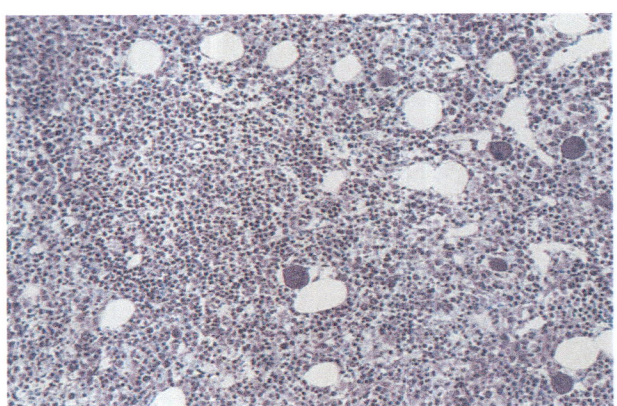

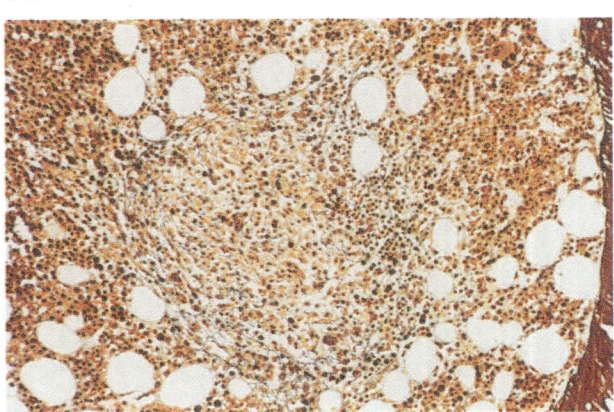

Figs. 6.49–6.54 Bone marrow manifestations in AIDS: stromal changes

Fig. 6.50 Lymphoid nodule separated from the haematopoietic tissue by a rim of fat cells. Gomori

Fig. 6.49 Large lymphoid nodule (upper left) within hypercellular marrow. Giemsa

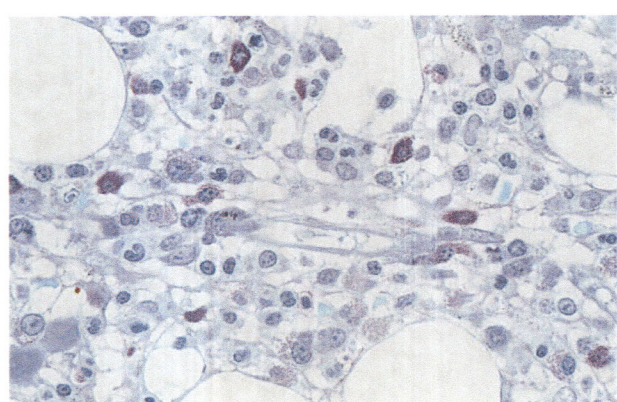

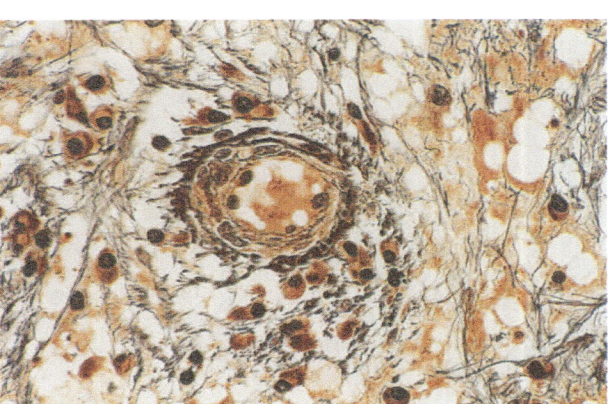

Fig. 6.51 Inflammatory reaction around a capillary, with increased mast cells, eosinophils and plasma cells. Giemsa

Fig. 6.52 Perivascular plasmacytosis and fibrosis in oedematous, hypercellular area. Gomori

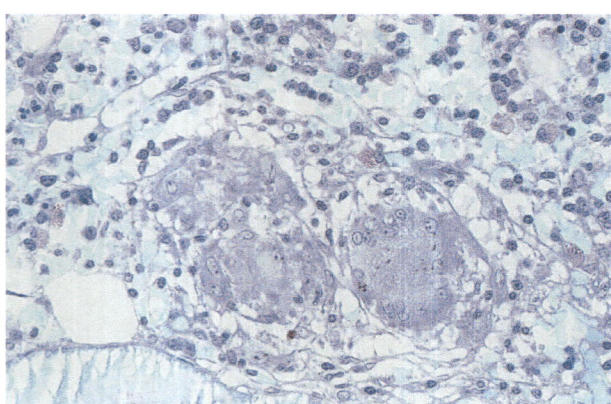

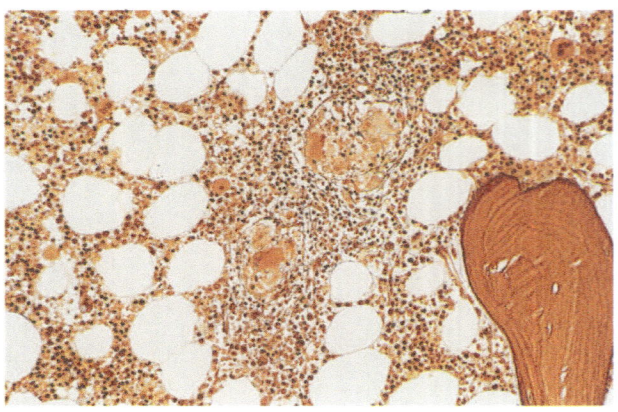

Fig. 6.53 Granuloma with giant cells, epithelioid cells and outer rim of lymphoid cells and eosinophils. Giemsa

Fig. 6.54 Larger granuloma with giant cells and broad rim of lymphoid cells, surrounded by fat cells. Gomori

14. Delacretaz F., Perey L., Schmidt P. M., Chave J. P. and Costa J. (1987). Histopathology of bone marrow in human immunodeficiency virus infection. *Virch. Arch. A*, **411**, 543

15. Dequeker J. and Geusens P. (1990). Osteoporosis and arthritis. *Ann. Rheum. Dis.*, **49**, 276

16. D'Angelo A., Fabris A. and Sartori L. (1985). Mineral metabolism and bone mineral content in rheumatoid arthritis. Effect of corticosteroids. *Clin. Exp. Rheumatol.*, **3**, 143

17. El-Naggar A. M., Hanna I. R. A., Chanana A. D., Carsten A. L. and Cronkite E. P. (1980). Bone marrow changes after localized acute and fractionated X irradiation. *Radiat. Res.*, **84**, 46

18. Epps C. H., Bryant D. D., Coles M. J. M. and Castro O. (1991). Osteomyelitis in patients who have sickle-cell disease. *J. Bone Jt Surg.*, **73A**, 1281

19. Esolen L. M., Fasano M. B., Flynn J., Burton A. and Lederman H. M. (1992). Brief report: pneumocystis carinii osteomyelitis in a patient with common variable immunodeficiency. *N. Engl. J. Med.*, **326**, 999

20. Frisch B. and Bartl R. (1990). *Atlas of Bone Marrow Pathology*. Dordrecht: Kluwer

21. Frisch B., Bartl R. and Goebel F.-D. (1989). Bone marrow manifestations in the acquired immune deficiency syndrome (AIDS). A study of 40 patients and review of the literature. *Haematol. Rev.*, **3**, 177

22. Frisch B., Lewis S. M., Burkhardt R. and Bartl R. (1985). *Biopsy Pathology of Bone and Marrow*. London: Chapman & Hall

23. Geller S. A., Muller R. and Greenberg M. L. (1985). Acquired immunodeficiency syndrome. Distinct features of bone marrow biopsies. *Arch. Pathol. Lab. Med.*, **109**, 138

24. Gillespie W. J. and Allardyce R. A. (1990). Mechanisms of bone degradation in infections: a review of current hypothesis. *Orthopedics*, **13**, 407

25. Howland W. J., Loeffler R. K., Starchman D. E. and Johnson R. G. (1975). Post irradiation atrophic changes of bone and related complications. *Radiology*, **117**, 667

26. Krech R. and Thiele J. (1985). Histopathology of the bone marrow in toxic myelopathy. A study of drug-induced lesions in 57 patients. *Virch. Arch. (Pathol. Anat.)*, **405**, 225

27. Leskinen R. H., Scrifvars B. V., Laasonen L. S. and Edgren K. J. (1984). Bone lesions in systemic lupus erythematodes. *Radiology*, **153**, 349

28. Maeda M., Bryant M. H., Yamagata M., Li G., Earle J. D. and Chao E. Y. S. (1988). Effects of irradiation on cortical bone and their time-related changes: a biomechanical and histomorphological study. *J. Bone Jt Surg.*, **70A**, 392

29. Magyar E., Talerman A., Feher M. and Wouters H. W. (1974). Giant bone cysts in rheumatoid arthritis. *J. Bone Jt Surg.*, **56B**, 121

30. Martini M. (1988). *Tuberculosis of the Bones and Joints*. Berlin: Springer

31. Mbuyi-Muamba J. M., Dequeker J. and Burssens A. (1983). Case report: massive osteolysis in a case of rheumatoid arthritis: clinical, histologic and biochemical findings. *Metab. Bone Dis. Rel. Res.*, **5**, 101

32. Milani S., Herbst H., Schuppan D., Stein H. and Surrenti C. (1991). Transforming growth factors $\beta 1$ and $\beta 2$ are differentially expressed in fibrotic liver disease. *Amer. J. Pathol.*, **139**, 1221

33. Miskew D. B. W., Lorenz M. A., Pearson R. L. and Pankowich A. M. (1983). *Pseudomonas aeruginosa* bone and joint infection in drug abusers. *J. Bone Jt Surg.*, **65A**, 829

34. Montemurro L., Fraioli P. and Rizzato G. (1991). Bone loss in untreated longstanding sarcoidosis. *Sarcoidosis*, **8**, 29

35. Mundy G. R. (1991). Inflammatory mediators and the destruction of bone. *J. Peridont. Res.*, **26**, 213

36. Murray T. M. (1989). Disorders of serum calcium homeostasis. Tam C. S., Heersche J. N. M. and Murray T. M., *Metabolic Bone Disease: Cellular and Tissue Mechanisms* (p. 91). Boca Raton: CRC Press

37. Namiki T. S., Boone D. C. and Meyer P. R. (1987). A comparison of bone marrow findings in patients with acquired immunodeficiency syndrome (AIDS) and AIDS related conditions. *Hematol. Oncol.*, **5**, 99

38. Osborne B. M., Guardia L. A. and Butler J. J. (1984). Bone marrow biopsies in patients with the acquired immunodeficiency sndrome. *Hum. Pathol.*, **15**, 1048

39. Piazza I. and Giunta G. (1991). Lytic bone lesions and polyarthritis associated with acne fulminans. *Brit. J. Rheumatol.*, **30**, 387

40. Ralston S. H., Urquart G. D. K., Brzeski M. and Sturrock R. D. (1990). Prevalence of vertebral compression fractures due to osteoporosis in ankylosing spondylitis. *Brit. Med. J.*, **300**, 563

41. Rees R. C. (1992). Cytokines as biological response modifiers. *J. Clin. Pathol.*, **45**, 93

42. Resnick D., Pineda C. and Trudell D. (1985). Widespread osteonecrosis of the foot in systemic lupus erythematodes: radiographic and gross pathologic correlation. *Skelet. Radiol.*, **13**, 33

43. Revell P. A. (1986). *Pathology of Bone*. Berlin: Springer

44. Sambrook P. N., Eisman J. A., Champion G. D., Yeates M. G., Pocock N. A. and Eberl S. (1987). Determinants of axial bone loss in rheumatoid arthritis. *Arthritis Rheum.*, **30**, 721

45. Schlag R., Burkhardt R., Bartl R. and Kettner G. (1984). Acute and chronic inflammatory changes in the bone marrow. Lennert K. and Hübner K., *Pathology of the Bone Marrow* (p. 411). Stuttgart: Fischer

46. Shenoy C. M. and Lin J. H. (1986). Bone marrow findings in acquired immunodeficiency syndrome (AIDS). *Amer. J. Med. Sci.*, **292**, 372

47. Silverman F. N. (1948). Skeletal lesions in leukemia: clinical and roentgenographic observations in 103 infants and children with review of the literature. *Amer. J. Radiol.*, **59**, 819

48. Slavin R. E., Welsh J. J. and Pollack A. D. (1980). Late generalized tuberculosis: a clinical pathologic analysis and comparison of 100 cases in the preantibiotic and antibiotic eras. *Medicine*, **59**, 352

49. Sponseller P. D., Malech H. L., McCarthy E. F., Horowitz S. F., Jaffe G. and Gallin J. I. (1991). Skeletal involvement in children who have chronic granulomatous disease. *J. Bone Jt Surg.*, **73A**, 37

50. Stern P. H. and Bell N. H. (1989). Disorders of vitamin D metabolism-toxicity and hypersensitivity. Tam C. S., Heersche J. N. M. and Murray T. M., *Metabolic Bone Disease: Cellular and Tissue Mechanisms* (p. 203). Boca Raton: CRC Press

51. Sugimoto M., Takahashi S., Toguchida T., Kotoura Y., Shibamoto Y. and Yamamuro T. (1991). Changes in bone after high-dose irradiation: biomechanics and histomorphology. *J. Bone Jt Surg.*, **73B**, 492

52. Tavassoli M. (1987). Structural alterations of marrow during inflammation. *Blood Cells*, **13**, 251

53. Thomas L. B., Forkner C. E., Frei E., Besse B. E. and Stabenau J. R. (1961). Skeletal lesions of acute leukaemia. *Cancer*, **14**, 608

Necrosis, grafts and healing in bone

7

BONE NECROSIS AND HEALING

The most common site of osteonecrosis is the femoral head due to deprivation of its blood supply, often because of a femoral neck fracture. Non-traumatic bone death is called *'idiopathic (primary) necrosis'*, which may be associated with various factors[49]. This also occurs mostly in the femur, although the humerus, tibia and radius may likewise be affected. However, bone necrosis is rarely observed in the iliac crest, probably due to its abundant blood supply. Furthermore, osteonecrosis of non-weight-bearing skeletal sites is often clinically silent and painless.

'Avascular necrosis' belongs to the 'aseptic' variants of osteonecrosis[3,31,43], and according to the literature four pathogenic groups are distinguished (Table 7.1):

1. traumatic,
2. marrow compartment syndromes,
3. small vessel occlusion, and
4. idiopathic.

Table 7.1 Basic disorders underlying necrosis of bone

Iatrogenic	*Rheumatic*
Thermal injuries	Systemic lupus
Fat embolism	erythematosus[39,56,67]
Caisson disease[47]	Periarteritis (vasculitis)
Radiation	Various mixed collagen disorders
Alcohol abuse	Scleroderma
Endotoxins[15]	
Cytotoxic chemotherapy[28]	*Gastrointestinal*
Steroid therapy[12,20,28,61]	Pancreatitis
Non-steroidal anti-inflammatory	Anorexia nervosa
agents	
	Renal
Haematological	Renal transplantation[19,29,33]
Sickle cell disease[8,54,66]	Renal osteodystrophy[44]
Acute leukaemias[5,42,63,65]	
Metastatic bone disease	*Infectious*
Polycythaemia vera	Tuberculosis
Chronic leukaemias[32,65]	Bacterial endocarditis[17,62]
	Disseminated intravascular
Metabolic	coagulation[15,27]
Cushing's syndrome	AIDS[23]
Diabetes mellitus[21]	
Gaucher's disease[2]	
Gout	

Necrosis of an area of marrow and bone (Plate 7.A)[9,10] is followed by proliferation and ingrowth of repair tissue. Especially vulnerable to interruption of the blood flow in the short term (hours) are the sinusoids and the small capillaries, as shown by disruption of their thin endothelial layer, with oedema and extravasation of erythrocytes into the surrounding marrow. This is followed by necrosis of haematopoietic and fat cells[41]. The hallmark of osseous necrosis is the loss of osteocytes (*osteocyte death*)[34]. Loss of nuclear staining of bone cells may be detected within a few days, but empty osteocytic lacunae in the affected trabeculae are rarely seen until a week after the ischaemic or toxic event. However, the mineral density and trabecular structure may remain unaltered for weeks so that radiological alterations do not occur during this time. The repair reaction begins with the removal by phagocytosis of necrotic tissue from the marrow spaces.

The macrophages are of variable size, depending on the quantity of debris they engulfed. Proliferating capillaries and fibroblasts, stimulated by factors released by the disintegrating elements, reconstitute the marrow stroma. Some of the necrotic bone may be resorbed directly by osteoclasts. In addition some of the non-viable trabeculae may be re-lined by a layer of living bone cells and lamellae of new bone before the osteoclasts become active. The phagocytic removal of necrotic bone tends to be limited to sites unprotected by lining cells or osteoblasts. Some woven bone is formed in the intertrabecular spaces near the necrotic areas.

The *aetiology* of bone/bone marrow necrosis is known only in rare cases. There are several reviews on the subject and a summary of related conditions is given in Table 7.1. It has been ascribed to radiation[13], chemotherapy[28] and especially to steroids[12,20], either as long-term or as short-term high-dose treatment[61]. Bone/bone marrow necrosis has also been described in severe infections[17,62], septic shock[15] as well as in hyperparathyroidism[60]. Intramedullary haemorrhage and ischaemia due to vascular obstruction may be important factors in its pathogenesis[50,55]. These may be caused by microthrombosis, emboli or other obstructions of small vessels. The clinical importance of bone necrosis is unknown; in patients with acute leukaemia it has been related to an ominous prognosis and a markedly shortened survival (Plate 7.B)[5,42,63,65].

BONE FRACTURES AND HEALING

Trauma to bone may cause extensive injury with displacement, haemorrhage and clot formation, or may affect only a small number of trabeculae without spectacular displacement or pain. Minor breaks or cracks (microfractures) occur chiefly in weight-bearing bones, especially the vertebrae, usually after the total quantity of bone has been reduced as in osteoporosis[38,40,48]. Sometimes only a single trabecula is involved. Microfractures are rare in iliac crest biopsies; their recognition may be difficult.

Major fractures are always accompanied by bleeding and subsequent organization of the clot is an integral part of the unique and highly complex healing process[57]. Indeed, adequate clot formation is followed by invasion of vessels and granulation tissue with direct formation of bone.

In brief, the main sequence of events in normal fracture healing is (Fig. 7.S1)[6,11]:

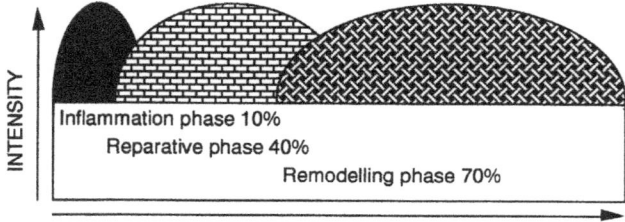

Fig. 7.S1 Diagram of the relative periods of time of the inflammatory, reparative and remodelling phases in fracture healing. Modified from Cruess R. L. (1984) Healing of bone, tendon and ligament. Rockwood C. A. and Green D. P., *Fractures in Adults* (p. 147). Philadelphia: Lippincott

Plate 7.A

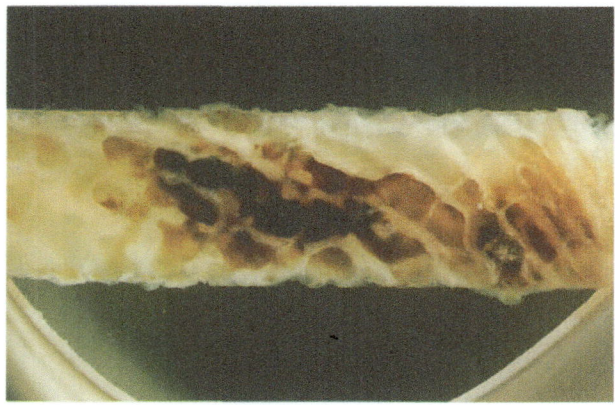

Figs 7.1–7.6 Necrosis and repair in bone

Fig. 7.1 Necrotic area and haemorrhage in the centre of an iliac crest biopsy (surface of trimmed plastic block) of a patient with acute leukaemia, at initial diagnosis

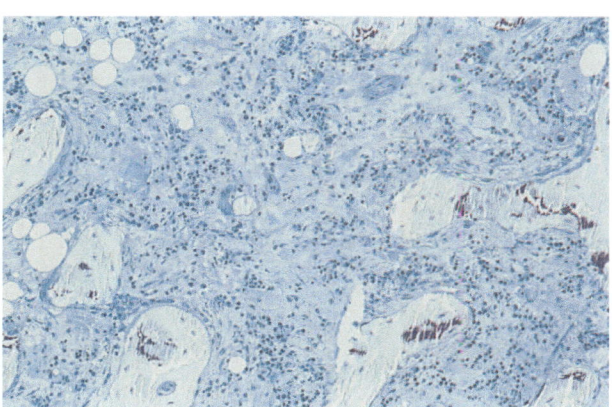

Fig. 7.2 Low magnification of bone marrow necrosis showing degenerating cells within oedematous stroma. Giemsa

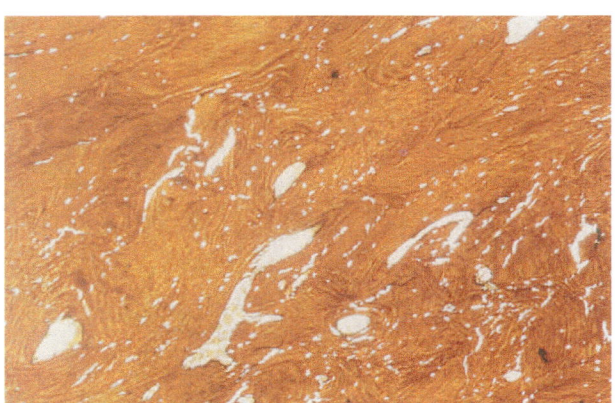

Fig. 7.3 Necrotic bone as evidenced by empty osteocytic lacunae as well as canals devoid of vessels. Gomori

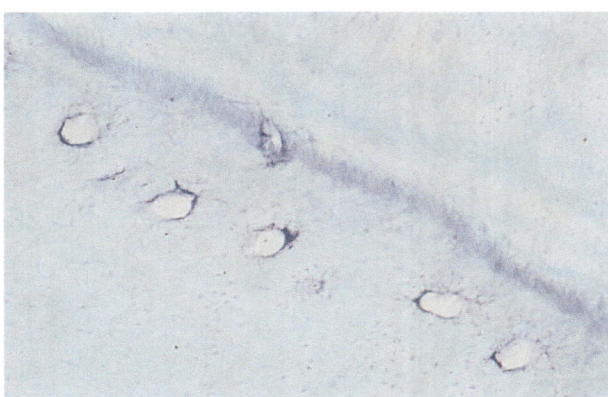

Fig. 7.4 Lamellae of newly formed osteoid separated by cement line from necrotic bone, with empty osteocytic lacunae. Giemsa

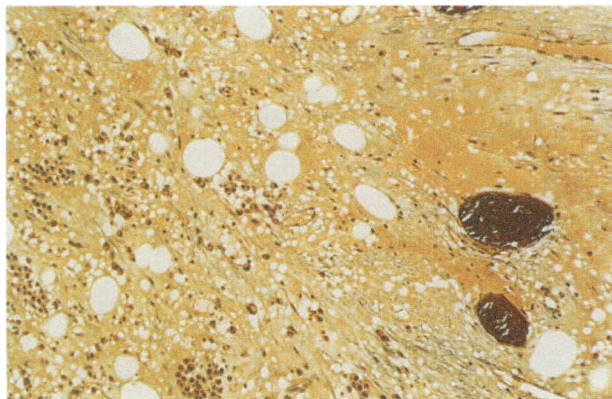

Fig. 7.5 Phase of inflammation with residual haematopoiesis and inflammatory cells (left), as well as oedema and haemorrhage (right). Gomori

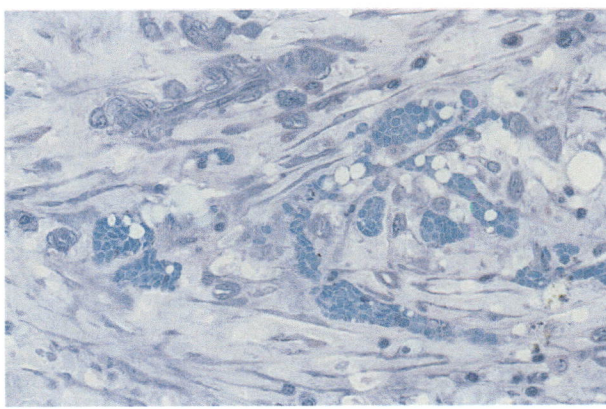

Fig. 7.6 Phase of repair with histiocytes, macrophages and plasma cells. Giemsa

Plate 7.B

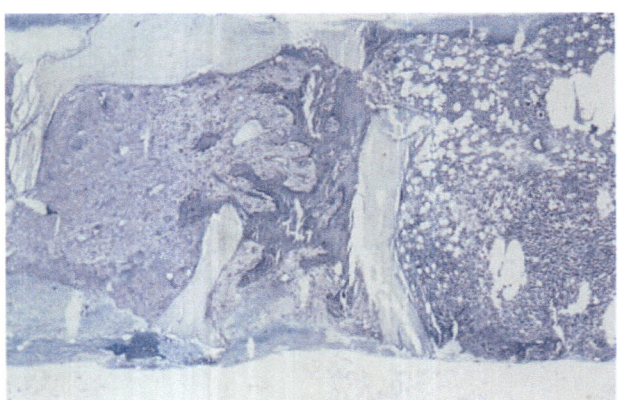

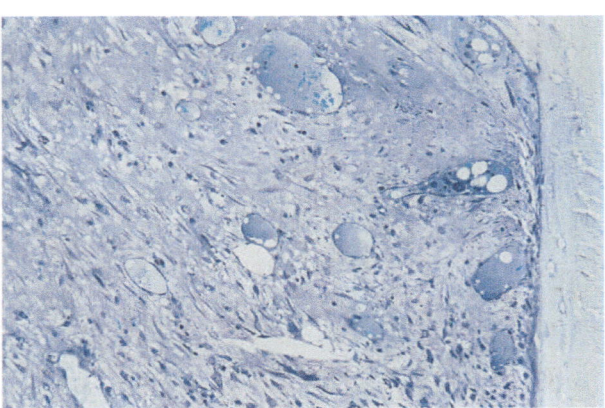

Figs 7.7–7.12 Iliac crest biopsy of patient with acute leukaemia and necrotic changes under chemotherapy

Fig. 7.7 Overview of biopsy with necrotic area of blastic infiltration (left), osseous reaction with production of primitive bone (centre) and normocellular haematopoiesis (right). Giemsa

Fig. 7.8 Higher magnification of Fig. 7.7 with bone marrow necrosis and marked oedematous reaction. Note loose residual infiltration by small blast cells. Giemsa

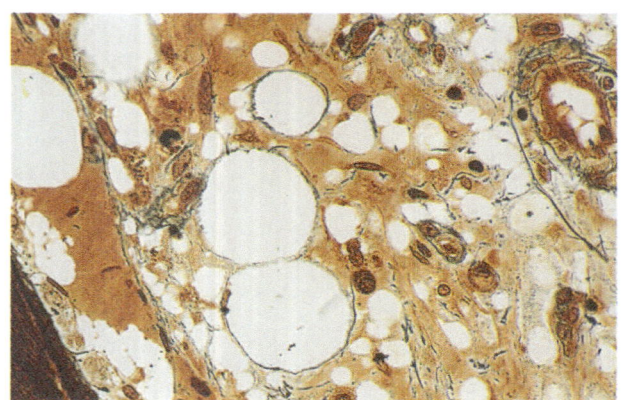

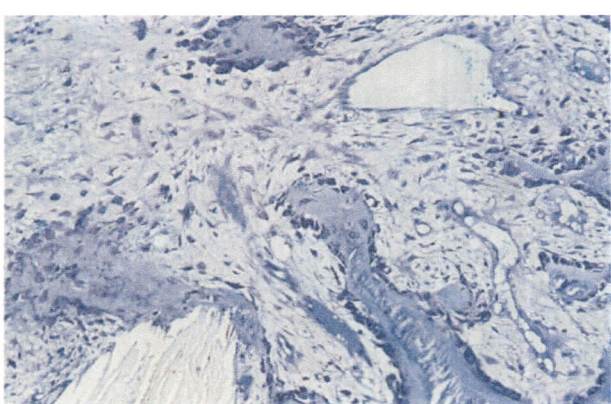

Fig. 7.9 Higher magnification of biopsy from Fig. 7.7, with oedematous stroma, fine fibrosis and some plasma cells adjacent to the necrotic area. Note broad endosteal sinusoid (left). Gomori

Fig. 7.10 Production of woven bone partly attached to lamellar ossicle and embedded in connective tissue. Note high vascularity

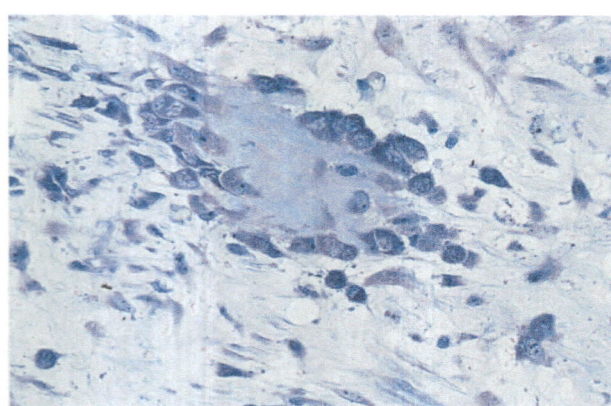

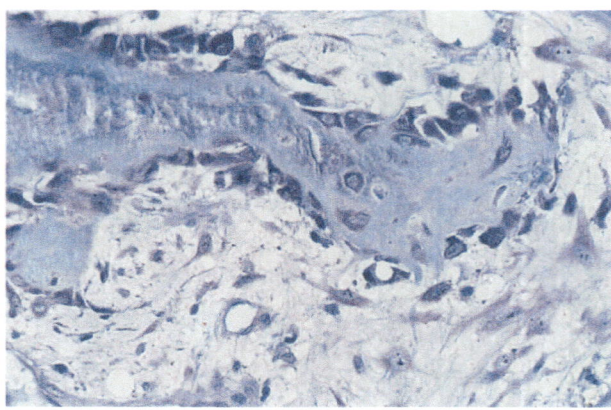

Fig. 7.11 Fibroblast and osteoblasts producing primitive bone (centre). Giemsa

Fig. 7.12 Maturation of woven bone covered by cuboidal oseoblasts. Note fibrocytes and vessels in the surrounding reparative tissue. Giemsa

1. *Inflammatory phase*, with an immediate and intense inflammatory response to the necrotic material: haemorrhage, vasodilatation and exudation of plasma. Tissue degeneration is due to injury, ischaemia and toxic products. For a period of days the fracture haematoma organizes – it has been shown to have osteogenic potential[46] – and the necrotic tissue is removed by phagocytosis and lysosomal breakdown.
2. *Reparative phase*, characterized by formation of callus, a complex tissue composed of fibrous, cartilaginous and osseous elements, derived from mesenchymal cells. The matrix produced consists of collagen (type III rather than type I) and proteoglycans. At about the same time, within a week, blood vessels begin to proliferate, bringing nutrients, hormones and growth factors. The progression of soft, fibrous callus to hard, bony callus (woven bone) occurs by mineralization of the matrix (osteoid) and by enchondral ossification. Within 3–6 weeks the new bone has acquired a trabecular pattern, which may be observed in bone histology.
3. *Remodelling phase*, characterized by conversion of the woven to the lamellar bone over a period of months or even years. The repaired bone tends slowly to regain its original shape and strength. Resorption of the callus is primarily due to the osteoclasts which in turn are controlled by mechanical and electrical phenomena responsible for stimulating cellular proliferation and activity, and morphological changes.

In a recent publication, Joyce and co-workers emphasize the role of the subsequent transforming growth factor-β (TGF-β) in the regulation of fracture healing[35]. They describe four distinct histological stages of fracture healing, characterized by cellular features, extracellular matrix and time of appearance of the tissues:

Stage I: Immediate injury response,
Stage II: Intramembranous bone formation,
Stage III: Chondrogenesis, and
Stage IV: Enchondral ossification.

Identification of different bone morphogenic proteins (BMP) at sequential stages of fracture healing suggest that a cascade of BMP may be needed to regulate both fracture healing and normal bone formation.

One further point that should be mentioned is the presence of mast cells. The mechanism of their formation is at present quite unknown, although their distribution suggests that the stimulus for their formation is related to the stimuli that activate the formation of vessels and repair tissue, and their localization near or on the trabecular surface suggests participation in both resorption and formation of bone.

PATHOLOGICAL FRACTURES

Throughout life, patterns of fracture frequency in general are rather characteristic, with peaks at the extremes of life and differences between the sexes[25,45]. The most common fractures are those of the hip, vertebrae and distal radius, although fractures at any skeletal site may occur in systemic osteoporosis and metastatic bone disease. The main factors thought to affect fracture risk are summarized in Table 7.2. Analogous to the use of blood pressure measurement for cerebrovascular risk, recent data have confirmed the usefulness of bone mass measurement for fracture risk stratification. However, one must be aware that changes in bone mass cannot usually be extrapolated from the measured to other sites (see Chapter 2).

Table 7.2 Factors that may increase fracture risk[25,45]

Age and sex	*Capacity to resist trauma*
Propensity to fall	Fat and muscle mass
Weight	Muscle conditioning
Balance	Speed of reflexes
Sensory capacity	Physical activity
Cognitive impairment	
Gait	*Increased bone fragility*
Neurological and psychiatric disorders	Osteoporosis
	Localized osteopenia
Foot problems	Undermineralization
Genetic factors?	Osteolytic lesions
Environmental factors (uneven surfaces)	Osteosclerotic lesions
	Unbalanced bone remodelling
	Drugs
	Alcohol
	Sedatives
	Antihypertensives

A pathological fracture has been described as one occurring after minor trauma or during normal physical activity. Both osseous and extraosseous factors contribute to fractures in patients with diseases affecting the bones. The osseous factors include insufficient bone mass, altered trabecular architecture and reduced strength of the skeletal material. The fracture site is influenced by the age and sex of the patient as well by the nature of the disease (for example 'diabetic fractures'); the incidence of fractures of the forearm rises steeply in women after the menopause, while that of fractures of the proximal femur reaches a peak in old age in both sexes. Decreased skeletal mass as a consequence of age-related bone loss is probably the most important determinant in these fractures. Moreover, there is a complex interplay of factors influencing the functions of bone cells in or near fracture sites, as some activities are stimulated while others may be depressed[13].

Although bones affected by Paget's disease usually have an increased mineral content, they are structurally weak because of the disorganized lamellar architecture. Likewise the bones of patients with fluorosis may be abnormally thick, but this does not protect them from fracture: defective mineralization of bone (osteomalacia) contributes to fragility. The increased risk of fracture is also related to alterations of trabecular architecture. Two patterns of trabecular bone loss have now been identified. In one, commonly found in patients with vertebral crush fractures, the number of ossicles and their connections is reduced. In the second the cancellous network remains, but the trabeculae are thinner. This pattern is typical of the age-related bone loss that occurs in men. For identical bone mass, the second pattern is mechanically stronger. Reduced strength may also ensue from a variety of changes in the mineral/matrix composition of bone. Inadequate repair of microfractures and fatigue damage appear to result in weakened bone, particularly in weight-bearing bones such as the vertebrae and femoral head and neck. Normally microscopic defects are restored by local bone resorption and subsequent deposition of fresh bone. There is growing evidence that this phenomenon is more common than generally recognized.

Metastases from carcinomas primary bone tumours and multiple myeloma all cause osteolyses with collapse and fracture of bone. Many other developmental, metabolic, inflammatory, neoplastic, genetic, nutritional and iatrogenic disorders increase bone fragility and lead to a high fracture risk.

BONE GRAFTS AND SUBSTITUTES

Bone grafting is a central problem in reconstructive surgery of the skeleton[26,37,59], and bone grafts are the second most common type of grafts after blood products[16]. It is used to accelerate osteogenesis between adjacent bones and to bridge cavities, gaps or defects in bones (for example after curettage or tumour resection)[1].

It would appear relatively simple to transfer vascularized bone from the iliac crest to a bone defect. A cancellous *autograft* in a well-vascularised bed is rapidly incorporated, new bone appears on the transplanted spongy bone and dead bone is slowly resorbed by osteoclasts. There is also evidence that the graft matrix contains proteins ('bone morphogenic proteins') which stimulate bone induction in the surrounding mesenchyme[64].

Bone *allografts*, though always dead tissues, are to some extent still immunogenic and behave somewhat differently[18,22,30,36]. They have two main functions: mechanical support and osteoinduction, though this function is still controversial. Deep-frozen or heat-treated allografts initially induce more or less pronounced osteoclastic and inflammatory reactions[7]. The subsequent osteoinduction is believed to be due to 'Urist's bone morphogenic protein' of bone matrix[64]. Mesenchymal cells are recruited from the surrounding host tissue; these cells then differentiate to produce vessels and bone-forming cells[51,52]. The irregular woven bone is later replaced by well-organized lamellar bone, which remodels in response to mechanical forces. Occasionally bone bridges between host and allograft have been detected in microscopic sections. Recently, coral recovered from the sea, treated to kill the organism and to convert calcium carbonate to hydroxyapatite, has proved to be an excellent substitute for bone in reconstructive surgery[53,58]. It is not rejected by the body.

Goldberg and Stevenson described five stages of bone graft incorporation[24], though they overlap and form a continuum. They are: inflammation and osteoclastic resorption, osteogenesis, revascularization and finally remodelling; the outcome is a mechanically efficient structure. Cancellous grafts are usually completely resorbed. Ripamonti investigated the morphogenesis of bone in a porous hydroxyapatite substratum, recommending its use as a biological alternative to autogenous bone grafts for the controlled initiation of bone formation in humans[53].

We investigated experimentally the mode of integration of bone allografts and bone substitutes (Fig. 7.S2) (in collaboration with Dr J.-H. Kühne, Orthopaedic Department, Klinikum Großhadern, University of Munich). Rabbit femoral condyle drill holes (diameter 6 mm) were filled with

1. deep-frozen cancellous allografts,

2. heat-treated cancellous allografts,

3. coralline hydroxyapatite (200 μm pore size), and

4. coralline hydroxyapatite (500 μm pore size).

For comparison, and for studying healing of bone defects, empty drill holes were also assessed. Radiological, microradiographic and histological examinations were performed over a period of up to 12 months. The most striking results and differences between the transplants tested are given in Plates 7.C–E and in Figs. 7.S3 and S4.

As pointed out by Atrah (1992), selecting the right bone donor is as important as selecting the right blood donor and subject to the same exclusion criteria. This has led to the steadily increasing establishment of *bone banks* (analogous to blood banks)[4].

[continued on p. 96]

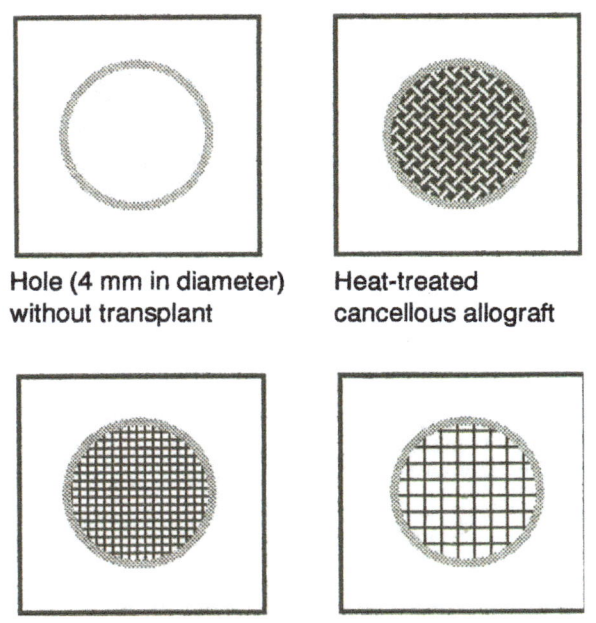

Fig. 7.S2 Diagram of bone allograft and substitutes used in experimental investigation of graft integration in rabbit femoral condyles

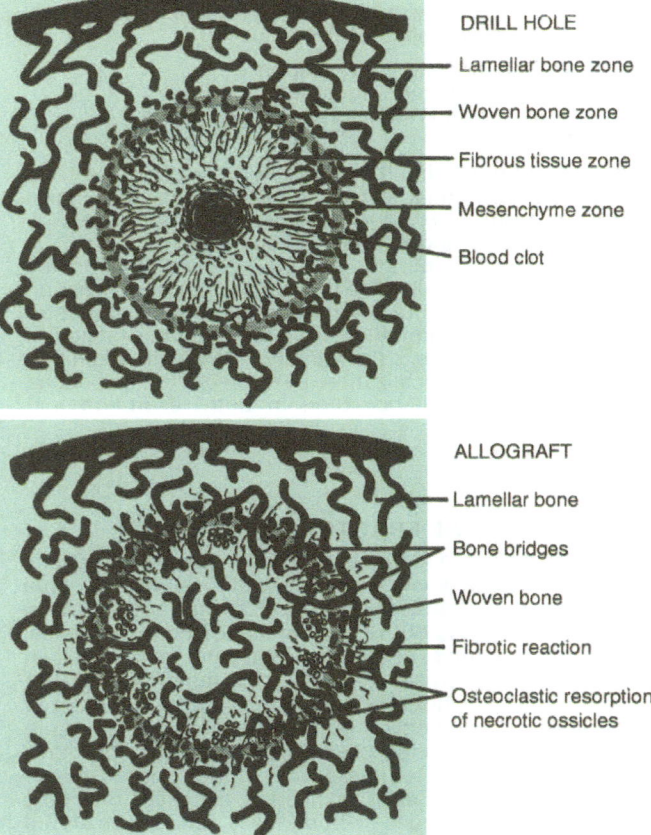

Fig. 7.S3 Sequence of bone repair of biopsy hole and of integration of bone allograft

Plate 7.C

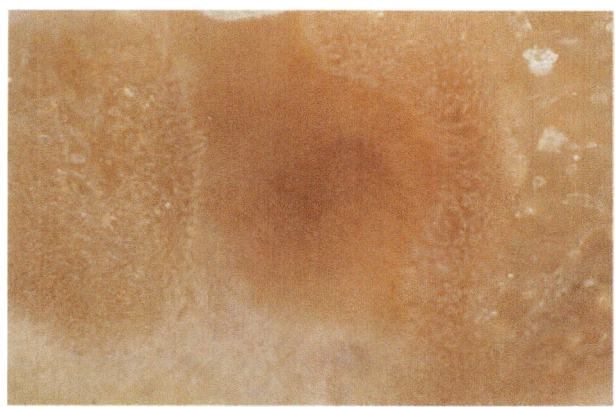

Figs. 7.13–7.30 Sequence of integration of bone allografts and substitutes I. Experimental study on rabbit femoral condyles, in collaboration with Dr J.-H. Kühne, Orthopaedic Department, Klinikum Großhadern, Munich

Figs. 7.13–7.18 Repair of drill hole in the absence of any transplant

Fig. 7.13 Surface of trimmed plastic block showing 6 mm hole filled with blood clot

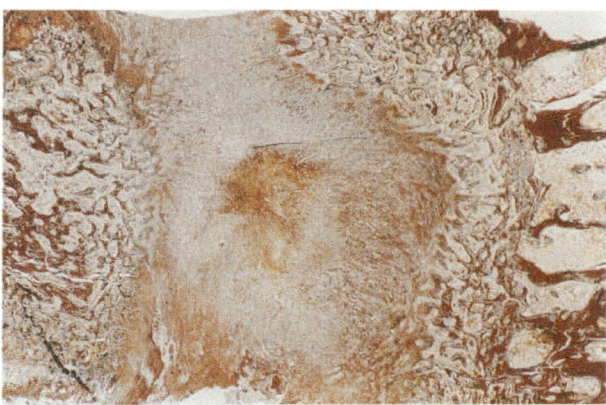

Fig. 7.14 Section showing connective tissue invading the clot from the edges of the hole (2 weeks later). Gomori

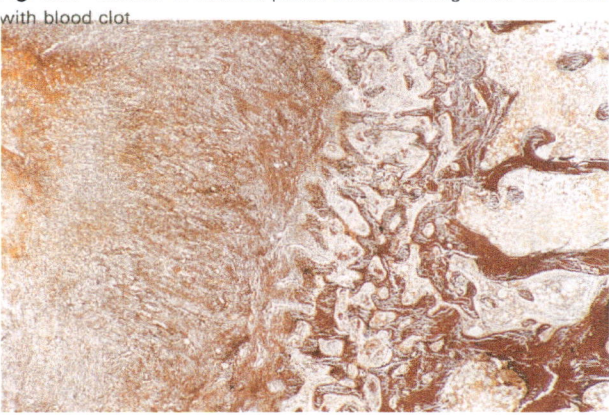

Fig. 7.15 Higher magnification of section through drill hole and adjoining tissues. Five zones can be recognized from left to right: (a) remains of blood clot; (b) zone containing fibres, inflammatory cells and blood vessels; (c) mesenchymal tissue with newly formed blood vessels; (d) zone of woven bone; and (e) trabecular bone of host. Gomori

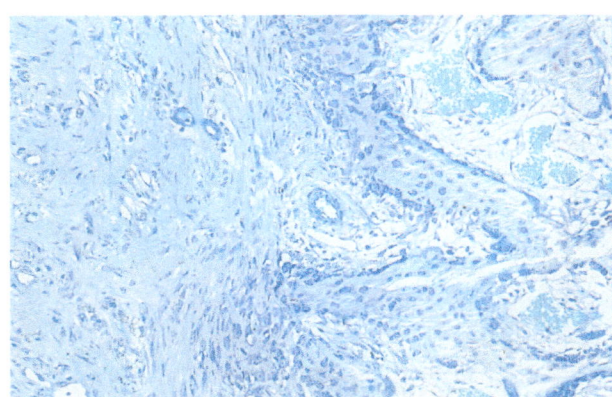

Fig. 7.16 Higher magnification of Fig. 7.15, illustrating the densely cellular mesenchymal zone with blood vessels (left) and transition to woven bone (right). Giemsa

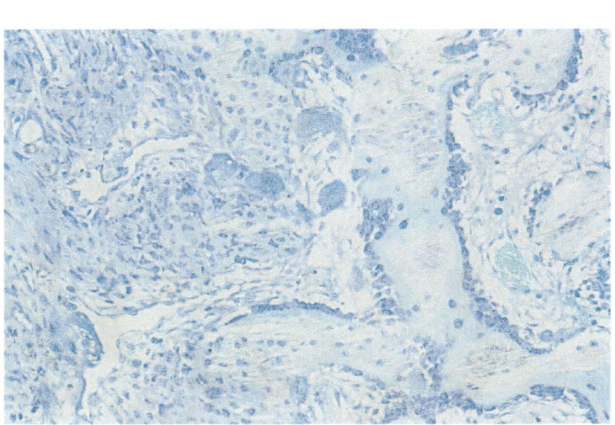

Fig. 7.17 Osteoblastic/osteoclastic remodelling in the zone of woven bone, 3 weeks later. Giemsa

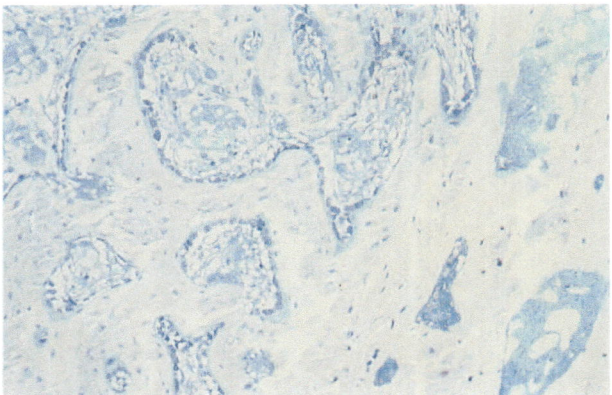

Fig. 7.18 Edge of the horizontal drill hole (right); trabecular bone now occupies the hole (left), 4 weeks later. Giemsa

Plate 7.D

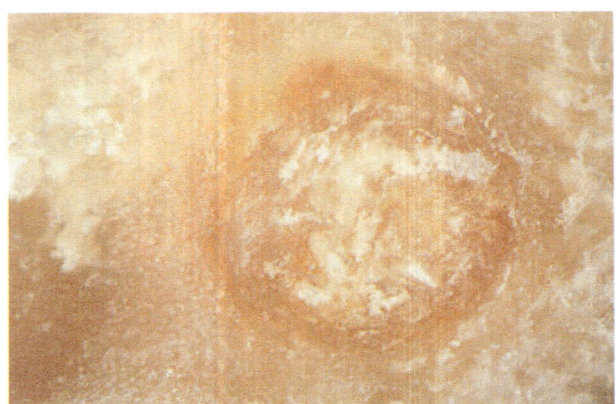

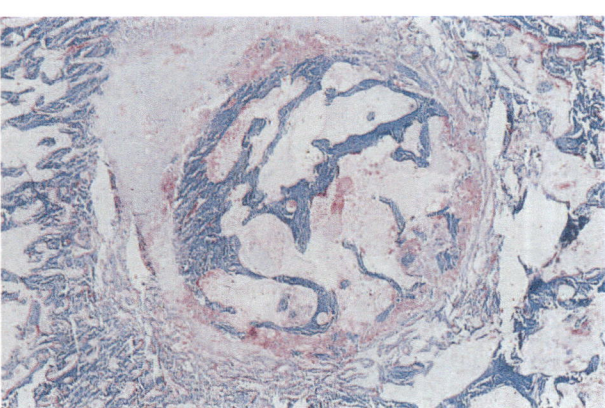

Figs. 7.19–7.24 Sequence of integration of allografts and bone substitutes II

Fig. 7.19 Surface of trimmed plastic block showing heat-treated allografts of cancellous bone in the drill hole, 2 weeks later

Fig. 7.20 Section from block in Fig. 7.19 illustrating allograft surrounded by mesenchymal reaction with patchy incipient new bone formation (lower left), 4 weeks later. Ladewig

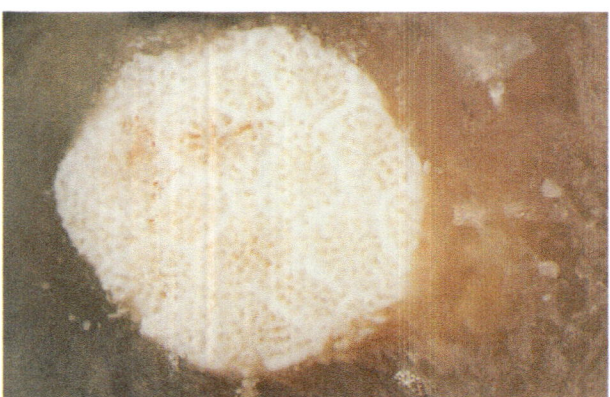

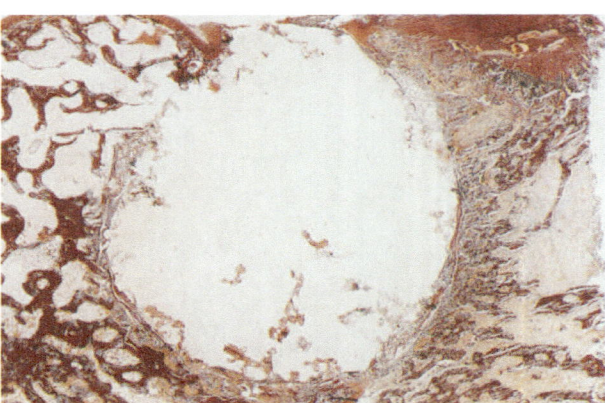

Fig. 7.21 Surface of trimmed plastic block showing coralline hydroxyapatite (200 μm pore size) graft

Fig. 7.22 Section from block in Fig. 7.21 demonstrating sharp delineation between host tissue and coralline transplant which has dropped out during processing; 4 weeks later. Gomori

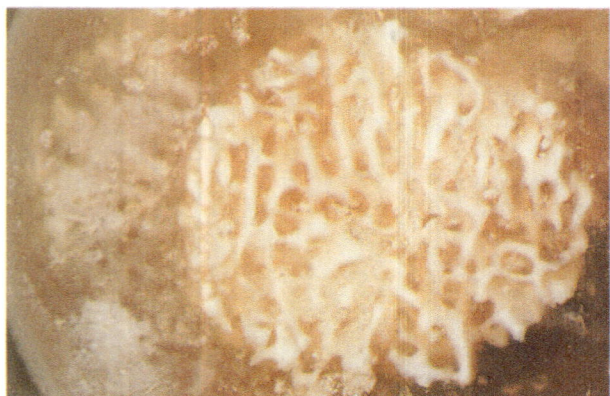

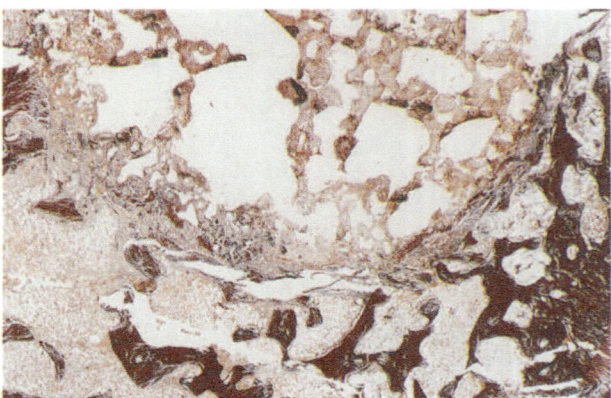

Fig. 7.23 Surface of trimmed plastic block showing coralline hydroxyapatite (500 μm pore size) graft

Fig. 7.24 Section from block in Fig. 7.23; the honeycomb of the graft has been filled by mesenchyme containing cells and blood vessels. These have grown in from the edges of the graft which has dropped out during cutting; 4 weeks later. Gomori

Plate 7.E

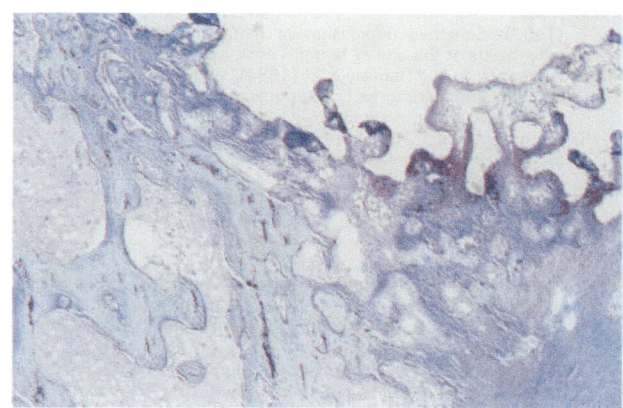
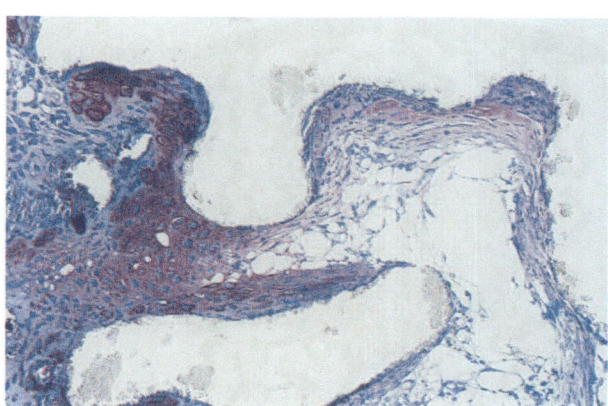

Figs. 7.25–7.30 Sequence of integration of allografts and bone substitutes III

Fig. 7.25 Section from block shown in Fig. 7.23 depicting the villous-like ingrowth of connective tissue into the graft (upper right). Giemsa

Fig. 7.26 Higher magnification of area in Fig. 7.25. The walls of the hydroxyapatite graft have dropped out, while the cavities between them have been filled by mesenchymal tissue, cartilage and newly formed bone (left). Giemsa

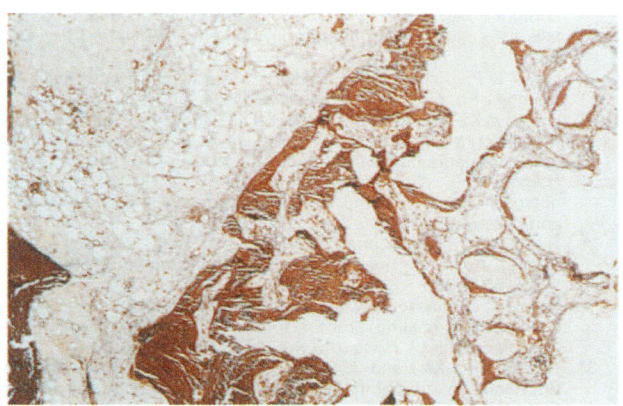
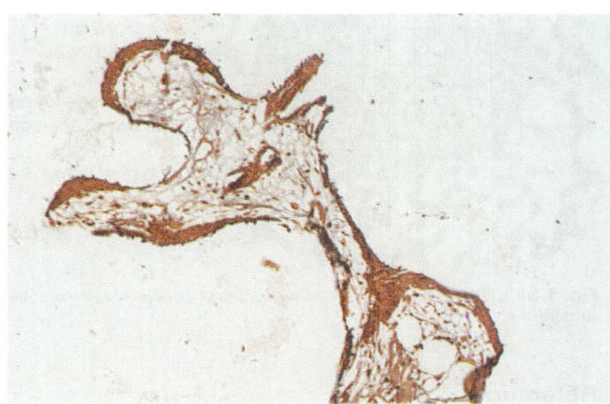

Fig. 7.27 Section from block shown in Fig. 7.23 demonstrating a marginal zone of newly formed bone around the graft and multiple small foci of new bone within the cavities in direct apposition to the walls of the graft which has fallen out. Giemsa

Fig. 7.28 Higher magnification of area from Fig. 7.27 demonstrating an intercavitary villous structure almost completely surrounded by a thin layer of bone. The walls of the graft have fallen out during cutting. Gomori

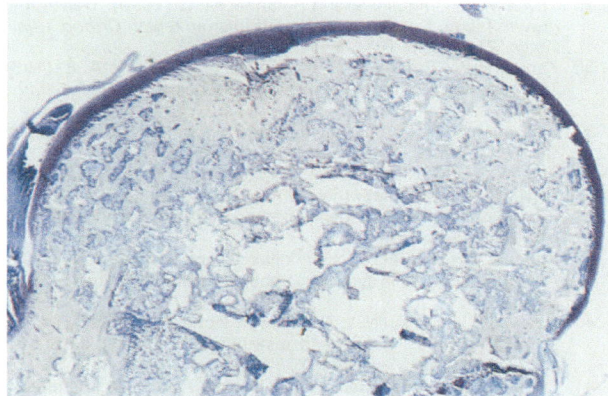
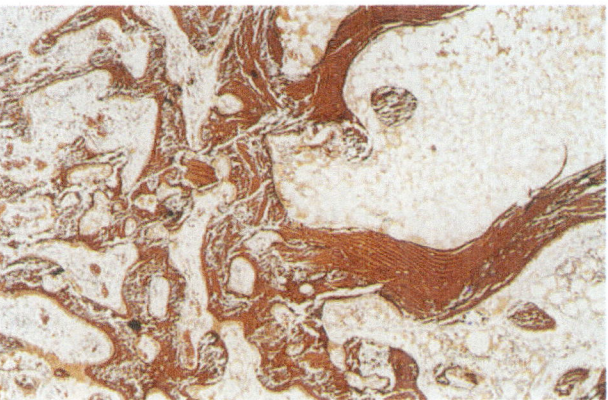

Fig. 7.29 Low magnification of section through graft (coralline hydroxyapatite 500 μm pore size) at 6 weeks. The original graft hole is bridged by trabecular bone. The empty spaces between the trabeculae were occupied by the graft which dropped out during cutting. Giemsa

Fig. 7.30 Section from grafted area at 12 weeks showing host trabeculae at right and newly formed trabeculae bridging the original drill hole on the left. Gomori

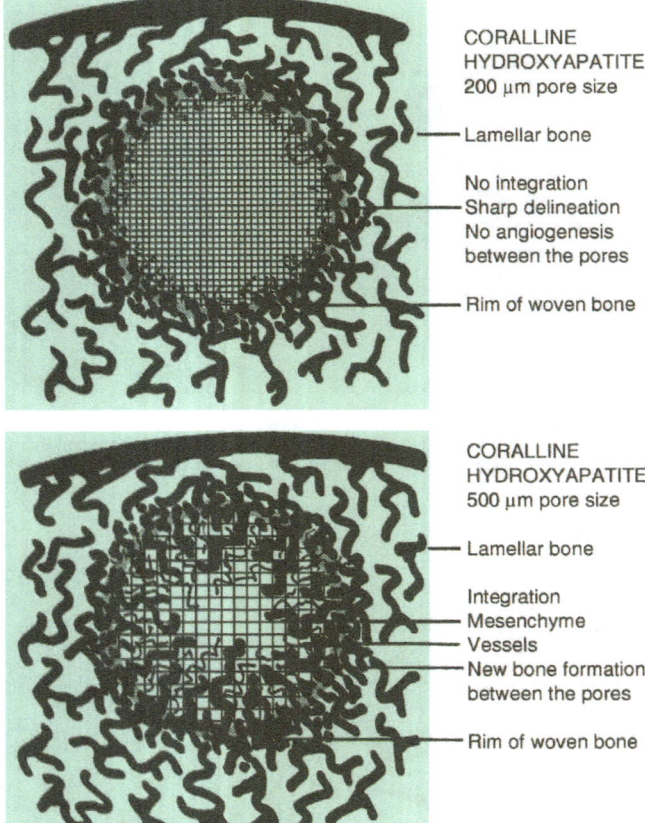

CORALLINE
HYDROXYAPATITE
200 μm pore size

— Lamellar bone

— No integration
— Sharp delineation
No angiogenesis
between the pores

— Rim of woven bone

CORALLINE
HYDROXYAPATITE
500 μm pore size

— Lamellar bone

— Integration
— Mesenchyme
— Vessels
— New bone formation
between the pores

— Rim of woven bone

Fig. 7.S4 Different integration of two types of coralline hydroxyapatite substitutes

References

1. Aebi M. and Regazzoni P. (1989). *Bone Transplantation*. Berlin: Springer
2. Amstutz H. C. and Carey E. J. (1966). Skeletal manifestations and treatment of Gaucher's disease. *J. Bone Jt Surg.*, **48A**, 670
3. Arlot M. E., Bonjean M., Chavassieux P. M. and Neunier P. J. (1983). Bone histology in adults with aseptic necrosis of bone. *J. Bone Jt Surg.*, **65A**, 1319
4. Atrah H. I. (1992). Bone banks: could be held by regional transfusion centres. *Brit. Med. J.*, **304**, 68
5. Bevilacqua G., Abadessa A., Consolini R., Frijia M., Nardi M. and Macchia P. (1985). Bone marrow necrosis foreshadowing acute lymphoid leukemia. *Amer. J. Pediatr. Hematol. Oncol.*, **7**, 228
6. Brand R. A. and Rubin C. T. (1990). Fracture healing. McCollister-Evarts C., *Surgery of the Musculoskeletal System* (p. 93). New York: Churchill Livingstone
7. Burchardt H. (1983). The biology of bone graft repair. *Clin. Orthop.*, **174**, 28
8. Charache S. and Page D. L. (1967). Infarction of bone marrow in the sickle cell disorders. *Ann. Intern. Med.*, **67**, 1195
9. Conrad M. E. and Carpenter J. T. (1979). Bone marrow necrosis. *Amer. J. Hematol.*, **7**, 181
10. Cowan J. D., Rubin R. N., Kies M. S. and Cerazo L. (1980). Bone marrow necrosis. *Cancer*, **46**, 2168
11. Cruess R. L. (1984). Healing of bone, tendon, and ligament. Rockwood C. A. and Green D. P., *Fractures in Adults* (p. 147). Philadelphia: Lippincott
12. Cruess R. L. and Crawshaw E. (1975). The etiology of steroid-induced avascular necrosis of bone. *Clin. Orthop.*, **113**, 178
13. Delaere O., Orloft S., Autrique J. C., Nyssen-Behets C., Dambrain R. and Dhem A. (1991). Long term sequelae of pelvis irradiation: histological and microradiographic study of a femoral head. *Clin. Rheumatol.*, **10**, 206
14. Dodds R. A., Emery R. J., Klenerman L., Chayen J. and Bitensky L. (1990). Selective depression of metabolic activities in cortical osteoblasts at the site of femoral neck fractures. *Bone*, **11**(3), 157
15. Duncan J. S. and Ramsay L. E. (1984). Widespread bone infarction complicating meningococcal septicaemia and disseminated intravascular coagulation. *Brit. Med. J.*, **288**, 111
16. Editorial. (1992). New bone? *Lancet*, **339**, 463
17. Eide J. (1982). Bone infarcts in bacterial endocarditis. *Hum. Pathol.*, **13**, 631
18. Enneking W. F. and Mindell E. R. (1991). Observations on massive retrieved human allografts. *J. Bone Jt Surg.*, **73A**, 1123
19. Evarts C. M. and Phalen G. S. (1971). Osseous avascular necrosis associated with renal transplantation. *Clin. Orthop.*, **78**, 330
20. Fisher D. E. and Bickel W. H. (1971). Corticosteroid-induced avascular necrosis. *J. Bone Jt Surg.*, **53A**, 859
21. Foss A. and Markus H. (1988). Osteolytic lesions in elderly diabetic woman. *Brit. Med. J.*, **296**, 280
22. Friedlaender G. E. (1991). Bone allografts: the biological consequences of immunological events (Editorial). *J. Bone Jt Surg.*, **73A**(8), 119
23. Frisch B., Bartl R. and Goebel F.-D. (1989). Bone marrow manifestations in the acquired immune deficiency syndrome (AIDS). A study of 40 patients and review of the literature. *Haematol. Rev.*, **3**, 177
24. Goldberg V. M. and Stevenson S. (1990). Bone transplantation. McCollister-Evarts C., *Surgery of the Musculoskeletal System* (p. 115). New York: Churchill Livingstone
25. Grisso J.-A., Kelsey J. L., Strom B. L., Chiu G. Y., Maislin G., O'Brian L. A., Hoffman S. and Kaplan F. (1991). Risk factors for falls as a cause of hip fracture in women. *N. Engl. J. Med.*, **324**, 1326
26. Gross T. P., Jinnah R. H., Clarke H. J. and Cox Q. G. (1991). The biology of bone grafting. *Orthopedics*, **14**, 563
27. Harigaya K., Watanabe S., Watanabe Y., Kageyama K. and Nakazawa K. (1977). Multiple bone marrow necrosis and disseminated intravascular coagulation. *Arch. Pathol. Lab. Med.*, **101**, 652
28. Harper P. G., Trask C. and Souhami R. L. (1984). Avascular necrosis of bone caused by combination chemotherapy without corticosteroids. *Brit. Med. J.*, **288**, 267
29. Harrington K. D., Murray W. R., Kountz S. L. and Belzer F. O. (1971). Avascular necrosis after renal transplantation. *J. Bone Jt Surg.*, **53A**, 203
30. Heiple K. G., Chase S. W. and Herndon C. H. (1963). A comparative study of the healing process following different types of bone transplantation. *J. Bone Jt Surg.*, **45A**, 1593
31. Hiehle J. F., Kreeland J. B. and Dalinka M. K. (1991). Magnetic resonance imaging of the hip with emphasis on avascular necrosis. *Rheum. Dis. Clin. N. Amer.*, **17**, 669
32. Hughes R. G., Islam A., Lewis S. M. and Catovsky D. (1981). Spontaneous remission following bone marrow necrosis in chronic lymphocytic leukaemia. *Clin. Lab. Haematol.*, **3**, 173
33. Ibels L. S., Alfrey A. C., Huffer W. E. and Weil R. (1978). Aseptic necrosis of bone following renal transplantation. *Medicine*, **57**, 25
34. James J. and Steijn-Myagkaya G. L. (1986). Death of osteocytes: electron microscopy after in vitro ischaemia. *J. Bone Jt Surg.*, **68B**, 620
35. Joyce M. E., Jingushi S. and Bolander M. E. (1990). Transforming growth factor-β in the regulation of fracture repair. *Orthop. Clin. N. Amer.*, **21**(1), 199
36. Kandel R. A., Pritzker K. P. H., Langer F. and Gross A. E. (1984). The pathologic features of massive osseous grafts. *Hum. Pathol.*, **15**, 141
37. Katthagen B.-D. (1986). *Bone Regeneration with Bone Substitutes*. Berlin: Springer
38. Kleerekoper M., Villanueva A. R., Stanciu J., Rao D. S. and Parfitt A. M. (1985). The role of three dimensional trabecular microstructure in the pathogenesis of vertebral compression fractures. *Calcif. Tissue Int.*, **37**, 594
39. Klippel J. H., Gerber L. H., Pollak L. and Decker J. L. (1979). Avascular necrosis in systemic lupus erythematodes. *Amer. J. Med.*, **67**, 83
40. Koszyca B., Fazzalari N. L. and Vernon-Roberts B. (1989). Trabecular microfractures: nature and distribution in the proximal femur. *Clin. Orthop. Rel. Res.*, **244**, 208
41. Kricun M. E. (1985). Red-yellow marrow conversion: its effect on the location of some solitary bone lesions. *Skelet. Radiol.*, **14**, 10
42. Kundel D. W., Brecher G., Bodey G. P. and Brittin G. M. (1964). Reticulin fibrosis and bone infarction in acute leukemia. Implication for prognosis. *Blood*, **23**, 526
43. Lagier R. (1989). Case report 552: Post-traumatic remodelling of

the distal tibial epiphysis: a form of aseptic osteonecrosis. *Skelet. Radiol.*, **18**, 331

44. Marry S. G., Bluestone R., Linenberg J. R. and Coburn J. W. (1975). Abnormalities of the musculoskeletal system in hemodialysis patients. *Semin. Arthritis Rheum.*, **4**, 321

45. Melton L. J. (1988). Epidemiology of fractures. Riggs B. L. and Melton L. J., *Osteoporosis: Etiology, Diagnosis, and Management* (p. 133). New York: Raven Press

46. Mizuno K., Mineo K., Tachibana T., Sumi M., Matsubara T. and Hirohata K. (1990). The osteogenic potential of fracture haematoma. Subperiosteal and intramural transplantation of the haematoma. *J. Bone Jt Surg.*, **72B**, 829

47. Ohta Y. and Matsunaga H. (1974). Bone lesions in divers. *J. Bone Jt Surg.*, **56B**, 3

48. Parfitt A. M. (1987). Trabecular bone architecture in the pathogenesis and prevention of fracture. *Amer. J. Med.*, **82**(Suppl 1B), 68

49. Petty W. (1986). Osteonecrosis. *J. Bone Jt Surg.*, **68A**, 1311

50. Phemister D. B. (1940). Changes in bones and joints resulting from interruption of circulation: non-traumatic lesions in adults with bone infarction: arthritis deformans. *Arch. Surg.*, **41**, 1455

51. Ray R. D. (1972). Vascularisation of bone grafts and implants. *Clin. Orthop.*, **87**, 43

52. Rhinelander F. W., Rouweyha M. and Milner J. C. (1971). Microvascular and histogenic responses to implantations of a porous ceramic in bone. *J. Biomed. Mater. Res.*, **5**, 81

53. Ripamonti U. (1991). The morphogenesis of bone in replicas of porous hydroxyapatite obtained from conversion of calcium carbonate exoskeletons of coral. *J. Bone Jt Surg.*, **73A**, 692

54. Rowe C. N. and Haggars M. E. (1957). Bone infarcts in sickle cell anemia. *Radiology*, **68**, 661

55. Saito S., Inoue A. and Ono K. (1987). Intramedullary hemorrhage as a possible cause of avascular necrosis of the femoral head. *J. Bone Jt Surg.*, **69B**, 346

56. Siemsen J. K., Brook J. and Meister L. (1962). Lupus erythematosus and avascular bone necrosis: a clinical study of 3 cases and review of the literature. *Arthritis Rheum.*, **5**, 452

57. Simmons D. J. (1985). Fracture healing perspectives. *Clin. Orthop. Rel. Res.*, **200**, 100

58. Soballe K., Gotfredsen, K., Brockstedt-Rasmussen H., Nielsen P. T. and Rechnagel K. (1991). Histologic analysis of a retrieved hydroxyapatite coated femoral prosthesis. *Clin. Orthop.*, **272**, 255

59. Solomon L. (1991). Bone grafts (Editorial). *J. Bone Jt Surg.*, **73B**, 706

60. Tavassoli M. (1983). Bone marrow necrosis secondary to hyperparathyroidism. *J. Miss. State Med. Assoc.*, **24**, 39

61. Taylor L. J. (1984). Multifocal avascular necrosis after short-term high-dose steroid therapy. *J. Bone Jt Surg.*, **66B**, 431

62. Terheggen H. G. and Lampert F. (1979). Acute bone marrow necrosis caused by streptococcal infection. *Eur. J. Paed.*, **130**, 53

63. Thomas L. B., Forkner C. E., Frei E., Besse B. E. and Stabenau I. R. (1961). The skeletal lesions of acute leukemia. *Cancer*, **14**, 608

64. Urist M. R. and Strates B. S. (1970). Bone formation in implants of partially and wholly demineralized bone matrix. *Clin. Orthop.*, **71**, 271

65. Vesterby A. and Jensen O. M. (1985). Aseptic bone/bone marrow necrosis in leukaemia. *Scand. J. Haematol.*, **35**, 354

66. Ware H. E., Brooks A. P., Toye R. and Berney S. I. (1991). Sickle cell disease and silent avascular necrosis of the hip. *J. Bone Jt Surg.*, **73B**, 947

67. Zizic T. M., Hungergord D. S. and Stevens M. B. (1990). Ischemic bone necrosis in systemic lupus erythematodes: the early diagnosis of ischemic necrosis of bone. *Medicine*, **67**, 83

The following recent review article includes a scheme for classifying the mechanisms of death of bone. The article deals mainly with non-traumatic osteonecrosis with onset in adulthood, and the pathogenic mechanisms.

Mankin H. J. (1992). Non-traumatic necrosis of bone (osteonecrosis). *N. Engl. J. Med.*, **326**, 1473

See also:
Sissons H, Nuovo M. A. and Steiner G. C. (1992). Pathology of osteonecrosis of the femoral head. *Skel. Radiol.*, **21**, 229

The following reference describes the materials used in bone grafting and a novel approach to enhance the osteogenic potential of demineralized bone.

Nolan P. C., Mollan R. A. B. and Wilson D. J. (1992). Living bone grafts. Cell culture may overcome the limitations of allografts. *Br. Med. J.*, **304**, 1520

Continuing efforts are being made to ensure the safety of bone grafts:
Kühne J.-H., Bartl R., Hammer C., Refior H. J., Jansson V. and Zimmer M. (1993). Moderate heat treatment of bone allografts: Experimental results of osteointegration. *Arch. Orthop. Trauma Surg.*, **112**, 1

Osteoporosis

8

Osteoporosis is by far the most common metabolic disorder of bone[1,2,94], but is still one of the least well understood and when established the most difficult to treat as witnessed by the many different treatments which are advocated[1,6,21,41,84,88,93,105,109,112,117,119,134,135,140,143]. It is defined as a condition in which decreased bone mass and strength lead to an increased incidence of fractures caused by minimal trauma or even occurring without[25,34,40,58,97]. Clinically we tend to make a diagnosis of osteoporosis when fractures and deformities have already occurred. The terms 'osteopenia' or 'asymptomatic osteoporosis' have been used to describe individuals who have a decreased bone mass but have not yet sustained a fracture. Bone density at any time during adult life is the result of peak bone mass achieved in early adulthood and subsequent bone loss[22]. In women at the menopause, 2 SD range is ±18% for the lumbar spine and ±24% for the femoral neck. Typically, postmenopausal bone loss is about 2% per year and gradually increases over 5–10 years after menopause[38,53,73,104,105]. The loss in bone mass is considerably greater in trabecular than in cortical bone[69].

But where is the borderline between 'normal' and 'excessive' bone loss, between 'physiological' osteopenia and 'accelerated' osteoporosis? The more widespread use of bone mass measurements has led to the following definition of osteoporosis: less than the 5th centile (i.e. − 2SD) of the bone mass at maturity of that population. The actual incidence of fractures in subjects with osteoporosis defined in this way is not known, and there is still controversy in the literature concerning the relationship between reduced bone mass and risk and rate of fracture[26].

The main causes of osteoporosis are shown in Table 8.1. Osteoporosis is called *primary*, if no other disease causing bone loss can be found. It occurs most commonly in postmenopausal and elderly women, and is then classified as *'age-related bone loss'*. Osteoporosis not clearly related to age can be grouped under the heading of *'accelerated bone loss'* and may occur as a result of a large number of underlying conditions (Table 8.1) with emphasis on their pathogenic mechanisms. Osteoporosis may coexist with osteomalacia, particularly in the elderly (poromalacia) and usually with nutritional deficiencies. However, other factors are also involved – e.g. which population groups are investigated; their age, and social status[45,78].

Patients with osteoporotic fractures have, on average, 30–50% less bone mass than normal young adults. The lower limit of bone mass for healthy young adults is usually taken as the fracture threshold, since 'physiological' reductions in bone mass with ageing are considered to reflect 'historic' bone loss and increased risk of fracture over the past. A valid test is still required for the only diagnostic criterion of osteoporosis, i.e. the low bone mass. Conventional X-rays cannot be used to determine the degree of bone loss at which fractures are likely to occur (Figs 8.R1–3)[63,96]. Over the past 20 years many methods for quantitation of bone mass have been developed (Table 8.2 and Fig. 8.R4)[38,60,61,146]. The number of procedures advocated is indicative of the need for such a measurement, but also reflects uncertainty about their respective accuracy and diagnostic value[69], and different methods may be suitable for different conditions[30,81]. No

Table 8.1 Main causes of osteopenia

Primary	*Haematopoietic*
Postmenopausal (type I)	Haemolytic anaemias
Senile (type II)	Aplastic anaemia
Juvenile	Myelodysplastic syndrome
Idiopathic	Chronic myeloproliferative disorders
	Acute leukaemias
Congenital	Chronic lymphoproliferative disorders
Osteogenesis imperfecta	Multiple myeloma
Marfan syndrome	Systemic mastocytosis
Ehlers–Danlos syndrome	
Homocystinuria	*Metabolic*
	Diabetes mellitus
Endocrine	Gaucher disease
Hyperparathyroidism	
Hyperthyroidism	*Metastatic*
Cushing syndrome	Diffuse bone metastasis
Hypogonadism	
Hyperprolactinaemia	*Drugs/toxins*
	Corticosteroids
Nutritional	Heparin
Malnutrition	Anticonvulsants
Scurvy	Excess of thyroid hormone replacement
Anorexia nervosa	Methotrexate
	Excess of alcohol
Gastrointestinal	
Gastrectomy	*Miscellaneous*
Primary biliary cirrhosis	Rheumatic and autoimmune disorders
Liver transplantation	Renal disease
Pancreatic disease	
Immobilization	
Bed rest	
Paraplegia	
Space flight	

technique has yet been widely accepted for the routine diagnosis of osteopenia. Osteoporotic bone loss affects preferentially the more metabolically active trabecular bone, and fractures occur at sites composed predominantly of trabecular bone. Thus measurements of the hand or the radius, which quantitate cortical bone, do not reflect the status of trabecular bone. Inaccuracies of up to 30% have been reported in vertebral measurements by CT (Fig. 8.R5). But with this method bone mass may be measured repeatedly at the same site in vertebrae in which fractures frequently occur[77].

Like osteomalacia, osteoporosis belongs to the group of 'metabolic' bone diseases. The common denominator of these diseases is their generalized distribution throughout the skeleton[31]. Consequently a sample of bone taken from

Table 8.2 List of techniques and skeletal sites measured

Methods of quantitating bone mass	
Technique	Site
Radiogrammetry	Metacarpals
Photon absorptiometry	Distal radius/ulna; femoral neck
Dual X-ray absorptiometry	Spine
Computed tomography	Spine
Neutron activation analysis	Total body calcium
Ultrasound	Patella; calcaneus
Iliac crest biopsy	Anterior iliac crest; posterior iliac crest

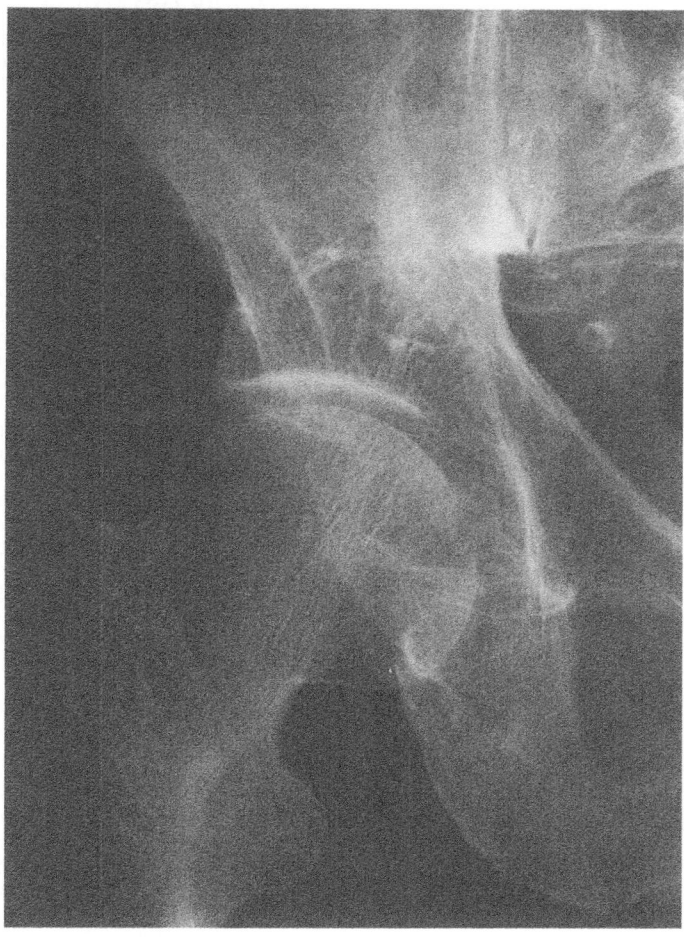

Fig. 8.R1   Marked osteopenia of pelvis and femur

one site should reflect changes occurring in the cancellous bone of the skeleton at large. This realization led to the use of the random bone biopsy in the histological evaluation of the osteopenic skeleton. The *iliac crest* is the preferred site for biopsy of patients with generalized disorders of bone[9,55,57]. A major advance in the histological evaluation of the osteopenic skeleton has been the development of techniques to prepare well-preserved, undecalcified semithin sections.

In young adults the iliac crest contains a fairly dense trabecular network with uniform ossicles regularly arranged[114]. There is no significant difference in iliac crest bone volume between young women and young men; both have a mean of about 27 vol% with a lower normal limit (mean minus 2 SD) of about 16 vol%. Trabecular changes in the different age groups are given in the chapter 'Ageing and bone structure' (Chap. 5). Autopsy studies indicate that 30–40 vol% of bone is lost during ageing in 'normal' men and women[114]. Loss of cortical bone is generally slower, with a peak in advanced age. Osteoporosis is characterized by trabecular bone loss and by cortical thinning[97].

Though there is no sharp distinction between 'normal' and excessive bone loss, patients with less than 16 vol% trabecular bone are defined as osteopenic in our biopsy reports. Evaluation of 400 biopsies of patients with primary osteopenia revealed four different *histological patterns of osteopenia* (Fig. 8.S1, Plate 8.A):

1. an irregular rarefaction of the cancellous bone volume, thickness and number, with marked differences in the various regions of the biopsy, ranging from normal structure to complete disappearance of trabeculae (44%),
2. an overall reduction in the thickness of the trabeculae (25% of the cases),
3. an overall reduction in the number of trabeculae, with coarse, broad ossicles and wide marrow spaces (15%), and
4. in severe osteopenia, presence of small discrete islands of bone (button phenomenon) rather than rods or spicules (16%).

These four histological patterns can be combined into two main histological types A and B (see Fig. 8.S2).

Histological heterogeneity in bone turnover has also been reported in osteoporosis. In our series 14% of the patients had only increased resorption, with active osteoclasts, deep resorption lacunae or even completely transected trabeculae, 26% had increased resorption and formation, while 60% of the patients had balanced remodelling or reduced bone turnover. Correlations between rates of bone formation and biochemical markers have

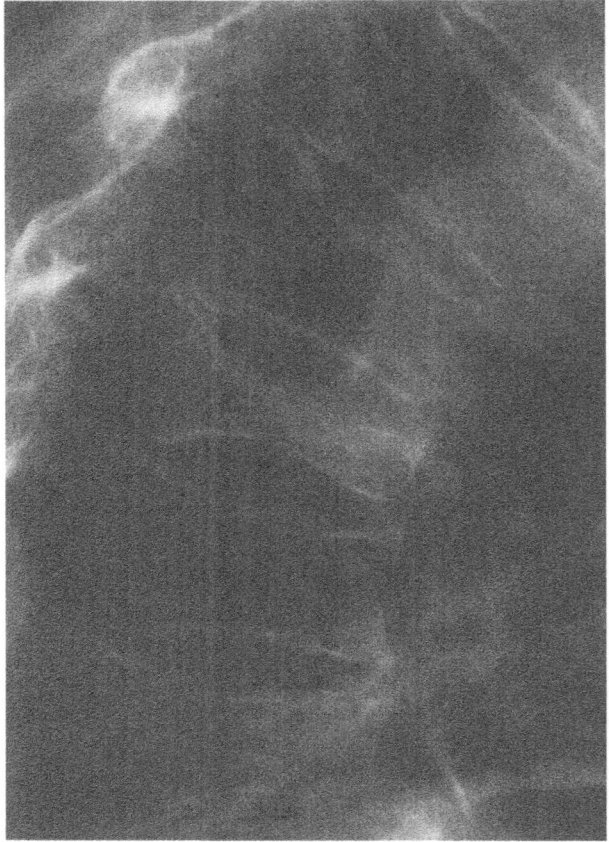

Fig. 8.R2 Marked osteopenia of the spine with 'pancake' vertebra

been published by Arlot[2,3] and by Delmas[30]. These variations in bone turnover, as either transient or long-lasting states, are used to describe the dynamics of the osteoporotic condition[101]: *'low turnover'* (inactive) and *'high turnover'* (active, accelerated) groups (Plates 8.B and C). Patients with a high remodelling activity also had significantly higher values for osteoid volume and surface (poromalacia). The relationship between haematopoiesis, bone remodelling and osteopenia has so far received very little attention and this could well be a promising area for future investigation[31,47,56]. Increase of the fatty tissue volume was observed in 60% of the cases, with four different topographic patterns of fatty tissue (Fig. 8.S3 and Plate 8.B):

1. diffuse (48%),
2. patchy (31%),
3. peritrabecular (4%), and
4. complete (7%).

Quantitative evaluation of the marrow in the osteopenic patients showed a reduction in haematopoiesis and sinusoids[31], and an increase in fatty and oedematous volumes (Fig. 8.S4). The main qualitative changes in the haematopoietic marrow were inflammatory, comprising increases in plasma cells, mast cells and lymphoid nodules[145]. Thickening and sclerosis of the walls of small arteries, capillaries and sinusoids were additional characteristics. Mast cell proliferation has been reported in postmenopausal osteoporosis[48].

PRIMARY OSTEOPOROSIS

Although there is considerable overlap, it is useful to divide age-related primary osteoporosis into two syndromes:

1. Type I osteoporosis

Type I osteoporosis, or the vertebral crush fracture syndrome, generally begins about 10 years after menopause and is also termed *postmenopausal osteoporosis* (approximately 85% of the cases are women). Loss of trabecular bone is the major underlying pathological change, with vertebral crush fractures and Colles' fractures of the wrist. Some patients have chronic back pain and show height loss and deformity. It is not clear, however, whether decreased trabecular bone mass occurs because their peak mass at maturity was lower[76] or because of rapid loss, particularly shortly after the menopause; or a combination of the two[68]. However, it has recently been shown that significant amounts of bone may be lost before the menopause.

Age-related osteoporosis is systemic and a bone biopsy is generally diagnostic, showing trabecular osteopenia[83]. Increased osteoclastic activity in the iliac crest indicates an active, progressive course[66]. It is likely, however, that bone loss is not inevitably progressive. Intermittent periods of loss may be separated by variable periods of a steady-state condition, or even by some degree of improvement, i.e. bone formation. Thus, age-related bone loss can be modified by many other factors, and there is considerable heterogeneity of osteoporotic syndromes and their response to calcitonin therapy[5,62].

Type II osteoporosis

This is a term recently applied to older patients with fractures of the proximal femur (*senile* or *involutional osteoporosis*)[118,130]. Loss of both trabecular and cortical bone is involved. As a general rule, senile osteoporosis corresponds to bone atrophy (involution), with inactive osteopenia in the biopsy. Increased osteoid (poromalacia) is relatively rare in these patients[24]. There is cortical thinning, together with increased porosity and a severe reduction in trabecular volume resulting in loss of the normal microarchitecture. Alterations in the lamellar arrangement of the trabeculae are frequent and may contribute to increased bone fragility. Fewer bone cells per unit of bone, hypocellularity of the marrow as well as degenerative changes of vasculature characterize the atrophic process of ageing[23].

Idiopathic osteoporosis

This is a term applied to premenopausal women or relatively young men with localized osteoporosis for which there does not appear to be a cause[129]. Usually bone loss is confined to the spine, and an iliac crest biopsy is not diagnostic[121]; it shows normal trabecular structure and turnover. Only a few patients had histological evidence of increased bone resorption. Hills *et al.* have demonstrated by double tetracycline labelling that the osteoclastic and osteoblastic numbers were normal in the group of patients with young adult osteoporosis but that the metabolic activity of osteoblasts was impaired[71].

Juvenile osteoporosis

Juvenile osteoporosis, a rare disorder, develops at the time of the pubertal growth spurt and predominantly involves the axial skeleton (vertebrae, ribs and, less pronounced, the pelvis)[13,79]. In these patients there may be a dissociation between linear growth and the ability

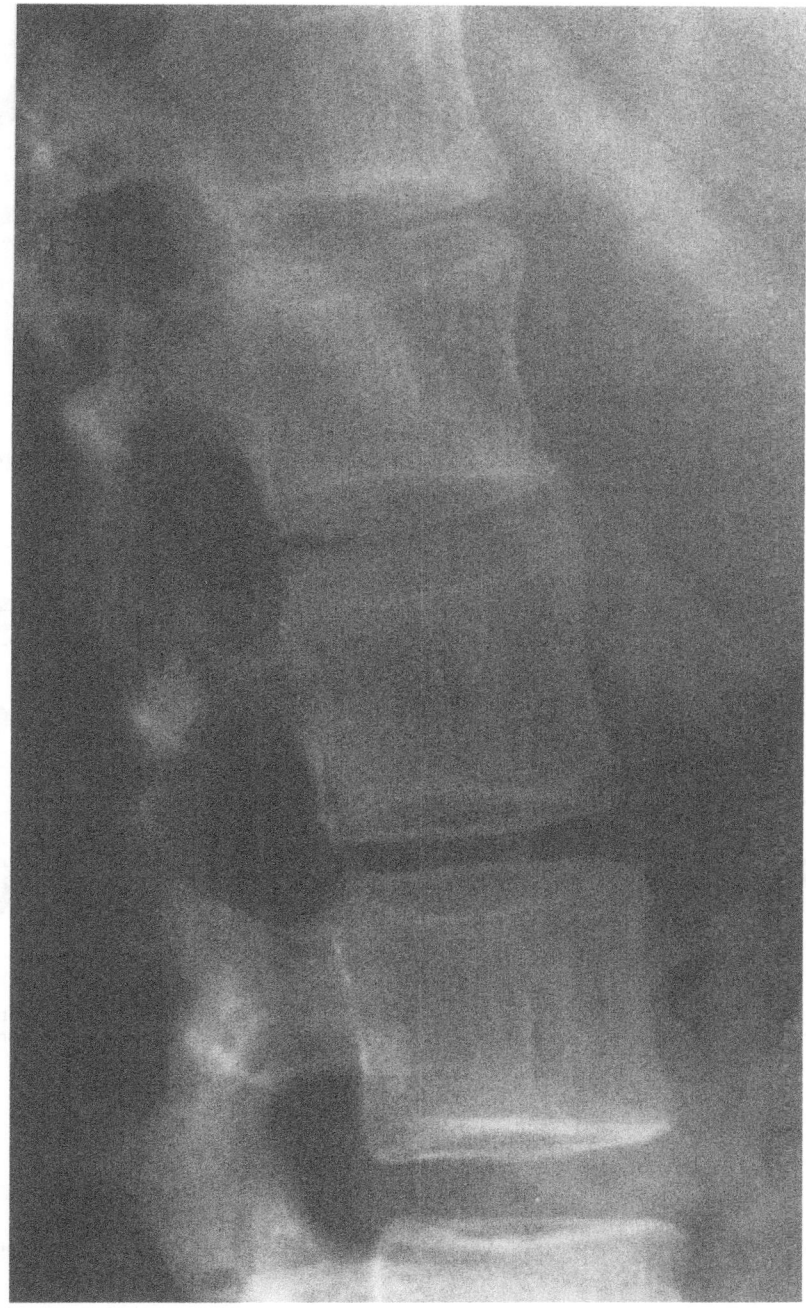

Fig. 8.R3 Juvenile osteopenia. Note relative preservation of the stress-bearing vertical trabeculae

to consolidate and strengthen the skeleton. Thus vertebral or other fractures may occur. The disease appears to be self-limited and as puberty progresses, bone mass and strength gradually return to normal. The condition from which it is most difficult to distinguish is mild osteogenesis imperfecta.

ENDOCRINE OSTEOPOROSIS

The skeleton is affected by many hormones and growth factors[53,59,69,73,91,111], and metabolic bone disease is fre-

quent in patients with endocrine disorders[82]. It is important to recognize this because most of these underlying disorders are treatable. Moreover, subtle endocrine abnormalities may exist in patients with age-related osteoporosis and aggravate their clinical problems. In a recent review, underlying medical conditions were identified in 20% of the women and in 40% of men presenting with osteoporotic fractures. Osteoporosis associated with *pregnancy and lactation* has also been reported[65,131]. These patients did not have osteomalacia or high-turnover osteoporotic features, and it is possible that this type of

[continued on p. 106]

Plate 8.A

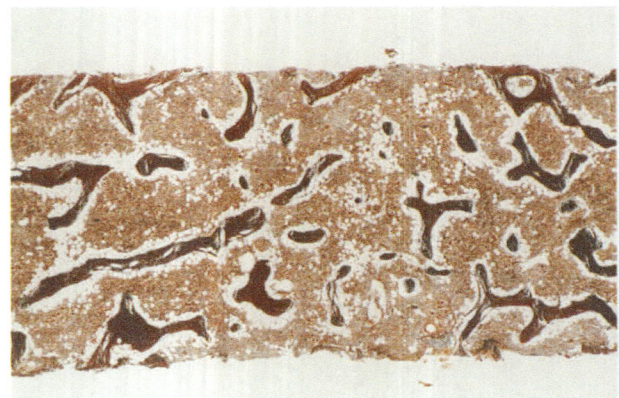

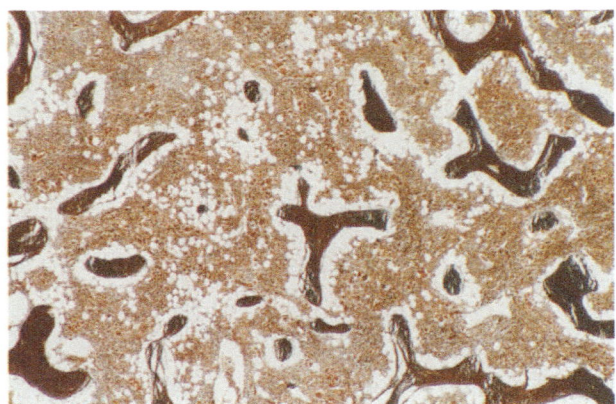

Figs. 8.1–8.6   Different histological patterns of osteopenia I

Fig. 8.1   Minimal reduction in trabecular bone volume, but overall reduction in trabecular width. Gomori

Fig. 8.2   Note rim of fat cells surrounding the ossicles which possibly represents an incipient phase in the atrophy of trabecular bone ('low-turnover' osteopenia). Gomori

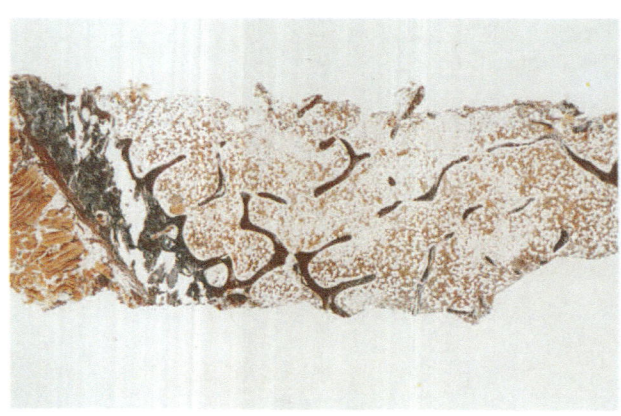

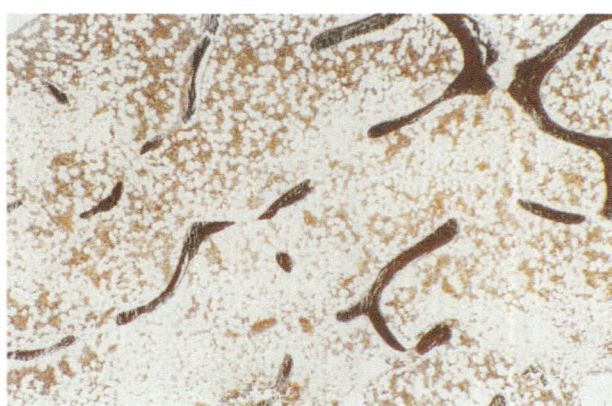

Fig. 8.3   Overview of iliac crest biopsy showing overall reduction in the width of trabecular plates. Note that there is no decrease in cortical bone thickness. Gomori

Fig. 8.4   Higher magnification showing thin trabeculae and patchy increase in fat cells with uneven distribution: osteoporosis, histological type A. Gomori

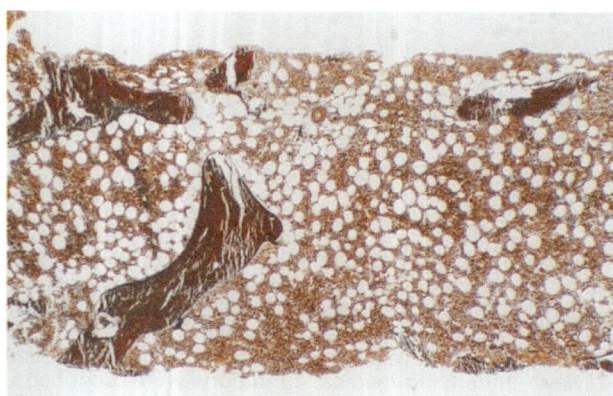

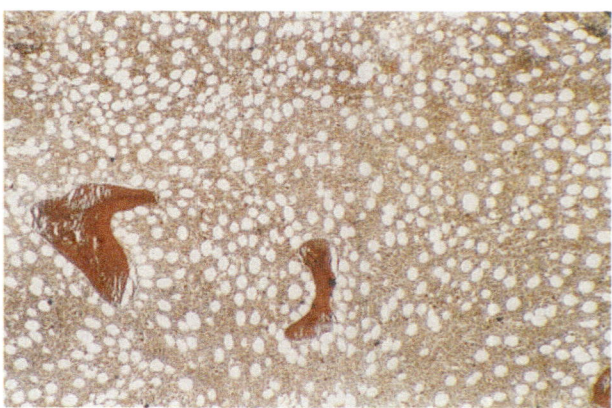

Fig. 8.5   Overall reduction in trabecular number with residual broad ossicles in subcortical region (left). Gomori

Fig. 8.6   Central and deeper part of same biopsy. Few trabeculae and wide marrow spaces corresponding to osteoporosis, histological type B. Gomori

Plate 8.B

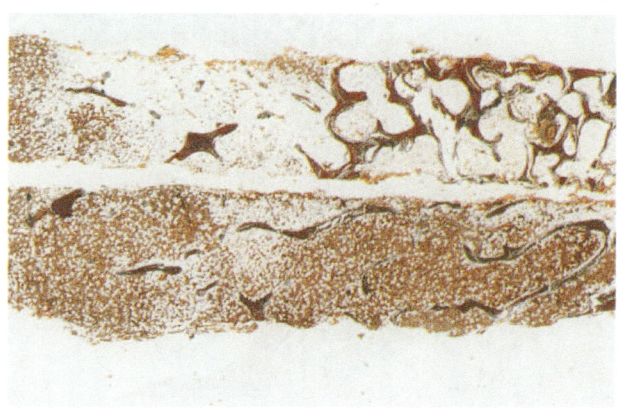

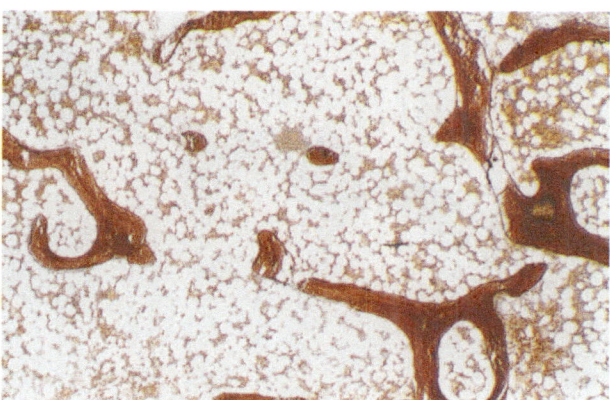

Figs. 8.7–8.12 Histological patterns of osteopenia II

Fig. 8.7 Overview showing irregular, patchy reduction in trabecular bone and haematopoiesis. In this biopsy there is no correlation between trabecular bone volume and marrow cellularity. Gomori

Fig. 8.8 Higher magnification of hypocellular area with patchy osteopenia (small 'buttons'). Note small lymphoid nodule (centre). Gomori

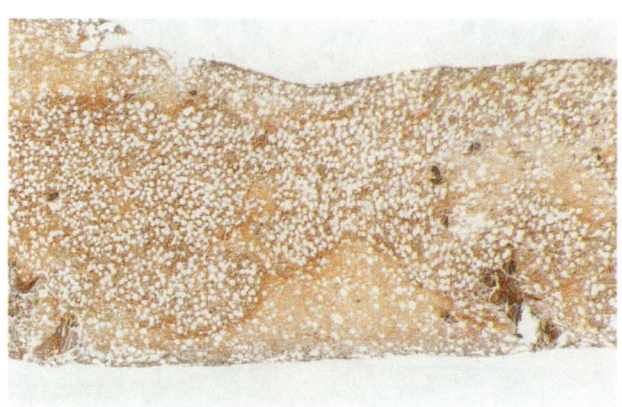

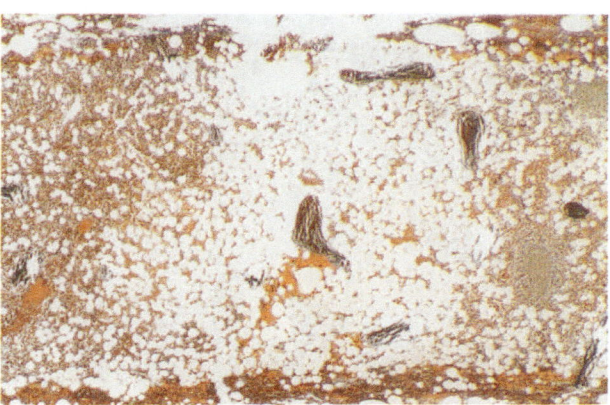

Fig. 8.9 Severe osteopenia with only small islands of bone (button phenomenon). Gomori

Fig. 8.10 Biopsy section illustrating drastic reduction in trabecular bone, hypocellular bone marrow and two small lymphoid nodules (right). Gomori. Benign lymphoid hyperplasia in iliac crest biopsy of older individuals has been associated with osteoporosis

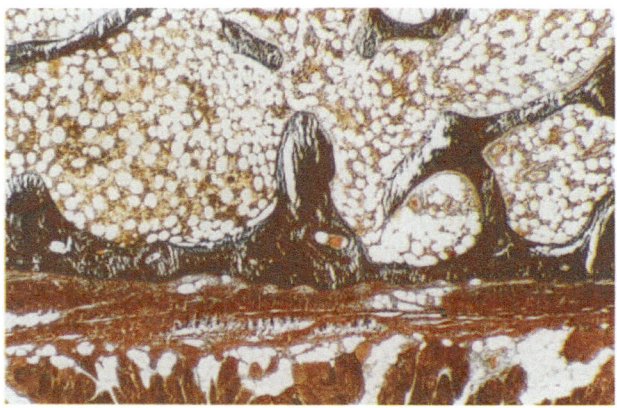

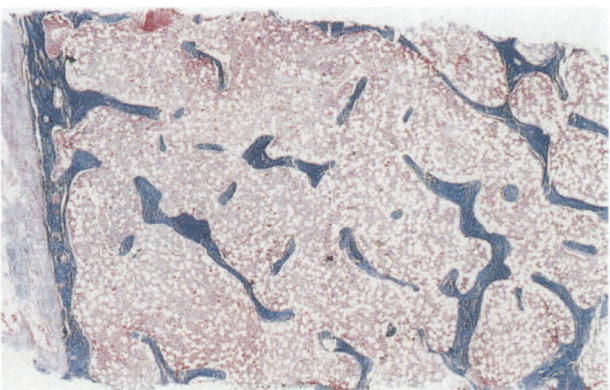

Fig. 8.11 Bone biopsy section with thin cortex. Gomori

Fig. 8.12 Biopsy with attenuated cortex and greater trabecular rarefaction in the subcortical zone than in the central area (left). Ladewig

Plate 8.C

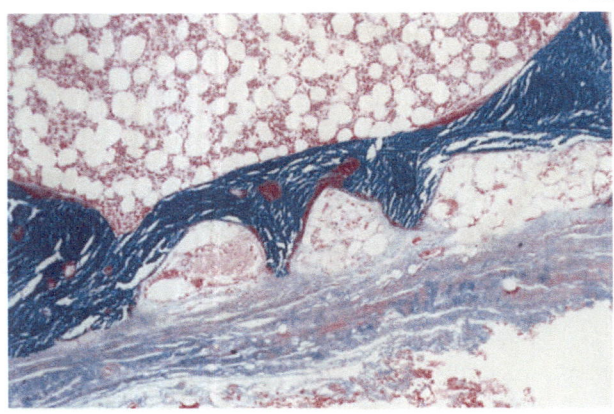

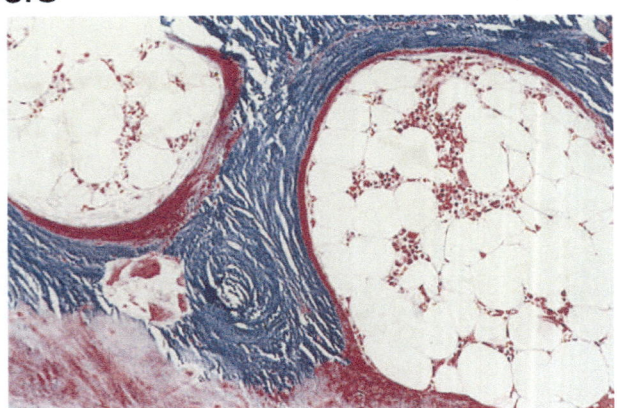

Figs. 8.13–8.18 High- and low-turnover osteopenia

Fig. 8.13 Cortex of bone biopsy with osteopenia (not shown in this figure). Note increased porosity and several foci of remodelling. Ladewig

Fig. 8.14 Higher magnification of biopsy in Fig. 8.13 with osteoid seam extending into cortex (= incipient osteoporomalacia) and osteoclasts in resorption cavity – 'dissecting osteoclasia'. Ladewig

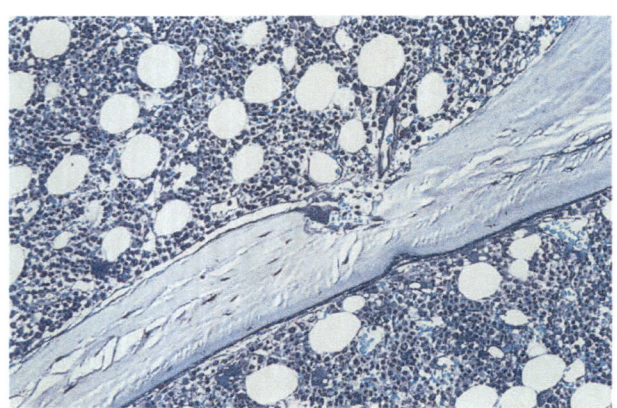

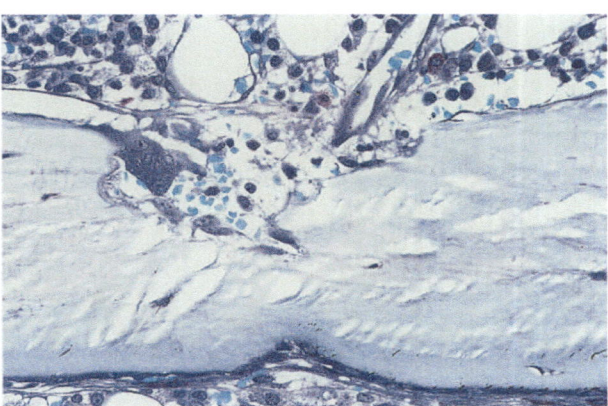

Fig. 8.15 Ossicle in iliac crest biopsy of patient with osteoporosis. Note cellular bone marrow and superficial bone remodelling. Giemsa

Fig. 816 Higher magnification of Fig. 8.15 illustrating deep osteoclastic resorption cavity, and osteoid seam lined by osteoblasts on opposite side of the trabecula. Giemsa. Similar deep resorption cavities – 'transsecting osteoclasia' – would predispose to trabecular microfractures in weight-bearing bones such as the vertebrae

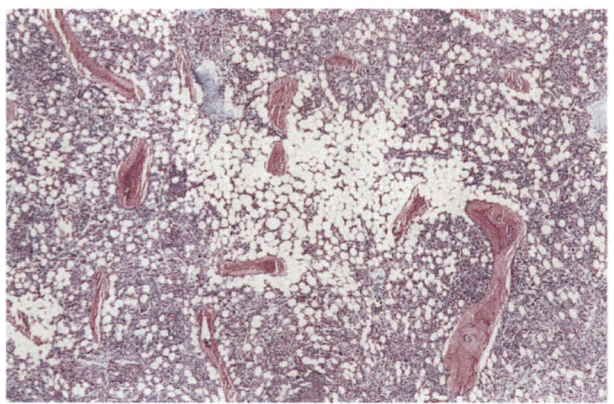

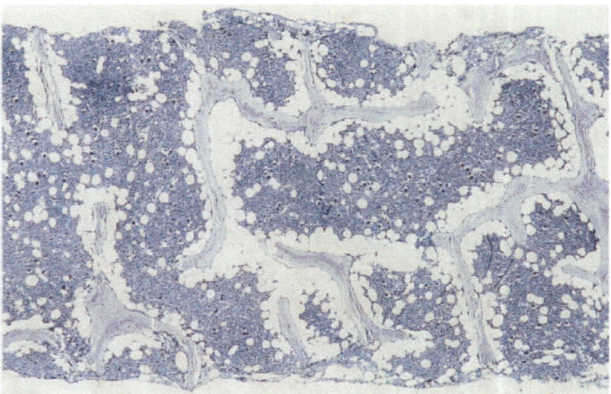

Fig. 8.17 Low-turnover osteopenia with patchy replacement of marrow by fat cells. H&E

Fig. 8.18 Low-turnover osteopenia with paratrabecular localization of fat cells. No osseous remodelling seen in these sections. Giemsa

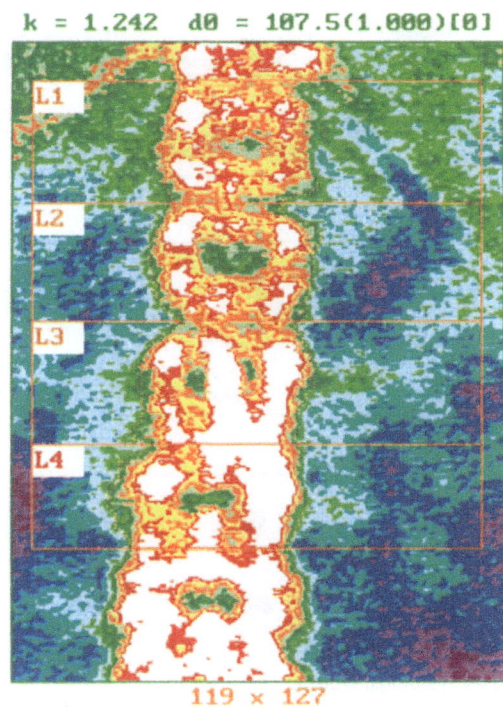

k = 1.242   d0 = 107.5(1.000)[0]

119 × 127

A10109103   Thu 10 Oct 1991 11:25
Name:
Comment:
I.D.:   91 / 46   Sex: F
S.S.#:   - -   Ethnic: W
ZIPCode: Height: 65.00 cm
Scan Code: Weight: 78.00 kg
BirthDate: Age: 59
Physician:

TOTAL BMD CV FOR L1 - L4 1.0%

C.F.   1.003   1.074   1.000

Region	Area (cm2)	BMC (grams)	BMD (gms/cm2
L1	11.52	6.90	0.599
L2	12.40	9.42	0.760
L3	13.50	13.96	1.034
TOTAL	37.42	30.29	0.809

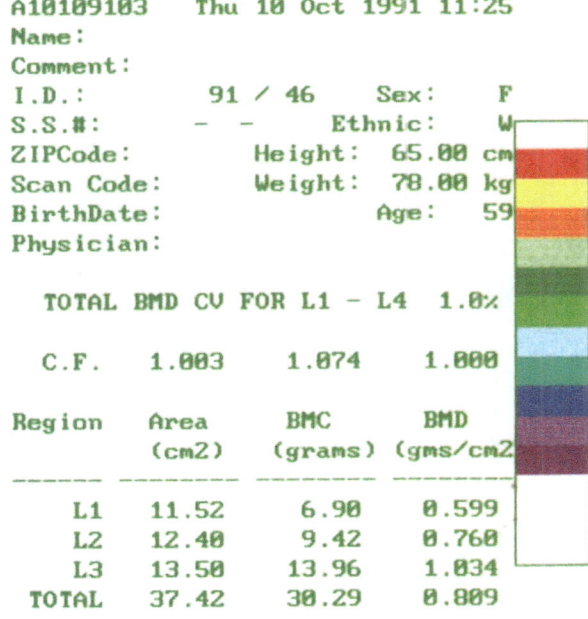

Reference Database *

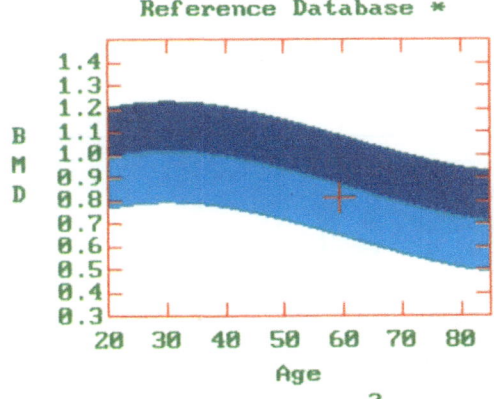

$BMD(L1-L3) = 0.809 \ g/cm^2$

Region	BMD	T(30.0)		Z	
L1	0.599	-2.96	65%	-1.76	76%
L2	0.760	-2.44	74%	-1.10	86%
L3	1.034	-0.45	95%	+0.96	111%
N/A					
L1-L3	0.809	-1.90	79%	-0.57	93%

* Age and sex matched
Reference Curve for Females
                    TK   13 Oct 89

Reference Database *

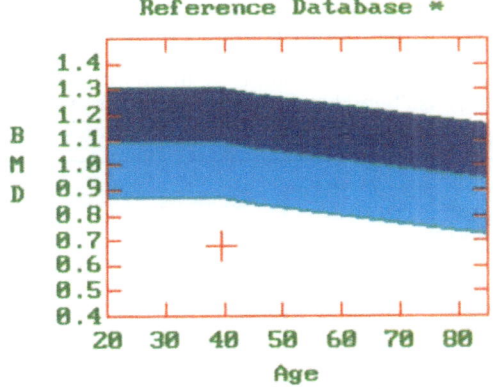

$BMD(L1-L4) = 0.676 \ g/cm^2$

Region	BMD	T(30.0)		Z	
L1	0.637	-3.37	63%	-3.37	63%
L2	0.671	-3.85	61%	-3.85	61%
L3	0.640	-4.21	58%	-4.21	58%
L4	0.741	-3.67	65%	-3.67	65%
L1-L4	0.676	-3.77	62%	-3.77	62%

* Age and sex matched
Reference Curve for Males
                    TK   13 Oct 89

Fig. 8.R4 Dual X-ray absorptiometry (DXA) of the lumbar spine in anteroposterior projection: the different vertebral levels L1 to L4 are elevated separately. AP measurements integrate areas of purely trabecular bone located within the vertebral body as well as zones of predominantly compact bone located in the vertebral endplates and the posterior spinal elements. Diagram of normal density in a femal individual (lower left) and diagram of decreased density in a male patient (lower right).

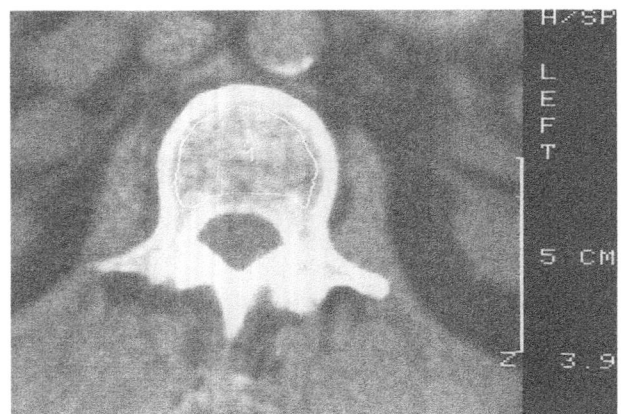

Fig. 8.R5 Assessment of vertebral bone mass by CT. Slice at the level of L2. The trabecular bone within the area delineated ('centrum' CT) is measured volumetrically

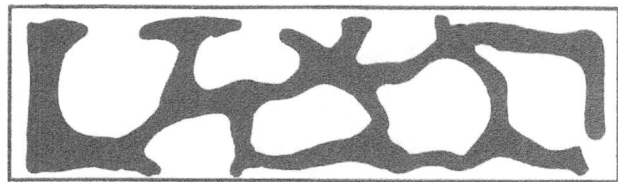

Normal compacta and trabecular bone

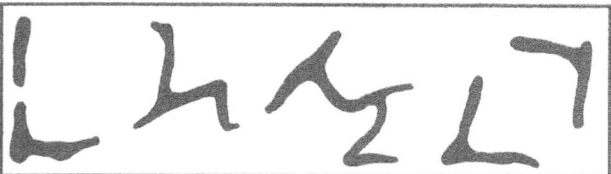

Osteoporosis, histologic type A

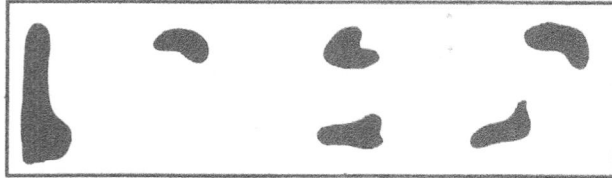

Osteoporosis, histologic type B

Fig. 8.S2 Comparison of normal cortical and trabecular bone in iliac crest biopsy with osteoporosis, histological types A and B

osteoporosis may be somewhat self-limiting depending on any adaptive lifestyle changes introduced by the patients. Men with a history of *delayed puberty* may also be at increased risk for osteoporotic fractures when they are older. This correlation demonstrates that the peak bone mass achieved during young adulthood is a major determinant of bone density in later life[51].

Two common endocrine conditions, hyperthyroidism and hypercorticosteroidism, have direct effects on bone.

Endogenous thyroid hormone affects bone by directly activating osteoclasts to resorb bone, which results in decreased bone mineral content[102]. In *thyrotoxicosis*, bone histology is 'hyperkinetic' with increases in both

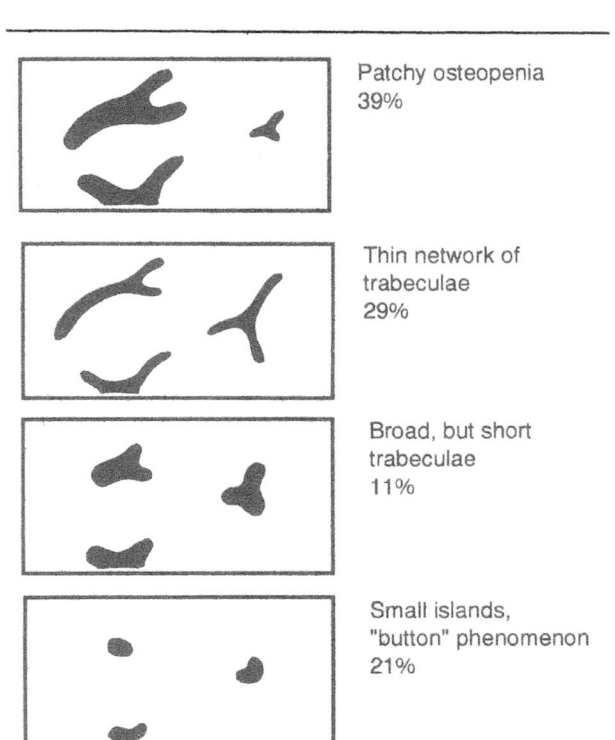

Patchy osteopenia
39%

Thin network of trabeculae
29%

Broad, but short trabeculae
11%

Small islands, "button" phenomenon
21%

Fig. 8.S1 Diagram of the four histological patterns of osteopenia

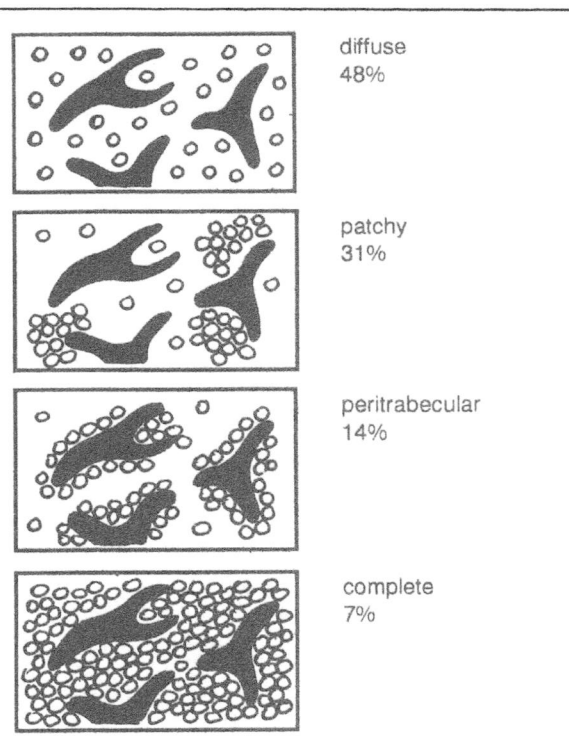

diffuse
48%

patchy
31%

peritrabecular
14%

complete
7%

Fig. 8.S3 Patterns of distribution and extent of fatty tissue in iliac crest biopsies of patients with osteoporosis

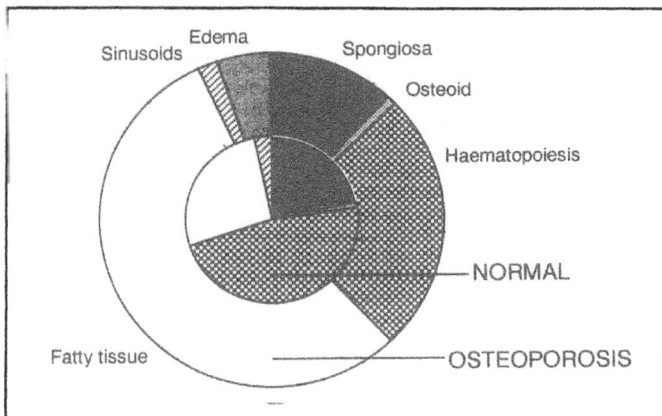

Fig. 8.S4 Volumetric comparison of components of iliac crest biopsy in normal (*n* = 100) and osteoporotic (*n* = 400) patients

osteoclast and osteoblast activities[4]. Bone resorption is more pronounced than bone formation and accelerates the bone loss associated with ageing and menopause. Mineralization is normal. Hyperthyroidism should be considered in all cases with obscure accelerated osteoporosis. The influence of *long-term L-thyroxine replacement therapy* on bone mass is of growing interest because of the large number of women receiving thyroid hormone therapy[54,64]. However, a recent study could demonstrate that the changes in bone density in women receiving long-term L-thyroxine therapy in the physiological range are minimal at most and should not be a contraindication to therapy[123].

The effects of *corticosteroids* differ from those of thyroxine. They appear to stimulate bone resorption and, simultaneously, to inhibit osteoid synthesis[72]. This combination is likely to cause rapid bone loss. The impairment of calcium absorption might also be expected to lead to impaired mineralization and osteomalacia. However, histological examination does not reveal wide osteoid seams, probably because the formation of matrix is also decreased. The altered formation of bone could also be due to reduced replication of osteoblast precursors and to an effect of corticosteroids on local prostaglandin synthesis. Osteoporosis has been observed in more than 80% of patients with Cushing's disease. Glucocorticoid excess is associated with an increased frequency of aseptic bone necrosis. The most common form of glucocorticoid-induced osteopenia is that due to long-term steroid therapy. An iliac crest bone biopsy confirms a striking reduction in trabecular and cortical bone, a low turnover, a marked increase in fatty tissue and inflammatory vascular changes. Because many patients receiving long-term steroid therapy suffer from inflammatory disorders that result in prolonged immobilization or produce local bone loss (e.g. rheumatoid arthritis or spondylarthritis), osteoporosis may be due in part to the primary disease and in part to glucocorticoid therapy. In contrast to the situation in thyrotoxicosis, the bone remains osteopenic after treatment for Cushing's disease or reduction of the steroid dose (in the absence of additional therapy aimed at improving the status of the bones). Whether inhaled corticosteroids do adversely affect skeletal growth in asthmatic children remains unclear. But recently Teelucksingh *et al.* (1991) demonstrated reduced formation in adults at what may be regarded as a standard paediatric dose[139].

Additional endocrine causes of osteoporosis are acromegaly[35], post-oophorectomy[52], hypogonadism, hypo-pituitarism, anorexia nervosa[7,120,141], hyperprolactinaemia[74] and disorders associated with secretion of calcitonin. Especially amenorrhoea in young women should be investigated and treated to prevent bone mineral loss[29,110,137]. However, the effect of intensive exercise may partially compensate for the adverse effect of amenorrhoea[37]. Also in women with anorexia nervosa, a high level of physical activity has been reported to protect the skeleton, as in athletes[145].

NUTRITIONAL OSTEOPOROSIS

This is frequently caused by inadequate dietary calcium[82]; other nutritional and gastrointestinal factors have also been implicated, although their relative importance is unclear. Moreover, excessive dietary protein, caffeine, alcohol[11,19,32,115], nicotine, lifestyle[106] as well as drugs[42,122] have all been considered as additional risk factors for osteoporosis[78,90,98,134].

Four main causes of malnutrition may be involved in the development of osteoporosis:

1. impaired dietary intake[10], including anorexia nervosa[7,120,137,141],
2. impaired absorption,
3. increased dietary loss of nutrients, and
4. hepatobiliary and pancreatic disorders associated with intestinal malabsorption.

Demineralization of the skeleton following gastric surgery has frequently been reported and both osteoporosis and osteomalacia can be complications of gastrectomy[12].

In summary, metabolic bone disease related to malnutrition is usually a combination of osteoporosis, osteomalacia and secondary hyperparathyroidism, and bone biopsy is a useful tool to quantitate each of these variants (Plate 8.D).

HEPATIC OSTEOPOROSIS

There are many bone biopsy studies concerning 'hepatic osteodystrophy' in *chronic liver disease*[33,70,125,128]. Osteoporosis and osteomalacia have both been described, but as is now realized, bone loss is the main clinical problem and impaired bone mineralization is rare[132]. Diminished bone formation is linked to impaired osteoblastic activity due to liver disease itself or to direct toxic effects of alcohol and excess of iron, aluminium, fluoride[92] or copper.

In *primary biliary cirrhosis* (PBC) bone loss results from trabecular plate thinning rather than from removal of whole ossicles, since the mean trabecular thickness is decreased in histomorphometry[133,144]. Total resorption surfaces are also significantly increased in PBC, suggesting that increased osteoclastic resorption may also contribute to bone loss in hepatic osteoporosis[28].

A further considerable bone loss occurs during the first 3 months after *liver transplantation*, frequently resulting in vertebral fractures[67,99]. The pathogenesis is likely to be multifactorial, although immobilization and corticosteroid therapy appear to be important causes.

IMMOBILIZATION OSTEOPOROSIS (Plate 8.E)

It is well established that the maintenance of bone mass is dependent on skeletal stress through muscle contraction and weight-bearing[43,44,86,87,106,142]. Thus, reduction in physical activity and weight-bearing may be major factors in age-related bone loss[17]. In healthy volunteers complete bed rest has been associated with bone loss of about 4% of bone mass per month[36], and osteoclasts have been implicated[18]. This bone loss affects primarily the weight-bearing parts of the skeleton[89,136]. With return to normal

[continued on p. 110]

Plate 8.D

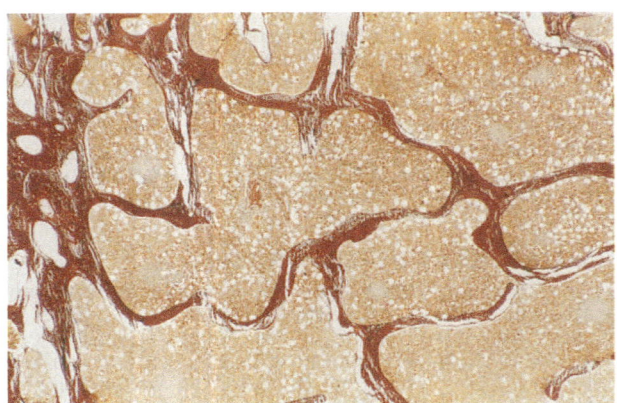

Figs. 8.19–8.24 Iliac crest biopsies of patients with osteoporosis due to various underlying conditions I

Fig. 8.19 Iliac crest biopsy of patient with osteoporosis. Note porosity of cortex and overall attenuation in trabecular width, but preservation of continuity of trabecular network. Multiple small lymphoid nodules. Gomori

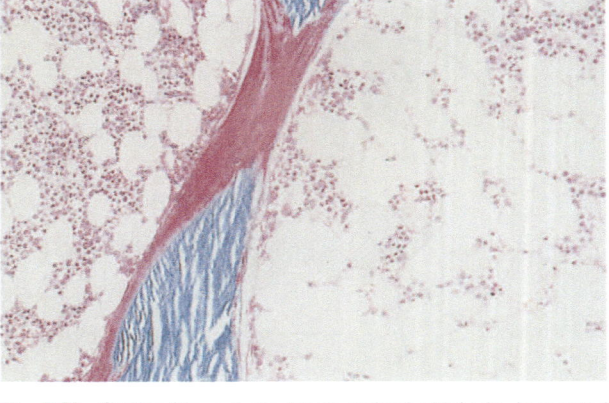

Fig. 8.20 Section from a similar biopsy stained with Ladewig revealed many foci of unmineralized bone demonstrating 'poromalacia'. Note osteoid spanning trabecular width. Ladewig

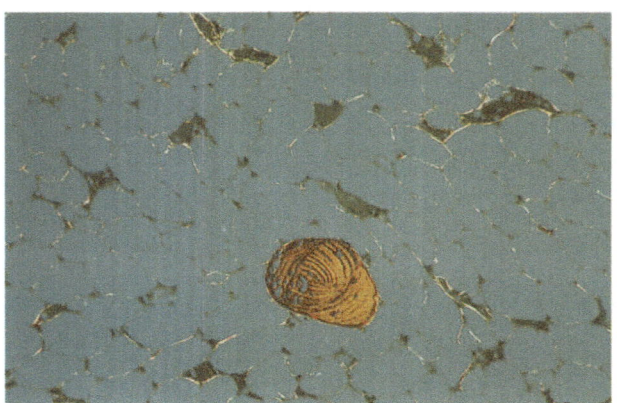

Fig. 8.21 Iliac crest biopsy section of patient with aplastic anaemia and osteoporosis. Note replacement of marrow fat cells and 'button phenomena'. Gomori, polar.

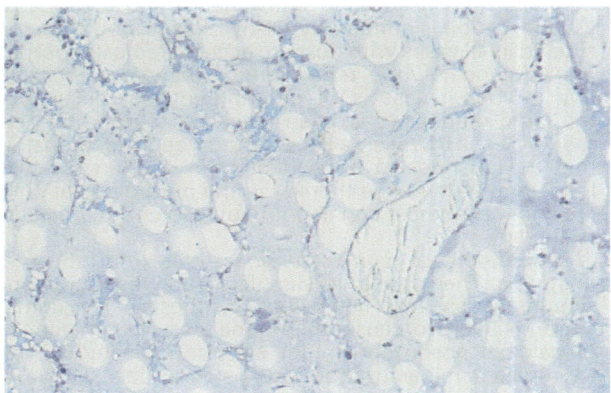

Fig. 8.22 Iliac crest biopsy of patient with anorexia nervosa. Replacement of marrow by serous atrophy, marked osteopenia and absence of osseous remodelling. Similar pictures may be seen in iliac crest biopsies of patients with malnutrition of whatever cause. Giemsa

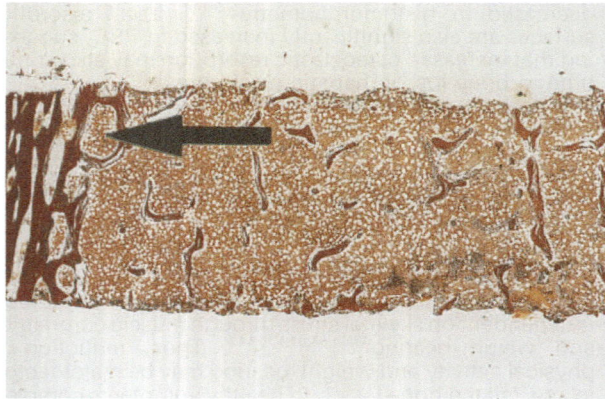

Figs. 8.23 and **8.24** Section of iliac crest biopsy of patient with 'typical' postmenopausal osteoporosis documented by X-ray, CT and DXA

Fig. 8.23 Note porosity of cortical bone and extreme reduction in trabecular bone volume (osteoporosis, histological type A), cellular marrow. Gomori

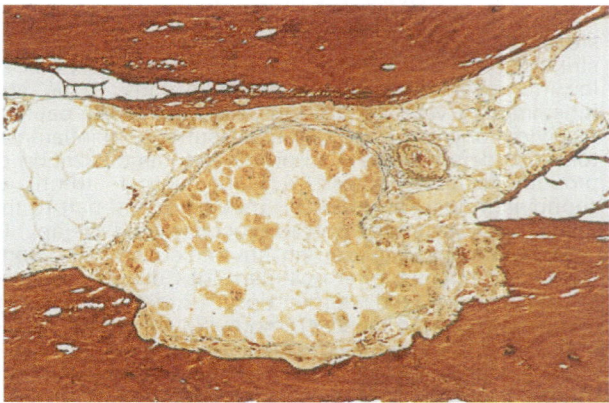

Fig. 8.24 However, higher magnification revealed metastatic carcinoma, 'micrometastasis', in the subcortical region (at arrow in Fig. 8.23), with erosion of bone (lower centre). Gomori

Plate 8.E

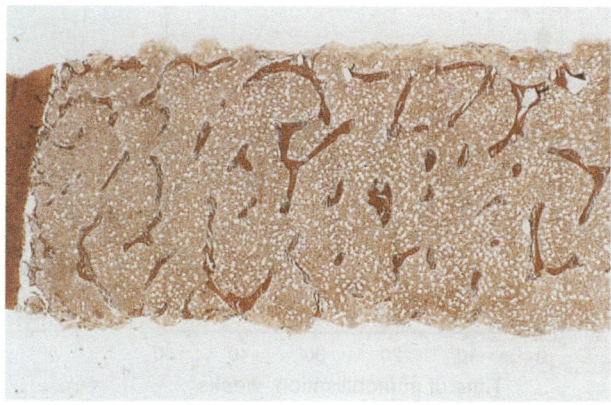

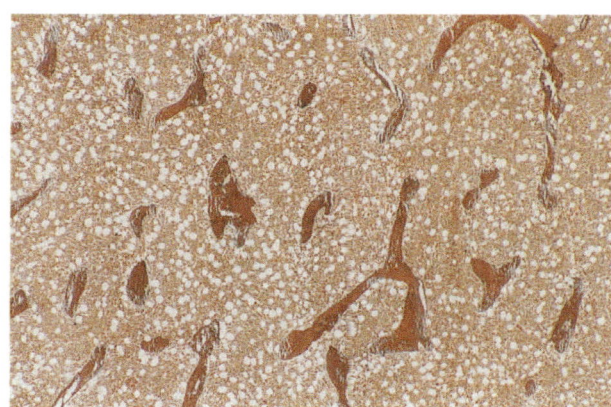

Figs. 8.25–8.30 Iliac crest biopsies of patients with osteoporosis due to various underlying conditions II

Figs. 8.25 and 8.26 Low and high magnification of iliac crest biopsy of child demonstrating immobilization osteoporosis

Fig. 8.25 Note growth plate. Gomori

Fig. 8.26 Cellular bone marrow and reduction in trabecular bone volume with attenuated trabeculae. Gomori

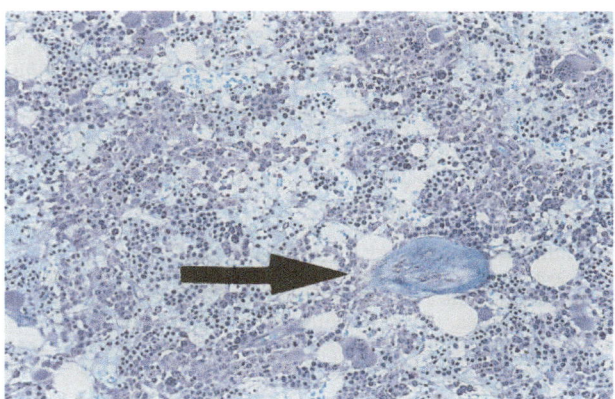

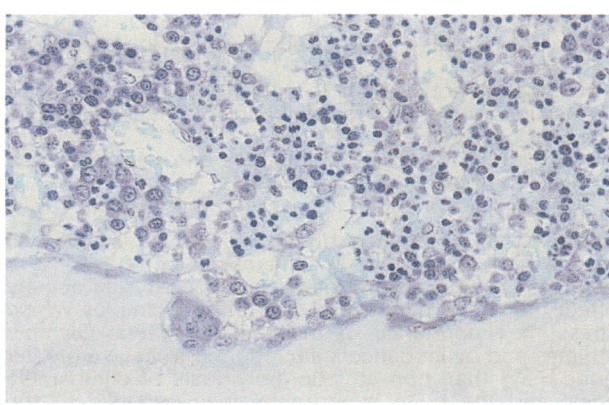

Fig. 8.27 Osteoporosis in iliac crest biopsy of patient with congenital haemolytic anaemia, showing 'button phenomenon' with osteoid seam (arrow). Giemsa

Fig. 8.28 Osteoporosis in iliac crest biopsy of patient with acquired haemolytic anaemia, showing hyperplastic erythropoiesis and osteoclastic bone resorption. Giemsa

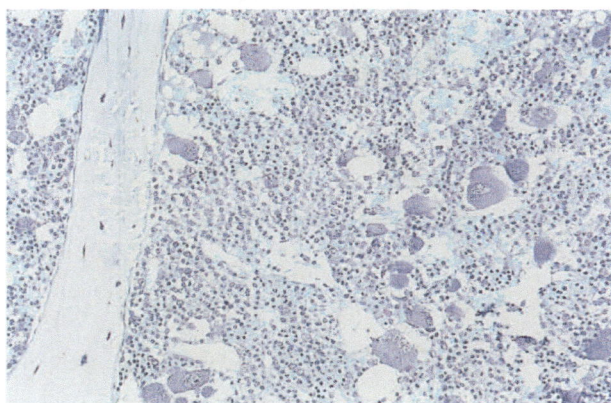

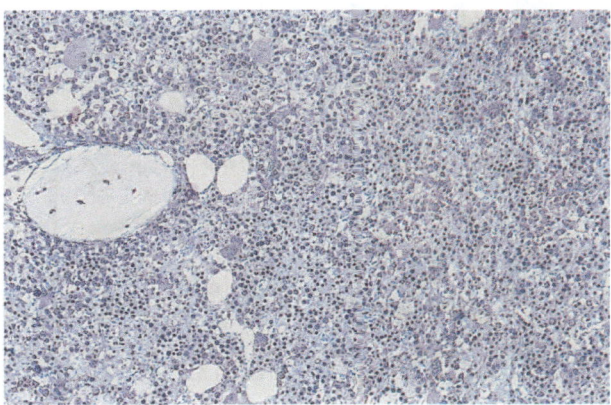

Fig. 8.29 Osteoporosis in iliac crest biopsy of patient with polycythaemia vera. Note thin ossicle with no remodelling; hypercellular bone marrow due to the myeloproliferation. Giemsa

Fig. 8.30 Osteoporosis in iliac crest biopsy of patient with chronic myeloid leukaemia. Note cross-section of ossicle at left and hypercellular bone marrow with few residual fat cells. Giemsa

activity the bone mass is restored over comparable periods of time. The bone tissue of childhood with its high modelling and remodelling activity is particularly susceptible to muscular inactivity (Fig. 8.S5).

In a prospective study we investigated the influence of immobilization on the bone structure of children (age 5–15 years). Iliac crest biopsies were taken at the beginning of immobilization predominantly caused by fractures of the lower extremities or by other traumata. Sequential biopsies were taken during the immobilization period, with a maximum interval of 35 weeks. The main results of this histomorphometric study were (Fig. 8.S6):

1. The trabecular volumes before immobilization ranged from 27 to 32 vol%, with a mean of 29 vol%.
2. Immobilization caused a rapid bone loss in all patients, and after 6 weeks the trabecular bone volume had dropped to < 20 vol%, with a minimum of 14 vol%. There were no morphological changes in the epiphyseal growth plate, and the osteoblastic and osteoclastic indices were not increased.
3. After an immobilization period of 10 weeks bone mass was reduced to about half of the initial volume (mean of 15 vol%), and longer periods of rest did not lead to further reductions ('lower plateau level').
4. There was a correlation between the duration and the degree of immobilization and bone loss. Complete disuse (i.e. paralysis) caused profound bone loss (Fig. 8.S6).
5. During immobilization a marked hypercalciuria was observed in 90% of the children, but hypercalcaemia never occurred.
6. With return to normal activity the bone mass increased over the period of observation (maximum of 12 months), but not quite to the pre-immobilization levels.

Sustained weightlessness during space flight is now well recognized as resulting in generalized bone loss[126]. In contrast, changes in bone mass relating to physical activity affect individual bones, and it is these examples which stress the importance of mechanical effects. Olympic athletes and ballet dancers are reported to have a greater bone mass than non-athletic individuals of comparable ages, and the bone hypertrophy was localized to the

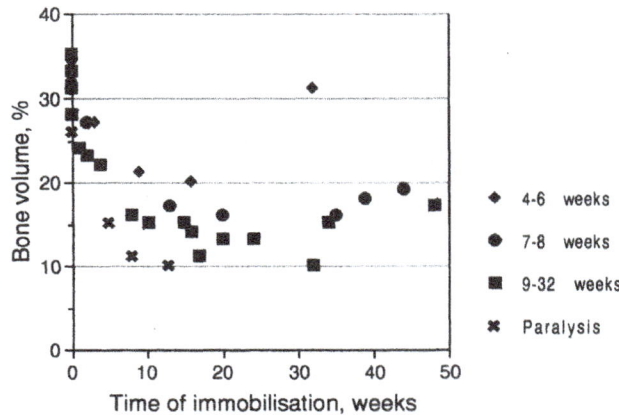

Fig. 8.S6 Reduction in trabecular bone volume in iliac crest biopsies of children correlated with length of time of immobilization

stressed parts of the skeleton[69]. The cortical thickness of the humerus of tennis players is greater on the playing side than on the non-playing side.

DIABETIC OSTEOPOROSIS

Osteoporosis is not generally considered to be a major complication of diabetes mellitus, but the bone mass is reduced, and this is associated with an increased risk of fracture. Mechanisms of bone loss include decreased bone formation due to insulin insufficiency[116], the loss of calcium in the urine due to glycosuria, decreased physical activity, or increased bone resorption for other reasons. Recently, more attention has been paid to bone disease in diabetes mellitus[15,127].

To address the question of the occurrence of diabetic osteomyelopathy as a distinct entity, we investigated iliac crest biopsies of 120 patients with manifest diabetes mellitus. Histomorphometry of the vascular system (Fig. 8.S7), bone and marrow was performed. In our study

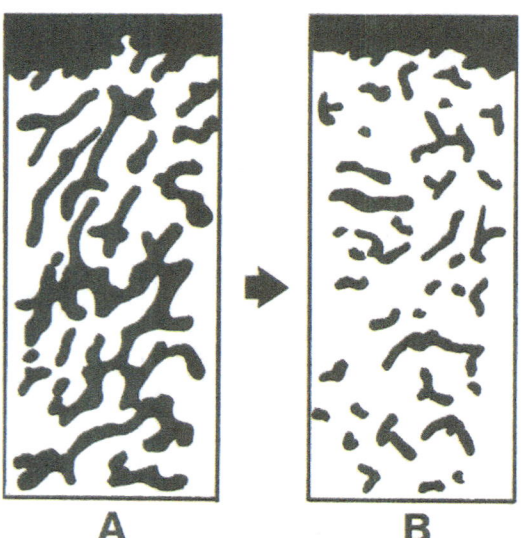

Fig. 8.S5 Iliac crest biopsy of child before (**A**) and after (**B**) a period of 17 weeks of immobilization. There is a marked reduction in trabecular volume

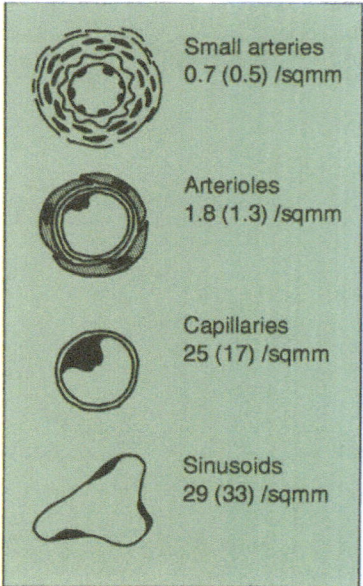

Fig. 8.S7 Histomorphometry of the vascular system in iliac crest biopsy of patients with diabetes mellitus. Note that arterioles and capillaries are increased, while the sinusoids are decreased (normal mean values in brackets)

diabetic microangiopathy was found in 82% of the biopsies as shown by degenerative changes of the vessel walls, perivascular increase in fibres (collagen type III) as well as in plasma cells and mast cells[8]. Possibly an increased vascular permeability caused by diabetic subendothelial changes induced these vascular and stromal reactions, which have a detrimental influence on the sinusoidal capillaries, on erythropoiesis and on osseous remodelling (Fig. 8.S8)[16]. The marked inflammatory reaction of the bone marrow stroma correlated with serological parameters of inflammation and may contribute significantly to bone marrow atrophy and the 'anaemia of chronic disorders' in diabetes mellitus. Atrophic reduction of trabecular bone mass was significantly higher in patients with diabetes mellitus, but bone remodelling was normal or slightly decreased. Insulin-dependent patients had a lower loss than orally adjusted diabetics. These results demonstrate the occurrence of a more or less specific 'diabetic osteomyelopathy' comprising

1. degenerative changes and deposits in the walls of the marrow vasculature,
2. inflammatory reactions with plasmacytosis and fibrosis,
3. marrow atrophy and exudative changes, and
4. osteopenia with slightly decreased bone remodelling (bone atrophy).

Hyperparathyroid bone disease may also occur in diabetic renal failure[27].

RHEUMATIC OSTEOPOROSIS

In rheumatoid arthritis, *generalized osteoporosis* may be a prominent feature of the polyarticular cases[95], and *localized osteoporosis* may be distinctive in pauciarticular cases. Superimposed bone loss due to long-term steroid therapy may aggravate the osteoporotic state[49,75].

Vertebral osteoporosis is a recognized feature of ankylosing spondylitis, and vertebral compression fractures due to osteoporosis are a common but frequently unrecognized complication. They may contribute to the pathogenesis of spinal deformity and back pain. There is resorption of the bone bordering the involved joints, and cystic cavities filled with granulation tissue may occur. Reactive *sclerosis* of bone occurs under progression of ankylosis.

The appearance of *bone erosions* on radiographs is most typically a feature of rheumatoid arthritis[39], but they have also been described in psoriatic arthropathy, Reiter's disease, systemic lupus erythematosus and mixed connective tissue disease. Since production of IgG antibodies is under T-lymphocyte control, and T-lymphocytes produce osteoclast activation factor and affect osteoclastic func-

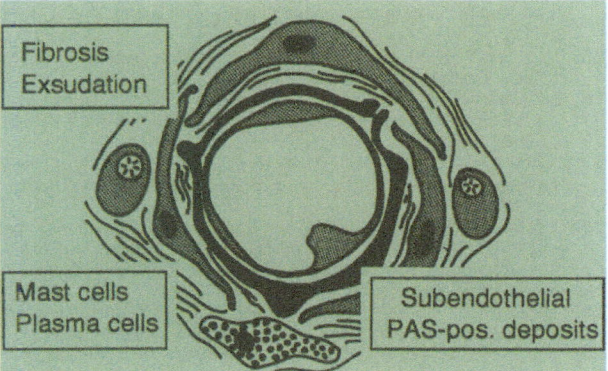

Fig. 8.S8 Diagram of small artery in iliac crest biopsy showing characteristic features of diabetic microangiopathy

tion by other means, it has been concluded that IgG rheumatoid factor may reflect osteoclastic activity[39].

HAEMATOPOIETIC OSTEOPOROSIS (Plate 8.E)

Bone and marrow are closely interrelated organs[55,57]. They share the same vascular system, and there are many interrelations between stromal elements and cellular lineages (e.g. monocytes and osteoclasts). Therefore it is not astonishing that disorders of the one invariably affect the other to a lesser or greater degree. The haematological conditions in which alterations in trabecular bone have been observed are listed in Table 8.1. The term 'haematic osteodysplasia' was first introduced by Gänsslen in 1938 to describe the effects on the skull caused by congenital haemolytic anaemia, i.e. the typical 'hair on end' appearance of the cranial bones. Subsequently, Rohr in 1940 and Markoff in 1942 used the terms *'myelogenous osteopathy'* and *'osteogenous myelopathy'* for the osteolysis and osteosclerosis occurring in myelogenous disorders and the suppression of haematopoesis due to diseases of the bones respectively.

There are different histological patterns in trabecular osteopenia depending on the underlying conditions of the bone marrow:

'Low-turnover' versus 'high-turnover' osteopenia

When the marrow is hypoplastic or aplastic there is a marked decrease in the number of sinusoids and of stromal elements including the bone-lining cells; this may be the main cause of the osteopenia. Thin trabeculae surrounded by fat cells, with virtual absence of endosteal sinusoids, osteoblasts and osteoclasts are characteristic of this type of cancellous bone atrophy. When the marrow is hypercellular, as in haemolytic anaemias and myeloproliferations, the endosteal sinusoids, the bone lining cells and the adjacent mesenchyme are also hypoplastic, corresponding to inactive osteopenia. 'High-turnover' osteopenia, particularly in the axial skeleton, is found in haematopoietic malignancies with diffuse spread (acute leukaemias, diffuse type of myelomatosis). Activation of the BRU has been ascribed to the production of osteoclast-activating factors (OAF) by myeloma, lymphoma or leukaemia cells; production of osteoblast-inhibiting factors has also been postulated.

'Thin-trabeculae' versus 'coarse trabeculae' osteopenia

Not only the degree of marrow cellularity but also the different proliferating haematopoietic cell lines influence osseous reactions. While in polycythaemia vera the trabeculae are attenuated but with normal microarchitecture and connections, a coarsening of the trabecular network with fewer connections and correspondingly large marrow spaces is characteristic of chronic myeloid leukaemia.

'Generalized' versus 'focal' osteopenia[108]

The mode of spread of marrow infiltrations is a major parameter determining the pattern of osseous lesions. Processes with diffuse marrow infiltration are characterized by a systemic osteopenia in bones which otherwise contain a trabecular network and red marrow, while in patients with focal, nodular or patchy infiltrations (granulomatous disorders, Hodgkin's disease, hairy cell leukaemia, nodular types of multiple myeloma and lymphomas) local osteopenia or even circumscribed osteolytic lesions are found.

TRANSIENT OSTEOPOROSIS

Transient osteoporosis (*TO*) may be defined as a rapidly developing, painful osteopenia in periarticular bone areas, of benign nature and as yet unexplained pathyphysiology[124]. Localized immobilization osteoporosis and Sudeck's atrophy should be ruled out. Klier *et al.* (1988) described two major clinical subtypes[85]:

1. *regional TO*[103,138], with the hip joint affected, including cases occurring during pregnancy, and
2. *migratory TO*, affecting multiple joints in a migratory fashion.

Neural, mechanical and circulatory pathomechanisms have all been discussed[147].

POTENTIAL OF BONE BIOPSY IN OSTEOPOROSIS

There is still uncertainty regarding the significance of changes in bone mass at the different skeletal sites which are usually studied by means of both non-invasive and invasive techniques; and no consensus concerning unselected screening for osteoporosis by bone mass measurement[100,107]. Although there are biological relationships between the spine, wrist, iliac crest and total skeleton as to the bone mass present, it unfortunately appears that changes in bone mass are specific for the site measured and cannot be extrapolated to others. In young adult osteoporosis, for example, we found marked differences in bone mass between the axial and appendicular skeleton; some cases had considerable osteopenia with fractures in the vertebrae, but normal trabecular values in the iliac crest biopsy. Consequently a normal bone mass in an iliac crest biopsy does not exclude an osteoporotic syndrome at other sites, while Charnley and co-workers (1989) demonstrated that metacarpal morphometry cannot predict histological osteoporosis of the iliac crest[20]. *To determine bone mass and changes therein with acceptable accuracy at any site, one must measure that site!*

A recent application of bone biopsy in osteoporosis has been in the assessment of the mechanisms of bone loss at the microarchitectural and lamellar levels, the results of which may partly explain discrepancies between bone mass measurements and bone fragility[14,50,113]. Iliac crest biopsies are also useful to detect occult osteomalacia in a clinically osteoporotic patient (for which the term 'poromalacia' has been used). We believe that bone biopsy including histomorphometry should be performed whenever possible in men with apparently idiopathic osteoporosis or with unusually progressive variants of primary osteoporosis. The finding of increased bone turnover in such patients should stimulate a thorough re-evaluation for secondary causes of accelerated bone loss such as hyperparathyroidism or hyperthyroidism which may remain clinically occult for considerable periods of time before the occurrence of osteoporotic features. Simultaneous assessment of the bone marrow permits recognition of myelogenous disorders with secondary osteopenia.

The pretreatment histomorphometric profile of high- and low-turnover osteopenia will also influence the appropriate choice of therapy[74]; and response to treatment may be followed by serial biopsies: effects on compact as well as trabecular bone[80]. Double tetracycline labelling allows quantitative assessment of structural elements as well as dynamic indices of bone remodelling (formation and resorption), complementing the histomorphometric manifestations of high- and low-turnover osteopenia.

References

1. Aitken M. (1984). *Osteoporosis in Clinical Practice*. Bristol: Wright
2. Arlot M. E., Delmas P. D., Chappard D. and Meunier P. J. (1990). Trabecular and endocortical bone remodelling in postmenopausal osteoporosis: comparison with normal postmenopausal women. *Osteoporosis Int.*, **1**(1), 41
3. Arlot M., Eduard C., Meunier P. J., Neer R. M. and Reeve J. (1984). Impaired osteoblastic function in osteoporosis: comparison between calcium balance and dynamic histomorphometry. *Brit. Med. J.*, **289**, 517
4. Auwerx J. and Bouillon R. (1986). Mineral and bone metabolism in thyroid disease: a review. *Q. J. Med.*, **60**, 737
5. Avioli L. V. (1991). Heterogeneity of osteoporotic syndromes and the response to calcitonin therapy. *Calcif. Tissue Int.*, **49**, S16
6. Avioli L. V. (1987). *The Osteoporotic Syndrome: Detection, Prevention and Treatment*. Orlando: Grune & Stratton
7. Bachrach L. K., Katzman D. K., Litt I. F., Guido D. and Marcus R. (1991). Recovery from osteopenia in adolescent girls with anorexia nervosa. *J. Clin. Endocrinol. Metab.*, **72**, 602
8. Bartl R., Moser W., Burkhardt R., Sandel P., Kampke W., Mähr G. and Adelmann B. C. (1978). Diabetische Osteomyelopathie: Histobioptische Befunde am Knochen und Knochenmark bei Diabetes mellitus. *Klin. Wschr.*, **56**, 743
9. Beck J. S. and Nordin B. E. C. (1960). Histological assessment of osteoporosis by iliac crest biopsy. *J. Pathol. Bacteriol.*, **80**, 391
10. Beresteijn E. C. H., Hof M. A., Waard H., Raymakers J. A. and Duursma S. A. (1990). Relation of axial bone mass to habitual calcium intake and to cortical bone loss in healthy early postmenopausal women. *Bone*, **11**, 7
11. Bikle D. D., Genant H. K., Cann C., Recker R. R., Halloran B. P. and Strewler G. J. (1985). Bone disease in alcohol abuse. *Ann. Intern. Med.*, **103**, 42
12. Bisballe S., Eriksen E. F. and Melsen F. (1991). Osteopenia and osteomalacia after gastrectomy: interrelations between biochemical markers of bone remodelling, vitamin D metabolites and bone histomorphometry. *Gut*, **32**, 1303
13. Bordier P. J., Miravet L. and Hioco D. (1973). Young adult osteoporosis. *J. Clin. Endocrinol. Metab.*, **2**, 277
14. Boskey A. L. (1990). Bone mineral and matrix: are they altered in osteoporosis? *Orthop. Clin. N. Amer.*, **21**, 19
15. Bouillon R. (1991). Diabetic bone disease. *Calcif. Tissue Int.*, **49**, 155
16. Burkhardt R., Moser W., Bartl R. and Mahl G. (1981). Is diabetic osteoporosis due to microangiopathy? *Lancet*, **11**, 844
17. Chantraine A. (1977). Actual concept of osteoporosis in paraplegia. *Paraplegia*, **16**, 51
18. Chappard D., Alexandre C., Palle S., Vico L., Morukov B. V., Rodionova S. S., Minaire P. and Riffat G. (1989). Effects of a biphosphonate (1-hydroxy ethylidene-1,1 biphosphonic acid) on osteoclast number during prolonged bed rest in healthy humans. *Metabolism*, **38**, 822
19. Chappard D., Plantard B., Petitjean M., Alexandre C. and Riffat G. (1991). Alcoholic cirrhosis and osteoporosis in men: a light and scanning electron microscopic study. *J. Stud. Alcohol*, **52**, 269
20. Charnley R. M., Bickerstaff D. R., Wallace W. A. and Stevens A. (1989). The measurement of osteoporosis in clinical practice. *J. Bone Jt Surg.*, **71B**, 661
21. Chesnut C. H. (1992). Osteoporosis and its treatment. *N. Engl. J. Med.*, **326**, 406
22. Chesnut C. H. (1991). Theoretical overview: bone development, peak bone mass, bone loss, and fracture risk. *Amer. J. Med.*, **91** (Suppl. 5B), 2S
23. Compston J. E. and Croucher P. I. (1991). Histomorphometric assessment of trabecular bone remodelling in osteoporosis. *Bone Miner.*, **14**, 91
24. Compston J. E., Vedi S. and Croucher P. I. (1991). Low prevalence of osteomalacia in elderly patients with hip fracture. *Age Ageing*, **20**, 132
25. Courpron P. (1981). Bone tissue mechanisms underlying osteoporoses. *Orthop. Clin. N. Amer.*, **12**, 513
26. Cummings S. R., Kelsley J. L., Nevitt M. C. and O'Dowd K. J. (1985). Epidemiology of osteoporosis and osteoporotic fractures. *Epidemiol. Rev.*, **7**, 178
27. Cundy T. F., Humphreys S., Watkins P. J. and Parsons V. (1990). Hyperparathyroid bone disease in diabetic renal failure. *Diabetes Res.*, **14**, 191
28. Cuthbert J., Pak C. Y. C., Zerwekh J. E., Glass K. D. and Combes B. (1984). Bone disease in primary biliary cirrhosis: increased bone resorption and turnover in the absence of osteoporosis or osteomalacia. *Hepatology*, **4**(1), 1
29. Davies M. C., Hall M. L. and Jacobs H. S. (1990). Bone mineral loss in young women with amenorrhoea. *Brit. Med. J.*, **301**, 790
30. Delmas P. D. (1991). Biochemical markers of bone turnover: methodology and clinical use in osteoporosis. *Amer. J. Med.*, **91** (Suppl. 5B), 59S
31. Demmler K., Otte P., Bartl R., Burkhardt R., Frisch B. and Jahn A.

(1983). Osteopenie, Markatrophie und Kapillarversorgung. Vergleichende Untersuchungen am menschlichen Beckenkamm und 1. Lendenwirbelkörper. *Z. Orthop.*, **121**(3), 223

32. Diamond T., Stiel D., Luncer M., Wilkinson M. and Posen S. (1989). Ethanol reduces bone formation and may cause osteoporosis. *Amer. J. Med.*, **86**, 282

33. Diamond T., Stiel D., Luncer M., Wilkinson M., Roche J. and Posen S. (1990). Osteoporosis and skeletal fractures in chronic liver disease. *Gut*, **31**, 82

34. Dickenson R. P., Hutton W. C. and Stott J. R. R. (1981). The mechanical properties of bone in osteoporosis. *J. Bone Jt Surg.*, **63B**, 233

35. Diebold J., Batge B., Stein H., Muller-Esch G., Muller P. K. and Löhrs U. (1991). Osteoporosis in longstanding acromegaly: characteristic changes of vertebral architecture and bone matrix composition. *Virch. Archiv. B.*, **4**, 209

36. Donaldson C. L., Hulley S. B., Vogel J. M., Hattner R. S., Bayers J. H. and McMillan D. E. (1970). Effect of prolonged bed rest on bone mineral. *Metabolism*, **19**, 1071

37. Drinkwater B. L., Nilson K., Chesnut C. H., Bremner W. J., Shainholtz S. and Southworth M. B. (1984). Bone mineral content of amenorrheic and eumenorrheic athletes. *N. Engl. J. Med.*, **311**, 277

38. Eastell R. and Riggs B. L. (1988). Diagnostic evaluation of osteoporosis. *Endocrinol. Metab. Clin. N. Amer.*, **17**(3), 547

39. Editorial. (1987). Bone erosions in rheumatic disease. *Lancet*, **2**, 375

40. Editorial. (1990). Fracture patterns revisited. *Lancet*, **336**, 1290

41. Editorial. (1990). New treatments for osteoporosis. *Lancet*, **335**, 1065

42. Editorial. (1991). Thiazide diuretics and osteoporosis: time for a clinical trial? *Ann. Intern. Med.*, **115**, 64

43. Eisman J. A., Sambrook P. N., Kelly P. J. and Pocock N. A. (1991). Exercise and its interaction with genetic influences in the determination of bone mineral density. *Amer. J. Med.*, **91** (Suppl. 5B), 5S

44. Ellis K. J. and Chon S. H. (1975). Correlation between skeletal calcium mass and muscle mass in man. *J. Appl. Physiol.*, **38**, 455

45. Evans R. A., Marel G. M., Lancaster E. K., Evans M. and Wong S. Y. P. (1988). Bone mass is low in relatives of osteoporotic patients. *Ann. Intern. Med.*, **104**, 870

46. Eventov I., Frisch B., Alk D., Eisenberg Z. and Weisman Y. (1989). Bone biopsies and serum vitamin-D levels in patients with hip fracture. *Acta Orthop. Scand.*, **60**(4), 411

47. Eventov I., Frisch B., Cohen Z. and Hammel I. (1991). Osteopenia, hematopoiesis, and bone remodelling in iliac crest and femoral biopsies: a prospective study of 102 cases of femoral neck fractures. *Bone*, **12**, 1

48. Fallon M. D., Whyte M. P., Craig R. B. and Teitelbaum S. L. (1983). Mast-cell proliferation in postmenopausal osteoporosis. *Calcif. Tissue Int.*, **35**, 29

49. Felder M. and Ruegsegger P. (1991). Bone loss in patients with rheumatoid arthritis – effects of steroids measured by low dose quantitative computed tomography. *Rheumatol. Int.*, **11**, 41

50. Ferris B. D., Klenerman L. and Dodds R. A. (1987). Altered organisation of noncollagenous bone matrix in osteoporosis. *Bone*, **8**, 285

51. Finkelstein J. S., Neer R. M., Biller B. M. K., Crawford J. D. and Klibanski A. (1992). Osteopenia in men with a history of delayed puberty. *N. Engl. J. Med.*, **326**, 600

52. Fiore C. E., Falcidia E., Fotii R., Caschetto S. and Grimaldi D. R. (1987). Postoophorectomy bone loss is associated with reduced bone Gla protein serum levels: a possible effect of osteoblastic insufficiency. *Calcif. Tissue Int.*, **41**, 303

53. Francis R. M. (1990). *Osteoporosis: Pathogenesis and Management*. Dordrecht: Kluwer

54. Franklyn J. A. and Sheppard M. C. (1990). Thyroxine replacement treatment and osteoporosis: controversy continues about the optimum dosage. *Brit. Med. J.*, **300**, 694

55. Frisch B. and Bartl R. (1990). *Atlas of Bone Marrow Pathology*. Dordrecht: Kluwer

56. Frisch B. and Eventov I. (1986). Hematopoiesis in osteoporosis – preliminary report comparing biopsies of the femoral neck and iliac crest. *Isr. J. Med. Sci.*, **22**, 380

57. Frisch B., Lewis S. M., Burkhardt R. and Bartl R. (1985). *Biopsy Pathology of Bone and Bone Marrow*. London: Chapman & Hall

58. Frost H. M. (1987). The mechanostat: a proposed pathogenic mechanism of osteoporoses and the bone mass effects of mechanical and nonmechanical agents. *Bone Miner.*, **2**, 73

59. Frost H. M. (1985). The pathomechanism of osteoporoses. *Clin. Orthop. Rel. Res.*, **200**, 198

60. Genant H. K., Faulkner K. G. and Glüer C-C. (1991). Measurement of bone mineral density: current status. *Amer. J. Med.*, **91** (Suppl. 5B), 49S

61. Gillespy T. and Gillespy M. P. (1991). Osteoporosis. *Radiol. Clin. N. Amer.*, **29**(1), 77

62. Gonzales D., Ghiringhelli G. and Mautalen C. (1986). Acute antiosteoclastic effect of salmon calcitonin in osteoporotic women. *Calcif. Tissue Int.*, **38** 71

63. Grech P., Martin T. J., Barringtcn, N. A. and Ell P. J. (1985). *Diagnosis of Metabolic Bone Disease*. London: Chapman & Hall

64. Greenspan S. L., Greenspan F. S., Resnick N. M., Block J. E., Friedlander A. L. and Genant H. K. (1991). Skeletal integrity in premenopausal and postmenopausal women receiving long-term L-thyroxine therapy. *Amer. J. Med.*, **91**, 5

65. Gruber H. E., Gutteridge D. H. and Baylink D. J. (1984). Osteoporosis associated with pregnancy and lactation: bone biopsy and skeletal features in three patients. *Metab. Bone Dis. Rel. Res.*, **5**, 159

66. Gruber H. E., Ivey J. L., Thompson E. R., Chesnut C. H. and Baylink D. J. (1986). Osteoblast and osteoclast cell number and cell activity in postmenopausal osteoporosis. *Miner. Electrolyte Metab.*, **12**, 246

67. Haagsma E. B., Thijn C. J. P., Post J. G., Sloof M. J. H. and Gips C. H. (1988). Bone disease after orthotopic liver transplantation. *J. Hepatol.*, **6**, 94

68. Hansen M. A., Overgaard K., Riis B J. and Christiansen C. (1991). Role of peak mass and bone loss in postmenopausal osteoporosis: 12 year study. *Brit. Med. J.*, **303**, 961

69. Harrison J. E. (1989). Osteoporosis. Tam C. S., Heersche J. N. M. and Murray T. M., *Metabolic Bone Disease: Cellular and Tissue Mechanisms* (p. 239). Boca Raton: CRC Press

70. Hay J. E., Lindor K. D., Wiesner R. H., Dickson E. R., Krom R. A. and Larusso N. F. (1991). The metabolic bone disease of primary sclerosing cholangitis. *Hepatology*, **14**, 257

71. Hills E., Dunstan C. R., Wong S. Y. P. and Evans R. A. (1989). Bone histology in young adult osteoporosis. *J. Clin. Pathol.*, **42**, 391

72. Hodgson S. F. (1990). Corticoid-induced osteoporosis. *Endocrinol. Metab. Clin. N. Amer.*, **19**(1), 95

73. Jackson J. A. and Kleerekoper M. (1990). Osteoporosis in men: diagnosis, pathophysiology, and prevention. *Medicine*, **69**(3), 137

74. Jackson J. A., Kleerekoper M. and Parfitt A. M. (1986). Symptomatic osteoporosis in a man with hyperprolactinemic hypogonadism. *Ann. Intern. Med.*, **105**, 543

75. Joffe I. and Epstein S. (1991). Osteoporosis associated with rheumatoid arthritis: pathogenesis and management. *Sem. Arthritis Rheum.*, **20**, 256

76. Johnston C. C. and Longcope C. (1990). Premenopausal bone loss – a risk factor for osteoporosis. *N Engl. J. Med.*, **323**(18), 1271

77. Johnston C. C., Slemenda C. W. anc Melton L. J. (1991). Clinical use of bone densitometry. *N. Engl. J. Med.*, **324**, 1105

78. Johnston C. C. and Slemanda C. W. (1991). Risk prediction in osteoporosis: a theoretic overview. *Amer. J. Med.*, **91** (Suppl. 5B), 47S

79. Jowsey J. and Johnson K. A. (1972). Juvenile osteoporosis: bone findings in seven patients. *J. Pediatr.*, **81**, 511

80. Kanis J. A. (1991). The restoration of skeletal mass: a theoretical overview. *Amer. J. Med.*, **91** (Suppl. 5B), 29S

81. Karantanis A. N., Kalef E. J. and Glavos D. (1991). Limitations of quantitative CT in corticosteroid induced osteopenia. *Acta Radiol.*, **32**, 339

82. Kelly P. J., Pocock N. A., Sambrook P. N. and Eisman J. A. (1990). Dietary calcium, sex hormones, and bone mineral density in men. *Brit. Med. J.*, **300**, 1361

83. Kimmel D. B., Recker R. R., Gallagher J. C., Vaswani A. S. and Aloia J. F. (1990). A comparison of iliac bone histomorphometric data in post-menopausal osteoporotic and normal subjects. *Bone Mineral.*, **11**, 217

84. Kleerekoper M. and Balena R. (1991). Fluoride and osteoporosis. *Ann. Rev. Nutr.*, **11**, 309

85. Klier I., Zoldan J., Yosipovitch Z. and Gadoth N. (1988). Transient regional and migratory osteoporosis: a possible neural mechanism. *Isr. J. Med. Sci.*, **24**, 201

86. Krolner B. and Toft B. (1983). Vertebral bone loss: an unheeded side effect of therapeutic bed rest. *Clin. Sci.*, **64**, 537

87. Landry M. and Fleisch H. (1964). The influence of immobilisation on bone formation as evaluated by osseous incorporation of tetracycline. *J. Bone Jt Surg.*, **46B**, 764

88. Law M. R., Wald N. J. and Meade T. W. (1991). Strategies for prevention of osteoporosis and hip fracture. *Brit. Med. J.*, **303**, 459

89. LeBlanc A., Schneider V., Krebs J., Evans H., Jhingran S. and

Johnson P. (1987). Spinal bone mineral after 5 weeks of bed rest. *Calcif. Tissue Int.*, **41**, 259

90. Lindholm J., Steiniche T., Rasmussen E., Thamsborg G., Nielsen I. D., Brockstedt-Rasmussen H., Storm T., Hyldstrup L. and Schou C. (1991). Bone disorder in men with chronic alcoholism: a reversible disease? *J. Clin. Endocrinol. Metab.*, **73**, 118

91. Lindsay R. (1991). Estrogens, bone mass, and osteoporotic fracture. *Amer. J. Med.*, **91** (Suppl. 5B), 10S

92. Lindsay R. (1990). Fluoride and bone-quantity versus quality. *N. Engl. J. Med.*, **322**(12), 845

93. Lindsay R. (1988). Management of osteoporosis. Martin T. J., *Metabolic Bone Disease* (p. 103). London: Baillière Tindall

94. Lindsay R. and Cosman F. (1990). Epidemiology of osteoporosis. Drife J. O. and Studd J. W. W., *HTR and Osteoporosis* (p. 76). London: Springer

95. Magaro M., Tricerri A., Piane, D., Zoli A., Serra F., Altomonte L. and Mirone L. (1991). Generalised osteoporosis in non-steroid treated rheumatoid arthritis. *Rheumatol. Int.*, **11**, 73

96. Mayo-Smith W. and Rosenthal D. I. (1991). Radiographic appearance of osteopenia. *Radiol. Clin. N. Amer.*, **29**(1), 37

97. Mazess R. B. (1990). Fracture risk: a role for compact bone. *Calcif. Tissue Int.*, **47**, 191

98. Mazess R. B. and Barden H. S. (1991). Bone density in premenopausal women: effects of age, dietary intake, physical activity, smoking, and birth-control pills. *Amer. J. Clin. Nutr.*, **53**, 132

99. McDonald J. A., Dunstan C. R., Dilworth P., Sherbon K., Sheil A. G. R., Evans R. A. and McCaughan G. W. (1991). Bone loss after liver transplantation. *Hepatology*, **14**, 59

100. Melton L. J., Eddy D. M. and Johnston C. C. (1990). Screening for osteoporosis. *Ann. Intern. Med.*, **112**, 516

101. Meunier P. J. (1988). Assessment of bone turnover by histomorphometry in osteoporosis. Riggs B. L. and Melton L. J., *Osteoporosis: Etiology, Diagnosis, and Management* (p. 317). New York: Raven Press

102. Mosekilde L., Eriksen E. F. and Charles P. (1990). Effects of thyroid hormones on bone and mineral metabolism. *Endocrinol. Metab. Clin. N. Amer.*, **19**(1), 35

103. Naides S. J., Resnick D. and Zvaifler N. J. (1985). Idiopathic regional osteoporosis: a clinical spectrum. *J. Rheumatol.*, **12**, 763

104. Nordin B. E. C. (1987). The definition and diagnosis of osteoporosis (Editorial). *Calcif. Tissue Int.*, **40**, 57

105. Nordin B. E. C., Crilly R. G. and Smith D. A. (1984). Osteoporosis. Nordin B. E. C., *Metabolic Bone and Stone Disease* (p. 1). Edinburgh: Churchill Livingstone

106. Notelovitz M. (1990). Lifestyle, exercise and osteoporosis. Drife J. O. and Studd J. W. W., *HRT and Osteoporosis* (p. 323). London: Springer

107. Ott S. (1986). Should women get screening bone mass measurement? *Ann. Intern. Med.*, **104**, 874

108. Ozoh J. O., Onuigbo M. A. C., Nwankwo N., Ukabam S. O., Umerah B. C. and Emeruwa C. C. (1990). 'Vanishing' of vertebra in a patient with sickle cell haemaglobinopathy. *Brit. Med. J.*, **301**, 1368

109. Parfitt M. (1991). Use of biphosphonates in the prevention of bone loss and fractures. *Amer. J. Med.*, **91** (Suppl 5B), 42S

110. Prior J. C. Vigna Y. M., Schechter M. T. and Burgess A. E. (1990). Spinal bone loss and ovulatory disturbances. *N. Engl. J. Med.*, **323**, 1221

111. Raisz L. G. (1988). Local and systemic factors in the pathogenesis of osteoporosis. *N. Engl. J. Med.*, **318**(13), 818

112. Raisz L. G. and Smith L. (1987). Osteoporosis. Martin T. J. and Raisz L. G., *Clinical Endocrinology of Calcium Metabolism* (p. 201). New York: Marcel Dekker

113. Rális Z. A. (1983). Bone quality defect: a more significant factor than osteopenia in patients with fracture of the femoral neck. *J. Bone Jt Surg.*, **65B**, 365

114. Revell P. A. (1986). *Pathology of Bone*. Berlin: Springer

115. Rico H., Cabranes J. A., Cabello J., Gomex-Castresana F. and Hernandez E. R. (1987). Low serum osteocalcin in acute alcohol intoxication: a direct toxic effect of alcohol on osteoblasts. *Bone Miner.*, **2**, 221

116. Rico H., Hernandez E. R., Cabranes J. A. and Gomez-Castresana F. (1989). Suggestion of a deficient osteoblastic function in diabetes mellitus: the possible cause of osteopenia in diabetics. *Calcif. Tissue Int.*, **45**, 71

117. Riggs B. L., Hodgson S. F., O'Fallon W. M., Chao E. Y. S., Wahner H. W., Muhs J. M., Cedel S. L. and Melton L. J. (1990). Effect of fluoride treatment on the fracture rate in postmenopausal women with osteoporosis. *N. Engl. J. Med.*, **322**, 802

118. Riggs B. L. and Melton L. J. (1983). Evidence of two distinct syndromes of involutional osteoporosis. *Amer. J. Med.*, **75**, 899

119. Riggs B. L. and Melton L. J. (1988). *Osteoporosis: Etiology, Diagnosis, and Management*. New York: Raven Press

120. Rigotti N. A., Nussbaum S. R., Herzog D. B. and Neer R. M. (1984). Osteoporosis in women with anorexia nervosa. *N. Engl. J. Med.*, **311**, 1601

121. Rodin A., Murby B., Smith M. A., Caleffi M., Fentiman I., Chapman M. G. and Fogelman I. (1990). Premenopausal bone loss in the lumbar spine and neck of femur: a study of 225 caucasian women. *Bone*, **11**, 1

122. Ronin D. I., Wu, Y. C., Sahgal V. and MacLean I. C. (1991). Intractable muscle pain syndrome, osteomalacia and axonopathy in long-term use of phenytoin. *Arch. Phys. Med. Rehabil.*, **72**, 755

123. Ross D. S. (1991). Monitoring L-thyroxine therapy: lessons from the effects of L-thyroxine on bone density. *Amer. J. Med.*, **91**, 1

124. Schapira D., Israel O., Goldsher D., Nahir M. and Scharf Y. (1989). Transient osteoporosis of the hip: case report and review of the literature. *Isr. J. Med. Sci.*, **25**, 709

125. Schiwy K.-H., Kühn H. and Beyer W. F. (1991). Beitrag zur hepatogenen Osteopathie: Ergebnisse histomorphometrischer Untersuchungen. *Pathologe*, **12**, 89

126. Schultheis L. (1991). The mechanical control of bone in weightless spaceflight and in aging. *Exp. Gerontol.*, **26**, 203

127. Shao A. H., Wang F. G., Hu Y. F. and Zang L. M. (1991). Calcium metabolism and osteopathy in diabetes mellitus. *Contrib. Nephrol.*, **90**, 212

128. Shih M. and Anderson C. (1987). Does 'hepatic osteodystrophy' differ from peri- and postmenopausal osteoporosis? A histomorphometric study. *Calcif. Tissue Int.*, **41**, 187

129. Smith R. (1980). Idiopathic osteoporosis in the young. *J. Bone Jt. Surg.*, **62B**, 417

130. Smith R. (1990). Osteoporosis after 60. *Brit. Med. J.*, **301**, 452

131. Smith R., Stevenson J. C., Winearls C. G., Woods C. G. and Wordsworth B. P. (1985). Osteoporosis of pregnancy. *Lancet*, **2**, 1178

132. Steinberg K. K., Bonkovsky H. L., Candell S. P., Bernhardt R. K. and Hawkins M. (1991). Osteocalcin and bone alkaline phosphatase in the serum of women with liver disease. *Ann. Clin. Lab. Sci.*, **21**, 305

133. Stellon A. J., Webb A., Compston J. and Williams R. (1987). Low bone turnover state in primary biliary cirrhosis. *Hepatology*, **7**, 137

134. Stevenson J. C. (1988). Osteoporosis: pathogenesis and risk factors. Martin T. J., *Metabolic Bone Disease* (p. 87). London: Baillière Tindall

135. Storm T., Thamsborg G., Steiniche T., Genant H. and Sorensen O. H. (1990). Effect of intermittent cyclical edidronate therapy on bone mass and fracture rate in women with postmenopausal osteoporosis. *N. Engl. J. Med.*, **322**, 1265

136. Stout S. D. (1982). The effects of long-term immobilisation on the histomorphology of human cortical bone. *Calcif. Tissue Int.*, **34**, 337

137. Szmukler G. I. and Brown S. W. (1985). Premature loss of bone in chronic anorexia nervosa. *Brit. Med. J.*, **290**, 26

138. Takatan Y., Kokub T., Nimomiya S., Nakamuro T., Okutsu I. and Kamogawa M. (1991). Transient osteoporosis of the hip: magnetic resonance imaging. *Clin. Orthop.*, **271**, 190

139. Teelucksingh S., Padfield P. L., Tibi L., Gough K. J. and Holt P. R. (1991). Inhaled corticosteroids, bone formation and osteocalcin. *Lancet*, **338**, 60

140. Tilyard M. W., Spears G. F. S., Thomson J. and Dovey S. (1992). Treatment of postmenopausal osteoporosis with calcitriol or calcium. *N. Engl. J. Med.*, **326**, 357

141. Treasure J. L. and Russell G. F. M. (1987). Reversible bone loss in anorexia nervosa. *Brit. Med. J.*, **295**, 474

142. Unthoff H. K. and Jaworski Z. F. G. (1978). Bone loss in response to long-term immobilisation. *J. Bone Jt Surg.*, **60B**, 420

143. Vaananen H. K. (1991). Pathogenesis of osteoporosis. *Calcif. Tissue Int.*, **49** Suppl., 11

144. VanBerkum F. N. R., Beukers R., Birkenhäger J. C., Kooij P. P. M., Schalm S. W. and Pols H. A. P. (1990). Bone mass in women with primary biliary cirrhosis: the relation with histological stage and use of glucocorticoids. *Gastroenterology*, **99**, 1134

145. Vigorita V. J., Suda M. K. and Lane J. M. (1983). Osteoporosis with idiopathic nodular lymphoid hyperplasia of the marrow. *Arch. Pathol. Lab. Med.*, **107**, 276

146. Wasnich R. D. (1991). Bone mass measurements in diagnosis and assessment of therapy. *Amer. J. Med.*, **91** (Suppl. 5B), 54S

147. Wilson A. J., Murphy W. A., Hardy D. C. and Totty W. G. (1988). Transient osteoporosis: transient bone marrow edema? *Radiology*, **167**, 757

148. Wolman R. L., Clark P., McNally E., Harries M. and Reeve J. (1990). Menstrual state and exercise as determinants of spinal trabecular bone density in female athletes. *Brit. Med. J.*, **301**, 516

The following nine references demonstrate the intense ongoing efforts to elucidate the causes of osteoporosis and devise strategies for its diagnosis and prevention.

Johnston C. C. *et al.* (1982). Calcium supplementation and increases in bone mineral density in children. *N. Engl. J. Med.*, **327**, 82

Matkovic V. (1992). Calcium intake and peak bone mass. *N. Engl. J. Med.*, **327**, 119

Riggs B. L. and Melton L. J. (1992). Prevention and treatment of osteoporosis. *N. Engl. J. Med.*, **327**, 620

Anderson D. C. (1992). Osteoporosis in men. Hormonal protection eventually fades and prevention is the key. *Br. Med. J.*, **305**, 489

Overgaard K. *et al.* (1992). Effect of solcatonin given intranasally on bone mass and fracture rates in established osteoporosis: a dose–response study. *Br. Med. J.*, **305**, 556

Khaw K.-T., Sneyd M.-J. and Compston J. (1992). Bone density parathyroid hormone and 25-hydroxyvitamin D concentrations in middle aged women. *Br. Med. J.*, **305**, 273

Ashton-Key M. and Gallagher P. J. (1992). The value of simple morphometric techniques in the diagnosis of osteoporosis. *Path. Res. Pract.*, **188**, 616

Diebold J., Bätge B., Stein H., Müller-Esch G., Müller P. K. and Löhrs U. (1991). Osteoporosis in longstanding acromegaly; characteristic changes of vertebral trabecular architecture and bone matrix composition. *Virch. Arch. A*, **419**, 209

Christiansen C. (1991). *Hormone Replacement and its Impact on Osteoporosis*. London: Baillière Tindall

The following reference gives an official evaluation of the efficacy and cost–effectiveness of bone screening. based on a review of published studies, and concludes that its impact and cost–effectiveness have been over-estimated.

Noticeboard (1992). Is bone density screening worthwhile? *Lancet*, **339**, 174

References added in proof:

Slemenda C. W., Christian J. C., Reed T., Reister T. K., Williams C. J. and Johnston C. C. (1992). Long-term bone loss in men: effects of genetic and environmental factors. *Ann. Intern. Med.*, **117**, 286

Franklyn J. A., Betteridge J., Daykin J., Holder R., Oates G. D., Parle J. V., Lilley J., Heath D. A. and Sheppard M. C. (1992). Long-term thyroxine treatment and bone mineral density. *Lancet*, **340**, 9

Osteogenesis imperfecta

9

Osteogenesis imperfecta, also called *'brittle bone syndrome'*[20], is a heritable disorder of connective tissue that causes molecular and biochemical changes in the structure and function of collagen[2,4,8,15,23]. The overall incidence of osteogenesis imperfecta is between 1:20 000 and 1:50 000 of the population[16,18]. The disorder may affect different types of collagen, and so usually presents as a generalized connective tissue disease involving bone, tendon, ligament, dentin, skin, sclerae (Fig. 9.1), cornea and ear[16,18,25]. Both amount and structure of collagen type I, the only collagen in adult bone, are abnormal[7,12]; the severity of the disease reflects the degree of structural instability of the collagen helix[22]. Glycosaminoglycans and other matrix proteins are also involved[7]. In addition to inadequate bone formation the calcification rate is reduced. Osteogenesis imperfecta results in osteopenia with consequent recurrent fractures. However, the clinical severity is extremely variable and ranges from stillbirth to fractures beginning late in adulthood, so that some of these patients may be incorrectly diagnosed as having primary osteoporosis[3]. Currently, *four main types* are recognized, though many patients are difficult to classify[16,18,25]:

Type I (blue sclerae and autosomal dominant inheritance) (Plate 9.A),
Type II (lethal perinatal type),
Type III (progressively deforming type), and
Type IV (white sclerae with autosomal dominant inheritance) (Plate 9.B).

There is usually no difficulty in diagnosing severe osteogenesis imperfecta, and the presence of a positive family history, blue sclerae, skeletal deformities and brittle bones is diagnostic. In adolescents and in young adults late-onset osteogenesis imperfecta may be diagnosed as 'idiopathic osteoporosis', especially in cases without blue sclerae[25].

There may be evidence of abnormal *skeletal matrix*[7,12,22], *bone mineral*[13] and growth, even in mild variants of osteogenesis imperfecta. Morphological changes in growth plate cartilage have also been described[17] (Figs 9.2–9.6). Iliac crest biopsies from infants and young adults show normal cartilage in the epiphyseal growth plate; but the transitional region from cartilage to bone illustrates the magnitude of the genetic lesion (Plate 9.A). Islands of cartilage are surrounded by a rim of woven bone ('popcorn' calcification)[9] or even persist within thin trabeculae, which do not provide sufficient mechanical strength and support (Fig. 9.6). The thickness of the cortical bone is also decreased[5,21], though not in all our cases. At the electron microscopic level the osteoblasts may contain dilated rough endoplasmic reticulum which probably reflects an intrinsic abnormality in procollagen secretion[18]. In mild and moderate variants of osteogenesis imperfecta the *trabeculae* do show a lamellar structure, while in severely affected patients the lamellae contain residual areas of woven bone. The trabeculae are thin, partly without an organized microarchitecture, and the bone volume is diminished – trabecular and cortical[5,21].

Osteoclasts may be increased, though not in all cases, indicating an augmented osseous remodelling[1]. Resorption occurs mainly on trabecular surfaces (Figs 9.6 and 9.10). Though the numbers of *osteoblasts* per unit of bone are increased, their activity, or rather their effectivity is greatly reduced (Figs 9.4, 9.6, 9.7 and 9.10). The osteoid-covered surfaces are increased, but the osteoid seam thickness is normal[14]. Large numbers of *osteocytes*, with a high density in the trabeculae, are characteristic, reflecting the high number of transformed osteoblasts (Figs 9.5, 9.10 and 9.11). Falvo and Bullough (1973) have emphasized that *hyperosteocytosis* is a prominent histological feature of the older patients with osteogenesis imperfecta[5] (Plate 9.B).

Nevertheless, the rate of bone formation is apparently increased, as shown by tetracycline labelling, probably because the low activity of individual osteoblasts is offset by an increased number of these cells[11,14].

Osteogenesis imperfecta is characterized by a high tendency for bones to break, and a striking inability to repair the fractures adequately, suggesting some *failure of the modelling–remodelling system*[6]. The occurrence of collagen defects with impairment of fracture healing raises the possibility that collagen structure may influence the way that bone detects and responds to its mechanical environment. Indeed defects in collagen crosslinking, aggregation and packing may impair the transfer of mechanical signals to the bone and thus increase the

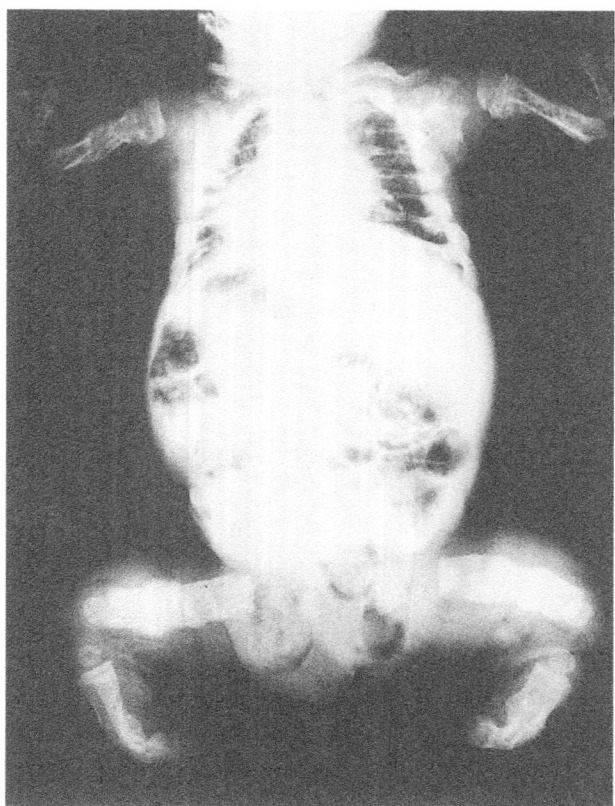

Fig. 9.R1 X-ray of infant with osteogenesis imperfecta type II showing multiple skeletal deformities

Plate 9.A

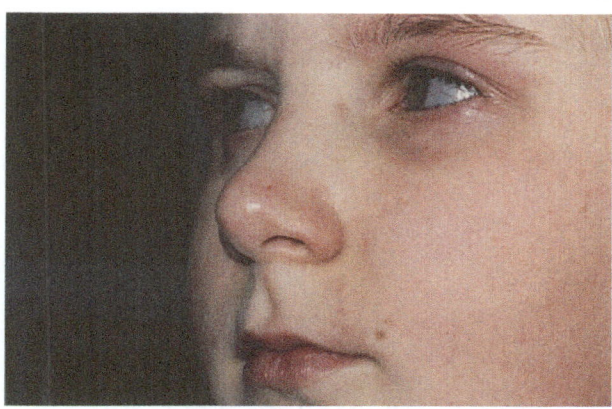

Fig. 9.1 Girl with osteogenesis imperfecta and multiple pathological fractures (see Fig. 9.R2), showing characteristic blue-grey sclerae

Figs. 9.2–9.6 Iliac crest biopsy of a 14-year-old girl with osteogenesis imperfecta, type I

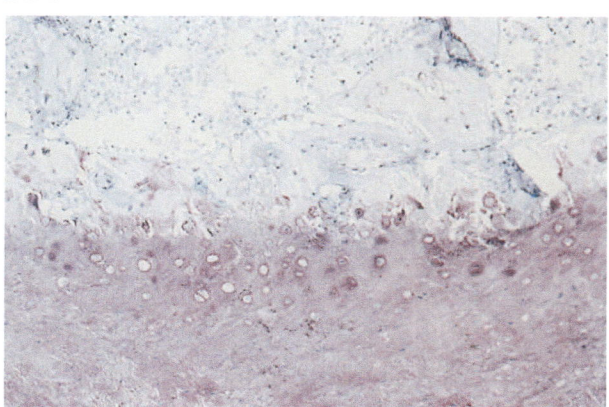

Fig. 9.2 Disorganization of growth plate in osteogenesis imperfecta: lack of columnar structure in the cartilaginous region and poorly defined calcification zone. Giemsa

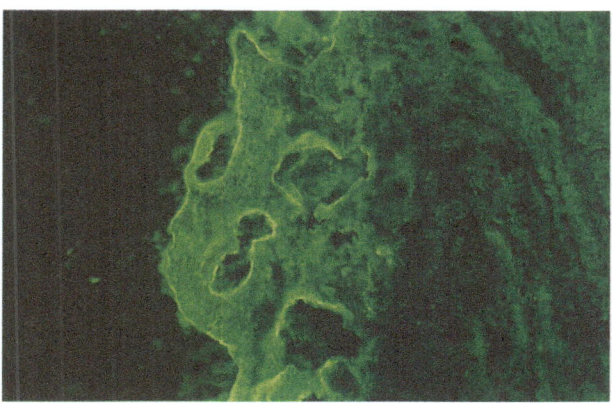

Fig. 9.3 Defective production and organization of collagen type I in osteogenesis imperfecta. Cryostat section of iliac crest biopsy

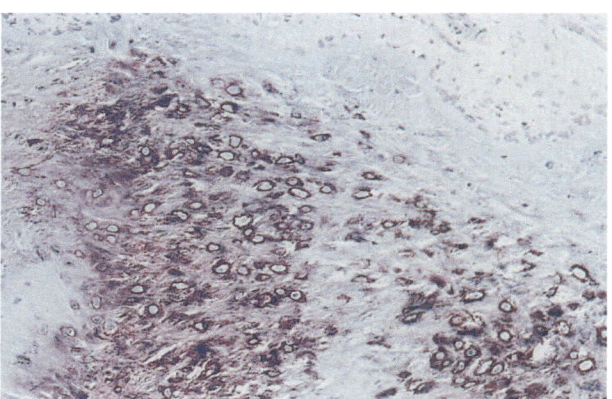

Fig. 9.4 Overview of growth plate of young patient with osteogenesis imperfecta illustrating topographic disorganization and irregularity of the different zones of cartilage. Thin cortex covered by a rim of osteoblasts upper right. Giemsa

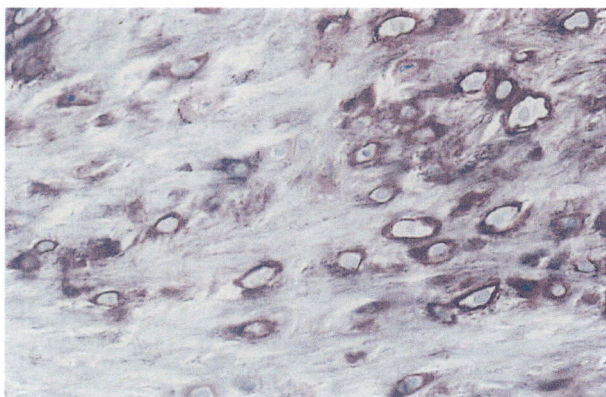

Fig. 9.5 Higher magnification of Fig. 9.4 showing lack of organization in transitional zone between cartilage and mineralized bone. Giemsa

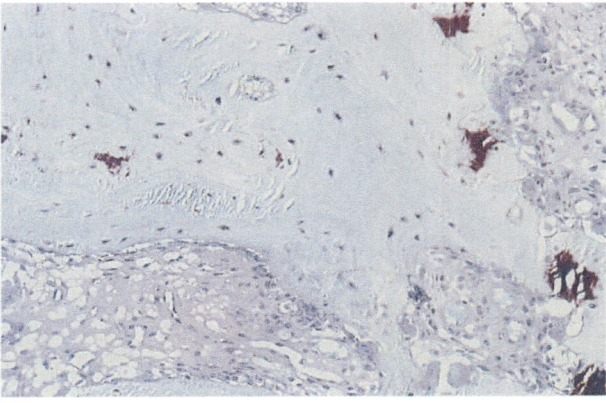

Fig. 9.6 Subcortical zone with broad ossicle, characterized by a high density of large osteocytes, some islands of residual cartilage as well as increased bone remodelling on the surface. Note oedematous reaction in the paratrabecular region. Giemsa

Plate 9.B

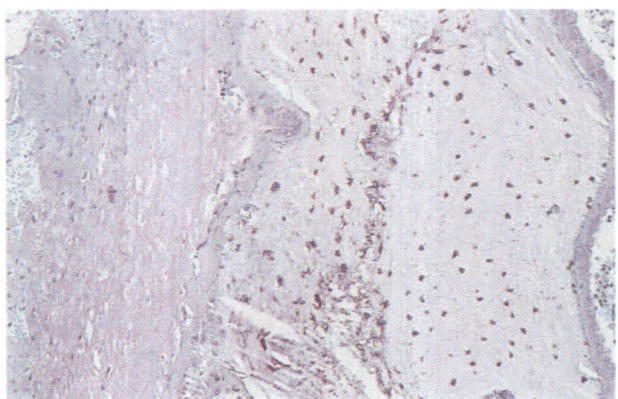

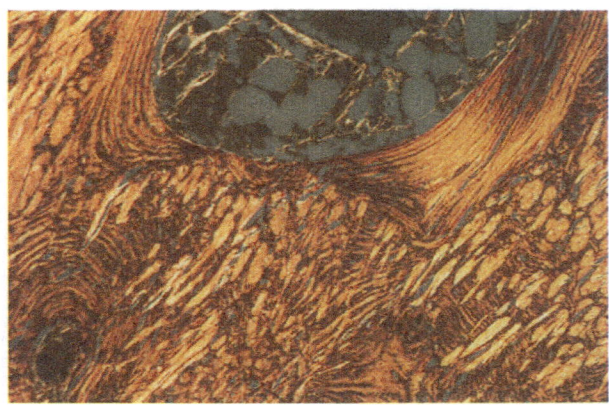

Figs. 9.7–9.11 Iliac crest biopsy of an adult patient with osteogenesis imperfecta, type IV

Fig. 9.7 Overview of broad cortex with high density of osteocytes and a broad endosteal seam of osteoid covered by osteoblasts (right). Periosteum at left. Giemsa

Fig. 9.8 Part of cortical bone with altered lamellar structure but without woven bone pattern. Gomori, polar.

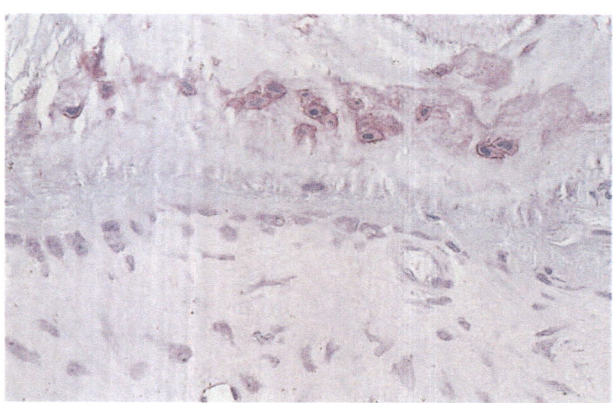

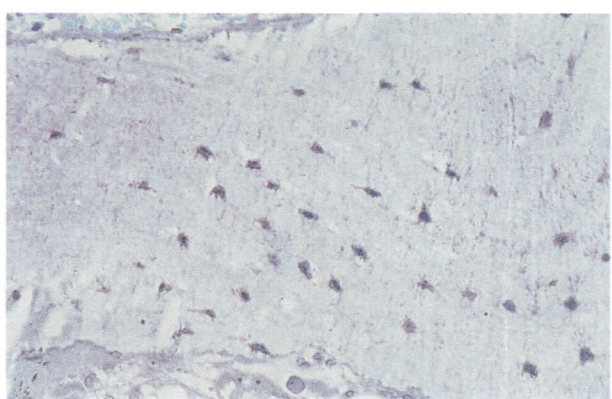

Fig. 9.9 Periosteal zone, from bottom up, showing: mesenchymal connective tissue (periosteum), a thin layer of cortical bone with seam of osteoblasts at the periosteal site, and a layer of osteocytes above which is a scalloped cement line (upper right). Giemsa

Fig. 9.10 Broad trabecula showing high density of osteoblasts within bone tissue, lamellar in type. Note increased osseous remodelling below. Giemsa

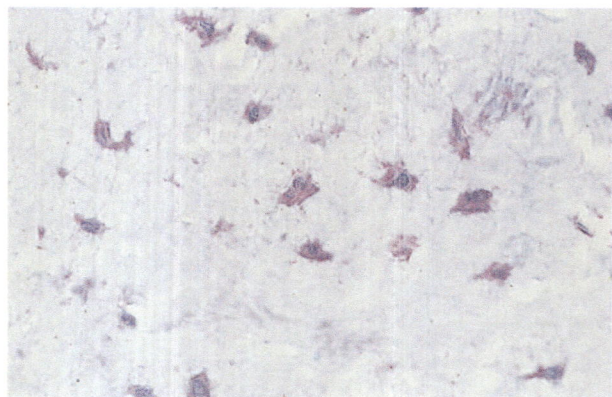

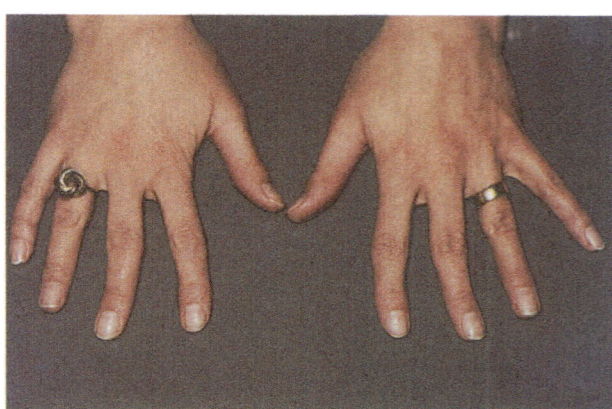

Fig. 9.11 Higher magnification of area from an ossicle in Fig. 9.10 showing disturbed lamellar structure and high density of osteocytes. Giemsa

Fig. 9.12 Spidery fingers (arachnodactyly) of a patient with Marfan syndrome

threshold to induce bone to model and remodel. The skeleton in osteogenesis imperfecta may sense an apparent disuse state and reduce bone mass[6]. This hypothesis (proposed by Frost) still has to be verified by experimental data.

Since most cases of osteogenesis imperfecta are caused by heritable molecular defects, medical *treatment* is largely ineffective[16,18,21,25]. In our departments three patients with

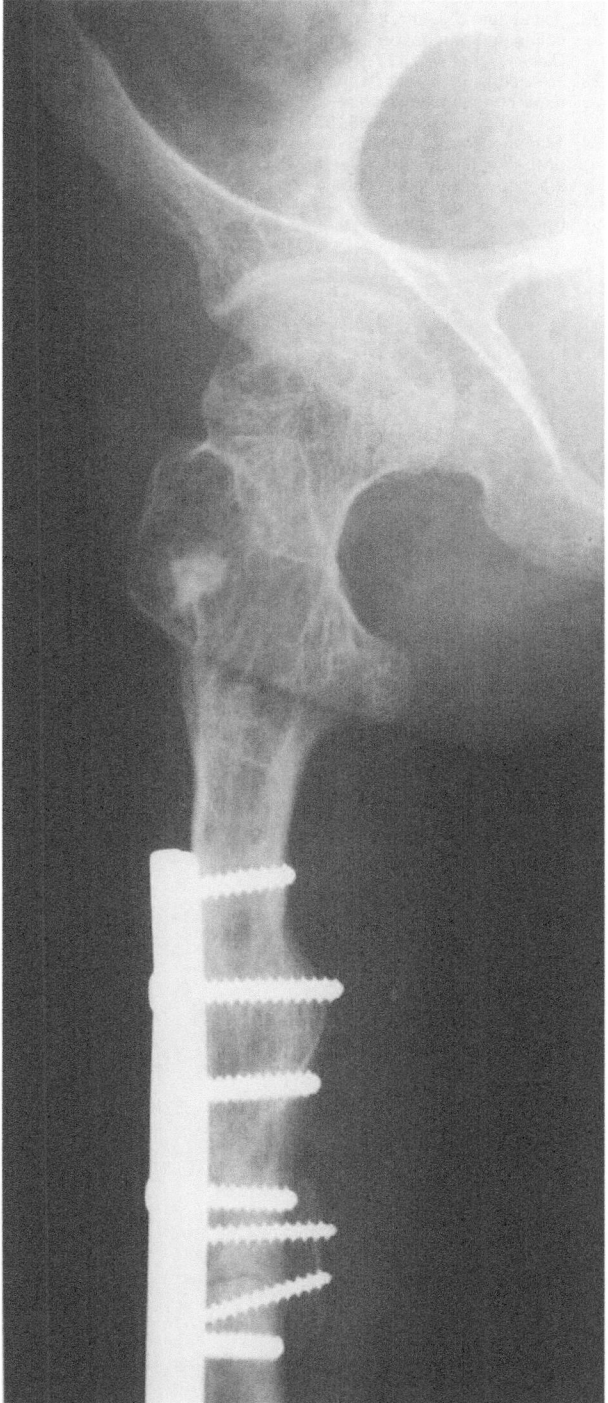

Fig. 9.R2 X-ray of girl with osteogenesis imperfecta showing thin cortices and poorly mineralized bone. Note old, healed and new fractures

osteogenesis imperfecta tarda were treated with fluoride, but the clinical results were disappointing. In sequential biopsies a further increase of osteoblasts and osteocytes was evident, but without improvement in the osteopenic state or decrease in the fracture rate.

EHLERS-DANLOS SYNDROME

This is another inherited connective tissue disorder characterized by articular hypermobility, dermal hyperelasticity and widespread tissue fragility[10]. At least 11 variants have been described. Specific biochemical defects have not been identified, and crosslink analysis has provided conflicting results. However, electron microscopy suggests abnormal collagen fibrillogenesis. Skeletal abnormalities include osteoporosis, defects in the radius and ulna, metacarpal fusion, and soft tissue calcification.

MARFAN SYNDROME

This is also an inherited connective tissue disorder, and collagen analysis showed impaired crosslink maturation leading to defective collagen fibre growth and bundle formation[24]. The multiple skeletal abnormalities (e.g. Fig. 9.12) suggest defective skeletal remodelling, though neither histomorphometry nor the mineral content of bone have been reported.

HOMOCYSTINURIA

Homocystinuria is a heritable disorder due to a deficiency of cystathionine β-synthase, demonstrable in cultured fibroblasts or lymphocytes. Unlike the Marfan syndrome, these patients suffer from generalized osteoporosis of early onset, with vertebral fractures. A similar mechanism may pertain in *lysinuric protein intolerance*[9] presenting in childhood osteoporosis; but these patients show an increase in bone mass under appropriate dietary management.

MENKES' SYNDROME

Menkes' (kinky hair) syndrome is an X-linked recessive disorder of copper metabolism, characterized by a fatal course in infancy. Skeletal morphology is reported to resemble rickets.

References

1. Baron R., Gertner J. M., Lang R. and Vignery A. (1983). Increased bone turnover with decreased bone formation by osteoblasts in children with osteogenesis imperfecta. *Pediatr. Res.*, **17**, 204
2. Bonadio J. and Byers P. H. (1985). Subtle structural alterations in the chains of type I procollagen produce osteogenesis imperfecta type II. *Nature*, **316**, 363
3. Byers P. H., Wallis G. A. and Willing M. C. (1991). Osteogenesis imperfecta: translation of mutation to phenotype. *J. Med. Genet.*, **28**, 433
4. Cole W. G. (1988). Osteogenesis imperfecta. *Clin. Endocrinol. Metab.*, **2**(1), 243
5. Falvo K. A. and Bullough P. G. (1973). Osteogenesis imperfecta: a histometric analysis. *J. Bone Jt Surg.*, **55A**, 275
6. Frost H. M. (1987). Osteogenesis imperfecta: the set point proposal (a possible causative mechanism). *Clin. Orthop. Rel. Res.*, **216**, 280
7. Fujii K. and Tanzer M. L. (1977). Osteogenesis imperfecta: biochemical studies of bone collagen. *Clin. Orthop. Rel. Res.*, **124**, 271
8. Gertner J. M. and Root L. (1990). Osteogenesis imperfecta. *Orthop. Clin. N. Amer.*, **21**(1), 151
9. Goldman A., Davidson D., Pavlov H. and Bullough P. G. (1980). 'Popcorn calcifications': a prognostic sign in osteogenesis imperfecta. *Radiology*, **136**, 351
10. Hoffman G. S., Filie J. D., Schumacher H. R., Ortiz-Bravo E., Tsokos M. G., Marini J. C., Kerr G. S., Ling Q. H. and Trentham D. E. (1991). Intractable vasculitis, resorptive osteolysis and immunity to type I collagen in type VIII Ehlers-Danlos Syndrome. *Arthritis Rheum.*, **34**, 1466

11. Jett S., Ramser J. R., Frost H. M. and Villanueva A. R. (1966). Bone turnover and osteogenesis imperfecta. *Arch. Pathol.*, **81**, 112

12. Kirsch E., Krieg T., Nerlich A., Remberger K., Meinecke P., Kunze D. and Muller P. K. (1987). Compositional analysis of collagen from patients with diverse forms of osteogenesis imperfecta. *Calcif. Tissue Int.*, **41**, 11

13. Kurtz D., Morrish K. and Shapiro J. R. (1985). Bone mineral content in osteogenesis imperfecta. *Calcif. Tissue Int.*, **37**, 14

14. Pirok D. J., Ramser J. R., Takahashi H., Villanueva A. R. and Frost H. M. (1966). Normal histological tetracycline and dynamic parameters in human mineralized bone sections. *Henry Ford Hosp. Med. Bull.*, **14**, 195

15. Ramirez F., Chu M. and DeWet W. (1984). Genetic defects and clinical manifestations in osteogenesis imperfecta. Butler W. T., *The Chemistry and Biology of Mineralized Tissue* (p. 391). Birmingham: Butler

16. Rowe D. W. and Shapiro J. R. (1990). Osteogenesis imperfecta. Avioli L. V. and Krane S. M., *Metabolic Bone Disease* (p. 659). Philadelphia: Saunders

17. Sanguinetti C., Greco F., DePalma L., Specchia N. and Falciglia F. (1990). Morphological changes in growth-plate cartilage in osteogenesis imperfecta. *J. Bone Jt Surg.*, **72B**, 475

18. Shapiro J. R. and Rowe D. W. (1987). Osteogenesis imperfecta. Martin T. J. and Raisz L. G., *Clinical Endocrinology of Calcium Metabolism* (p. 251). New York: Marcel Dekker

19. Siegel R. C. (1979). Lysyl oxidase. *Int. Rev. Connect. Tissue Res.*, **8**, 73

20. Smith R., Francis M. J. O. and Houghton G. R. (1983). *The Brittle Bone Syndrome: Osteogenesis Imperfecta*. London: Butterworths

21. Ste-Marie L. G., Charhon S. A., Edouard C., Chapuy M. C. and Meunier P. J. (1984). Iliac bone histomorphometry in adults and children with osteogenesis imperfecta. *J. Clin. Pathol.*, **37**, 1081

22. Teitelbaum S. L., Kraft W. J., Lang R. and Avioli L. V. (1974). Bone collagen aggregation abnormalities in osteogenesis imperfecta. *Calcif. Tissue Res.*, **17**, 75

23. Trelstad R. L., Rubin D. and Gross J. (1977). Osteogenesis imperfecta congenita. Evidence of a generalized molecular disorder of collagen. *Lab. Invest.*, **36**, 50

24. Tsipouras P., DelMastro R. and Sarfarazi M. (1992). Genetic linkage of the marfan syndrome, ectopia lentis, and congenital contractual arachnodactyly to the fibrillin genes on chromosomes 15 and 5. *N. Engl. J. Med.*, **326**, 905

25. Whyte M. P. (1990). Heritable metabolic and dysplastic bone disease. *Endocrinol. Metab. Clin. N. Amer.*, **19**, 133

Osteosclerosis

10

Osteosclerosis is characterized by an increase in skeletal mass (hyperostosis), usually involving both cortical and cancellous bone. In spite of the increase in density the affected bones are more fragile. Osteosclerosis is caused by increased bone formation, reduced bone resorption or both, and may be either inherited or acquired[13,40]. The osteoscleroses may be local, multifocal or generalized, and result from a variety of metabolic, inflammatory, toxic or neoplastic disorders in addition to the congenital forms[1,3,9]. The commoner syndromes which present with increased bone density are listed in Table 10.1. Those not related to metabolic and hereditary disorders will be discussed in the appropriate chapters. Increments in bone mass are manifest radiologically as increased osseous density, with variable alterations of the architecture of the bones involved[6,27].

Table 10.1 Main causes of osteosclerosis

Congenital disorders	Inflammatory disorders
Osteopetroses	'Sclerosing myelitis'
Carbonic anhydrase II deficiency	Sarcoidosis*
Pycnodysostosis	Radiation*
Progressive diaphyseal dysplasia*	Osteomyelitis* (followed by
Hyperphosphatasia	osteosclerosis)
Chemical poisoning	Haematopoietic disorders
Fluorosis	Sickle cell disease
Hypervitaminosis A, D	Osteomyelosclerosis
Heavy-metal poisoning	Malignant lymphomas*
Biphosphonate intoxication	Multiple myeloma (sclerotic
	variant)*
Endocrine disorders	Systemic mastocytosis*
Primary hyperparathyroidism	
Secondary hyperparathyroidism	Osteoblastic metastases
Acromegaly	Prostate carcinoma*
Hypothyroidism	Breast carcinoma*
Healing osteomalacia	
	Paget's disease (sclerotic phase)*

*May occur as widespread or as patchy osteosclerotic lesions

OSTEOPETROSIS (MARBLE BONE DISEASE)

This term is given to a number of inherited disorders characterized by a generalized increase in bone mass (Figs 10.R1 and 10.R2), in spite of which the bones fracture easily and the frequency of osteomyelitis is increased. It has now been demonstrated that osteopetrosis is due primarily to incompetent osteoclasts or their precursors, rendering them unresponsive to hormones and other regulatory factors, with consequent impairment of normal bone resorption[4,30]. Processes that rely on bone resorption, such as formation of adequate intertrabecular marrow spaces and bone modelling and remodelling, are either delayed or do not occur at all. This results in the delayed or inadequate formation or even the absence of marrow cavities, with signs of leukoerythroblastic anaemia and myelophthisis. Walker demonstrated that marble bone disease could be treated by early bone marrow transplantation[5,39]. However, it has since transpired that not all children were cured by this procedure, indicating the heterogeneity of the inherited osteopetroses[2,12,17,18].

There are *two main forms* of the disease:

1. an autosomal-dominant variant, less severe and usually manifest in adults[7], and

2. an autosomal-recessive variant affecting juveniles, often causing death from refractory anaemia because of the absence of marrow spaces and consequent haematopoietic failure[20].

Detailed histological studies have been made of *bone* from patients with congenital osteopetrosis by Shapiro *et al.*[35]. The volume of the marrow cavities was greatly reduced and the border between the cortex and cancellous bone was blurred or indistinguishable (Plate 10.A)[23]. The periosteal surface expands while decreased endosteal resorption inhibits remodelling of the marrow cavities

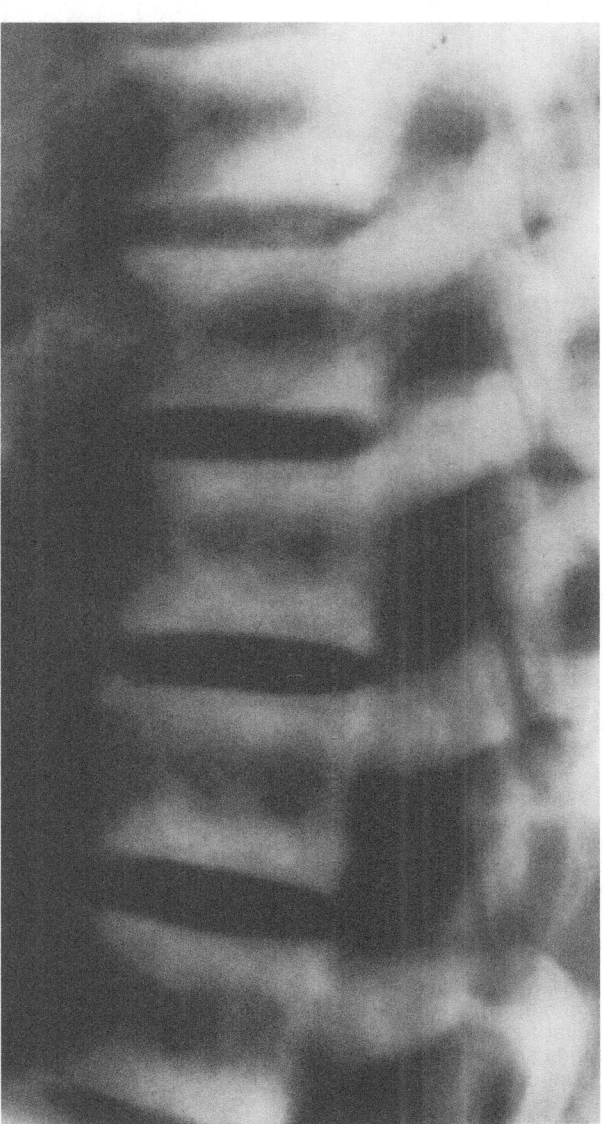

Fig. 10.R1 'Sandwich vertebrae' in osteopetrosis (Albers–Schönberg disease, 'marble bone disease')

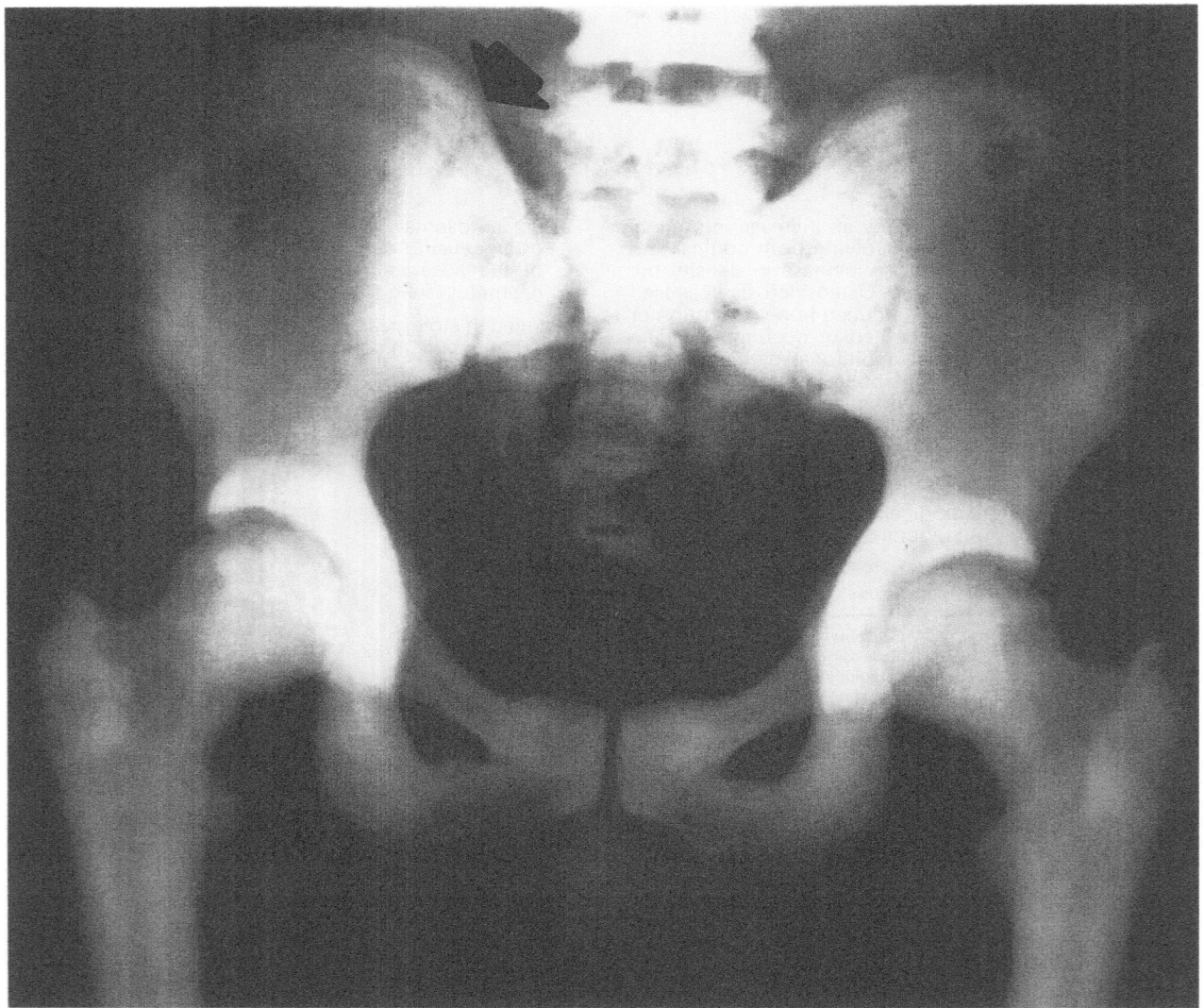

Fig. 10.R2 Osteopetrosis: overall increase in bone density in ilium and femur. Arrow indicates biopsy site

(Figs 10.7 and 10.8). These processes lead to a thick cortex indistinguishable from the compact 'trabecular bone' region (Plate 10.C). In general, the microscopic appearance indicated that little remodelling had occurred. The increased bone density is manifest predominantly as an architectural effect caused by reduced activation of remodelling: lamellar bone persists unremodelled.

The number of *osteoclasts*, however, has variously been reported to be decreased, normal or even increased[19,20,38]. In some cases bone resorption was absent even in the presence of twice the normal number of osteoclasts. In these patients the ruffled border of the osteoclasts was reduced in size, suggesting a defect in the system that signals them to start osseous resorption; but this abnormality was not found in all cases. In a few cases, osteoclasts have been shown to contain viral inclusions, similar to the nucleocapsides of Paramyxoviridae[26]. Their significance, however, is still unclear. Other possibilities of osteoclast failure are:

1. defects of the signals that mediate the recruitment and differentiation of progenitor cells[28],

2. failure of chemotactic factors responsible for cell migration,
3. lack of factors that cause osteoclasts to begin resorption, possibly mediated by osteoblasts, and
4. defect of the ability of osteoclasts to 'recognize' resorbable bone, though fully capable of its breakdown once recognized.

In summary, the *pathogenesis of inherited osteopetrosis* is heterogeneous and includes the following possibilities:

1. a morphological and biochemical abnormality that results in impaired bone resorption[30,36],
2. an abnormality in the haematopoietic system (defective monocytes, T- and B-lymphocytes), that impairs the differentiation of the osteoclast precursor[3,11,16,21,25,41],
3. an abnormality in the stromal system of bone and marrow,
4. abnormalities of humoral or non-marrow cellular factors,
5. hormonal abnormalities (e.g. vitamin D, calcitonin and parathyroid hormone)[8,24,32], and
6. a viral aetiology[26,37].

[continued on p. 126]

Plate 10.A

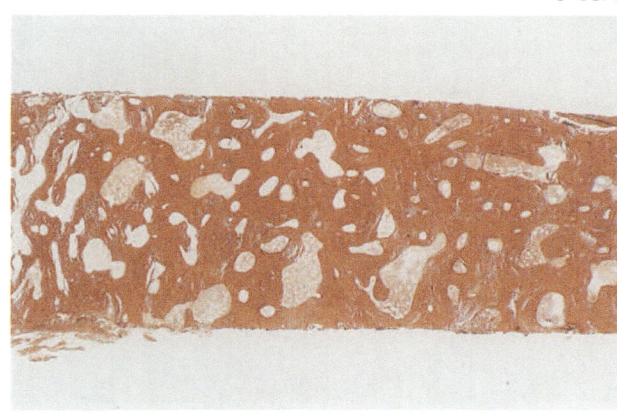

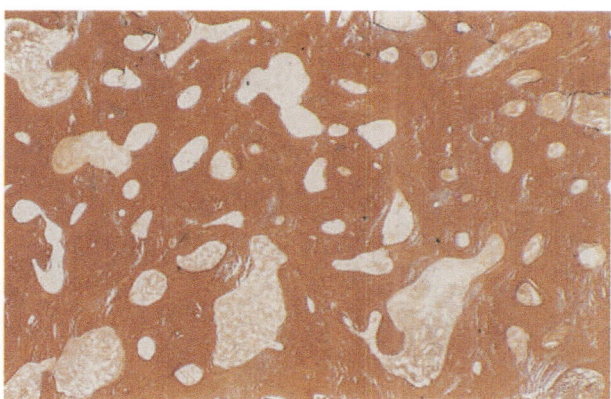

Figs. 10.1–10.6 Iliac crest biopsies in osteosclerosis I

Fig. 10.1 Iliac crest biopsy of young adult with osteoporosis. Note subcortical area (left) containing more marrow cavities than the more distal part of the biopsy (right). Gomori

Fig. 10.2 Higher magnification of the biopsy in Fig. 10.1. The trabecular network has been thickened to such an extent that the original structure has been obliterated. Gomori

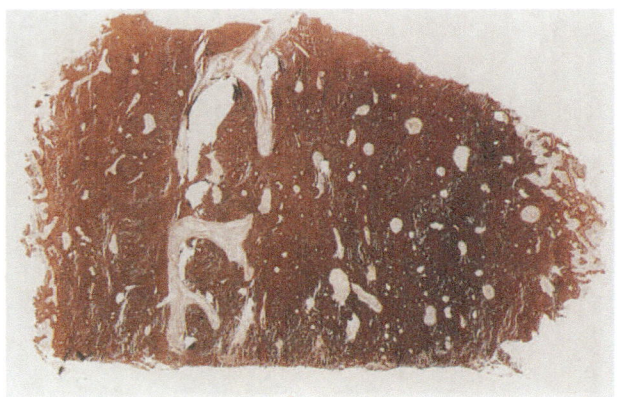

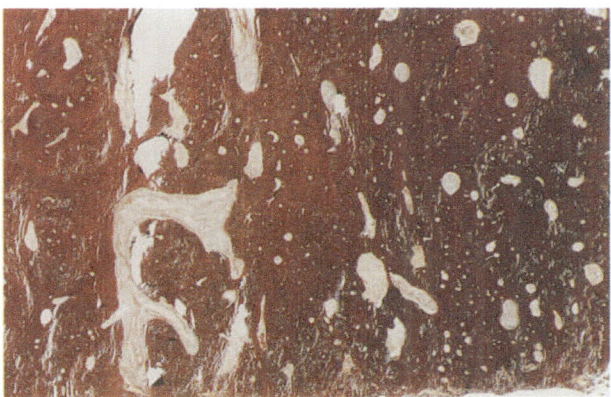

Fig. 10.3 Iliac crest biopsy of patient with osteosclerosis showing cortical bone and some residual bone marrow cavities in the subcortical region. Gomori

Fig. 10.4 Higher magnification of part of section shown in Fig. 10.3 illustrating almost complete obliteration of the marrow cavities. Gomori

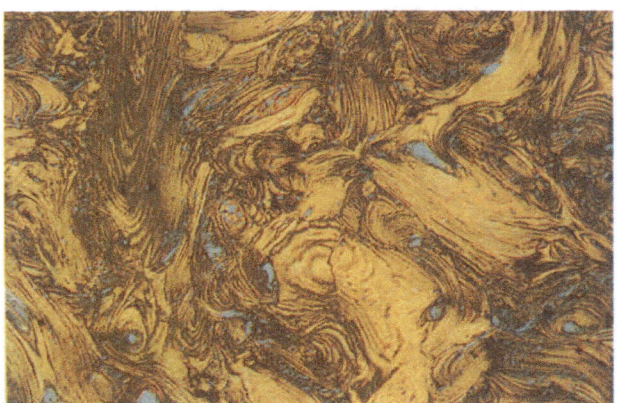

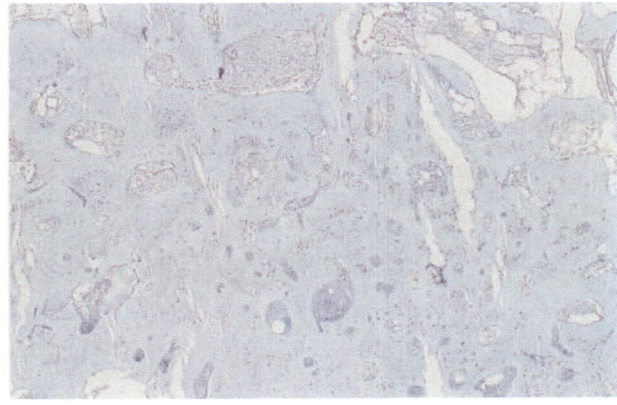

Fig. 10.5 Central part of biopsy section of patient with osteosclerosis. Altered lamellar structure in 'ivory bone'. Gomori, polar.

Fig. 10.6 Central part of biopsy section of patient with osteosclerosis. The bone shows numerous Haversian-like structures. Giemsa

Plate 10.B

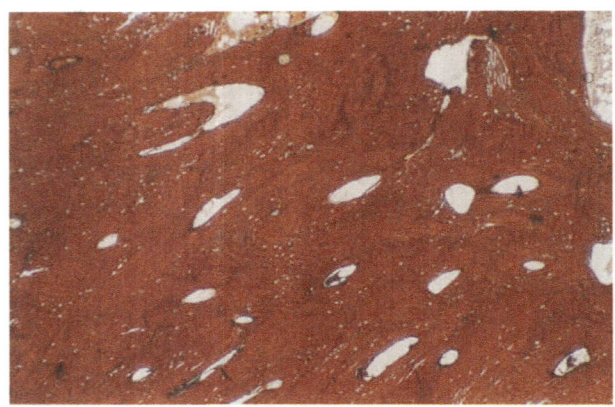

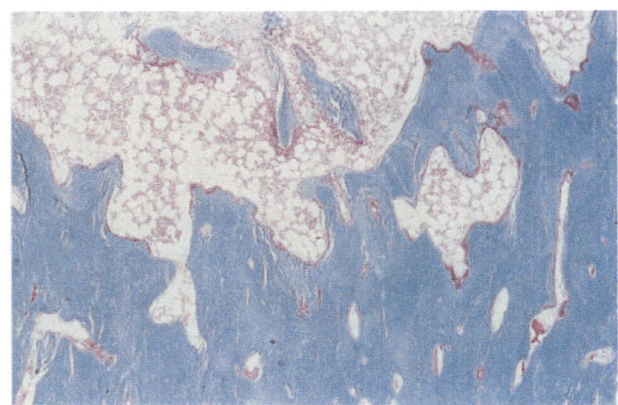

Figs. 10.7–10.12 Iliac crest biopsies in osteosclerosis II

Fig. 10.7 Iliac crest biopsy of a patient with osteosclerosis and bone marrow failure. Note multiple small residual marrow cavities but no haematopoietic cells. Gomori

Fig. 10.8 Iliac crest biopsy of a patient with osteosclerosis, milder form of disease. Note larger marrow spaces with some haematopoieic tissue and osteoid (red). Ladewig

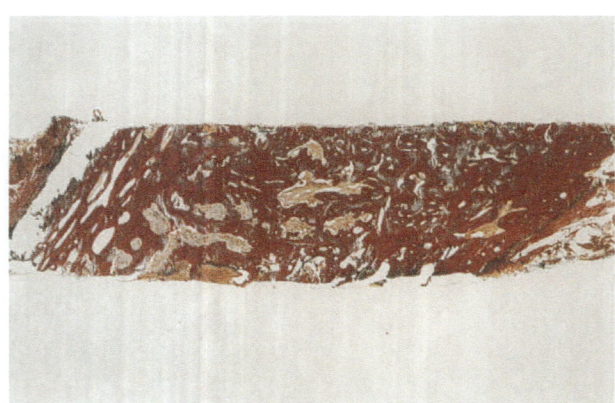

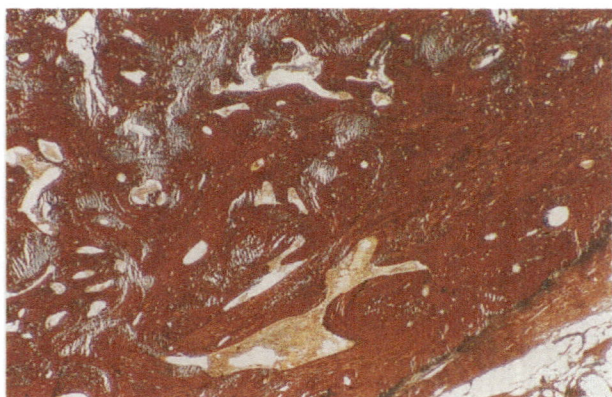

Fig. 10.9 Iliac crest biopsy of a patient with fluorosis. Tangential biopsy showing cortical bone at both ends. Gomori

Fig. 10.10 Higher magnification of biopsy in Fig. 10.9, with thickening of the trabecular bone and encroachment on the marrow spaces. Gomori

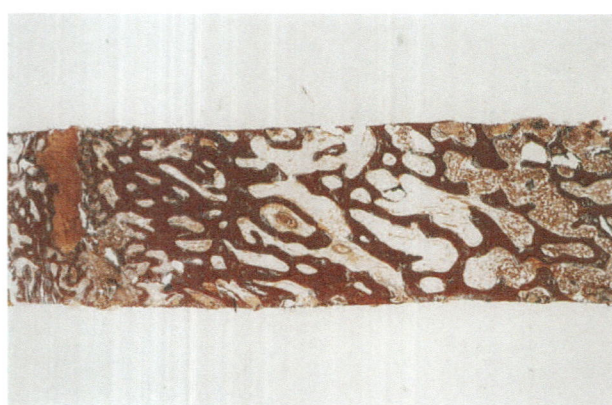

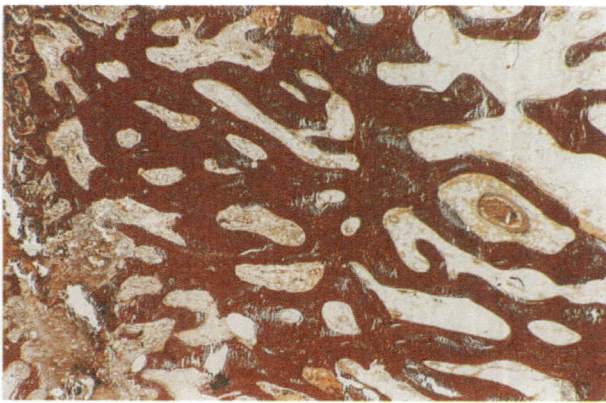

Fig. 10.11 Low magnification of iliac crest biopsy in fluorosis. Gomori. The biopsy was taken because of the incidental finding of osteosclerosis on routine X-ray of the skeleton

Fig. 10.12 Higher magnification of biopsy in Fig. 10.11. Note particularly subcortical thickening of trabecular network. Gomori

Plate 10.C

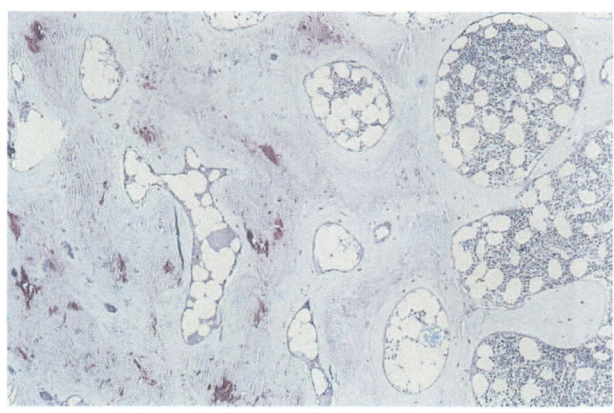

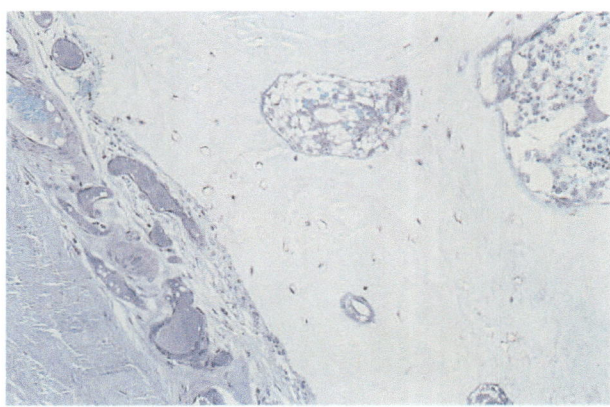

Figs. 10.13–10.18 Aspects of cortical thickening in osteosclerosis

Fig. 10.13 Iliac crest biopsy of a child with osteosclerosis: broad cortex and thickening of trabecular network in the subcortical zone. Note multiple islands of residual cartilage. Giemsa

Figs. 10.14 and **10.15** Iliac crest biopsy of young adult with osteosclerosis of unknown origin
Fig. 10.14 Broad cortex, but presence of bone remodelling and dissecting osteoclasia (centre). Note high vascularity of the periosteum. Giemsa

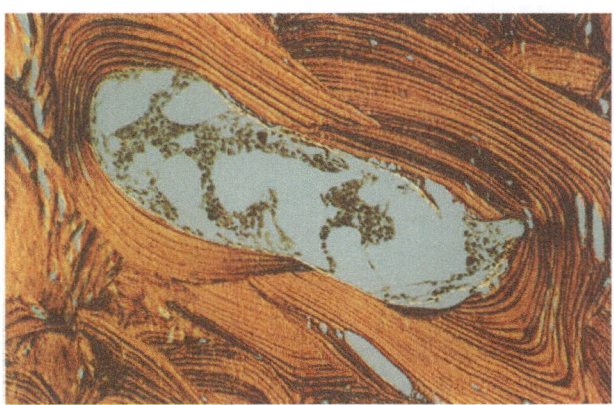

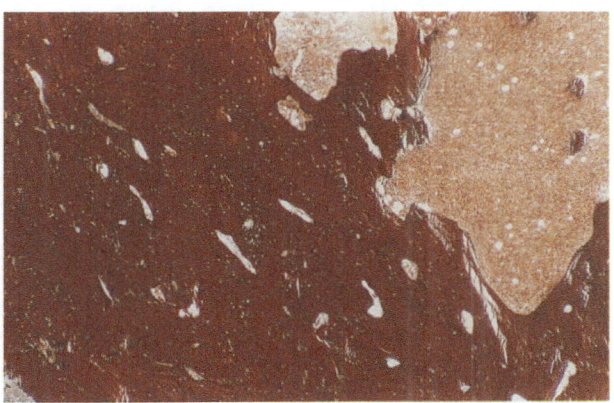

Fig. 10.15 Higher magnification of biopsy from Fig. 10.14 showing lamellar organization and signs of previous remodelling. Gomori, polar.

Figs. 10.16–10.18 Iliac crest biopsy of an older individual with osteosclerosis of unknown origin

Fig. 10.16 Thick cortex with only small Volkmann's canals. Gomori

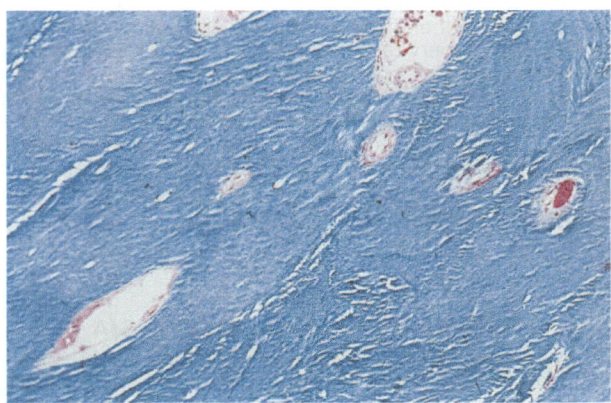

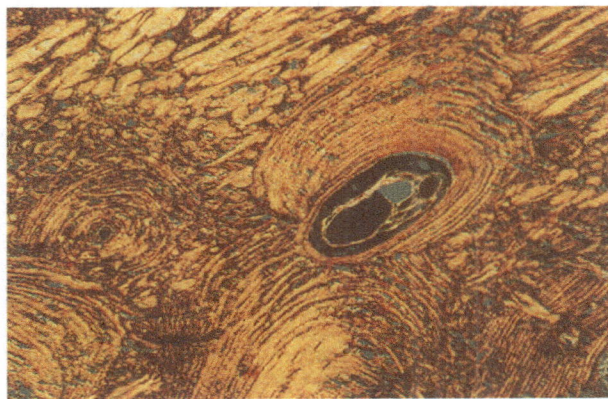

Fig. 10.17 Higher magnification illustrating absence of osteoid seams and bone formation. Presence of vessels in the Volkmann's canals. Ladewig

Fig. 10.18 Higher magnification with irregular and patchy orientation of lamellar structures. Gomori, polar.

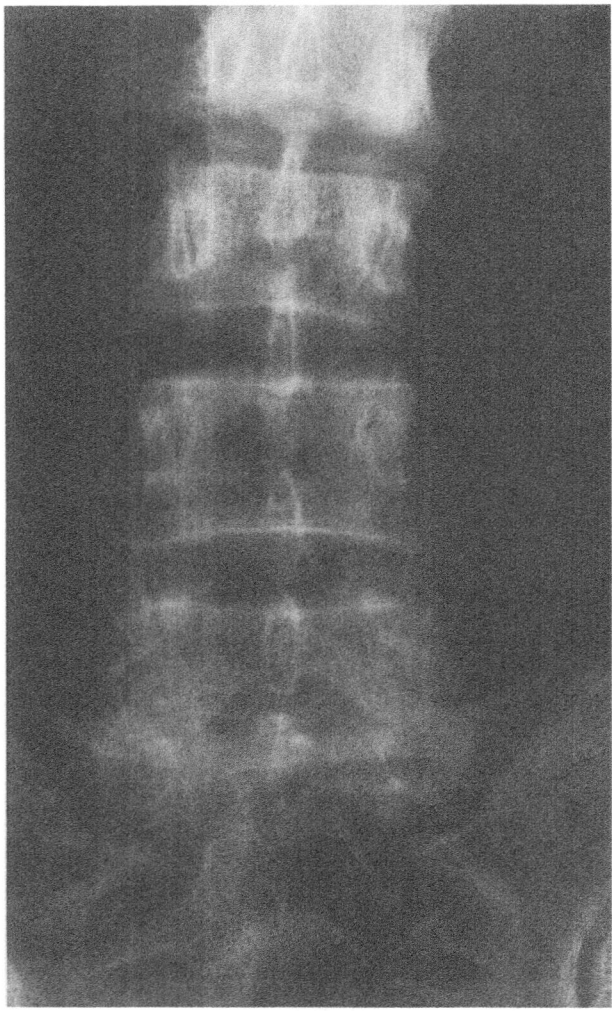

Fig. 10.R3 Fluorosis, with coarsening and thickening of the trabecular pattern

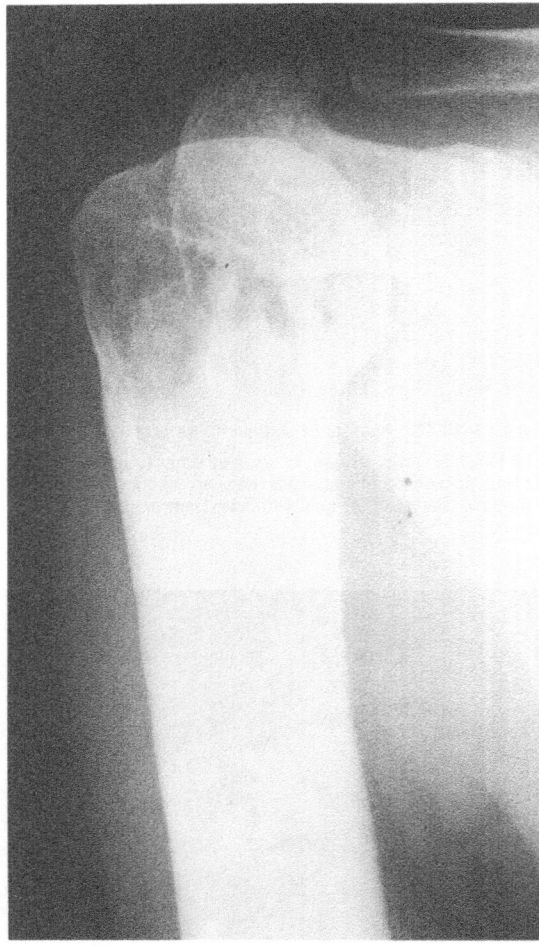

Figs. 10.R4 and **10.R5** Camurati–Engelmann's disease. X-rays kindly supplied by Dr D. Wuttge-Hannig, Technical University of Munich. The anterior iliac crest biopsy showed no abnormalities of bone structure, osseous remodelling and marrow architecture

Fig. 10.R4 Marked hyperostosis of the diaphyses of long bones (humerus). The metaphyses and epiphyses are spared

FLUOROSIS

Fluoride is incorporated into bone matrix and stimulates osteoblastic activity[10,14,42]. Fluoride is lost from the skeleton at a very low rate; only about 50% decrease in skeletal fluoride content after 20 years. Prolonged exposure to high concentrations of fluoride during industrial processes, during therapeutic administration, or drinking of mineral water rich in fluoride may produce systemic osteosclerosis[22].

Radiographs show sclerosis throughout the skeleton, with the most pronounced changes in the vertebrae and pelvis (Fig. 10.R3). Bone histology reveals increases in values of remodelling, of trabecular bone and osteoid, and of osteoclastic activity (Figs. 10.9–10.12). There is disordered lamellar orientation and the overall histological appearance has some similarities to Paget's disease. The definite diagnosis of fluorosis is made by clinical history and by chemical analysis of a small piece of the iliac crest biopsy.

Other acquired osteopetroses may result from pharmacological reduction in bone resorption, such as treatment with diphosphonates. A number of other chemicals may also cause an increase in bone density as part of their effects on the body: lead, phosphorus, bismuth and mercury[3,29]. Generalized osteosclerosis may occur in children with hypervitaminosis A and D. Prolonged and intensive physical activity affect the stressed parts of the skeleton and cause osteosclerosis, though the trabecular structure and the bone remodelling proved to be normal in the cases examined so far. Dietary or even pharmacological influences must be excluded in patients with increased bone volume (even, for example, in olympic athletes) (Plate 10.D).

PROGRESSIVE DIAPHYSEAL DYSPLASIA

The generalized form of progressive diapyseal dysplasia, also called 'Camurati–Engelmann's disease', has received some attention because of its striking clinical features, in particular osteosclerotic lesions (woven bone) primarily confined to the diaphyses of long bones (Figs. 10.R4 and 10.R5). In severe cases, however, the osteosclerosis is widespread, and the skull and axial skeleton are also

Plate 10.D

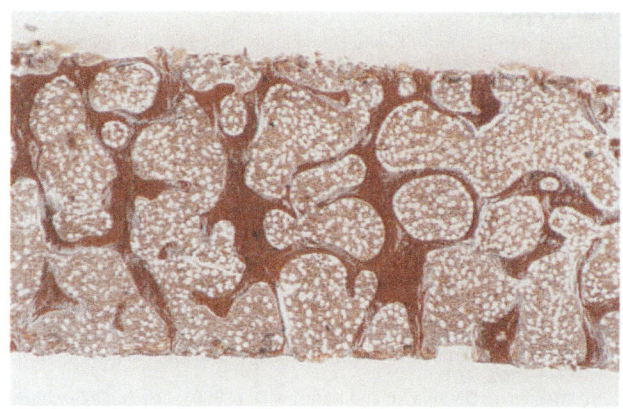

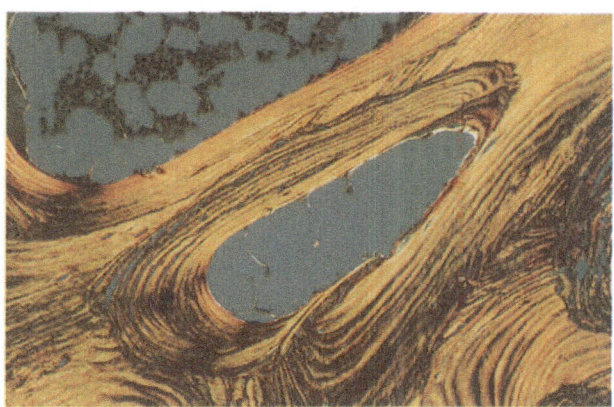

Figs. 10.19–10.21 Iliac crest biopsy of an adult athlete (decathlon)

Fig. 10.19 Overview of biopsy with thick, connected trabeculae and normocellular marrow. Gomori

Fig. 10.20 Higher magnification showing parallel orientation of lamellae. Gomori, polar.

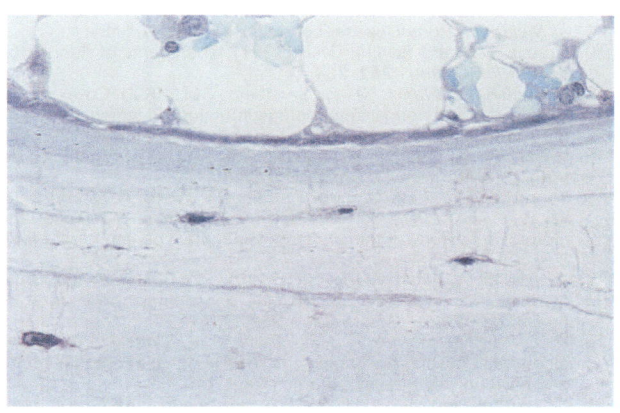

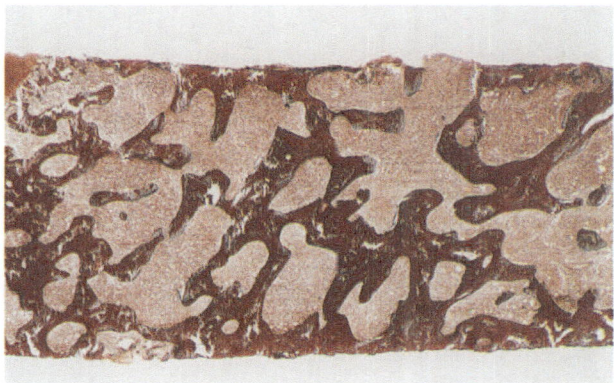

Fig. 10.21 Broad ossicle with seam of osteoid and a layer of flat osteoblasts. Note parallel cement lines and osteocytes with canaliculi. Giemsa

Figs. 10.22–10.24 Iliac crest biopsy of a 12-year-old athlete

Fig. 10.22 Overview of biopsy with increased trabecular bone volume, part of growth plate (upper left) and hypercellular marrow. Gomori

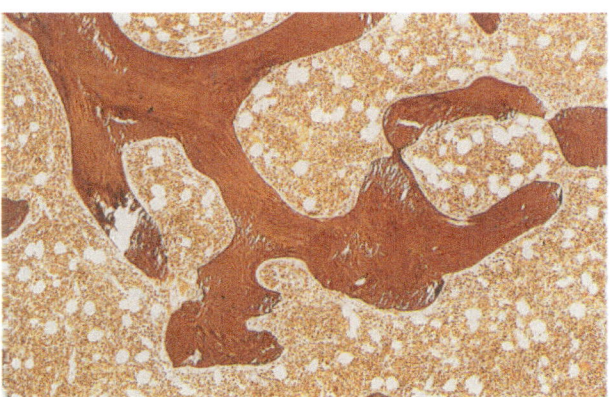

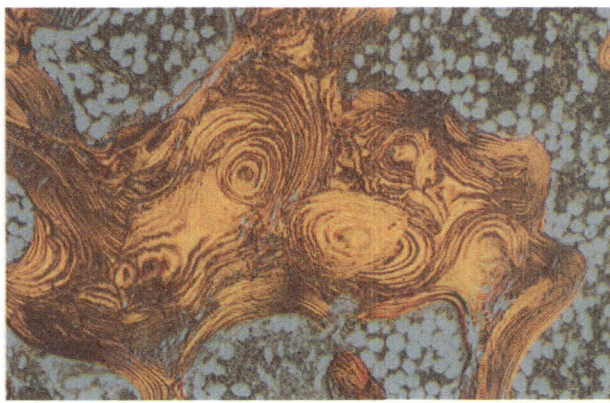

Fig. 10.23 Higher magnification showing increased trabecular width and surface. Gomori

Fig. 10.24 Broad junction of five trabeculae, with multiple osteons in the centre. Gomori, polar.

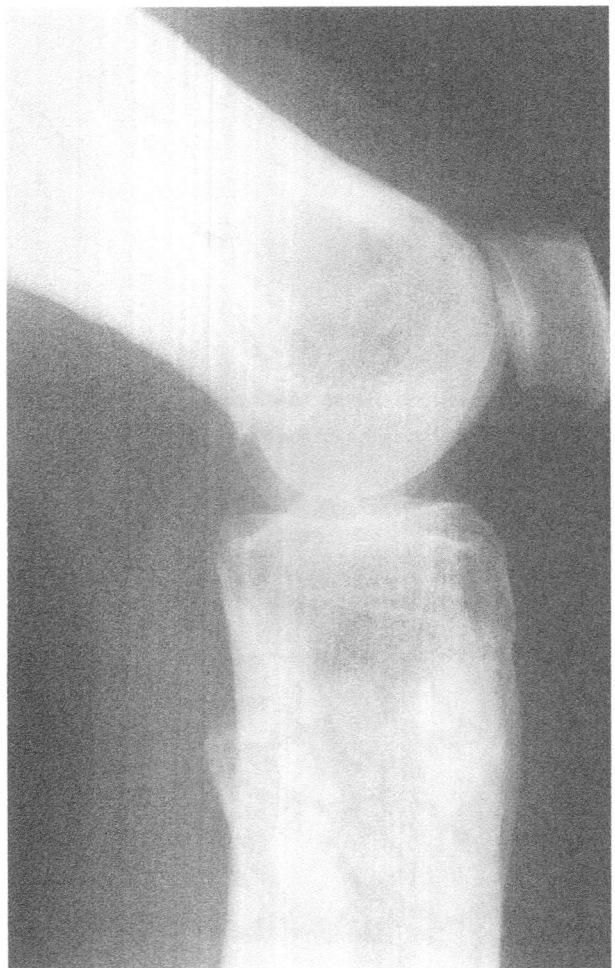

Fig. 10.R5 Marked hyperostosis of the diaphyses of femur and tibia. The metaphyses and epiphyses are spared

involved[15]. Sear reported increased bone density of the ilium, near the sacroiliac joints, and of the ischium, near the acetabulum. However, iliac crest biopsy examination in one case did not show any abnormalities of bone or marrow, at least in the anterior iliac crest area.

The clinical and laboratory manifestations of Engelmann's disease, together with its ready responsiveness to glucocorticoid treatment, account for the suggestion that it is a systemic inflammatory disorder of connective tissue.

OTHER SCLEROSING DISORDERS OF BONE

Hyperostosis is a term describing an abnormal increase in the ossification of the skeleton, but not applicable to adaptive changes such as those occurring as a result of physical exercise. Some local, unusual and obscure variants of hyperostosis are *ankylosing hyperostosis of spine, hyperostosis frontalis interna, melorheostosis* and *osteopoikilosis*. These are only mentioned here; further information can be obtained in several books and reviews on metabolic and dysplastic bone diseases[6,27,31,40].

References

1. Beighton P., Horan F. and Hammersma H. (1977). A review of the osteoscleroses. *Postgrad. Med. J.*, **53**, 507
2. Bollerslev J., Nielsen H. K., Storm T. and Mosekilde L. (1988). Serum vitamin D metabolites and nuclear uptake of (3H)-1,25-dihydroxyvitamin D 3 in monocytes from patients with autosomal dominant osteopetrosis: a study of two radiological types. *Calcif. Tissue Int.*, **43**(2), 67
3. Bowley N. B. (1984). Osteosclerosis. Nordin B. E. C., *Metabolic Bone and Stone Disease* (p. 234). Edinburgh: Churchill Livingstone
4. Burr D. B. and Martin R. B. (1988). Errors in bone remodeling: toward a unified theory of metabolic bone disease. *Amer. J. Anat.*, **186**, 186
5. Coccia P. F., Krivit W., Cervenka J., Clawson C., Kersey J., Kim T. H., Nesbit M. E., Ramsay M. K. C., Warkentin P. I., Teitelbaum S. L., Kahn A. J. and Brown D. M. (1980). Successful bone marrow transplantation for infantile malignant osteopetrosis. *N. Engl. J. Med.*, **302**, 701
6. Edeiken J., Dalinka M. and Karasick D. (1990). *Edeiken's Roentgen Diagnosis of Diseases of Bone*. Baltimore: Williams & Wilkins
7. Evans R. A., Hughes W. G., Dunstan C. R., Lennon W. P., Kohan L., Hills E. and Wong S. Y. P. (1983). Adult osteopetrosis. *Metab. Bone Dis. Rel. Res.*, **5**, 111
8. Glorieux F. H., Pettifor J. M., Marie P. J., Delvin E. E., Travers R. and Shepard N. (1981). Induction of bone resorption by parathyroid hormone in congenital malignant osteopetrosis. *Metab. Bone Dis. Rel. Res.*, **3**, 143
9. Grech P., Martin T. J., Barrinton N. A. and Ell P. J. (1985). *Diagnosis of Metabolic Bone Disease*. London: Chapman & Hall
10. Gruber H. E. and Baylink D. J. (1991). The effects of fluoride on bone. *Clin. Orthop.*, **267**, 264
11. Hochmann N., Wahl L. M. and Sandberg A. L. (1982). Co-existence of defective and normal immunologic functions in lymphocytes and macrophages from osteopetrotic (op) rats. *J. Immunol.*, **129**, 278
12. Horton W. A., Schimke R. N. and Iyama T. (1980). Osteopetrosis: further heterogeneity. *J. Pediatr.*, **97**, 580
13. Johnston C. C., Lavy N., Lord T., Vellios F., Merrit A. D. and Deiss W. P. (1968). Osteopetrosis: a clinical, genetic, metabolic, and morphologic study of the dominantly inherited, benign form. *Medicine*, **47**, 149
14. Khoker M. A. and Dandona P. (1990). Fluoride stimulates (3D) thymidine incorporation and alkaline phosphatase production by human osteoblasts. *Metabolism*, **39**(11), 1118
15. Kumar B., Murphy W. A. and Whyte M. P. (1981). Progressive diaphyseal dysplasia (Engelmann disease): scintigraphic–radiographic–clinical correlations. *Radiology*, **140**, 87
16. Labat M.-L. and Milhaud G. (1986). Osteopetrosis and the immune deficiency syndrome. Peck W. A., *Bone and Mineral Research*, vol. 4 (p. 131). Amsterdam: Elsevier
17. Marks C. R., Seifert M. F. and Marks S. C. (1984). Osteoclast populations in congenital osteopetrosis: additional evidence of heterogeneity. *Metab. Bone Dis. Rel. Res.*, **5**, 259
18. Marks S. C. (1987). Osteopetrosis – multiple pathways for the interception of osteoclast function. *Appl. Pathol.*, **5**, 172
19. Marks S. C. (1973). Pathogenesis of osteopetrosis in the ia rat: reduced bone resorption due to reduced osteoclast function. *Amer. J. Anat.*, **138**, 165
20. Marks S. C. and McGuire J. L. (1989). Primary bone cell dysfunction II-osteopetrosis. Tam C. S., Heersche J. N. M. and Murray T. M., *Metabolic Bone Disease: Cellular and Tissue Mechanism* (p. 49). Boca Raton: CRC Press)
21. Marks S. C. and Walker D. G. (1981). The hematogenous origin of osteoclasts: experimental evidence of osteopetrotic (microphthalmic) mice treated with spleen cells from beige mouse donors. *Amer. J. Anat.*, **161**, 1
22. Meunier P. J., Femenias M., Duboeuf F., Chapuy M. C. and Delmas P. D. (1989). Increased vertebral bone density in heavy drinkers of mineral water rich in fluoride. *Lancet*, **45**(1), 152
23. Milgram J. W. and Jasty M. (1982). Osteopetrosis: a morphological study of twenty-one cases. *J. Bone Jt Surg.*, **64A**, 912
24. Milhaud G., Labat M. L., Litwin I., Moricard Y., Moutier R., Rimbaut C., Buffe D. and Juster M. (1981). Osteopetro-rickets: a new congenital bone disorder. *Metab. Bone Dis. Rel. Res.*, **3**, 91
25. Milhaud G. and Labat M. L. (1978). Thymus and osteopetrosis. *Clin. Orthop.*, **135**, 260
26. Mills B.-G., Yake H. and Singer F. R. (1988). Osteoclasts in human osteopetrosis contain viral nucleocapsid-like nuclear inclusions. *J. Bone Miner. Res.*, **3**(1), 101
27. Murray R. O., Jacobson H. G. and Stoker D. J. (1990). *The Radiology of Skeletal Disorders*. Edinburgh: Churchill Livingstone

28. Nisbet N. W., Menage J. and Loutit J. F. (1982). Osteogenesis in osteopetrotic mice. *Calcif. Tissue Int.*, **34**, 37

29. Pounds J. G., Long G. J. and Rosen J. F. (1991). Cellular and molecular toxicity of lead in bone. *Environ. Health Perspect.*, **91**, 17

30. Reeves J., Arnaud S., Gordon S., Subryan B., Block M., Huffer W., Arnaud C., Mundy G. and Haussler M. (1981). The pathogenesis of infnatile malignant osteopetrosis: bone mineral metabolism, and complications in five infants. *Metab. Bone Dis. Rel. Res.*, **3**, 135

31. Revell P. A. (1986). *Pathology of Bone*. Berlin: Springer

32. Rouleau M., Warshawsky H., Marks S. C. and Goltzman D. (1986). Calcitonin receptor binding as a marker of osteoclast heterogeneity in osteopetrotic rodents. *J. Bone Miner. Res.*, **1**, 543

33. Schneider G. B. (1978). The role of lymphoid cells in bone resorption. Cellular immunologic competence in ia rats. *Amer. J. Anat.*, **153**, 305

34. Sear H. R. (1948). Engelmann's disease. *Brit. J. Radiol.*, **21**, 236

35. Shapiro F., Glimcher M. J., Holtrop M. E., Tashjian A. H., Brickley-Parsons D. and Kenzora J. E. (1980). Human osteopetrosis. *J. Bone Jt Surg.*, **62A**, 384

36. Sly W. S., Whyte M. P. and Sundaram V. (1985). Carbonic anhydrase II deficiency in 12 families with the autosomal recessive syndrome of osteopetrosis with renal tubular acidosis and cerebral calcification. *N. Engl. J. Med.*, **313**, 139

37. Smith R. E. and Morgan J. H. (1984). Pathogenesis of osteopetrosis induced by rapid and slow onset plaque isolated of an avian osteopetrosis virus. *Metab. Bone Dis. Rel. Res.*, **5**, 289

38. Volker G. (1981). Diagnosis of osteopetrosis (Albers-Schönberg) by Jamshidi needle biopsy. *Hum. Pathol.*, **12**, 198

39. Walker D. G. (1975). Control of bone resorption by hematopoietic tissue. The induction and reversal of congenital osteopetrosis in mice through use of bone marrow and splenic transplants. *J. Exp. Med.*, **142**, 651

40. Whyte M. P. (1990). Heritable metabolic and dysplastic bone disease. *Endocrinol. Metab. Clin. N. Amer.*, **19**(1), 133

41. Wiktor-Jedrzejczak W., Ahmed A., Szczylik C. and Skelly R. R. (1982). Hematological characterization of congenital osteopetrosis in op/op mouse. Possible mechanism for abnormal macrophage differentiation. *J. Exp. Med.*, **156**, 1516

42. Zerwekh J. E., Morris A. C., Padalino P. K., Gottschalk F. and Pak C. Y. (1990). Fluoride rapidly and transiently raises intracellular calcium in human osteoblasts. *J. Bone Miner. Res.*, **5**(1), 131

The following reference describes a modern and unusual cause of osteosclerosis:

Villareal D. T., Murphy W. A., Teitelbaum S. T., Arens M. Q. and Whyte M. P. (1992). Painful diffuse osteosclerosis after intravenous drug abuse. *Amer. J. Med.*, **93**, 371

Osteomalacia

11

Osteomalacia (soft bone) is the skeletal manifestation of various metabolic abnormalities which result in defective bone formation[1,2,14,16,33,34,39]: the lag time between bone formation and mineralization is increased, generally by more than 100 days. Histomorphometrically, this results in a high osteoid volume greater than 10% of the total bone volume. Because the rate of bone turnover is greater in trabecular bone, the most prominent manifestation in osteomalacia occurs along the trabecular surface characterized by extensive and thick osteoid seams. Severe osteomalacia also results in patchy periosteocytic and intratrabecular areas of demineralization. For the full expression of a mineralization defect, an adequate amount of bone matrix must be formed by the osteoblasts (matrix synthesis). When osteomalacia occurs in children, it is called *rickets*, which includes the epiphyseal effects of defective skeletal mineralization (Figs 11.R1 and 11.R2). The 'softness' of bone results in progressive deformity and pain under normal stresses. The overall reduction in skeletal density and, more helpful, the *Looser's zones* constitute the typical radiological features in adults (Fig. 11.R3)[2,37]. When the diagnosis is considered, selected biochemical investigations are essential for confirmation of the underlying abnormality. The combination of low plasma calcium (hypocalcaemia, Table 11.1) and phosphate concentrations with a high level of osseous alkaline phosphatase generally points to the diagnosis of osteomalacia. Plasma levels of 25-OH vitamin D and of PTH are useful for the main differential diagnosis of nutritional[10], gastrointestinal (Fig. 11.S1)[11,13,19,43,45] and renal[12] variants. The main causes of osteomalacia and rickets are summarized in Table 11.2.

To understand the evolution of osteomalacic bone diseases one must consider the complex process of *mineralization*[24,27,28,31]. Approximately 90% of bone matrix is composed of collagen, while the remaining 10% consists primarily of organic non-collagenous proteins, proteoglycans and lipids. Several of these important constituents (e.g. osteonectin) appear to control the orientation and growth of mineral crystals in osteoid. Osteoblasts produce bone matrix and play a role in its maturation, which occurs during the 8–20 days after synthesis and before mineral is deposited at the mineralization front (matrix maturation time). At present this maturation process is not clearly understood, but alterations of these matrix events can lead to the occurrence of osteomalacia. The most critical portion of the osteoid seam is an area about 3 μm wide at the osteoid–mineralized bone interface, known as the *mineralization front* (Fig. 11.S2)[27]. This is the site of primary mineralization, still under the influence of osteoblasts and 'nearly-osteoid-osteocytes', where approximately 80% of mineral is deposited in a short period of 3–4 days. In the following 3–4 months, mineral accumulates more slowly distal to the mineralization front until a maximal calcification level of approximately 95% is reached. During this phase of secondary mineralization, which appears to be independent of any significant influence emanating from the osteoblasts covering the osteoid seam, bone crystal growth slowly displaces crystal-bound water. At the mineralization front an amorphous calcium complex transforms into crystal calcium hydroxyapatite. The mineralization front is also the site of tetracycline binding, a phenomenon which has

aided the study of remodelling in osteomalacia and other metabolic disorders of bone.

Though in some patients a presumptive *diagnosis* can be obtained from results of biochemistry and radiology, mineralized bone histology provides the only reliable means of diagnosing all cases of osteomalacia (Plate 11.A), especially the mild forms. The iliac crest is the

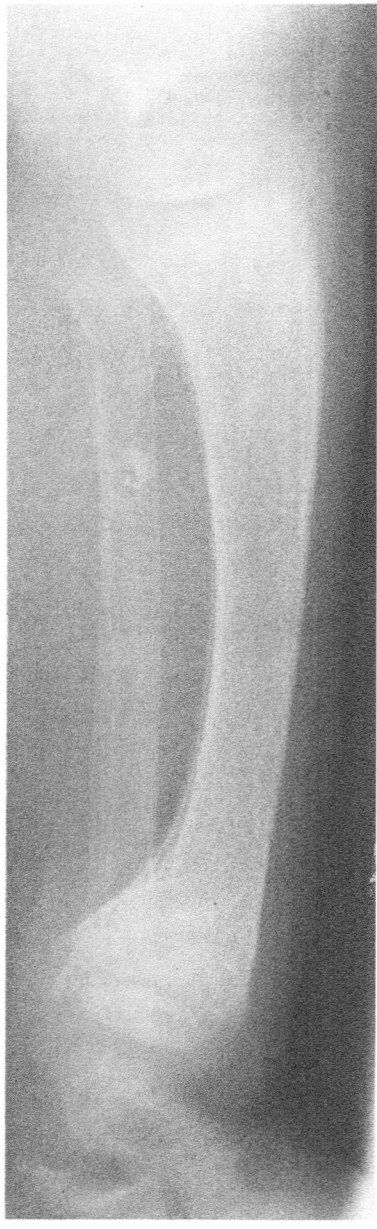

Fig. 11.R1   Juvenile osteomalacia (rickets) in a 3-year-old child, with marked anterior bowing of the tibia

Plate 11.A

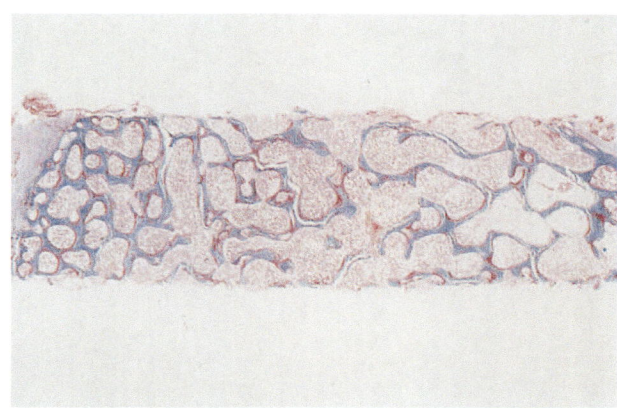

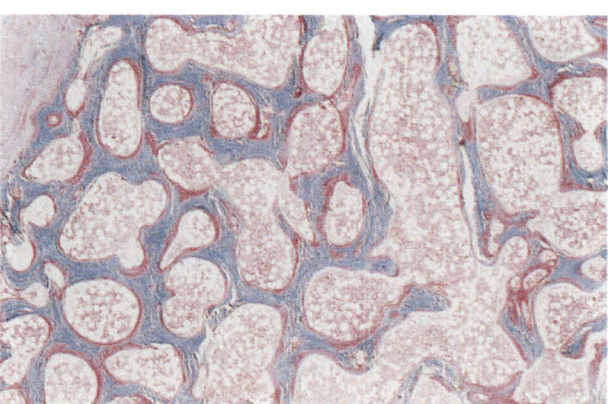

Figs. 11.1–11.4 Iliac crest biopsy of patients with osteomalacia

Fig. 11.1 Overview showing preservation of normal trabecular bone structure, though there are architectural variations in the different zones of the biopsy. Ladewig

Fig. 11.2 Higher magnification demonstrating denser trabecular network in subcortical region and revealing increased extent of osteoid surfaces on the trabecular bone. Ladewig

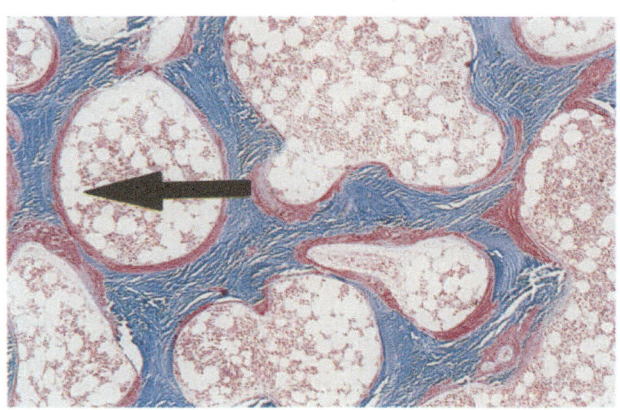

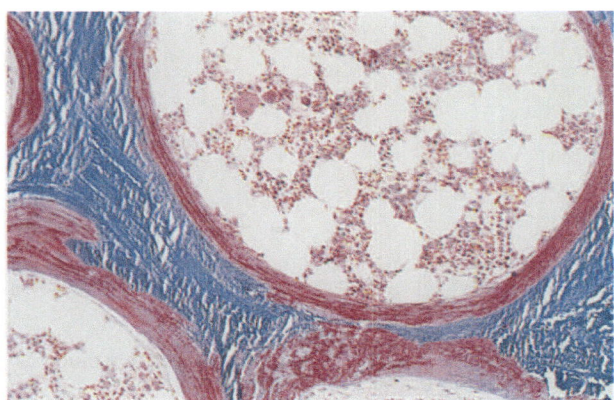

Fig. 11.3 Higher magnification of area of Fig. 11.2 illustrates that nearly all trabecular surfaces are covered by a layer of osteoid. Ladewig

Fig. 11.4 Higher magnification of area from Fig. 11.3 (arrow) shows layer of osteoid as well as patchy, irregular demineralization of trabecular bone. Ladewig

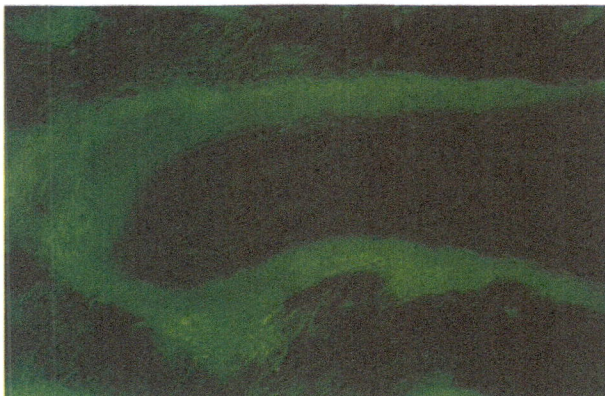

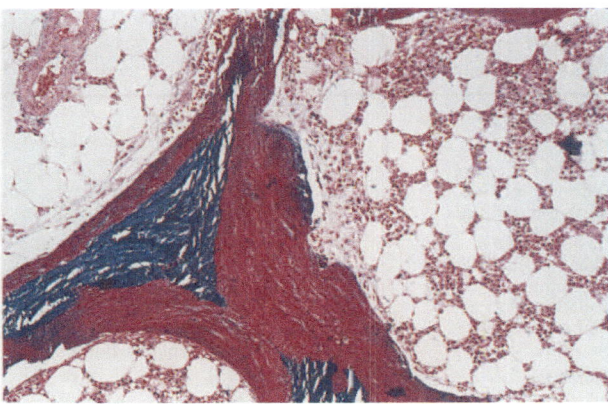

Fig. 11.5 Tetracycline labelling shows diffuse, broad fluorescence surrounding a trabecular surface (= osteoid layer as seen in Ladewig stain)

Fig. 11.6 Iliac crest biopsy of patient with osteomalacia showing osteoid spanning the trabecular width, a phenomenon characteristic of marked osteomalacia. Ladewig

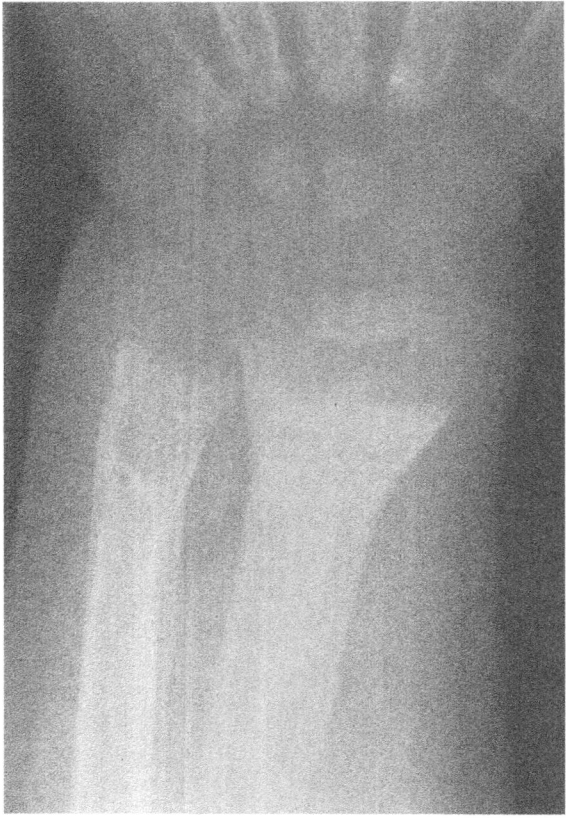

Fig. 11.R2 Juvenila osteomalacia (rickets), same patient as in Fig. 11.R1: metaphyses with wide bands of translucency and irregularities of the metaphyseal margins

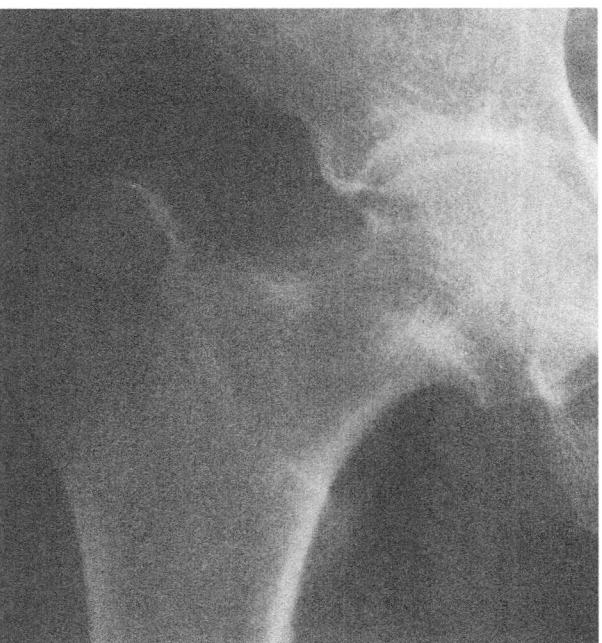

Fig. 11.R3 Looser zone of the femoral neck: a transverse band about 3 mm thick at right angle to the cortex and involving mainly the cortex with slight periosteal reaction. The Looser's zones are the radiological hallmark of osteomalacia and are found mainly in bones responsible for bearing the major mechanical stresses. They are often multiple, bilateral and can be related anatomically to the arterial supply of the bone (sites of entrance of nutrient arteries). They may progress to complete fractures and may heal very slowly even under therapy. (Kindly supplied by Prof. M. Kessler, Department of Radiology, Klinikum Großhadern, University of Munich)

most commonly used site of biopsy. Two simple diagnostic criteria apply in the vast majority of cases:

1. increased extent of osteoid surfaces (> 50% of the trabecular surface), and
2. increased width of the osteoid seams (> 15 μm),

so that the overall effect is an increased osteoid volume (> 10% of the trabecular bone volume). Islands of non-mineralized bone matrix within the trabeculae and in the periosteocytic area are highly characteristic (Plate 11.B) and are also important criteria in distinguishing osteoma-

lacia from high-turnover states without defective mineralization (e.g. Paget's disease, pHPT). In minor and in 'mixed' variants of osteomalacia refinements can be added to these criteria, including the demonstration of decreased extent of calcification fronts and prolonged mineralization lag time by double tetracycline labelling (> 100 days). Two examples are the osteomalacia associated with the use of diphosphonates in Paget's disease and that occurring with aluminium toxicity in patients with chronic renal failure[3,12,25,26,36]. Analogous to the situation in osteoporosis it is not clear whether high-turnover and low-turnover variants of osteomalacia represent distinct enti-

Table 11.1 Causes of hypocalcaemia

Hypoparathyroid	*Neoplastic*
Renal	Osteoblastic metastases
Acute renal failure	
Chronic renal failure	*Infectious*
Nephrotic syndrome	Measles
Gastrointestinal	*Drugs*
Vitamin D deficiency	Calcitonin
Malnutrition	Diphosphonates
Malabsorption	Chelating agents
Acute pancreatitis	Aminoglycosides
Hepatic disease	Anticonvulsant drugs
	Antineoplastic drugs
Metabolic	
Alkalosis	*Postsurgical*
Magnesium deficiency	Acute tissue necrosis
Phosphate administration	Massive blood transfusions
	Toxic shock syndrome
	Pregnancy

Table 11.2 Main causes of osteomalacia and rickets

Congenital	*Renal*
Hypophosphataemic rickets	Chronic renal failure
Hypophosphatasia	Dialysis bone disease
Vitamin D-dependent rickets,	Renal tubular acidosis
types I and II	Nephrotic syndrome
Primary renal tubular defects	
Axial osteomalacia	*Tumour-associated*
	Mesenchymal tumours
Nutritional	Metastatic carcinomas
Low dietary intake	Acute leukaemias
Lack of exposure to sun	Malignant lymphomas
Parenteral alimentation	Multiple myeloma
Gastrointestinal	*Drugs/toxins*
Postgastrectomy	Fluoride
Malabsorption syndrome	Biphosphonates
Hepatobiliary diseases	Anticonvulsants
Chronic pancreatic insufficiency	Barbiturates
	Cholestyramine
	Aluminium
	Lead

Plate 11.B

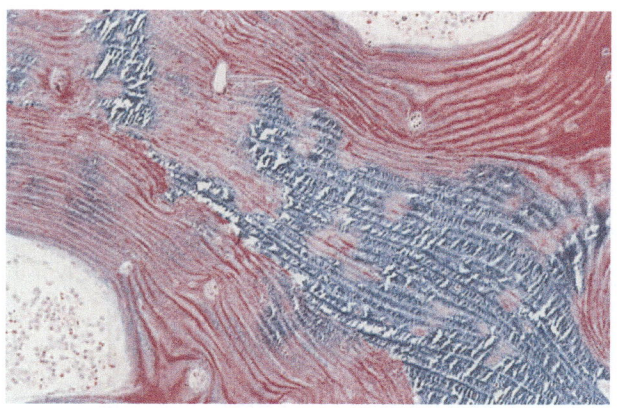

Figs. 11.7–11.12 Structural details of demineralization in osteomalacia

Fig. 11.7 Broad bands of demineralized lamellae (red), with patchy extensions into the centre of the trabeculae. Ladewig

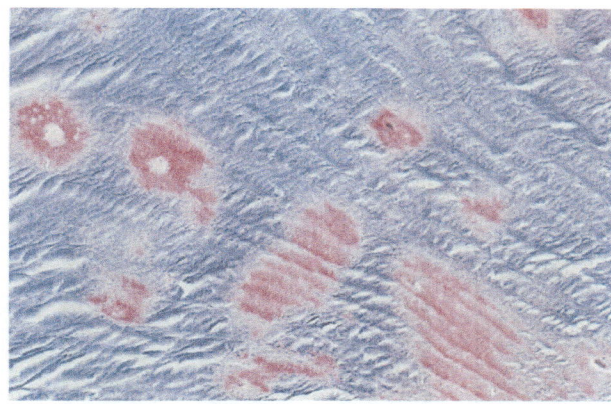

Fig. 11.8 Isolated foci of demineralization within the trabecula — pathognomonic for osteomalacia. Ladewig

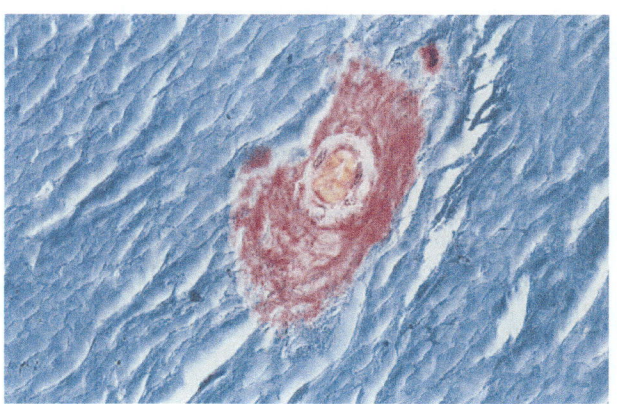

Fig. 11.9 Broad perivascular area of demineralization. Ladewig

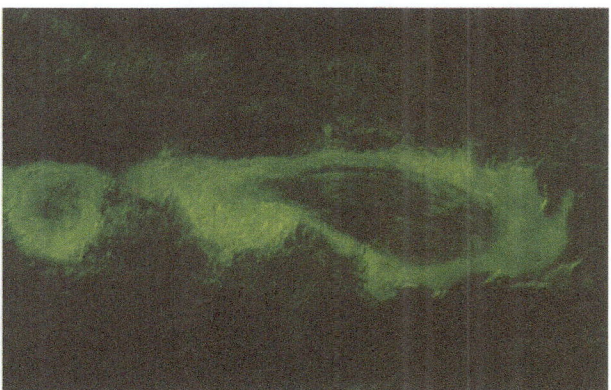

Fig. 11.10 Tetracycline labelling illustrating fluorescence of perivascular area of Haversian systems in cortex

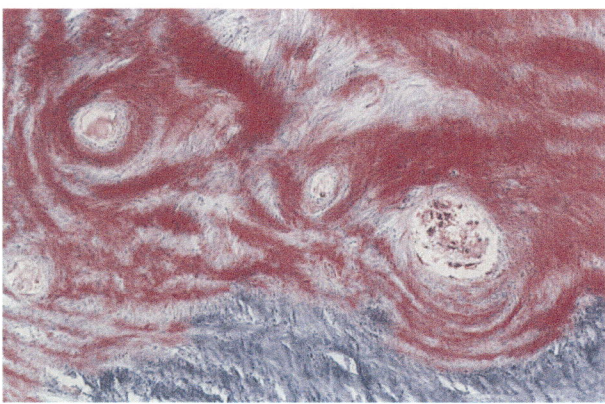

Fig. 11.11 Confluent areas of demineralization of the concentric lamellae of Haversian systems in cortex. Ladewig

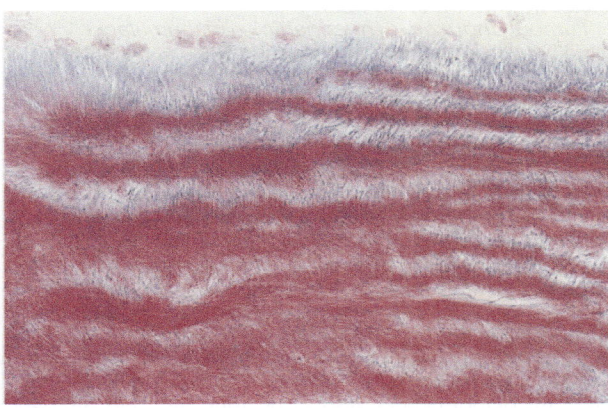

Fig. 11.12 Osteoid lamellae lined by a layer of osteoblasts. Note pale-blue collagen fibrils beneath the osteoblasts. Ladewig

| ☐ Fatty tissue | ▨ Haematop. | ▨ Osteoid |
| ▨ Edema | ⧅ Fibrosis | ■ Bone |

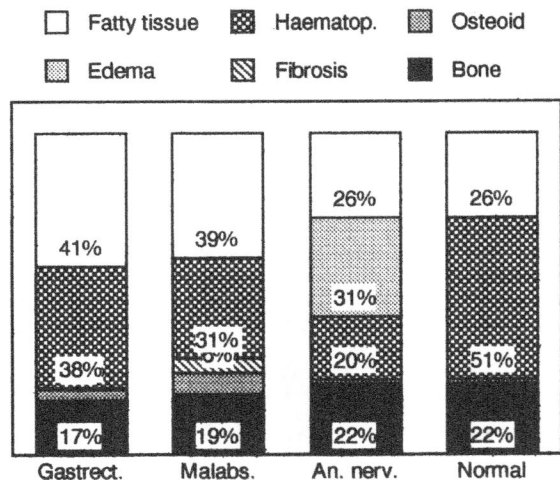

Fig. 11.S1 Histomorphometry of iliac crest biopsies in malnutrition, due to different aetiologies

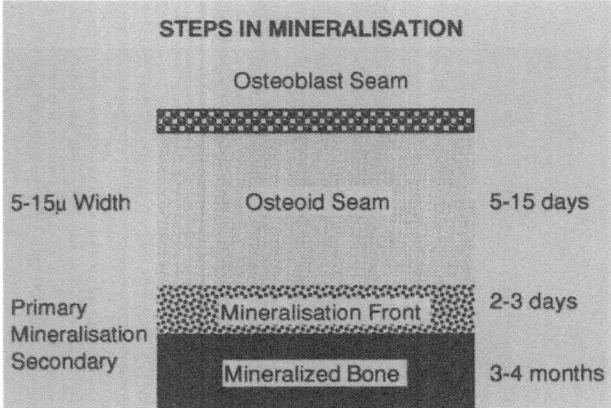

Fig. 11.S2 Zones and duration of the various steps in mineralization

ties or merely phases of the same process. Osteomalacia may be associated with osteosclerosis (Figs 11.14–11.17) and with secondary hyperparathyroidism (Fig. 11.18), especially in the younger age groups. Atypical *axial osteomalacia* is a rare disorder involving only the axial skeleton and affecting adult men[8,15,46].

Tumour-induced (oncogenic) osteomalacia[29,30,32,42] usually accompanies benign tumours of mesenchymal origin. Three pathophysiological events have been reported: increased renal excretion of phosphate, impaired production of 1,25-OH vitamin D and increased osteoclastic bone resorption[7]. Recently PTH receptor-mediated adenylate cyclase stimulating activity (PTH-like substances acting via PTH receptors) have been isolated from tumours of patients with oncogenic osteomalacia. Excision of the tumour is followed by rapid disappearance of the osteomalacia. Increased osteoid may also be found in osteoblastic metastases of prostatic carcinoma: mineralization cannot keep up with the intensive production of woven bone matrix. Recently, Ryan and Reiss pointed out that tumour-induced osteomalacia might account for a substantial number of cases of adult-onset vitamin D-resistant osteomalacia, and often there is a lag between the diagnosis of osteomalacia and the discovery of the tumour[40].

Anticonvulsant[5,35], *toxic* and *acidosis*[9] induced osteomalacia are not rare and the clinical spectrum ranges

from asymptomatic individuals to clinically apparent bone disease with fractures. In *'aplastic'* aluminium bone disease, aluminium appears to cause inhibition of matrix synthesis as well as of mineralization, so that broad osteoid seams do not develop[3,41].

Treatment of osteomalacia[14] is usually effective, if the underlying pathogenic mechanism is correctly diagnosed and reversed: histological improvement in the structural parameters of bone is seen within 6 months of therapy. Repeat biopsies 1–2 years after institution of vitamin D therapy may be necessary to demonstrate that the mineralization defect has been rectified, particularly if the underlying disease remains active[23].

X-LINKED HYPOPHOSPHATAEMIA (XLH)

This variant of 'vitamin D-resistant' rickets is the most common inherited form of rickets[4,6,17,18,20–22]. In the study by Reid *et al.* (1991), about half of the 14 patients who underwent transiliac bone biopsy had an elevated cancellous bone volume (osteoid and mineralized bone) and the group's mean value was above normal[38]. Axial bone mass tends to be increased in adults with XLH, and this is only partially attributable to hyperosteoidosis. Peripheral bone mass, however, tends to be diminished. These findings suggest that 'osteoporotic' fractures are unlikely to develop as a late complication of XLH in adults; but other skeletal complications have been described[44].

HYPOPHOSPHATASIA

The term describes an unusual heritable form of rickets, characterized by a general defect of the tissue-non-specific (bone/liver/kidney) alkaline phosphatase isoenzyme (TNSALP)[47]. This inborn error of metabolism demonstrates that this type of ALP must have an important role in the mineralization of the skeleton and in dentition.

The clinical expression ranges from profound disease *in utero* to asymptomatic hypophosphatasaemia in adults. Four clinical types of hypophosphatasia are noted:

1. perinatal (lethal),
2. infantile,
3. childhood, and
4. adult.

Traditional therapies for osteomalacia, e.g. vitamin D and mineral supplementation, are important to avoid, since serum levels of calcium, phosphate and 1,25-(OH)$_2$ vitamin D$_3$ are not reduced. Prognosis appears to become more favourable after infancy.

References

1. Balsan S. and Garabedian M. (1991). Rickets, osteomalacia and osteopetrosis. *Curr. Opin. Rheumatol.*, **3**, 496
2. Bilezikian J. P. (1987). Clinical disorders of vitamin D. Martin T. J. and Raisz L. G., *Clinical Endocrinology of Calcium Metabolism* (p. 97). New York: Marcel Dekker
3. Bloom W. J. and Flinchum D. (1960). Osteomalacia with pseudofractures caused by ingestion of aluminium hydroxide. *J. Amer. Med. Assoc.*, **174**, 1327
4. Brooks M. H., Bell N. H. and Love L. (1978). Vitamin D dependent rickets type II, resistance of target organs to 1,25 dihydroxyvitamin D. *N. Engl. J. Med.*, **293**, 996
5. Brunet J. A. (1986). Drug-induced osteomalacia. Uhthoff H. K. and Stahl E., *Current Concepts of Bone Fragility* (p. 271). Berlin: Springer
6. Brunette M. G. (1985). The X-linked hypophosphatemic vitamin D resistant rickets: old and new concepts. *Int. J. Pediatr. Nephrol.*, **6**, 55
7. Cheng C. L., Ma J. and Wu P. C. (1989). Osteomalacia secondary to osteosarcoma. *J. Bone Jt Surg.*, **71A**, 228
8. Condon J. R. and Nassim J. R. (1971). Axial osteomalacia. *Postgrad. Med. J.*, **47**, 817

Plate 11.C

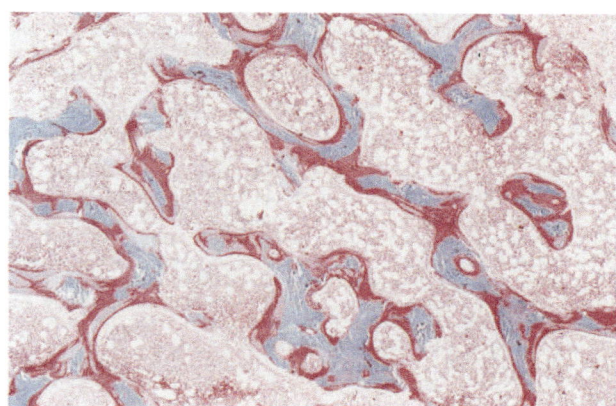

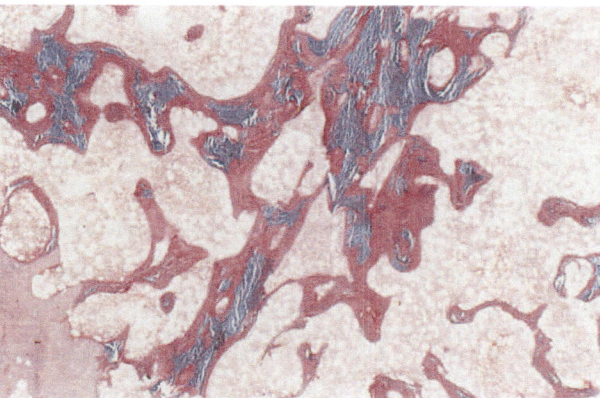

Figs. 11.13 and **11.14** Trabecular structure and volume in osteomalacia

Fig. 11.13 Normal trabecular network and volume, but increased volume percentage of osteoid. Ladewig

Fig. 11.14 Irregular trabecular structure and increased trabecular volume as well as increased amount of osteoid. Note focus of new cartilage in apposition to the trabeculae (lower left). Ladewig

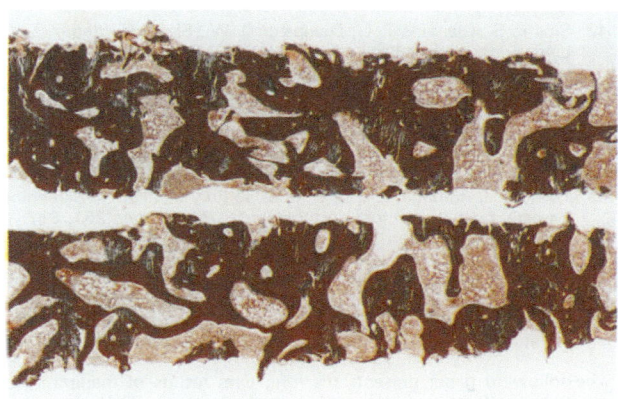

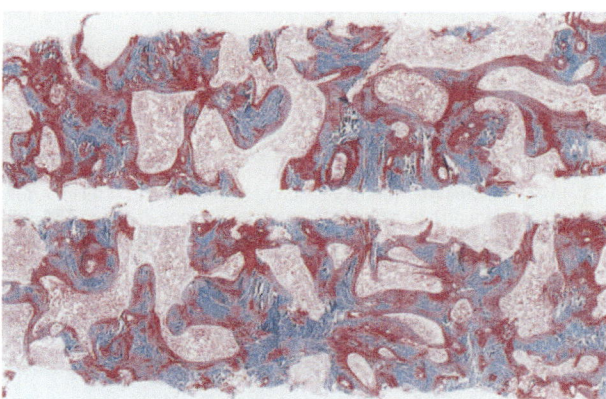

Fig. 11.15 Iliac crest biopsy showing marked osteosclerosis. Gomori

Fig. 11.16 Parallel section of biopsy in Fig. 11.15 shows high percentage of osteoid indicating osteomalacia. Ladewig

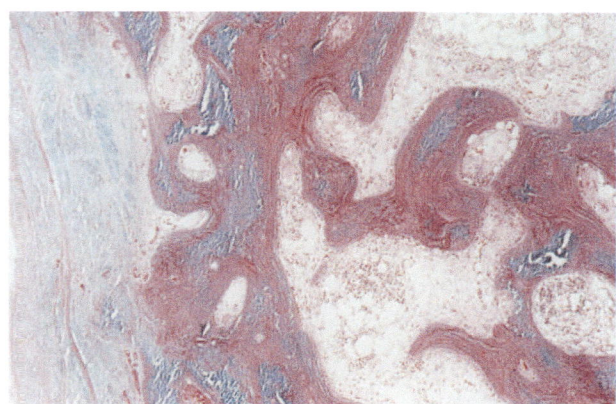

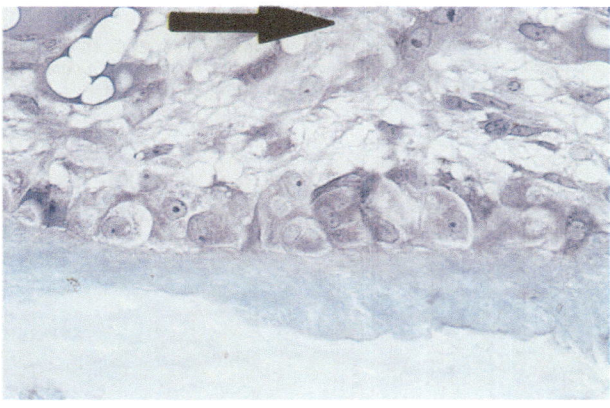

Fig. 11.17 Iliac crest biopsy of patient with osteomalacia. Periosteal tissues at left, cortical bone shows porosity and consists mainly of osteoid. Ladewig

Fig. 11.18 Iliac crest biopsy of patient with osteomalacia and accompanying secondary hyperparathyroidism. Osteoblastic new bone formation with paratrabecular connective tissue, fibrosis and osteoprogenitor cells at arrow. Giemsa

9. Cunningham, H., Frazer L. J. and Clemens T. L. (1982). Chronic acidosis with metabolic bone disease. Effect of alkali on bone morphology and vitamin D metabolism. *Amer. J. Med.*, **73**, 199

10. Dent C. E. (1970). Rickets (and osteomalacia) nutritional and metabolic (1919–1969). *Proc. Roy. Soc. Med.*, **63**, 401

11. Driscoll R. H., Meredith S. C. and Sitrin M. (1982). Vitamin D deficiency and bone disease in patients with Crohn's disease. *Gastroenterology*, **83**, 1252

12. Drueke T. and Cournot-Witmer G. (1985). Dialysis osteomalacia: clinical aspects and physiopathological mechanisms. *Clin. Nephrol.*, **24** (Suppl. 1), S26

13. Eddy R. L. (1971). Metabolic bone disease after gastrectomy. *Amer. J. Med.*, **50**, 442

14. Eisman J. A. (1988). Osteomalacia. *Clin. Endocrinol. Metab.*, **2**(1), 125

15. Frame B., Frost H. M. and Ormond R. S. (1961). Atypical osteomalacia involving the axial skeleton. *Ann. Intern. Med.*, **55**, 632

16. Frame B. and Parfitt A. M. (1978). Osteomalacia: current concepts. *Ann. Intern. Med.*, **89**, 982

17. Fraser D. and Scriver C. R. (1976). Familial forms of vitamin D-resistant rickets revisited: X-linked hypophosphatemia and autosomal recessive vitamin D dependency. *Amer. J. Clin. Nutr.*, **29**, 1315

18. Frymoyer J. W. and Hodgkin W. (1977). Adult-onset vitamin D-resistant hypophosphatemic osteomalacia. *J. Bone Jt Surg.*, **59A**, 101

19. Garrick R., Ireland A. W. and Posen S. (1971). Bone abnormalities after gastric surgery. *Ann. Intern. Med.*, **75**, 221

20. Hanna J. D., Niimi K. and Chan J. C. (1991). X-linked hypophosphatemia. Genetic and clinical correlates. *Amer. J. Dis. Child*, **145**, 865

21. Harrison N. A., Bateman J. M., Ledingham J. G. and Smith R. (1991). Renal failure in adult onset hypophosphatemic osteomalacia with Fanconi Syndrome: a family study and review of the literature. *Clin. Nephrol.*, **35**, 148

22. Hughes M. R., Macloy P. J., O'Malley B. W., Pike J. W. and Feldman D. (1991). Genetic defects of the 1,25-dihydroxyvitamin D3 receptor. *J. Receptor Res.*, **11**, 699

23. Itoi E., Sakurai M., Honma T., Sato K. and Kasama F. (1991). Adult-onset vitamin D-resistant osteomalacia. *J. Bone Jt Surg.*, **73A**, 932

24. Liberman U. A. and Marx S. J. (1989). Disorders of vitamin D metabolism – deficiency and resistance. Tam C. S., Heersche J. N. M. and Murray T. M., *Metabolic Disease: Cellular and Tissue Mechanisms* (p. 173). Boca Raton: CRC Press

25. Mankin H. J. (1974). Rickets, osteomalacia and renal osteodystrophy. *J. Bone Jt Surg.*, **56A**, 101

26. Mankin H. J. (1990). Rickets, osteomalacia, and renal osteodystrophy: an update. *Orthop. Clin. N. Amer.*, **21**(1), 81

27. Marel G. M., McKenna M. J. and Frame B. (1986). Osteomalacia. Peck W. A., *Bone and Mineral Research*, vol. 4 (p. 335). Amsterdam: Elsevier

28. Marx S. J. (1989). Disorders of vitamin D metabolism – basic aspects. Tam C. S., Heersche J. N. M. and Murray T. M., *Metabolic Bone Disease: Cellular and Tissue Mechanisms* (p. 157). Boca Raton: CRC Press

29. McClure J. and Smith P. S. (1987). Oncogenic osteomalacia. *J. Clin. Pathol.*, **40**, 446

30. McGuire M. H., Merenda J. T. and Etzkorn J. R. (1989). Oncogenic osteomalacia. *Clin. Orthop.*, **244**, 305

31. Murray T. M. (1989). PTH-like substances. Tam C. S., Heersche J. N. M. and Murray T. M., *Metabolic Bone Disease: Cellular and Tissue Mechanisms* (p. 125). Boca Raton: CRC Press

32. Nuovo M. A., Dorfman H. D. and Chen-Chih J. (1989). Tumor-induced osteomalacia and rickets. *Amer. J. Surg. Pathol.*, **13**, 588

33. Parfitt A. M. (1990). Osteomalacia and related disorders. Avioli L. V. and Krane S. M., *Metabolic Bone Disease* (p. 329). Philadelphia: Saunders

34. Peacock M. (1984). Osteomalacia and rickets. Nordin B. E. C., *Metabolic Bone and Stone Disease* (p. 71). Edinburgh: Churchill Livingstone

35. Pierides A. M., Ellis H. A., Ward M., Simpson W., Peart K. M., Alvares-Ude F., Uldall P. R. and Kerr D. N. S. (1976). Barbiturate and anticonvulsant treatment in relation to osteomalacia with haemodialysis and renal transplantation. *Brit. Med. J.*, **1**, 190

36. Pierides A. M., Skillen A. W. and Ellis H. A. (1979). Serum alkaline phosphatase in azotemic and hemodialysis osteodystrophy: a study of isoenzyme patterns, their correlation with bone histology and their changes in response to treatment with 1 OH D3 and 1,25 (OH)2 D3. *J. Lab. Clin. Med.*, **93**, 899

37. Pitt M. J. (1991). Rickets and osteomalacia are still around. *Radiol. Clin. N. Amer.*, **29**(1), 97

38. Reid I. R., Murphy W. A., Hardy D. C., Teiltelbaum S. L., Bergfeld M. A. and Whyte M. P. (1991). X-linked hypophosphatemia: skeletal mass in adults assessed by histomorphometry, computed tomography, and absorptiometry. *Amer. J. Med.*, **90**, 63

39. Revell P. A. (1986). *Pathology of Bone*. Berlin: Springer

40. Ryan E. A. and Reiss E. (1984). Oncogenous osteomalacia. Review of the world literature of 42 cases and report of two new cases. *Amer. J. Med.*, **77**, 501

41. Sherrard D. J. (1986). Aluminium and renal osteodystrophy. *Semin. Nephrol.*, **6**, 5

42. Siris E. S., Clemens T. L., Dempster D. W., Shane E., Segre G. V., Lindsay R. and Belizikian J. P. (1987). Tumor-induced osteomalacia. *Amer. J. Med.*, **82**, 307

43. Sitrin M., Meredith S. and Rosenberg I. H. (1978). Vitamin D deficiency and bone disease in gastrointestinal disorders. *Arch. Intern. Med.*, **138**, 886

44. Taylor H. G. and Hothersall T. E. (1991). Hypophosphatemic rickets and pyrophosphate arthropathy. *Clin. Rheumatol.*, **10**, 155

45. Tovey F. I., Karamanolis D. G. and Godfrey J. (1987). Screening for early post-gastrectomy osteomalacia. *Practitioner*, **231**, 817

46. White M. P., Fallon M. D. and Murphy W. A. (1981). Axial osteomalacia. *Amer. J. Med.*, **71**, 1041

47. Whyte M. P., Teitelbaum S. L., Murphy W. A., Bergfeld M. A. and Avioli L. V. (1979). Adult hypophosphatasia, clinical, laboratory and genetic investigation of a large kindred with review of the literature. *Medicine*, **58**, 329

The following paper presents the long term results of therapy in 24 children, its effects on growth, and the high incidence (79%) of therapy-related nephrocalcinosis:

Verge C. F., Lam A., Simpson J. M., Cowell C. T., Howard N. J. and Silink M. (1991). Effects of therapy in X-linked hypophosphatemic rickets. *N. Engl. J. Med.*, **325**, 1843-B

An update on Vitamin D and the immune system is provided in this article:

Hewison M. (1992). Vitamin D and the immune system. *J. Endocrinol.*, **132**, 173

Primary hyperparathyroidism

12

The widespread use of multi-channel biochemical analysers has led to the identification of increasing numbers of patients with *hypercalcaemia*. In large series, about 3% of patients screened were found to have plasma calcium values greater than 2.6 mmol/l. Although hypercalcaemia can be caused by a wide spectrum of conditions, the vast majority of cases are due to one of two disorders: primary hyperparathyroidism and malignancy. The former occurs more frequently in the outpatient setting while the latter is the most common cause in hospitalized patients. Isolated cases of hypercalcaemia due to vitamin D intoxication and thyrotoxicosis have been reported. Sarcoidosis may be accompanied by hypercalcaemia, apparently because of the unregulated production of 1,25-OH vitamin D and concomitant renal insufficiency. Table 12.1 lists the causes of hypercalcaemia and divides them into common and uncommon.

Hyperparathyroidism (HPT) refers to the clinical syndromes which result directly from the consequences of PTH secretion. A classification is given in Table 12.2. The prototype of hyperparathyroid syndromes is primary hyperparathyroidism, a disorder characterized by excessive production of PTH. The elevated PTH levels act on bone and kidney and indirectly on the intestine to cause hypercalcaemia[11,27]. Disturbances of vitamin D metabolism participate in determining the clinical presentation of hyperparathyroidism. Despite a number of new and exciting findings, the precise mechanisms by which PTH stimulates bone remodelling are not known[30]. PTH has been shown to increase the production of local growth factors such as TGF-β, PGE and IL-6[14]. Growth factors

are known to be important in mediating the effects of PTH and other systemic hormones on bone cells, and in 'coupling' bone resorption and formation. 1,25-$(OH)_2$ D_3 enhances the effectiveness of PTH, possibly in the differentiation of bone-resorbing cells. In patients with severe HPT, the rate of 25-(OH) vitamin D catabolism is most rapid, and explains the relation between overt parathyroid bone disease and low 25-(OH) vitamin D levels[11,12]. Therefore HPT associated with osteomalacia usually is not a consequence of vitamin D deficiency – the latter may, in part at least, be a consequence of the HPT. Other substances like PTH-related peptides, systemic hormones and even various drugs (e.g. corticosteroids[34], oestrogen[15], thyroid hormones) may cause changes in the osseous manifestations of HPT[20,21]. Furthermore the cellular mechanisms of osteoclastic stimulation, both in numbers and in activity, are not completely understood[22,30]. No direct effect of HPT on the osteoclast itself has yet been demonstrated[19]. The speculation has been made that stimulated osteoblasts produce local growth factors capable of osteoclast recruitment[24,28]. Another theory suggests that PTH causes endosteal lining cells to contract, thereby offering more trabecular surfaces for the resorbing activity of osteoclasts[33]. The anabolic effect of low doses of PTH is believed to be mediated by osteoblastic activation, with a net increase in bone production.

Primary hyperparathyroidism (pHPT) occurs mainly in adults between the ages of 20 and 40 and it is twice as common in females as in males. The symptomatology of pHPT is extremely varied, both in terms of the systems involved and in terms of the severity of the condition[1,5,21,23]. About 20% of patients with pHPT present with nephrolithiasis ('stone disease'); indeed, a symptomatic kidney stone may be the first manifestation of pHPT (Table 12.3). In these patients 1,25-OH vitamin D levels are greatly increased, resulting in intestinal hyperabasorption of calcium, though serum calcium and PTH levels are often only mildly elevated. Even metastatic calcifications in the walls of arteries (Fig. 12.35) and in the lung alveoli may occur. In a minority of patients, less than 10%, pHPT presents as 'bone disease' with greatly augmented bone remodelling, resulting in osteitis fibrosa cystica, the classic bone lesion (Table 12.3). However, this does not

Table 12.1 Causes of hypercalcaemia

Common	Uncommon
Malignant disease	Thyrotoxicosis
Primary hyperparathyroidism	Vitamin D intoxication
Artefactual	Sarcoidosis
	Tertiary hyperparathyroidism
	Haemodialysis
	Immobilization (not in the elderly)
	Addison's disease
	Phaeochromocytoma
	Milk alkali syndrome
	Thiazide diuretics
	Lithium therapy
	Parenteral nutrition
	Vitamin A intoxication
	Hypereosinophilic syndrome
	Berylliosis
	Tuberculosis

Table 12.2 Types of hyperparathyroid syndrome

Primary hyperparathyroidism	*Tertiary hyperparathyroidism*
Parathyroid adenoma(s)	
Parathyroid hyperplasia	*Ectopic hyperparathyroidism*
Parathyroid carcinoma	*PTH-like substances (oncogenic)*
	'Pseudohyperparathyroidism'
Secondary hyperparathyroidism	Oncogenic osteomalacia
Chronic renal failure	
Gastrointestinal diseases	
Pseudohypoparathyroidism	

Table 12.3 Clinical and histological data in patients with pHPT disease: bone versus stone disease

Variant of pHPT	Stone disease	Bone disease
Number of patients	43	36
Trabecular bone (vol%, BV/TV)	26	21
Osteoid (vol%)	2	11
Fibrosis (vol%)	0	31
Haematopoiesis (vol%)	45	21
Osteoclasts (no./mm²)	1	11
Osteoblasts (no./mm²)	3	19
Age of patients (years), median	44	55
Size of adenoma(s) (mm²)	90	143
Renal calculi	+++	0
Osteolyses (X-ray)	0	+++
Serum ALP, increased	normal	+++

necessarily occur in all parts of the skeleton – or even symmetrically, i.e. in the left and right sides of the ilium. The circulating levels of 25-(OH) vitamin D are decreased, possibly as a consequence of a rapid rate of 25-(OH) vitamin D catabolism[11,12]. In response to vitamin D treatment the bone lesions heal and frank hypercalcaemia is unmasked. In general, patients with bone disease have a more progressive course and higher serum calcium and PTH levels, but lower urine calcium values, than patients with kidney stones. Whether variations in clinical presentation result from differences in PTH metabolism, or in PTH receptors in different tissues, or from differences in vitamin D metabolism remains to be clarified. Currently, because of the early detection due to biochemical screening, as many as 60% of patients identified may have no symptoms at all ('asymptomatic variant').

In most cases (85%) pHPT is due to single, double or multiple adenomas[5]. In the remaining 15% of cases it is caused by diffuse hyperplasia of all four glands or, rarely, by parathyroid carinoma (Table 12.4). Secondary HPT develops in response to chronic hypocalcaemia, as in chronic renal failure or in intestinal malabsorption. With prolonged hypocalcaemia the hyperplastic glands may become autonomous, that is overactive, and cause normo- or hypercalcaemia. This tertiary HPT may be difficult to distinguish from the primary one[23,30].

Table 12.4 Parathyroid glands and osteoclastic activity in pHPT

Parathyroid glands*	Frequency (%)	Osteoclast number†
Hyperplasia	19	9
Single adenoma	68	14
Adenoma and hyperplasia	3	16
Multiple adenomata	9	24
Carcinoma	1	41

*Derived from 58 cases
†No./mm² bone area, mean value

Clinically evident bone disease in pHPT, which used to affect approximately 15% of the patient population, is now uncommon. Skeletal symptoms are now limited to those cases with the most severe forms of disease. The major radiological findings in pHPT reflect increased bone resorption (generalized osteopenia), although occasionally increased bone formation (osteosclerosis) is also apparent[17]. The classical radiological manifestations are subperiostal resorption (Fig. 12.R1) (10–20% of patients) and, generally seen only in advanced cases, bone cysts and 'brown tumours'[22]. A recent analysis of radiological findings in pHPT gave an incidence of mild osteopenia in 62%, vertebral compression in 53% and subperiosteal resorption in only 21%. Some studies using densitometric analysis suggest bone loss is greater at sites of predominantly trabecular bone, while others suggest there is greater loss at cortical sites[7,8,31]. However, in one study, measurements of total body calcium failed to demonstrate large overall deficits of bone mineral in pHPT.

In iliac crest *bone biopsies*[4,7,8,13,22], the most consistent feature is evidence of increased bone turnover, but without uncoupling. Histomorphometry suggests an increase in the 'birth rate' of new remodelling cycles under the influence of excess PTH, thus the skeletal consequences are probably due to the effects of PTH on cell recruitment rather than the activation of osteoblasts and osteoclasts already present[10,25,29]. There is a spectrum of histological changes in pHPT (Plates 12.A, B and D), and the mean values are given in Table 12.5.

Twenty per cent of the patients, particularly those with kidney stones and with asymptomatic hypercalcaemia, had no morphological abnormalities in the bone biopsy,

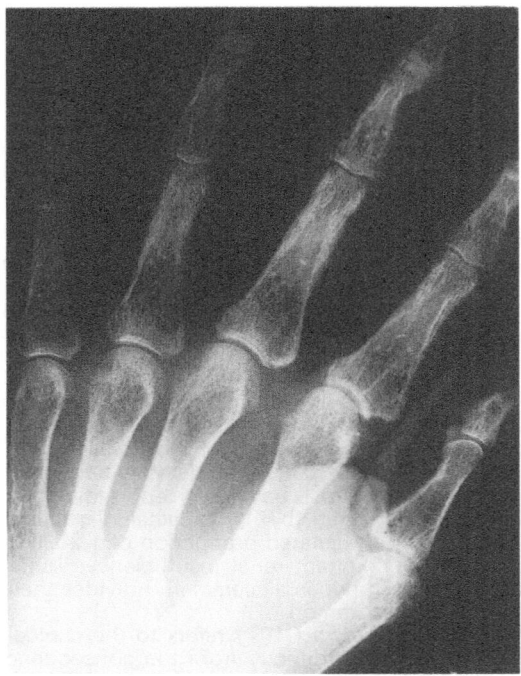

Fig. 12.R1 Radiological features of hyperparathyroid bone disease. Note the marked subperiosteal bone resorption involving the phalanges, as well as the cortical porosity. (Kindly supplied by Prof. M. Kessler, Department of Radiology, Klinikum Großhadern, University of Munich)

and histomorphometric values were within normal limits (Table 12.6)[2]. In *mild* cases there was a minimal increase in resorption and formation parameters, with focal activation of bone remodelling units. Small intracortical and intratrabecular burrows filled with active osteoclasts, blood vessels and mesenchymal cells are highly diagnostic. Although cement lines may be accentuated and irregular, the 'mosaic pattern' found in Paget's disease is not observed.

Table 12.5 Histomorphometry of iliac crest biopsies in pHPT

Parameters*	Units	pHPT mean (maximum)	Normal mean
Lamellar bone	LBV/TV, %	19 (62)	22
Woven bone	WBV/TV, %	5 (32)	–
Osteoid	OSV/TV, %	3 (24)	1
Howship's lacunae	HOV/TV,%	5 (29)	–
Osteoclasts	No./mm² bone area	16.3 (143)	1.0
Osteoblasts	No./mm² bone area	9.5 (34)	2.5
Haematopoiesis	HAV/TV, %	32 (61)	45
Fatty tissue	FAV/TV, %	22 (55)	28
Fibrous tissue	FIV/TV, %	6 (71)	–
Sinusoids	SIV/TV, %	4 (15)	3
Oedema	EDV/TV, %	4 (21)	1

*Derived from 139 cases

Table 12.6 Bone disease and nephrolithiasis in pHPT

Osteoclasts*	< 5	5–25	> 25
Nephrolithiasis	75%	38%	26%

*No./mm² bone area

[continued on p. 142]

Plate 12.A

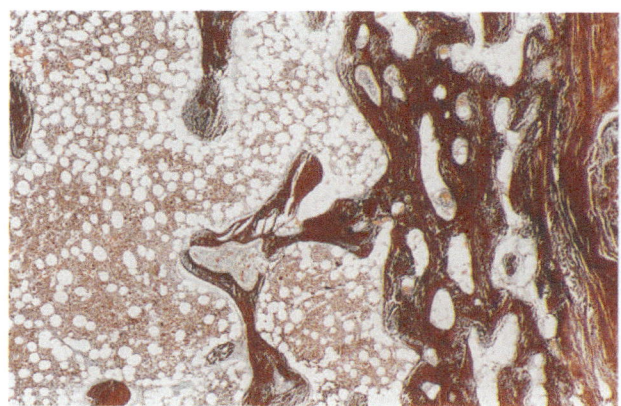

Figs. 12.1–12.6 Aspects of cortical bone in iliac crest biopsies in pHPT

Fig. 12.1 Marked porosity of cortex. Gomori

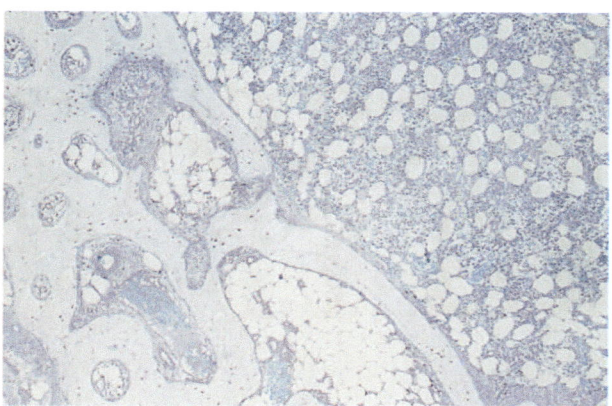

Fig. 12.2 Higher magnification of cortical area from Fig. 12.1 showing dissecting osteoclasia in cortex. Except in foci of osseous remodelling fibrosis is not increased and the marrow shows preservation of haematopoietic tissue and fat cells. Giemsa

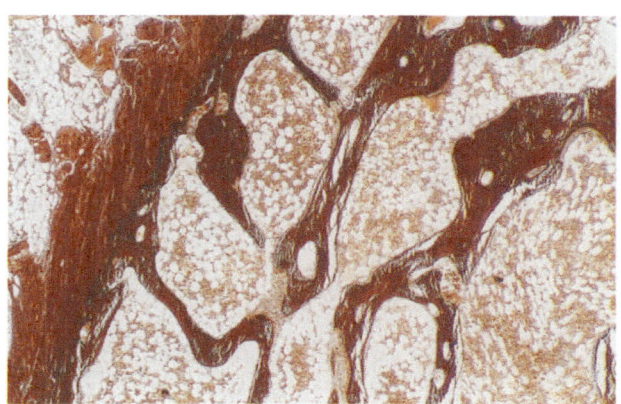

Fig. 12.3 Very thin cortex with multiple sites of dissecting osteoclasia. Gomori

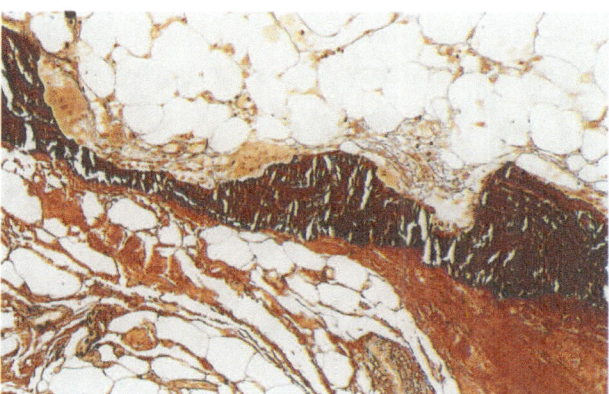

Fig. 12.4 Higher magnification of biopsy from Fig. 12.3: surface erosion of cortex by layers of multinucleated osteoclasts. Transection almost complete. Gomori

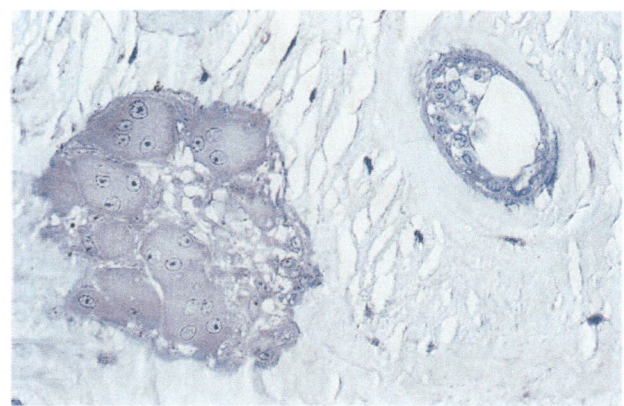

Fig. 12.5 Numerous osteoclasts in cross-sectioned tunnel through cortical bone, near a Haversian system with concentric lamellae. Giemsa

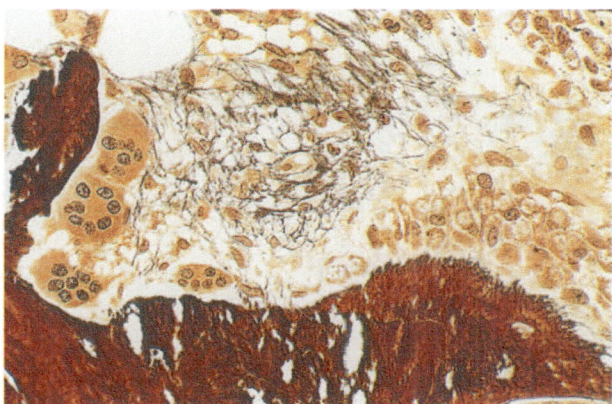

Fig. 12.6 Parallel section of the same biopsy at higher magnification showing multinucleated osteoclasts (left and centre), paratrabecular fibrosis (centre) and layers of osteoblasts (right). Gomori

Plate 12.B

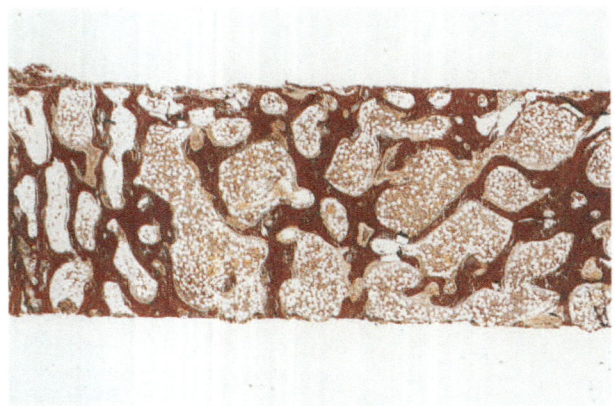

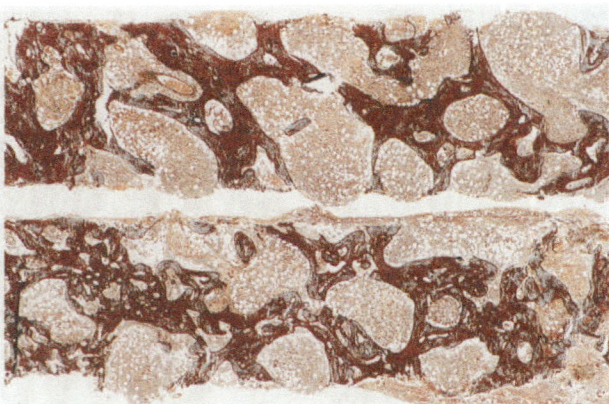

Figs. 12.7–12.12 Aspects of trabecular bone in iliac crest biopsies in pHPT

Fig. 12.7 Fairly homogeneous involvement of trabecular bone with overall preservation of its structure. Gomori

Fig. 12.8 Uneven involvement of trabecular bone with more pronounced remodelling in the lower than in the upper part of this biopsy. Gomori

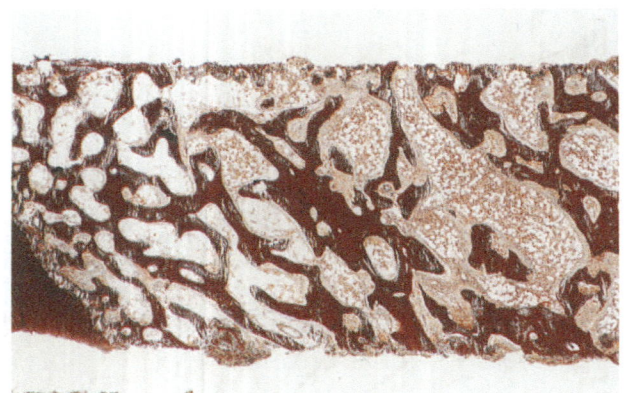

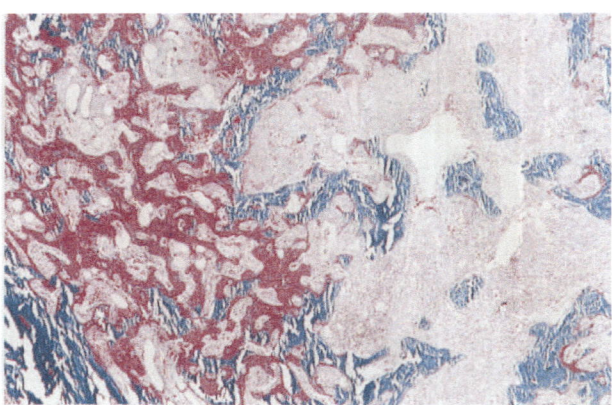

Fig. 12.9 Bone biopsy of a child with pronounced involvement of the central and deeper zones, but almost unaffected subcortical zone and growth plate (left). Gomori

Fig. 12.10 Patchy involvement in subcortical area with production of unmineralized primitive bone. Ladewig

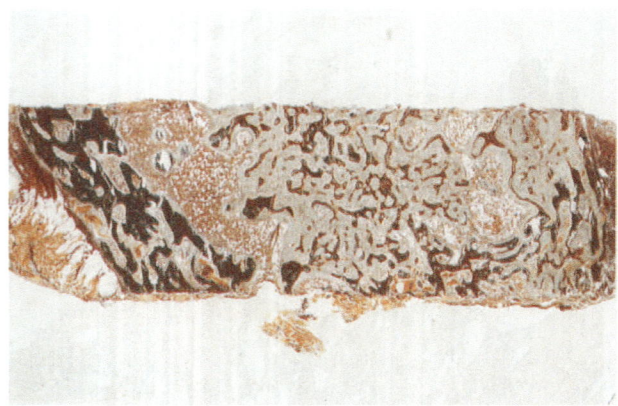

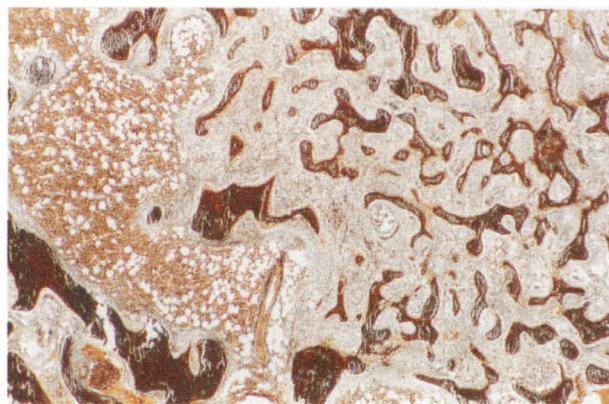

Fig. 12.11 Porous cortex, small area of haematopoietic marrow and large central area consisting mainly of woven bone. Gomori

Fig. 12.12 Higher magnification of Fig. 12.11 to show focus of woven bone in network of fibrous connective tissue. Gomori

Plate 12.C

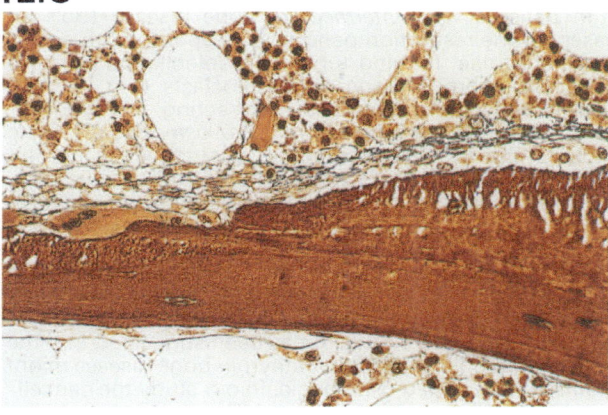

Figs. 12.13–12.18 Stages and types of trabecular resorption in pHPT

Fig. 12.13 Superficial erosion of ossicle on both sides, with seam of paratrabecular fibrosis. Giemsa

Fig. 12.14 Superficial erosion of ossicle. Note osteoclasts with Howship lacunae (left), osteoblasts (right) and paratrabecular fibrosis (upper side of trabecula). Note completely unaffected lower side. Gomori

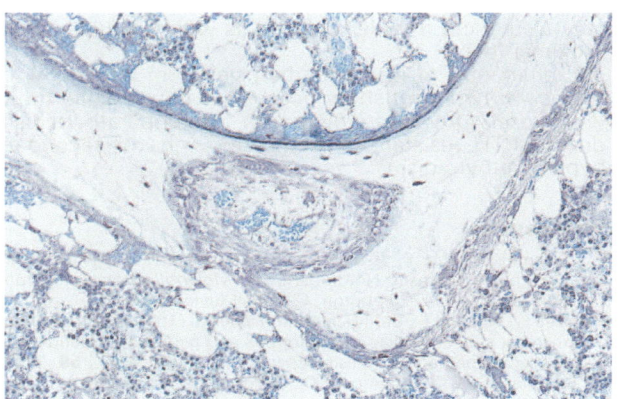

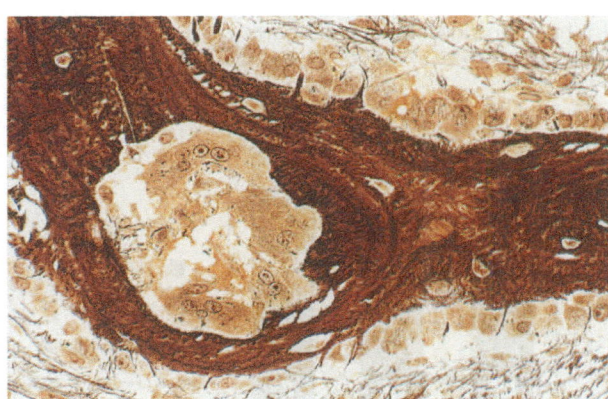

Fig. 12.15 Dissecting osteoclasia of ossicle, as well as minimal surface erosion (right). Giemsa

Fig. 12.16 Dissecting osteoclasia inside the trabeculae with osteoblastic activity on bone surface (both upper and lower side of the trabecula). Note paratrabecular fibrosis. Gomori

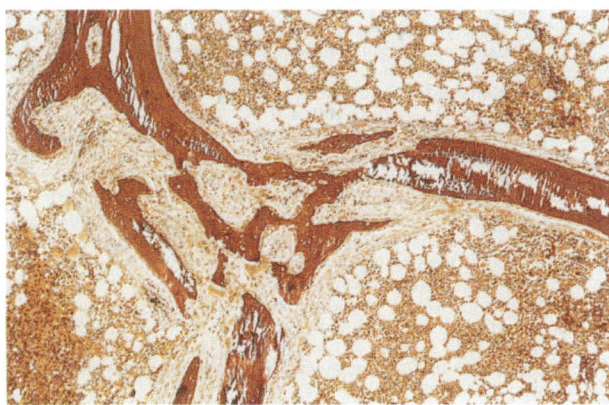

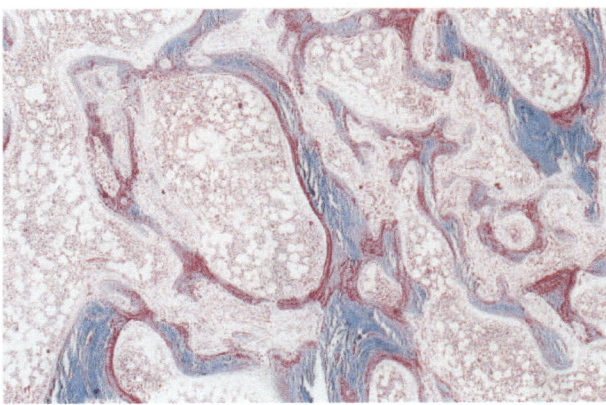

Fig. 12.17 Substitution of large part of trabecular network by fibrous connective tissue. Gomori

Fig. 12.18 Substitution of part of trabecular network by fibrous tissue, osteoid and woven bone, as yet unmineralized. Ladewig

In patients with *intermediate* bone disease (35% of cases), bone resorption penetrates deep into both cortex and trabeculae, forming tunnelling defects and burrows filled with fibrous tissue and osteoclasts (Fig. 12.S1). Terms used for this process are 'dissecting' and 'transecting' resorption or *'dissecting fibro-osteoclasia'* (Plate 12.D, E and F). The presence of paratrabecular fibrosis adjacent to resorption surfaces (Howship's lacunae) is pathognomonic, and in extreme cases trabeculae may be totally replaced by fibrous tissue. Increased osteoblastic activity is reflected in the raised plasma alkaline phosphatase levels[16]. Increases in osteoid volume, thickness and surface may be found, as well as in dynamic indices such as extent of double-labelled tetracycline surfaces and rate of bone formation[29]. While it has been suggested that the primary catabolic effect in parathyroid bone disease might result in widespread osteopenia, in our study the cancellous bone volume was maintained. Recent studies, moreover, support a preferential effect of PTH on cortical bone with substantial reductions in width, which, together with the large tunnelling defects, create a spongy appearance, or even splits in the cortices (Fig. 12.S2)[31]. The fact that the structure and turnover of cancellous and cortical bone are well reflected in a bone biopsy explains the superiority of bone histology over radiography for the early diagnosis of pHPT bone disease; previous reports have reviewed the histomorphometric findings in pHPT and compared them to those in other metabolic bone disorders[35].

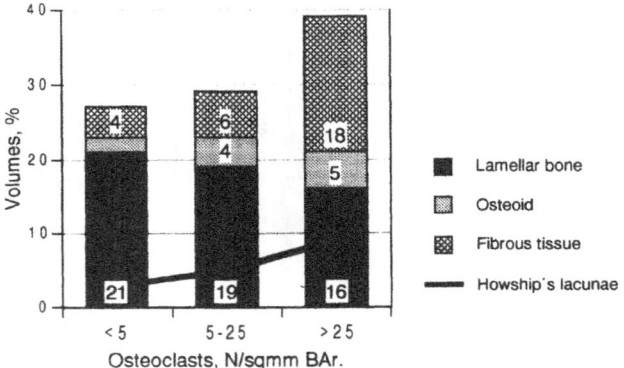

Fig. 12.S1 Histomorphometry of osseous remodelling in pHPT grouped according to number of osteoclasts

BIOPSY COMPACTA IN PRIMARY HYPERPARATHYROIDISM

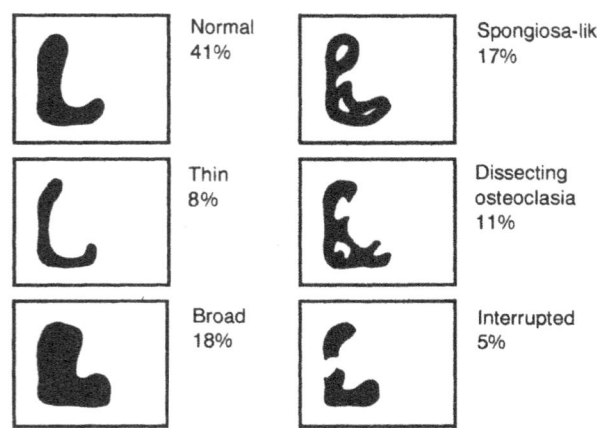

Normal 41%	Spongiosa-like 17%
Thin 8%	Dissecting osteoclasia 11%
Broad 18%	Interrupted 5%

Fig. 12.S2 Cortical bone in iliac crest biopsy in pHPT

Changes in trabecular bone remodelling following surgical treatment may also be evaluated by histomorphometry[9,18], and sequential iliac crest biopsies taken 3 months after parathyroid adenectomy showed restoration of bone and osseous remodelling, though residual disorganization of lamellar structure and cement lines were still remnants of previous osteoclasia and increased remodelling. Concomitant use of various drugs may cause changes in the osseous manifestations of pHPT, for example steroid hormones[24].

In the *severe* cases (10%) the classical skeletal manifestations of pHPT – osteitis fibrosa cystica – are seen, with massive osteoclastic resorption and diffuse fibrosis of the marrow in rare cases even causing bone marrow failure[6] (Plate 12.G). The trabecular network is replaced by deposits of poorly mineralized woven bone and fibrous tissue. Large foci of resorption appear as cystic areas filled with highly vascularized fibrous tissues, zones of haemorrhage and haemosiderin phagocytosed by macrophages (Fig. 12.42) and osteoclast-like multinucleated giant cells. These areas constitute the so-called *brown tumours* of pHPT bone disease which closely resemble a giant cell tumour (osteoclastoma) of bone[26,32]. 'Brown tumours' with spontaneous fractures are now uncommon clinically, as the diagnosis of pHPT is now made in the early stages of the disease. However, hyperparathyroidism may also occur in older individuals with fractures of the proximal femur[3].

Examination of iliac crest biopsies from patients with *hypoparathyroidism* show no abnormalities, while those with *pseudohypoparathyroidism* (hypoparathyroidism due to PTH resistance) may show signs of secondary hyperparathyroidism[30].

References

1. Adami S., Milroy E. J. G. and O'Riordan J. L. H. (1984). Primary hyperparathyroidism. Nordin B. E. C., *Metabolic Bone and Stone Disease* (p. 112). Edinburgh: Churchill Livingstone
2. Beil E., Prechtel K., Bartl R. and Kronseder A. (1974). Histomorphometrical studies of iliac crest biopsies and parathyroid glands with primary hyperparathyroidism. *Verh. Dtsch. Ges. Pathol.*, **58**, 344
3. Benhamow C. L., Chappard D., Ganvain J. B., Popelier M., Roux C., Picaper G. and Alexandre C. (1991). Hyperparathyroidism in proximal femur fractures: biological and histomorphometric study in 21 patients over 75 years old. *Clin. Rheumatol.*, **10**, 144
4. Bianco P. and Bonucci E. (1991). Endosteal surfaces in hyperparathyroidism: an enzyme cytochemical study on low-temperature processed, glycol methacrylate embedded bone biopsies. *Virch. Archiv. A*, **419**, 425
5. Bilezikian J. P. (1987). Clinical disorders of the parathyroid glands. Martin T. J. and Raisz L. G., *Clinical Endocrinology of Calcium Metabolism* (p. 53). New York: Marcel Dekker
6. Boxer M., Ellman L. and Geller R. (1977). Anemia in primary hyperparathyroidism. *Arch. Intern. Med.*, **137**, 588
7. Byers P. D. and Smith R. (1971). Quantitative histology of bone in hyperparathyroidism: its relation to clinical feature, x-ray, and biochemistry. *Q. J. Med.*, **160**, 471
8. Charon S. A., Edouard C. M., Arlot M. E. and Meunier P. J. (1982). Effects of parathyroid hormone on remodeling of iliac trabecular bone packets in patients with primary hyperparathyroidism. *Clin. Orthop. Rel. Res.*, **162**, 255
9. Christiansen P., Steinicke T., Mosekilde L., Hessov I. and Melsen F. (1990). Primary hyperparathyroidism: changes in trabecular bone remodeling following surgical treatment – evaluated by histomorphometric methods. *Bone*, **11**(2), 75
10. Delling G. (1987). Bone morphology in primary hyperparathyroidism. A qualititative and quantitative study of 391 cases. *Appl. Pathol.*, **5**, 147
11. Editorials. (1988). Acquired vitamin D deficiency and hyperparathyroidism. *Lancet*, **1**, 451
12. Editorials. (1991). Primary hyperparathyroidism and 1,25-dihydroxyvitamin D. *Lancet*, **337**, 768
13. Eriksen E. F., Mosekilde L. and Melsen F. (1986). Trabecular bone remodeling and balance in primary hyperparathyroidism. *Bone*, **7**, 213

Plate 12.D

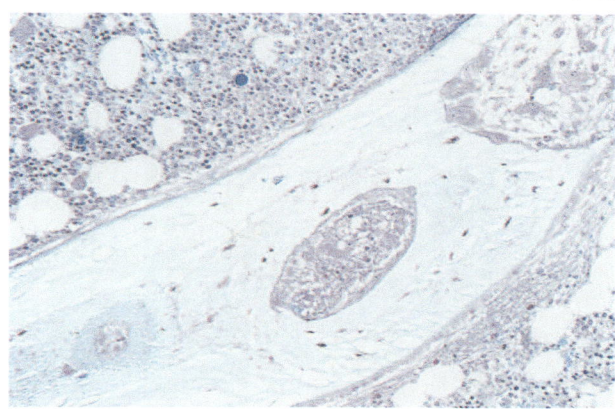

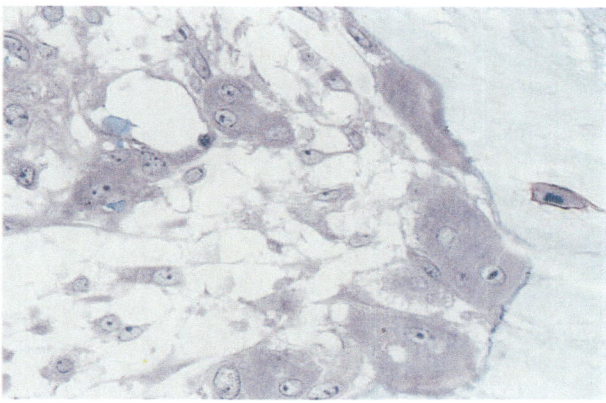

Figs. 12.19–12.24 Transecting osteoclasia in trabeculae and osteoblastic reaction

Fig. 12.19 Three steps in the sequence of dissecting osteoclasia: **(a)** narrow 'hole' in trabecular bone surrounded by osteoid and containing connective tissue elements (left), **(b)** larger excavation filled with connective tissue, small vessels and osteoprogenitor cells (centre), and **(c)** a still larger excavation which almost transects the trabecula (right). Giemsa

Fig. 12.20 Higher magnification of excavation (right) in Fig. 12.19 showing dissecting osteoclasia. Note two osteoclasts closely associated with a blood vessel. Giemsa

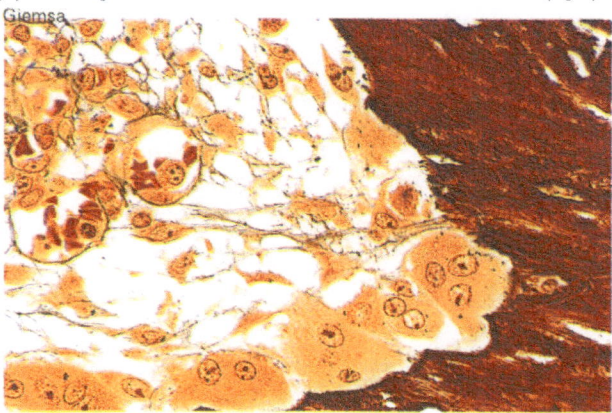

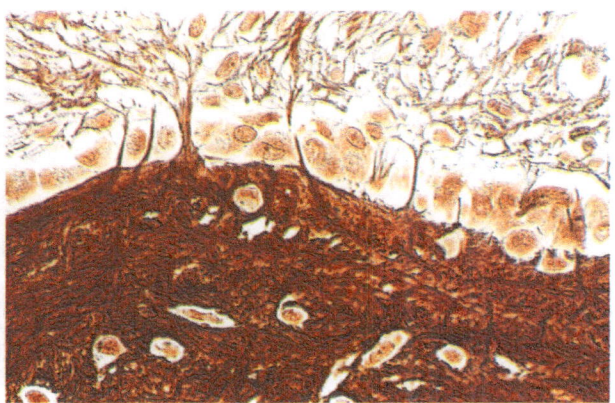

Fig. 12.21 Deep resorption cavity with multinucleated and nucleolated osteoclasts in Howship lacunae, associated with blood vessels, fibroblasts and fibres. Gomori

Fig. 12.22 Different area from the same biopsy section as in Fig. 12.21 showing trabecular surface with layer of osteoblasts and numerous large osteocytic lacunae with osteocytes. Note collagen fibres radiating out from trabecular surface between osteoblasts. Gomori

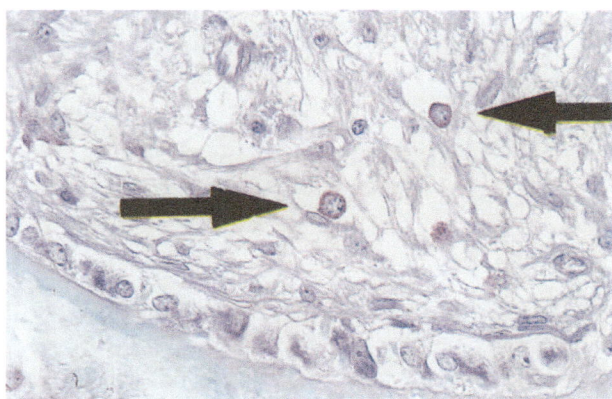

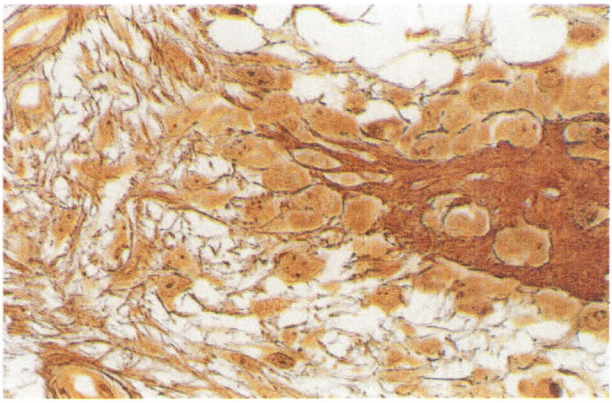

Fig. 12.23 Area adjacent to Fig. 12.22 showing trabecular surface, osteoblasts on layer of osteoid, cellular connective tissue containing fibroblasts and mast cells (at arrow). Giemsa

Fig. 12.24 Osteoblastic new bone formation. Note radiating collagen fibres between osteoblasts and large osteoblasts trapped within the bone (transformation to osteocytes). Gomori

Plate 12.E

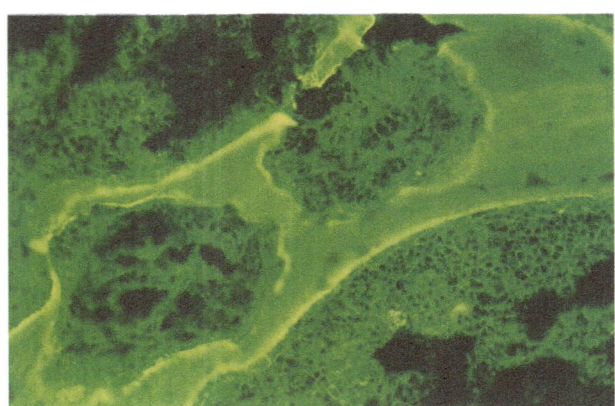

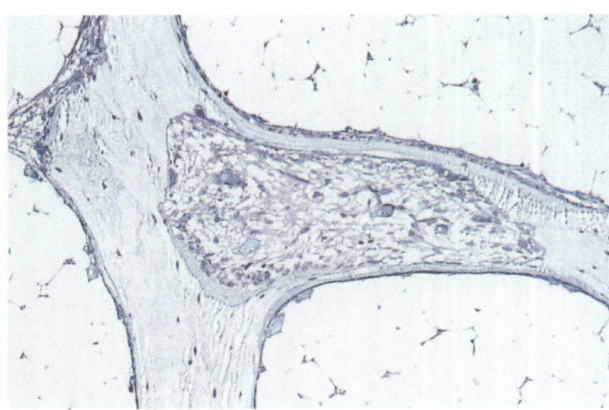

Figs. 12.25–12.30 Aspects of remodelling and fibrosis in pHPT

Fig. 12.25 Section incubated for demonstration of collagen type I; ossicle with two cavities caused by dissecting osteoclasia. Cryostat section

Fig. 12.26 Large excavation within trabecular bone surrounded by fatty marrow devoid of haematopoietic cells. Cavity filled with loose connective tissue, stromal cells and blood vessels, but few osteoclasts. The lowest part of the cavity is lined by osteoblasts with a thin seam of osteoid. Presumably the bone cells required for remodelling are supplied via the blood vessels within the cavity. Giemsa

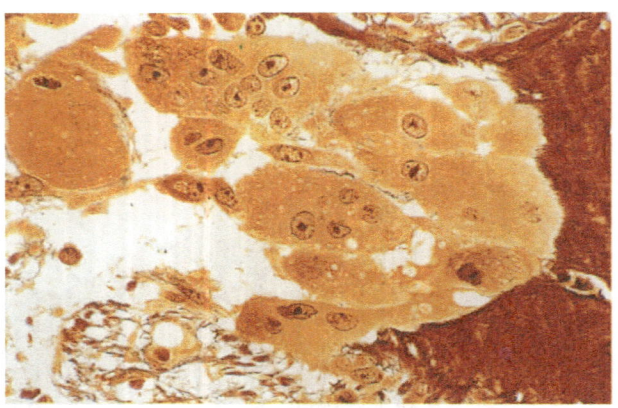

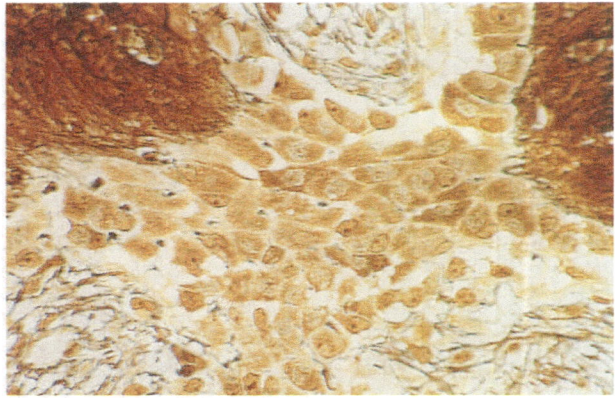

Fig. 12.27 Aggregate of large multinucleated osteoclasts within erosion cavity. Giemsa

Fig. 12.28 Apparently multilayered osteoblasts probably due to the cutting plane of the section in area close to that of Fig. 12.27. Gomori

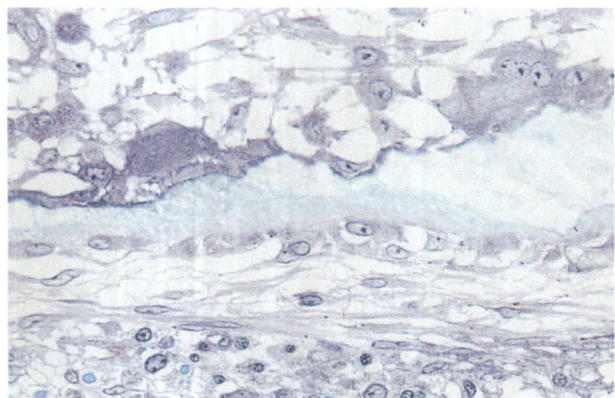

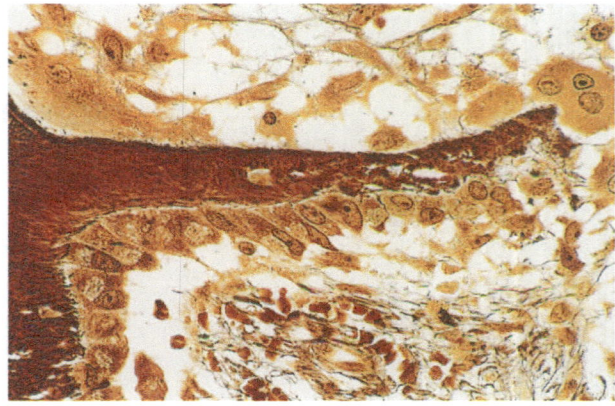

Fig. 12.29 'Coupled' osteoclastic (upper surface) and osteoblastic (lower surface) remodelling surrounded by highly cellular connective tissue. Giemsa

Fig. 12.30 Section parallel to that in Fig. 12.27 showing high columnar osteoblasts (lower surface): formation phase. Gomori

Plate 12.F

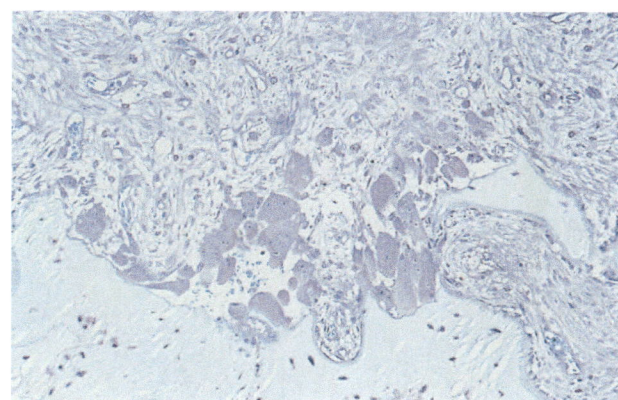

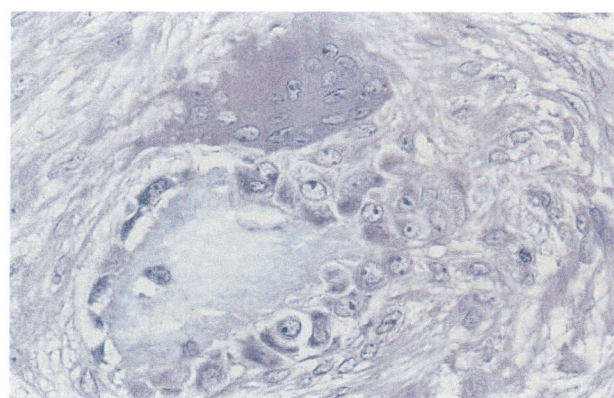

Figs. 12.31–12.34 Osteoclasts in pHPT

Fig. 12.31 Trabecular bone within cellular connective tissue with disproportionate numbers of osteoclasts on and near the trabecular surface. Giemsa

Fig. 12.32 Giant osteoclast within connective tissue, near a cross-sectioned ossicle surrounded by osteoblasts on a layer of osteoid. The osteoclast has no apparent connection to any bone surface. Giemsa

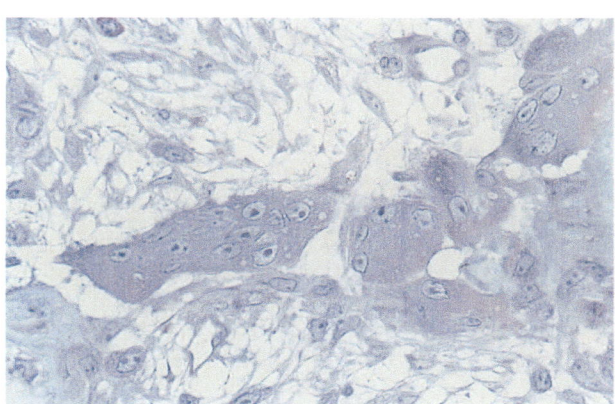

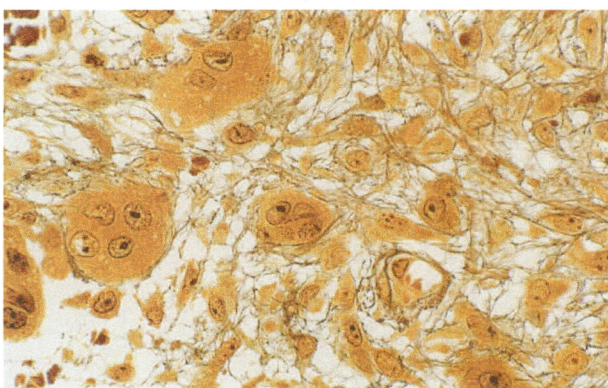

Fig. 12.33 Group of large, multinucleated and nucleolated osteoclasts within cellular connective tissue. Only two fragments of bone are visible (lower left and extreme right). Giemsa

Fig. 12.34 Cellular connective tissue containing fibres and blood vessels showing range of morphological stages in the development of osteoclast. No bone present. Gomori

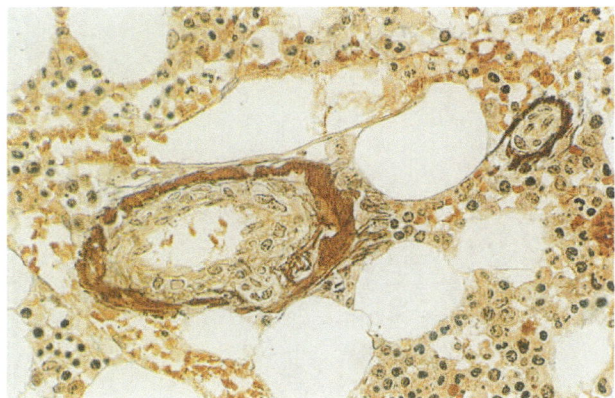

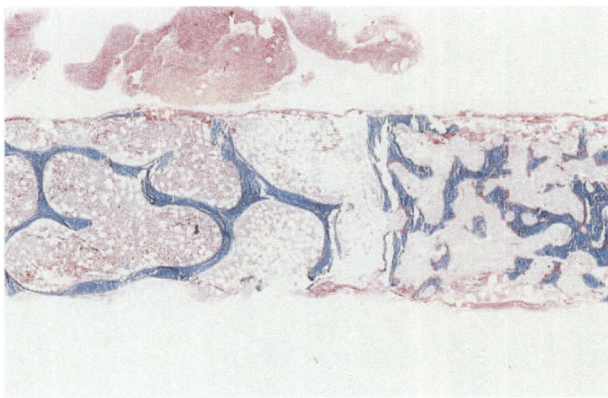

Fig. 12.35 Part of section of iliac crest biopsy of patient with pHPT showing calcification of the walls of a small (right) and a large (left) blood vessel. Gomori

Fig. 12.36 Overview of iliac crest biopsy illustrating uneven distribution of osseous manifestations in pHPT. Normal trabecular bone structure and bone marrow in the left half of the biopsy and typical derangement of trabecular network with woven bone formation (right). Ladewig

Plate 12.G

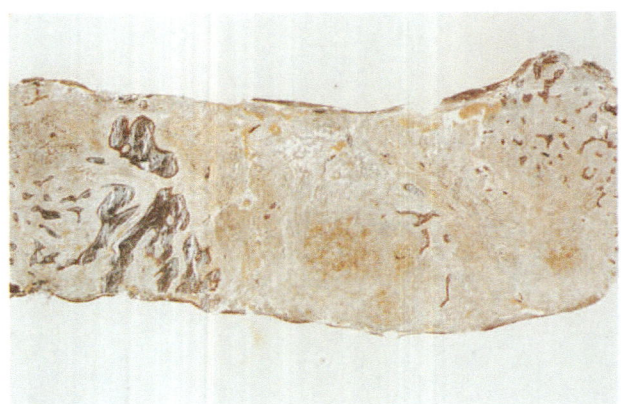

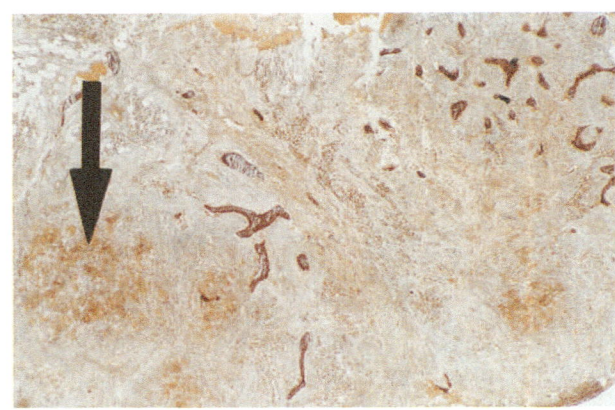

Figs. 12.37–12.42 'Brown tumour' of pHPT bone disease. Figs 12.38–12.42 illustrate different areas from the iliac crest biopsy shown in Fig. 12.37

Fig. 12.38 Large (arrow) and small aggregates of osteoclasts. Gomori

Fig. 12.37 Low-power view showing remains of trabecular bone in subcortical area (left) while the rest of the biopsy consists of dense connective tissue containing islands of woven bone and aggregates of osteoclasts. Gomori

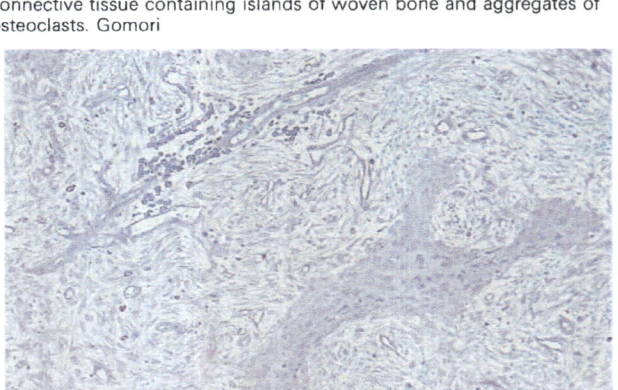

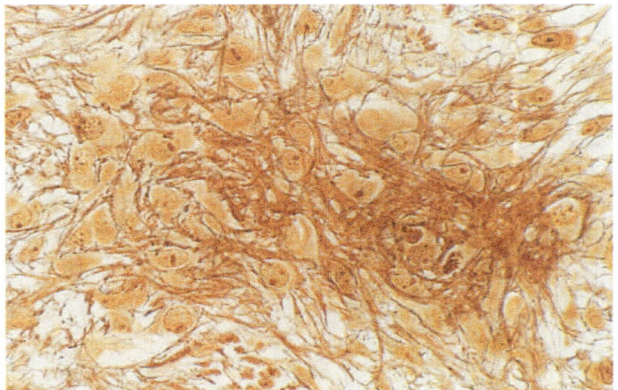

Fig. 12.39 Development of spicule of woven bone containing osteocytes within cellular connective tissue. Giemsa

Fig. 12.40 Ossification of fibrous tissue. Gomori

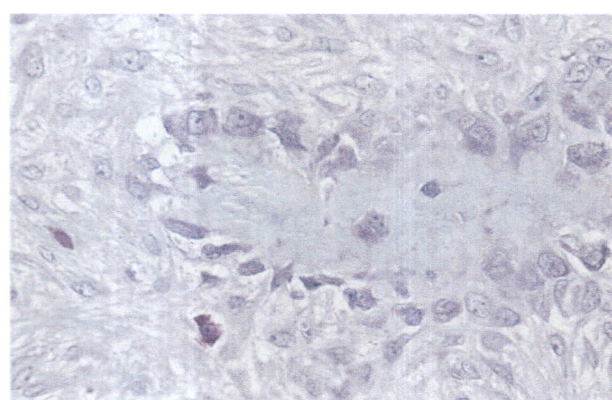

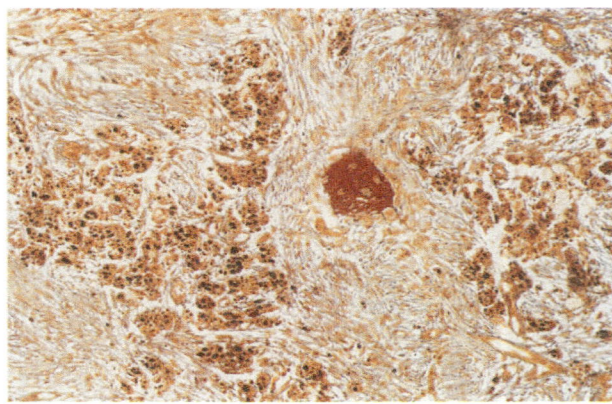

Fig. 12.41 Osteoblastic bone formation. Note two mast cells. Giemsa

Fig. 12.42 Residual fragments of bone undergoing remodelling, surrounded by aggregates of haemosiderin-containing cells. Gomori

14. Feyer J. H., Elford P., DiPadova F. E. and Trechsel V. (1989). Interleukin 6 is produced by bone and modulated by parathyroid hormone. *J. Bone Miner. Res.*, **4**(4), 633

15. Fukayama S. and Tashjian A. H. (1989). Direct modulation by estradiol of the response of human bone cells to human parathyroid hormone (PTH) and PTH-related protein. *Endocrinology*, **124**(1), 397

16. Fukayama S. and Tashjian A. H. (1990). Stimulation by parathyroid hormone of 45 Ca^{2+} uptake in osteoblast-like cells: possible involvement of alkaline phosphatase. *Endocrinology*, **127**(6), 2648

17. Genant H. K., Baron J. M., Straus F. H., Paloyan E. and Jowsey J. (1975). Osteosclerosis in primary hyperparathyroidism. *Amer. J. Med.*, **59**, 104

18. George D. C., Incavo S. J., Devlin J. T. and Kristiansen T. K. (1990). Histology of bone after parathyroid adenectomy. *J. Bone Jt Surg.*, **72A**, 1558

19. Grech P., Martin T. J., Barrington N. A. and Ell P. J. (1985). *Diagnosis of Metabolic Bone Disease*. London: Chapman & Hall

20. Habener J. F. and Potts J. T. (1990). Fundamental considerations in the physiology, biology, and biochemistry of parathyroid hormone. Avioli L. V. and Krane S. M., *Metabolic Bone Disease* (p. 69). Philadelphia: Saunders

21. Habener J. F. and Potts J. T. (1990). Primary hyperparathyroidism. Avioli L. V. and Krane S. M., *Metabolic Bone Disease* (p. 457). Philadelphia: Saunders

22. Hayes C. W. and Conway W. F. (1991). Hyperparathyroidism. *Radiol. Clin. N. Amer.*, **29**(1), 85

23. Heath D. A. (1991). Primary hyperparathyroidism and renal osteodystrophy. *Curr. Opin. Rheumatol.*, **3**, 490

24. Martin T. J. (1983). Drug and hormone effects on calcium release from bone. *Pharmacol. Ther.*, **21**, 209

25. Melsen F., Mosekilde L. and Kragstrup J. (1983). Metabolic bone diseases as evaluated by bone histomorphometry. Recker R. R., *Bone Histomorphometry: Techniques and Interpretation* (p. 265). Boca Raton: CRC Press

26. Mergenthaler H.-G., Fink M., Sauer H., Bartl R. and Wilmanns W. (1989). Multiple brown tumours in a patient with nutritional secondary hyperparathyroidism. *Klin. Wschr.*, **67**, 42

27. Minisola S., Scarnecchia L., Carnevale V., Bigi F., Romagnoli E., Pacitti M. T. and Mazzuoli G. F. (1989). Clinical value of the measurement of bone remodeling markers in primary hyperparathyroidism. *J. Endocrinol. Invest.*, **12**, 537

28. Morris C. A., Mitnick M. E., Weir E. C., Horowitz M., Kreider B. L. and Insogna K. L. (1990). The parathyroid-related protein stimulates human osteoblast-like cells to secrete a 9,000 dalton bone-resorbing protein. *Endocrinology*, **126**(3), 1783

29. Mosekilde L. and Melson F. (1973). A tetracycline-based histomorphometric evaluation of bone resorption and bone turnover in hyperthyroidism and hyperparathyroidism. *Acta Med. Scand.*, **204**(97),

30. Murray T. M. (1989). Parathyroid hormone and hyperparathyroidism. Tam C. S., Heersche J. N. M. and Murray T. M., *Metabolic Bone Disease: Cellular and Tissue Mechanisms* (p. 105). Boca Raton: CRC Press

31. Parisien M., Silverberg S. J., Shane E., Dempster D. W. and Bilezikian J. P. (1990). Bone disease in primary hyperparathyroidism. *Endocrinol. Metab. Clin. N. Amer.*, **19**(1), 19

32. Revell P. A. (1986). *Pathology of Bone*. Berlin: Springer

33. Rhodan G. A. and Martin T. J. (1981). Role of osteoblasts in hormonal control of bone resorption – a hypothesis. *Calcif. Tissue Int.*, **33**, 349

34. Silve C., Fritsch J., Grosse B., Tam C., Edelmann A., Dehnas P., Balsan S. and Garahedian M. (1989). Corticosteroid-induced changes in the responsiveness of human osteoblast-like cells to parathyroid hormone. *Bone Miner.*, **6**(1), 65

35. Vigorita V. J. (1984). The tissue metabolic features of metabolic bone disease. *Orthop. Clin. N. Amer.*, **15**, 613

An unusual presentation of pHPT is given in the following reference:

Hollenberg A. N. and Arnold A. (1991). Hypercalcemia with low-normal serum intact PTH; a novel presentation of primary hyperparathyroidism. *Amer. J. Med.*, **91**, 547

Renal bone disease

13

The term 'renal bone disease' or 'renal osteodystrophy' is used to describe osseous disorders occurring in patients with renal disease[21,33,43,49,53,71]. Abnormalities of bone are seen mainly in patients suffering from chronic renal failure (impaired glomerular filtration rate, GFR). Variants of metabolic bone disease may also occur in patients with a normal GFR, but with renal tubular acidosis, nephrotic syndrome, renal stone diseases and oxalosis. A wide spectrum of factors influences the skeleton in renal disorders: the type of renal disease, the degree of uraemia, the severity of secondary hyperparathyroidism, changes in vitamin D metabolism, accumulation of toxic products (e.g. aluminium, fluorine, iron)[11,51,68,70], the type and duration of dialysis therapy and of drugs, particularly corticosteroids[5,21,25,26,37,38,50]. Patients with renal disease are also subject to the same conditions that affect the skeleton in normal individuals: sex, age, activity, endocrine disturbances, ethanol intake, immobilization, diabetes mellitus[5] and so forth. For example, renal complications may occur in B-cell dyscrasias due to deposition of monoclonal immunoglobulins in the kidneys[34]. Of all these, three have been identified as dominant factors in the pathomechanism of renal bone disease: abnormalities of vitamin D metabolism, hyperparathyroidism and aluminium retention. And they in turn interact in a number of ways to induce the heterogeneity of renal osteodystrophy. The diagnostic situation becomes even more complex when one realizes that the blood tests and radiographic studies usually employed do not always reflect bone disease in renal patients. Therefore suspected osteodystrophy is one of the leading indications for bone biopsy which itself is the most accurate way to diagnose renal bone disease[52,64].

Bone biopsy shows abnormal features in virtually all cases of chronic renal failure[20,31,52,72]. The earliest histological changes are seen when the GFR is reduced to 50% of normal, but they are usually not associated with clinical symptoms. The osseous changes characteristic of chronic renal failure may occur singly or in various combinations. None is unique to impairment of kidney function or to particular treatment modalities, for example conservative therapy, haemodialysis or transplantation. There are differences among the patients and between different renal units. The variable frequencies and types of osseous disorders also reflect use of differing histological and radiological criteria for diagnosis as well as the patients' age, the type and duration of disease, the degree of renal insufficiency and the therapy administered (Table 13.1). Hence renal bone disease comprises a collection of metabolic disorders which may occur singly or in combinations.

There are three main components of renal osteodystrophy:

1. changes in *bone remodelling* (osteitis fibrosa cystica versus adynamic bone disease),
2. changes in *mineralization* (osteomalacia), and
3. changes in *bone mass* (osteoporosis versus osteosclerosis).

Every degree of osteomalacia and hyperparathyroidism may be observed and osteoporosis and osteosclerosis may even coexist in the same patient. In children with chronic renal failure *growth retardation* of the skeleton is a further and often a major problem.

Utilizing abnormalities in osseous remodelling, mineralization and bone mass, osteodystrophy in patients with reduced kidney function can be subdivided into two broad categories: high-turnover bone disease (e.g. secondary hyperparathyroidism, sHPT) and low-turnover bone disease (e.g. osteomalacia and osteopenia). Most investigators agree that sHPT is the most common endocrine disorder in renal failure, and the degree can range from mild (*mild bone disease*) to severe (*hyperparathyroid bone disease*) (McCarthy and Kumar)[57]. The next common lesion is *mixed uraemic bone disease*, with elements of both hyperparathyroidism and osteomalacia. *Osteomalacia* and *low-turnover bone disease* are relatively infrequent, though with a wide range of frequency in different dialysis centres. It is worthwhile to distinguish these groups because the patients' therapy can be tailored to the predominant histological pattern.

Transformations may occur and the frequency of the five groups varies depending on the patients, their age, aluminium exposure, therapy with vitamin D metabolites, dietary intake, parathyroidectomy, dialysis-related factors and renal transplantation. The five groups are briefly considered below.

HYPERPARATHYROID URAEMIC BONE DISEASE (Plate 13.A)

Increased secretion of parathormone (PTH) is considered to be of major importance in renal bone disease by increasing the numbers and activity of bone cells, and thereby all aspects of bone turnover. A number of studies has shown the relationship between bone biopsy parameters and serum PTH levels. One major factor that enhances PTH secretion is hypocalcaemia, and the main causes in uraemic patients are phosphate retention, altered vitamin D metabolism, skeletal resistance to the action of PTH and impaired degradation of PTH metabolites.

Table 13.1 Histomorphometry of osseous remodelling in renal osteodystrophy, the patients grouped according to creatinine values and duration of haemodialysis

Parameters	Units	Creatinine* 2–4	Creatinine* > 4–6	Creatinine > 6–	Haemodialysis†
Bone	BV/TV, %	24	20	23	23
Osteoid	OV/TV, %	3	4	4	4
Osteoclasts	No. per mm² bone area	5	14	18	14
Osteoblasts	No. per mm² bone area	6	11	8	9

*Serum creatinine, mg/dl
†Duration of haemodialysis > 1 year

Plate 13.A

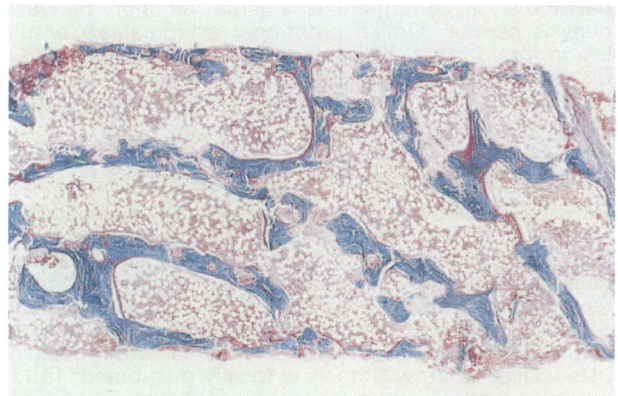

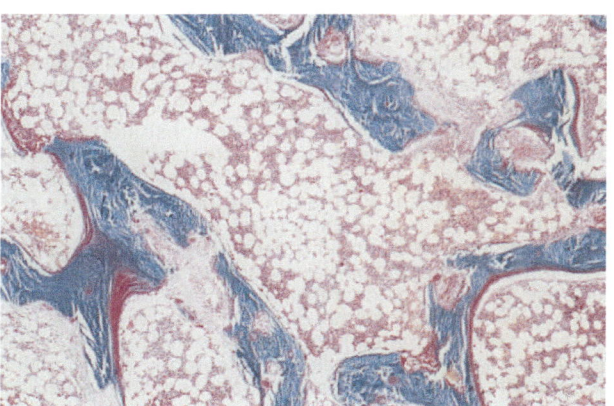

Figs. 13.1–13.6 Hyperparathyroid uraemic bone disease in iliac crest biopsies

Fig. 13.1 Low-power view illustrating preservation of overall trabecular network. Ladewig

Fig. 13.2 In higher magnification numerous foci of dissecting osteoclasia are evident. Also incipient demineralization (left). Ladewig

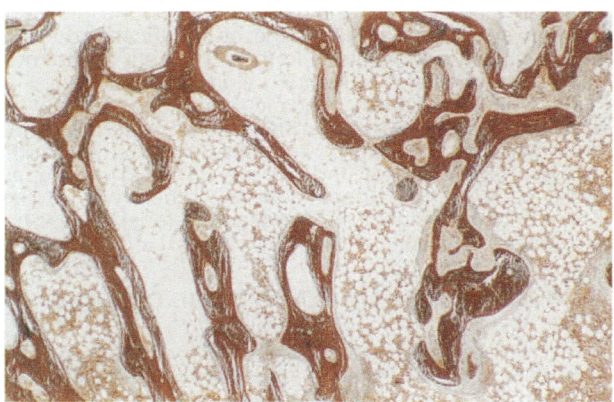

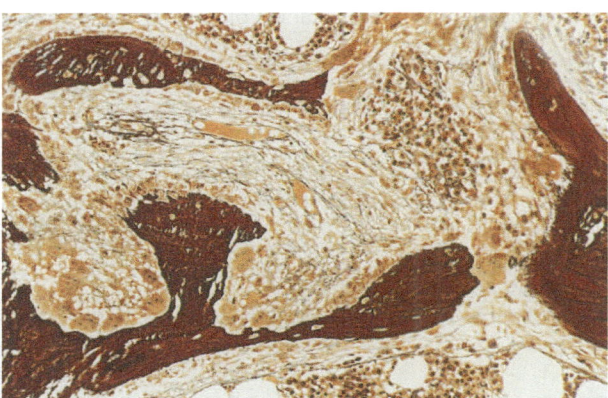

Fig. 13.3 Marked dissecting osteoclasia with strong fibrotic component. Note hypocellular bone marrow as frequently seen in renal osteodystrophy. Gomori

Fig. 13.4 Dissecting osteoclasia (at left, lower centre and right) and replacement of parts of the trabeculae by fibrous tissue. Gomori

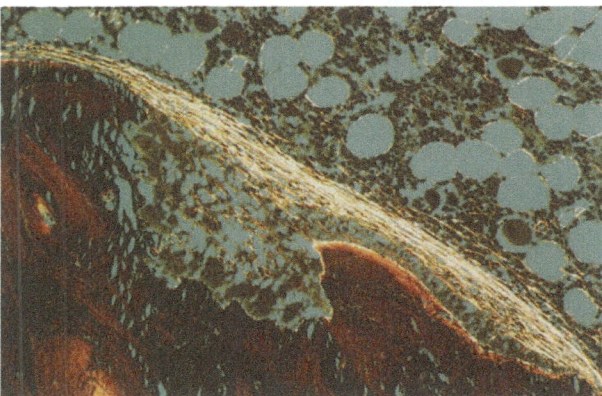

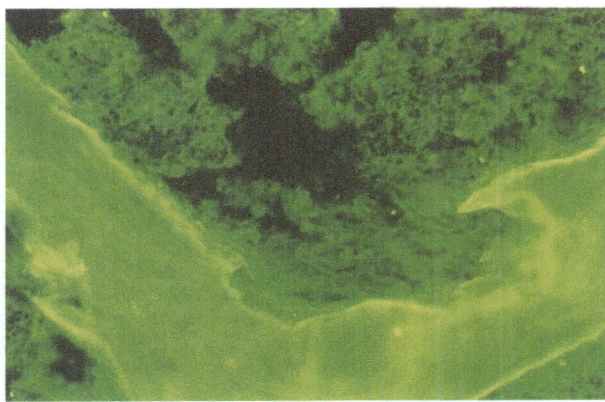

Fig. 13.5 High magnification of a trabecula showing deep osteoclastic excavation separated from haematopoietic marrow by paratrabecular band of fibres. Gomori, polar.

Fig. 13.6 Relatively shallow surface erosion and irregular staining of bone by antibodies to collagen type I. Cryostat section, immunofluorescence

Light microscopic examination of bone biopsy sections shows the effects of excessive PTH: increased surfaces of osteoclastic bone resorption and marrow fibrosis (*osteitis fibrosa cystica*). Dissecting and transecting osteoclasia of trabeculae are highly characteristic. The coupling of bone formation with bone resorption is demonstrated in these biopsies by the numerous active osteoblasts and osteocytes. The extent as well as the volume of osteoid is increased, while the formation of bone matrix is not lamellar, but fibrous in structure (primitive, or woven bone), as clearly seen under polarized light. This, together with *transecting osteoclasia*, impairs its strength and may give rise to serious mechanical consequences, particularly in the young. Tetracycline deposition shows normal or increased rates of mineral uptake. Excessive mesenchymal and osteoblastic activity result in disorderly arrangement of collagen, which is deposited not only at the trabecular surface (osteoid seam), but also into the marrow cavities near it, causing *peritrabecular fibrosis* as well as fibrotic replacement of resorbed trabeculae. Marrow fibrosis encroaches on the haematopoietic areas and may contribute to the anaemia of chronic renal failure, particularly in children. These events predominantly affect the cancellous bone, but *subperiosteal resorption* and *dissecting osteoclasia* may also be found in the cortical bone. There is a tendency for overall cancellous bone mass to rise with increasing levels of PTH, though osteopenic and even osteolytic lesions may be observed within the same biopsy. Most patients with this form of bone disease have minimum aluminium staining in their biopsy sections; Malluche and Faugere reported that 35% of patients do have stainable bone aluminium. Serum aluminium levels are highly variable in patients with severe HPT. Though there is a correlation between the serum concentrations of creatinine and of PTH and the histomorphometric values of bone turnover, a variety of factors may nevertheless modify the response of skeletal tissue to PTH. The most severe variants of hyperparathyroid bone disease were observed in children and in patients with tertiary HPT.

OSTEOMALACIC URAEMIC BONE DISEASE
(Plate 13.B)

The hallmark of this form is an excessive volume of osteoid. This occupies most of the trabecular surface and represents a considerable fraction of the trabecular bone volume (*hyperosteoidosis*), due to which the total cancellous bone mass may be increased. It may be that extensive seams of osteoid prevent resorption and therefore bone matrix tends to accumulate faster than it is removed, despite osteoclastic activity. The numbers and activity of the bone-forming and -resorbing cells vary, often in different areas in the same biopsy. An irregular interface between osteoid and mineralized bone reflects previous resorption. Tetracycline-based parameters demonstrate markedly impaired mineralization with a prolonged mineralization lag time. In most renal patients with osteomalacia, special stains demonstrate deposits of aluminium at the mineralization front[19,22,28,55,61]. Occasional demonstration of iron deposition may indicate that this metal is also capable of inducing a similar syndrome. Identification of aluminium along the mineralization front suggests that this metal prevents mineralization and inhibits hydroxyapatite crystal formation[8,59]. But aluminium also inhibits enzymes of the osteoblasts leading to reduced matrix synthesis[23,62]. Abnormal collagen synthesis[66] and defective bone crystal maturation[12,66,67] are additional causes of osteomalacia.

Osteomalacic uraemic bone disease is the one that most frequently causes bone pain and pathological fractures. The incidence of osteomalacia rises with time on haemodialysis, but there is a large variation between dialysis centres. Unlike nutritional osteomalacia or the lesion found in pre-dialysis patients, osteomalacia under dialysis is often associated with histological evidence of low turnover and low levels of serum alkaline phosphatase (low-turnover osteomalacia).

MIXED URAEMIC BONE DISEASE

Bone biopsy shows characteristics of both hyperparathyroidism and osteomalacia, which may coexist to varying degrees. The major histological findings are increased osteoid-associated parameters, and increased bone remodelling with numerous or many osteoclasts and resorbing surfaces. The numbers of osteoblasts may be disproportionately low when compared with those of osteoclasts. Marrow fibrosis is focally distributed. Tetracycline uptake is abnormal with a decrease in doubly labelled lamellar osteoid seams. Histochemical stains for aluminium will often disclose significant aluminium deposition, according to Malluche in approximately 50–70% of the cases. Other factors that may contribute to low bone formation rate and osteopenia are diabetes mellitus, immobilization, heparin therapy, acidosis, glucocorticoid therapy and altered collagen synthesis. The effects of iron overload and deposition on bone in dialysis patients are difficult to determine, as significant bone iron staining rarely occurs alone in these patients[56,74]. In most cases there was also significant aluminium staining.

Patients with mixed uraemic bone disease may be asymptomatic, or they may have the clinical features of both hyperparathyroidism and osteomalacia. McCarthy found no biochemical findings which could distinguish these patients from those with the other two entities. Functional assessment of osteoblasts in renal disease has also been reported.

LOW-TURNOVER URAEMIC BONE DISEASE
(Plate 13.C)

This type is characterized by markedly diminished bone remodelling, low osteoid-associated parameters and reduced bone mass (*osteopenia*). The dynamic tetracycline-based parameters demonstrate an impaired bone formation rate, which confirms the diagnosis of an adynamic aplastic bone disease. Aluminium deposition is very variable in patients with this pattern.

The treatment of low-turnover bone disease varies according to the aetiological factors present. However, post-parathyroidectomy- and steroid-induced variants are very difficult to treat.

MILD URAEMIC BONE DISEASE (Plate 13.C)

Bone biopsy shows slightly increased parameters of bone remodelling. The resorption surfaces are flat and dissecting bone resorption is rarely found. There is no evidence of a mineralization defect and the bone mass is within normal range.

This type of bone disease is found when proper medical attention has been given to correct the abnormalities of mineral metabolism seen in renal failure. The patients are asymptomatic from their bone disease, and radiographic studies are essentially normal.

DIALYSIS BONE DISEASE

Several long-term studies have shown that the incidence of low-turnover bone disease – osteomalacia as well as osteopenia – increases with duration of dialysis[16,44,54,65]. These patients usually fail to respond to treatment with vitamin D metabolites. Though various causes have been reported in the past, such as fluoride, phosphate depletion

Plate 13.B

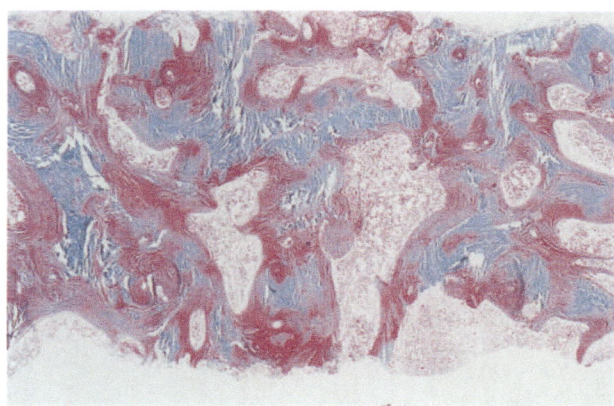

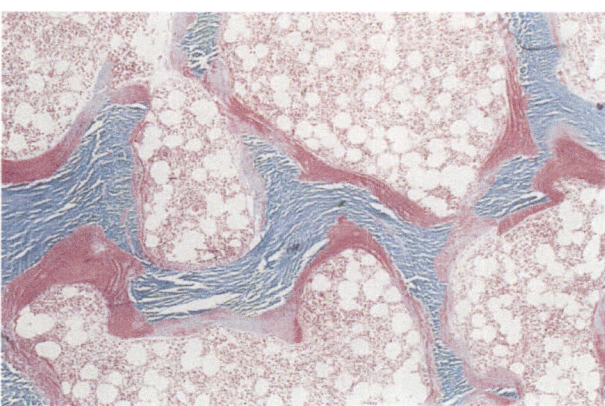

Figs. 13.7–13.12 Osteomalacic uraemic bone disease in iliac crest biopsies

Fig. 13.7 Increased cancellous bone volume ('osteosclerosis'), partly due to a large component of osteoid. Ladewig

Fig. 13.8 Fairly normal cancellous bone volume but with considerable increase in both extent and width of osteoid seams. Ladewig

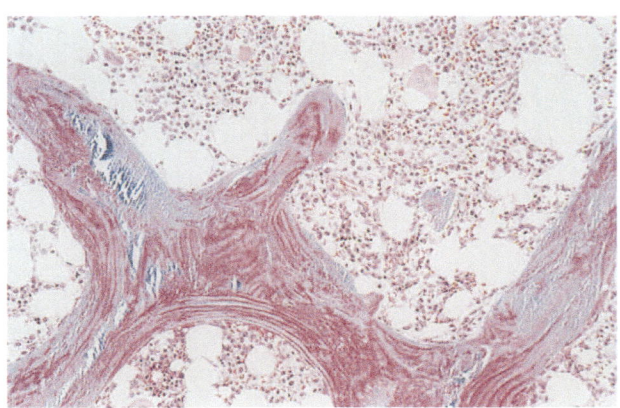

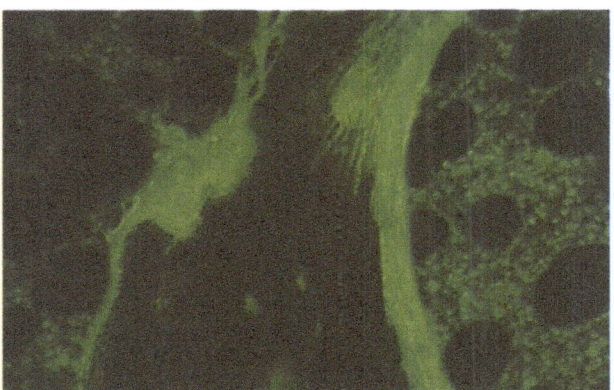

Fig. 13.9 Section showing almost complete demineralization of trabecular bone. Ladewig

Fig. 13.10 Irregular diffuse fluorescence after tetracycline administration in uraemic bone disease

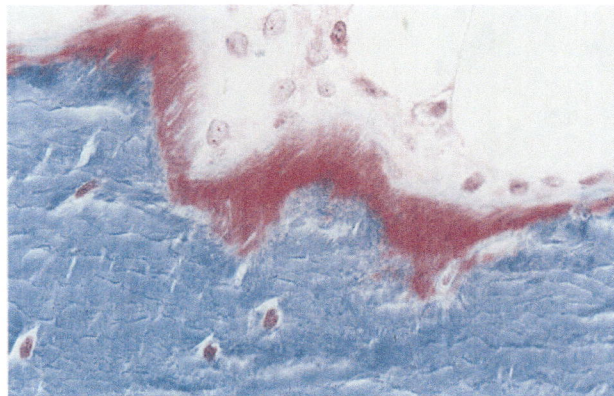

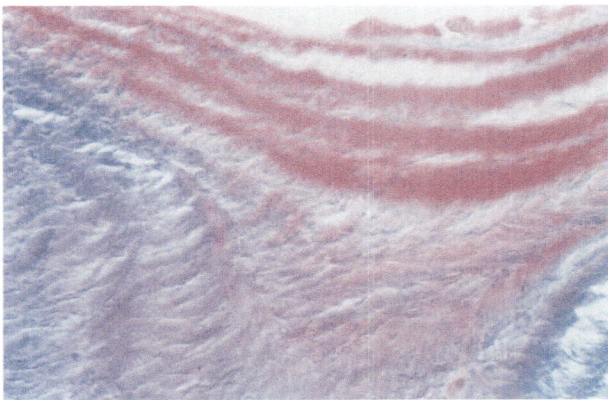

Fig. 13.11 Iliac crest biopsy of patient with long-standing renal failure. Note lack of parallel lamellae in mineralized bone as well as in osteoid. Ladewig

Fig. 13.12 In contrast to Fig. 13.11, well-defined lamellae in both osteoid and mineralized bone. Note incipient demineralization under the osteoid layer. Ladewig

Plate 13.C

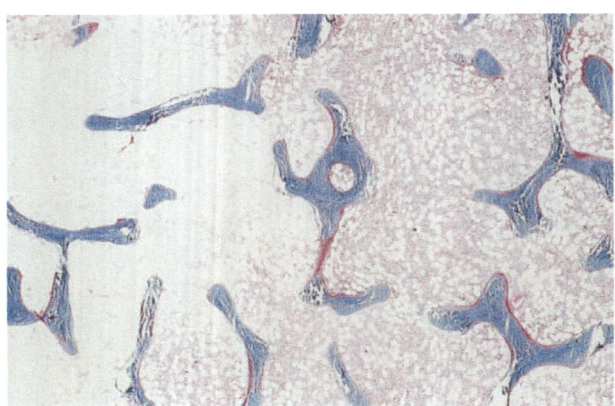

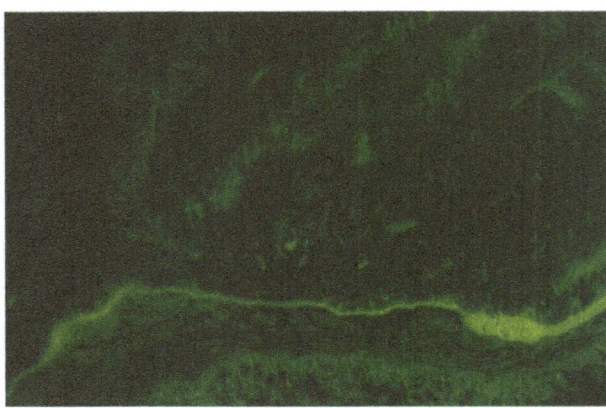

Figs. 13.13–13.18 Low turnover and mild uraemic bone disease in iliac crest biopsies

Fig. 13.13 Low magnification illustrating markedly diminished osseous remodelling, little osteoid and reduced cancellous bone volume (osteopenia). Note variable marrow cellularity. Ladewig

Fig. 13.14 Only a narrow band of fluorescence seen on trabecular surface after tetracycline administration, indicating the low bone formation rate

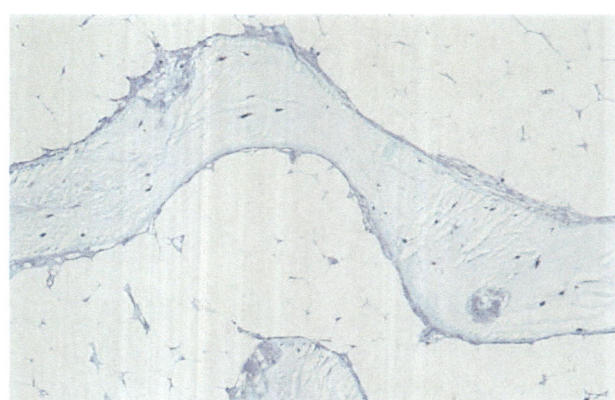

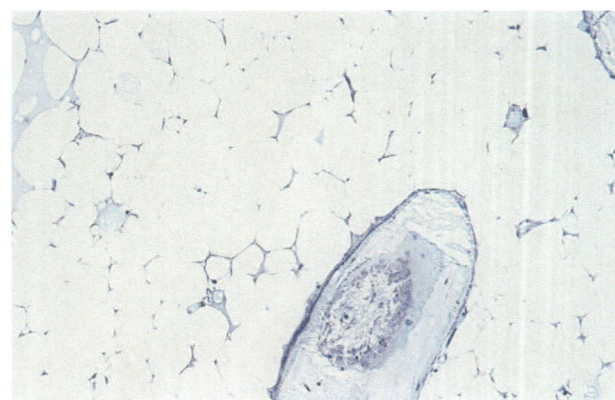

Fig. 13.15 Trabecular bone showing little superficial remodelling but an occasional surface erosion (upper left) as well as a small focus of dissecting osteoclasia (lower right), which distinguishes such biopsies from similar ones in aplastic anaemia and osteoporosis. Giemsa. Iliac crest biopsy of a patient with aluminium accumulation established by chemical analysis of a piece of the biopsy

Fig. 13.16 An example of somewhat larger dissecting osteoclasia in an iliac crest biopsy similar to that in Fig. 13.15. Giemsa

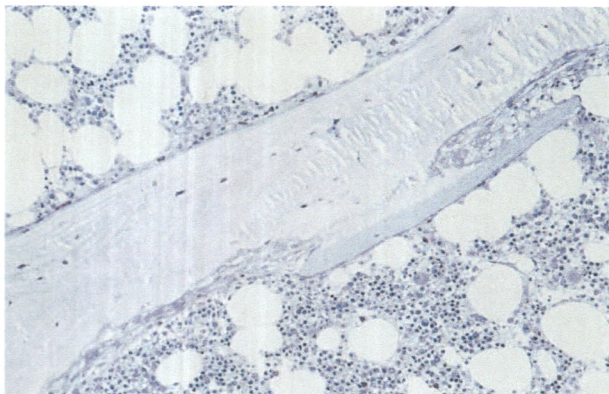

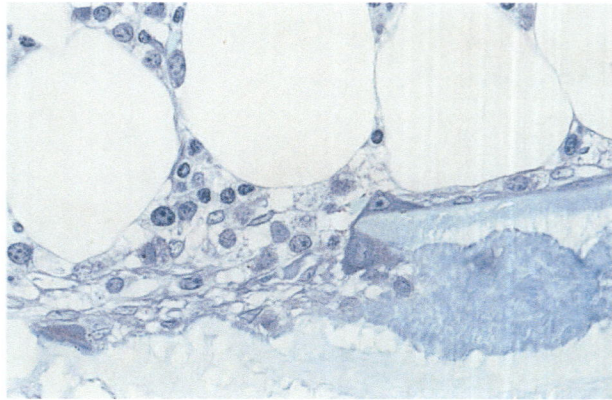

Figs. 13.17 and **13.18** Examples of uraemic bone disease in which there is slightly increased osseous remodelling, but dissecting bone resorption rarely occurs

Fig. 13.17 Superficial osteoclastic resorption as well as osteoblastic new bone formation. Note undermining of layer of osteoid by osteoclasts (upper right). Giemsa

Fig. 13.18 Higher magnification of section in Fig. 13.17 illustrating undermining of osteoid seam by osteoclasts (centre) and newly formed osteoid in the deep resorption hole. Note two 'young' osteocytes in the osteoid zone. Giemsa

and anticonvulsants, aluminium is now thought to be the major cause of *refractory osteomalacia*[1–3,24,46,58,60,63,75]. Also parathyroidectomized dialysis patients, characteristically presenting low-turnover bone disease, show a marked tendency to develop aluminium-related osteomalacia. Therefore the *treatment strategy* of dialysis osteodystrophy should include two steps:

1. treating aluminium-related low-turnover bone disease by removing high aluminium burden, e.g. with the chelating agent desferoxamine[4,18], and thereafter
2. treating hyperparathyroid bone disease, e.g. by vitamin D metabolites[32], bisphosphonates[42] or even by parathyroidectomy[17].

The variant of *osteoporomalacia* is mainly influenced by low dialysate calcium concentration[9,10], immobilization, long-term heparin treatment, diabetic microangiopathy, steroids and toxic–uraemic agents leading to inflammatory and atrophic reactions of the bone marrow.

Continuous ambulatory peritoneal dialysis (CAPD) is a relatively new technique, and follow-up studies of renal bone disease in CAPD-treated patients are rare and only with small numbers of patients, though recently several studies have been published[6,15,36,39,40]. Several reports have documented little progression of bone disease, with no significant differences between the two dialysis treatment modalities[69]. High dialysate concentrations had no influence on progressive bone loss.

The association between cystic bone changes, pathological fractures, scapulohumeral periarthritis and carpal tunnel syndrome has been described in patients with long-term dialysis[29,30,47]. Bone biopsies revealed amyloid deposits in the walls of the small arterial vessels and in the interstitium of the marrow: '*dialysis amyloidosis*'[30,41,45]. Immunohistological studies have shown that the amyloid protein is composed of β_2-microglobulin[35,48]. The cystic osseous lesions characteristically are caused by 'amyloidomas' eroding the bone[14].

BONE DISEASE AFTER RENAL TRANSPLANTATION (Plate 13.D)

Following successful transplantation, normal renal function is restored and one can expect an improvement in the pre-existing bone disease. Numerous histological and radiological studies have been carried out on these transplanted patients, and the results show that many of the metabolic abnormalities of renal failure are reversed, though some changes remain[13,27]. Features of hyperparathyroidism in the biopsy may persist in some patients and in others may disappear completely after some months. Aluminium-associated bone disease is rarely seen after renal transplantation because aluminium is rapidly excreted by the transplanted kidney.

However, the immunosuppressive treatment necessary in renal transplantation may effect bone metabolism. Cyclosporin has direct effects on bone cells *in vitro*[73]. Glucocorticoids inhibit intestinal absorption of calcium and decrease the bone formation rate, resulting in bone loss with the clinical features of progressive osteoporosis. Patients with parathyroidectomy before transplantation had a slower rate of bone loss.

References

1. Andress D. L., Kopp J. B., Maloney N. A., Coburn J. W. and Sherrard D. J. (1987). Early deposition of aluminium in bone in diabetic patients on haemodialysis. *N. Engl. J. Med.*, **316**, 292
2. Andress D. L., Maloney N. A., Endres D. B. and Sherrard D. J. (1986). Aluminium-associated bone disease in chronic renal failure: high prevalence in a long-term dialysis population. *J. Bone Miner. Res.*, **1**, 391
3. Andress D. L., Maloney N. A., Coburn J. W., Endress D. B. and Sherrard D. J. (1987). Osteomalacia and aplastic bone disease in aluminium-related osteodystrophy. *J. Clin. Endocrinol. Metab.*, **65**, 11
4. Andress D. L., Nebeker H. G. and Ott S. M. (1987). Bone histologic response to long-term treatment with deferoxamine for aluminium-related bone disease. *Kidney Int.*, **31**, 1344
5. Andress D. L., Pandian M. R., Endres D. B. and Kopp J. B. (1989). Plasma insulin-like growth factors and bone formation in uremic hyperparathyroidism. *Kidney Int.*, **36**, 471
6. Asai K., Miura S., Kawahara H., Toriyama T. and Kuzuya F. (1991). A comparative study of atherosclerosis and osteopenia in elderly and young hemodialysis patients. *Aging (Milano)*, **3**, 79
7. Avram M. M. (1980). Lower parathyroid hormone and creatinine in diabetic uremia. *Contrib. Nephrol.*, **20**, 4
8. Blumenthal N. C. and Posner A. S. (1984). *In vitro* model of aluminium-induced osteomalacia: inhibition of hydroxyapatite formation and growth. *Calcif. Tissue Int.*, **36**, 439
9. Bone J. M., Davison A. M. and Robson J. S. (1972). The role of dialysate calcium concentration in osteoporosis in patients on hemodialysis. *Lancet*, **1**, 1047
10. Bouillon R., Verberckmoes R. and DeMoor P. (1975). Influence of dialysate calcium concentration and vitamin D on serum parathyroid hormone during repetitive dialysis. *Kidney Int.*, **7**, 422
11. Boyce B. F., Fell G. S. and Elder H. Y. (1982). Hypercalcaemic osteomalacia due to aluminium toxicity. *Lancet*, **2**, 1009
12. Burnell J. M., Teubner E., Wegedal J. E. and Sherrard D. J. (1974). Bone crystal maturation in renal osteodystrophy in humans. *J. Clin. Invest.*, **53**, 52
13. Carroll R. N. P., Williams E. D., Aung T., Yeboah E. and Shackman R. (1973). The effects of renal transplantation on renal osteodystrophy. *Proc. Europ. Dialysis Transpl. Assoc.*, **10**, 446
14. Casey T., Stone W. J., DiRaimondo C. R., Brantley B. D., DiRaimondo C. V., Gorevic P. D. and Page D. L. (1986). Tumoral amyloidosis of bone of beta-2-microglobulin origin associated with long term hemodialysis: a new type of amyloid disease. *Hum. Pathol.*, **17**, 731
15. Cassidy M. J. D., Owen J. P. and Ellis H. A. (1985). Renal osteodystrophy and metastatic calcification on long-term continuous ambulatory peritoneal dialysis. *Q. J. Med.*, **54**, 29
16. Chan Y., Furlong T. J., Cornish C. J. and Posen S. (1985). Dialysis osteodystrophy. A study involving 94 patients. *Medicine*, **64**, 296
17. Charhon S. A., Berland Y. F. and Olmer M. J. (1985). Effects of parathyroidectomy on bone formation and mineralisation in hemodialysed patients. *Kidney Int.*, **27**, 426
18. Charhon S. A., Chavassieux P. and Boivin G. (1987). Desferrioxamine-induced bone changes in haemodialysis patients: a histomorphometric study. *Clin. Sci.*, **73**, 227
19. Charhon S. A., Chavassieux P. M., Chapuy M. C., Boivin G. Y. and Meunier P. J. (1985). Low rate of bone formation with or without histologic appearance of osteomalacia in patients with aluminium intoxication. *J. Lab. Clin. Med.*, **106**, 123
20. Charhon S. A., Delmas P. D. and Malaval L. (1986). Serum bone Gla-protein in renal osteodystrophy: comparison with bone histomorphometry. *J. Clin. Endocrinol. Metab.*, **63**, 892
21. Coburn J. W. and Slatopolsky E. (1991). The renal osteodystrophies. Brenner B. M. and Rector F. C., The Kidney, 4th edn (p. 2057). Philadelphia: Saunders
22. Connor M. O., Garrett P., Dockery M., Donohoe J. F., Doyle G. D., Carmody M. and Dervan P. A. (1986). Aluminium-related bone disease: correlation between symptoms, osteoid volume and aluminium staining. *Amer. J. Clin. Pathol.*, **86**, 168
23. Cournot-Witmer G., Plachot J. J. and Bourdeau A. (1986). Effect of aluminium on bone and cell localization. *Kidney Int.*, **29**(Suppl. 18), 37
24. Cournot-Witmer G., Zingraff J. and Plachot J. J. (1981). Aluminium localization in bone from haemodialyzed patients: relationship to matrix mineralisation. *Kidney Int.*, **20**, 375
25. Cundy T., Hamdy N., Gray R., Jackson B. and Kanis J. A. (1985). Hyperparathyroid bone disease in chronic renal failure. *Ulster Med. J.*, **54**, s34
26. Cundy T., Hand D. J. and Oliver D. O. (1985). Who gets renal bone disease before beginning dialysis? *Brit. Med. J.*, **290**, 271
27. Dalen N. and Alvestrand A. (1973). Bone mineral content in chronic renal failure and after renal transplantation. *Clin. Nephrol.*, **1**, 338
28. Denton F., Freemont A. J. and Ball J. (1984). Detection and distribution of aluminium in bone. *J. Clin. Pathol.*, **37**, 136
29. DiRaimondo C. R., Casey T. T., DiRaimondo C. V. and Stone W. J. (1986). Pathologic fractures associated with idiopathic amyloidosis of bone in chronic hemodialysis patients. *Nephron*, **43**, 22

Plate 13.D

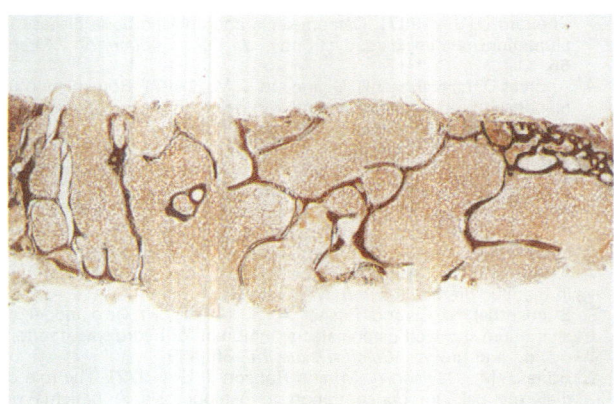

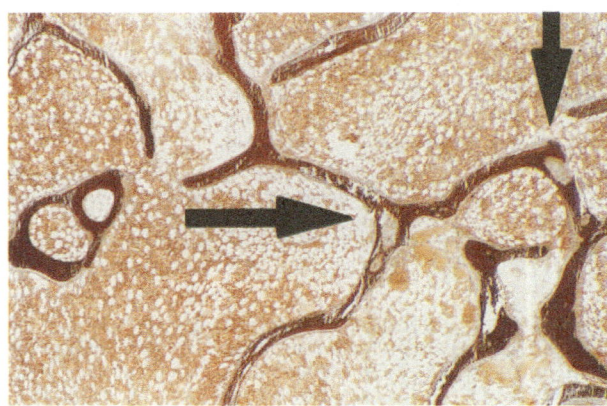

Figs. 13.19–13.24 Iliac crest biopsies after renal transplantation

Fig. 13.19 Tangentially taken biopsy showed marked trabecular osteopenia, histological type A. Gomori

Fig. 13.20 Higher magnification reveals residual dissecting osteoclasia (arrows). Gomori

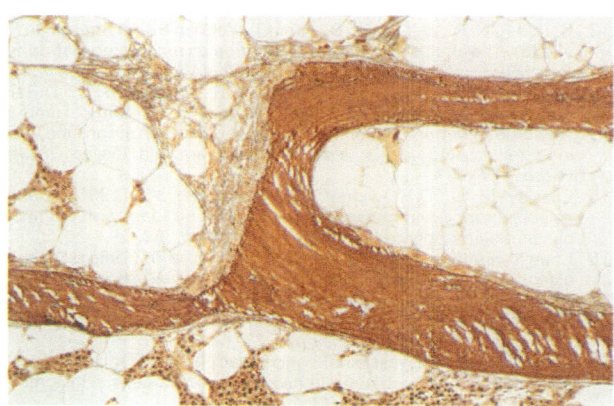

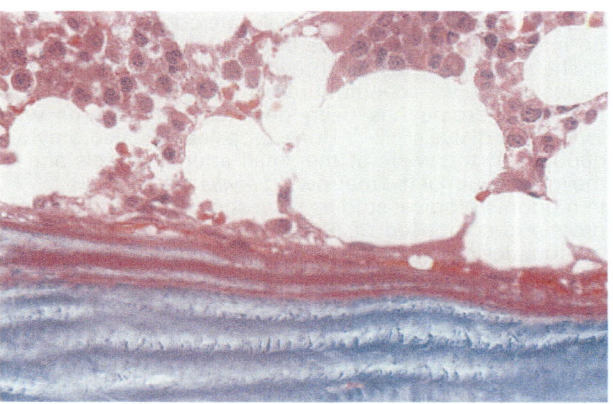

Fig. 13.21 Section showing residual paratrabecular and interstitial fibrosis. Gomori

Fig. 13.22 Presumably residual osteoid seam consisting of parallel lamellae. Note absence of surface layer of osteoblasts. Ladewig

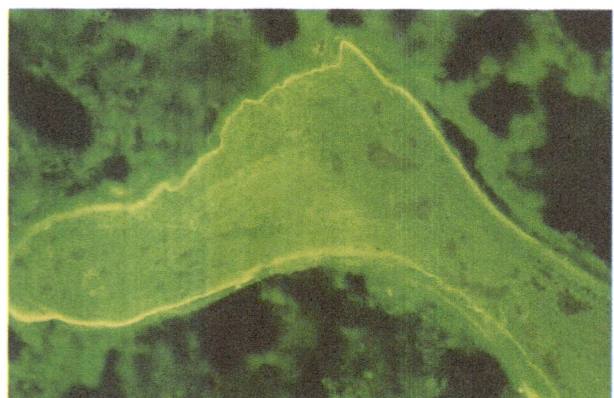

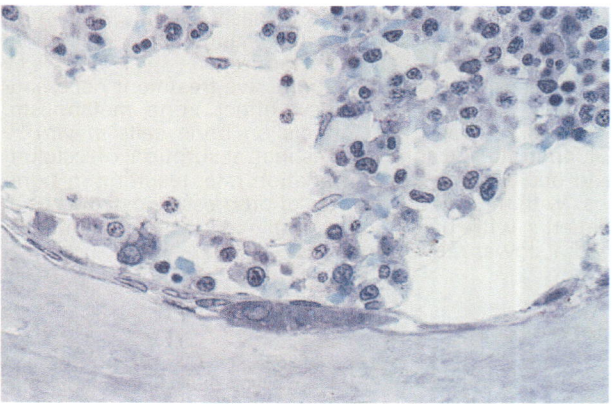

Fig. 13.23 Trabecular with scalloped upper edge (indicating previous osteoclastic remodelling) and multiple small staining defects as shown by antibodies to collagen type I. Cryostat section, immunofluorescence

Fig. 13.24 Flat osteoclast covered by endosteal lining cells. Giemsa

30. Editorials. (1991). Dialysis amyloidosis. *Lancet*, **338**, 349
31. Ellis H. A. and Peart K. M. (1973). Azotemic renal osteodystrophy, a quantitative study on iliac. *J. Clin. Pathol.*, **26**, 83
32. Ellis H. A., Pierides A. M., Feest T. G., Ward M. K. and Kerr D. N. S. (1977). Histopathology of renal osteodystrophy with particular reference to the effects of 1 alpha-hydroxyvitamin D3 in patients treated by long-term haemodialysis. *Clin. Endocrinol.*, **7**(Suppl.), 31
33. Feest T. G., Ward M. K., Ellis, H. A., Conceicao S., Pierides A. M., Aird E., Simpson W., Cook D. B. and Kerr D. N. S. (1977). Renal bone disease – what is it and why does it happen? *Clin. Endocrinol.*, **7**(Suppl.), 19
34. Gallo G. (1991). Renal complications of B-cell dyscrasias. *N. Engl. J. Med.*, **324**, 1889
35. Gejyo F., Yamada T. and Odani S. (1985). A new form of amyloid protein associated with chronic hemodialysis was identified as $\beta2$-microglobulin. *Biochem. Biophys. Res. Commun.*, **129**, 701
36. Gilmour J., Wu G., Khanna R., Schilling H., Mitwalli A. and Oreopoulos D. G. (1985). Long-term continuous ambulatory peritoneal dialysis. *Peritoneal Dial. Bull.*, **5**, 112
37. Grech P., Martin T. J., Barrington N. A. and Ell P. J. (1985). *Diagnosis of Metabolic Bone Disease*. London: Chapman & Hall
38. Hodgson S. F. (1986). Skeletal remodeling and renal osteodystrophy. *Semin. Nephrol.*, **6**, 42
39. Hutchinson A. J., Freemont A. J., Lumb G. A. and Gokal R. (1991). Renal osteodystrophy in CAPD. *Adv. Peritoneal Dial.*, **7**, 237
40. Joffe P., Podenphant J. and Haef J. G. (1989). Bone histology in CAPD patients: a comparison with haemodialysis and conservatively treated chronic uremics. *Adv. Peritoneal Dial.*, **5**, 171
41. Kachel H. G., Altmeyer P., Baldamus C. A. and Koch K. M. (1983). Deposition of an amyloid-like substance as a possible complication of regular dialysis treatment. *Contrib. Nephrol.*, **36**, 127
42. Kanis J. A. (1987). Clodronate – a new perspective in the treatment of neoplastic bone disease. *Bone*, **8**(Suppl. 1), 1
43. Kanis J. A., Cundy T. and Hamdy N. A. T. (1988). Renal osteodystrophy. *Clin. Endocrinol. Metab.*, **2**(1), 193
44. Kerr D. N. S., Walls J. and Ellis H. (1969). Bone disease in patients undergoing regular haemodialysis. *J. Bone Jt Surg.*, **51B**, 578
45. Kleinman K. S. and Coburn J. W. (1989). Amyloid syndromes associated with hemodialysis. *Kidney Int.*, **25**, 567
46. Kriegshauser J. S., Swee R. G., McCarthy J. T. and Hauser M. F. (1987). Aluminium toxicity in patients undergoing dialysis: radiographic findings and prediction of bone biopsy results. *Radiology*, **164**, 399
47. Kurer M. H. J., Baillod R. A. and Madgwick J. C. A. (1991). Musculoskeletal manifestations of amyloidosis: a review of 83 patients on haemodialysis for at least 10 years. *J. Bone Jt Surg.*, **73B**, 271
48. Linke R. P., Nathrath W. B. J. and Eulitz M. (1986). Classification of amyloid syndromes from tissue sections using antibodies against various amyloid fibril proteins: report of 142 cases. Glenner G. G., Osserman E. F., Benditt E. P., Calkins E., Cohen A. S. and Zucker-Franklin D., *Amyloidosis*. New York: Plenum
49. Llack F. (1991). Renal bone disease. *Transplant. Proc.*, **23**, 1818
50. Lopez-Hilker S., Galceran T. and Chan Y. (1986). Hypocalcemia may not be essential for the development of secondary hyperparathyroidism in chronic renal failure. *J. Clin. Invest.*, **78**, 1097
51. Malluche H. H., Faugere M.-C., Smith A. J. and Friedler R. M. (1986). Aluminium intoxication of bone in renal failure – fact or fiction? *Kidney Int.*, **29**(Suppl. 18), 70
52. Malluche H. H. and Faugere M.-C. (1986). *Atlas of Mineralized Bone Histology*. Basel: Karger
53. Malluche H. H. and Faugere M.-C. (1989). Renal osteodystrophy. *N. Engl. J. Med.*, **321**, 317
54. Malluche H. H., Ritz E. and Lange H. P. (1976). Bone mass in maintenance haemodialysis. Prospective study with sequential biopsies. *Eur. J. Clin. Invest.*, **6**, 265
55. Maloney N. A., Ott S., Alfrey A. C., Miller L. N., Coburg J. W. and Sherrard D. J. (1982). Histologic quantitation of aluminium in iliac bone from patients with renal failure. *J. Lab. Clin. Med.*, **99**, 206
56. McCarthy J. T., Hodgson S. F., Fairbanks V. F. and Moyer T. P. (1991). Clinical and histological features of iron-related bone disease in dialysis patients. *Amer. J. Kidney Dis.*, **17**, 551
57. McCarthy J. T. and Kumar R (1990). Renal osteodystrophy. *Endocrinol. Metabol. Clin. N. Amer.*, **19**(1), 65
58. McCarthy J. T., Milliner D. S., Kurtz S. B., Johnson W. J. and Moyer T. P. (1986). Interpretation of serum aluminium values in dialysis patients. *Amer. J. Clin. Pathol.*, **86**, 629
59. Meyer J. L. and Thomas W. C. (1986). Aluminium and aluminium complexes. Effect of calcium phosphate precipitation. *Kidney Int.*, **29**(Suppl. 18), 20
60. Norfray J., Calenoff L., DelGreco F. and Krumlovsky F. A. (1975). Renal osteodystrophy in patients on hemodialysis as reflected in the bony pelvis. *Amer. J. Roentgenol.*, **125**, 352
61. Norris K. C., Goodman W. G. and Howard N. (1986). The iliac crest bone biopsy for the diagnosis of aluminium toxicity and a guide to the use of deferoxamine. *Semin. Nephrol.*, **6**(Suppl. 1), 27
62. Parisien M., Charhon S.A., Arlot M., Mainetti E., Chavassieux P., Chapuy M.-C. and Meunier P. J. (1988). Evidence for a toxic effect of aluminium on osteoblasts: a histomorphometric study in hemodialysis patients with aplastic bone disease. *J. Bone Miner. Res.*, **3**(3), 259
63. Quarles L. D., Dennis V. W. and Gitelman H. J. (1984). Aluminium deposition in bone: an epiphenomenon of the osteomalacic state. *Clin. Res.*, **32**, 522
64. Revell P. A. (1986). *Pathology of Bone*. Berlin: Springer
65. Ritz E., Krempien B., Mehls O. and Malluche H. H. (1973). Skeletal abnormalities in chronic renal insufficiency before and during maintenance hemodialysis. *Kidney Int.*, **4**, 116
66. Russell J. E., Avioli L. V. and Mechanic G. (1975). The nature of the collagen cross-links in bone in the chronic uraemic state. *Biochem. J.*, **145**, 119
67. Russell J. E., Termine J. D. and Avioli L. V. (1973). Abnormal bone mineral maturation in the chronic uremic state. *J. Clin. Invest.*, **52**, 2848
68. Sherrard D. J. (1991). Aluminium – much ado about something. *N. Engl. J. Med.*, **324**, 558
69. Shusterman N. H., Wasserstein A. G., Morrison G., Audet P., Fallon, M. D. and Kaplan F. (1987). Controlled study of renal osteodystrophy in patients undergoing dialysis. Improved response to continuous ambulatory peritoneal dialysis compared with hemodialysis. *Amer. J. Med.*, **82**, 1148
70. Slatoplsky E. (1987). The interaction of parathyroid hormone and aluminium in renal osteodystrophy. *Kidney Int.*, **31**, 842
71. Slatopolsky E. and Coburn J. W. (1990). Renal osteodystrophy. Avioli L. V. and Krane S. M., *Metabolic Bone Disease* (p. 452). Philadelphia: Saunders
72. Steiniche T., Mosekilde L., Christensen M. S. and Melsen F. (1989). A histomorphometric determination of iliac bone remodeling in patients with recurrent renal stone formation and idiopathic hypercalcuria. *Acta Pathol. Microbiol. Immunol. Scand.*, **97**, 309
73. Stewart P. J., Green O. C. and Stern P. H. (1986). Cyclosporine A inhibits calcemic hormone-induced bone resorption in vitro. *J. Bone Miner. Res.*, **1**, 285
74. VandeVyer F. L., Visser W. J., Haese P. C. and DeBroe M. E. (1990). Iron overload and bone disease in chronic dialysis patients. *Nephrol. Dial. Transplant.*, **5**, 781
75. Wills M. R. and Savory J. (1983). Aluminium poisoning: dialysis encephalopathy, osteomalacia, and anaemia. *Lancet*, **2**, 29

References added in proof:

Coe F. L., Parks J. H. and Asplin J. R. (1992). The pathogenesis and treatment of kidney stones. *N. Engl. J. Med.*, **327**, 1141

Paget's disease of bone

14

Synonym: osteitis deformans

Although generally grouped with metabolic bone disease, Paget's disease of bone is a unifocal or multifocal skeletal disorder, characterized by abnormally rapid turnover and disorganized structure at the involved sites[3,15,17,21,25,33,34,36,40,41]. Paget's disease occurs predominantly in middle and old age, though it may occur in young adults. It is usually slowly progressive. The most common complaints and complications are bone pain, skeletal deformities, pathological fractures[9,14] and neurological problems. An increased cardiac output caused by a shunting of blood may occur, when more than one-third of the skeleton is involved[18]. The X-ray appearance is far more striking than the symptomatology, and it is estimated that at least 90% of those affected are asymptomatic[5,23].

Based on radiological features several *stages* are distinguishable: an initial lytic phase, followed by a mixed phase and finally an advanced sclerotic, 'cold', 'burnt out' phase[23]. Bone scintigraphy provides the most sensitive method for localization of involved sites and has the advantage over radiography that the entire skeleton may be scanned[1,11]. Electron and light microscopic studies have revealed cytoplasmic and intranuclear inclusions in osteoclasts, and a *slow viral infection* has been held responsible[28,35,37]. Some workers favour the concept that there is a genetic basis for immunoregulatory dysfunction and susceptibility of osteoclasts to viral infection[37].

The radiological and biochemical findings generally indicate the *diagnosis*, particularly if there is extensive bone involvement. Bone tumours, metastases, severe HPT and fibrous dysplasia occasionally confuse the picture, in which case a bone biopsy is usually taken from an involved site[5]. However it is of interest that 12% of patients with Paget's disease who did not show pelvic involvement on X-ray or bone scan had positive iliac crest biopsies.

The incidence of *tumours*, benign and malignant, has been estimated as high as 10% in the generalized, severe forms of Paget's disease[16]. If all patients with pagetic bone are included the incidence is lower than 1%. The vast majority of malignant bone tumours are osteosarcomas, which are found most frequently in the pelvis[12,38]. In view of the excessive vascularization in pagetic lesions, it is surprising that carcinomatous metastases are not encountered more frequently in such bone. The pathophysiology and treatment of Paget's disease of bone has recently been extensively reviewed by Kanis[19]. Paget-like lesions in bone have also been reported in lymphoproliferative disorders (Fig. 14.24)[32].

Osteoclasts constitute the primary abnormality in Paget's disease (Plate 14.A)[4,6,13,26,30,31,37]. Data obtained from bone biopsies strongly point to this cell as being the initiation site for the series of pathological events which result in the biochemical, radiological and histological manifestations of Paget's disease (Table 14.1). Nuclear inclusions consistent with viral nucleocapsids were found in 20–40% of the osteoclasts, though not in osteocytes, osteoblasts or cells of the monocyte–macrophage lineage[28,37]. Pagetic osteoclasts are larger and contain more nuclei and nucleoli than their normal counterparts. In our biopsy study their number was only slightly increased, but the individual osteoclasts were large, together occu-

pying 2% of the total biopsy volume. Sixty per cent of the osteoclasts were multinucleated (osteoclasts with > 10 nuclei up to as many as 100) with prominent nucleoli (Fig. 14.S1). They resorbed bone in a relatively disorganized fashion (Figs 14.EM1 and 14.EM2) producing large cavities, enclosing huge osteoclasts, mast cells, blood vessels and fibrotic mesenchymal tissue ('osteitis deformans') (Plate 14.B).

Table 14.1 Histomorphometry of iliac crest biopsies in patients with Paget's disease (*n* = 100)

Parameters	Units	Paget's disease	Normal
Spongiosa	% TV	42	22
Osteoid	% TV	3	1
Fibrosis	% TV	12	0
Haematopoiesis	% TV	17	47
Fatty tissue	% TV	18	27
Sinusoids	% TV	5	3
Osteoclasts	% TV	2	0
Osteoclasts	per mm² B.Ar.	4	1
Osteoblasts	per mm² B.Ar.	6	2
Mast cells	per mm² M.Ar.	14	3
Arteries	per mm² M.Ar.	1.2	0.4
Arterioles	per mm² M.Ar.	6.5	1.3
Capillaries	per mm² M.Ar.	48	18
Sinusoids	per mm² M.Ar.	53	34

Abreviations and units: see Table 3.1

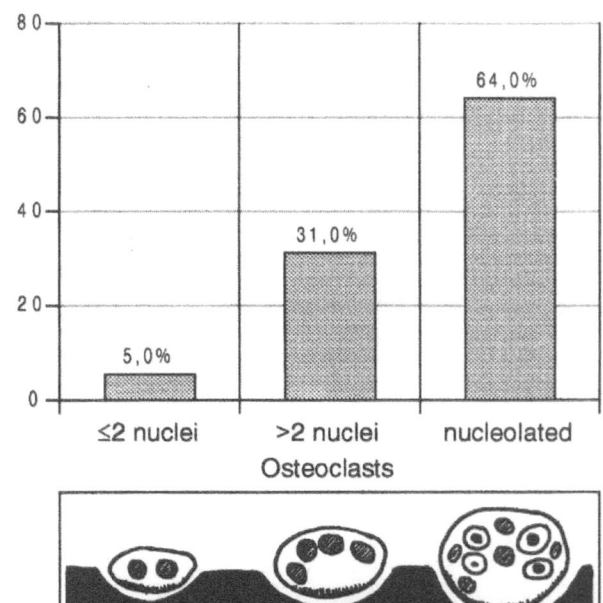

Fig. 14.S1 Frequency of types of osteoclasts in iliac crest biopsies of patients with Paget's disease (*n* = 100)

Plate 14.A

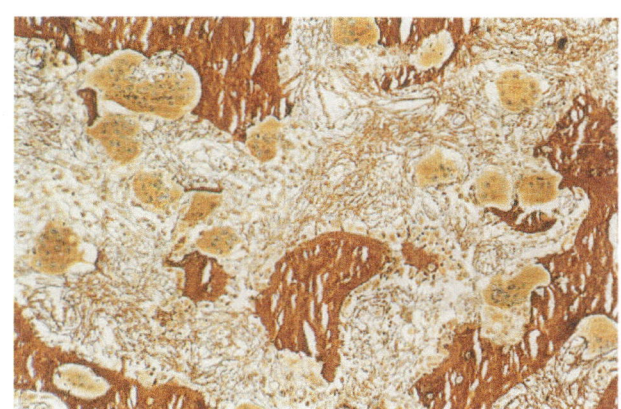

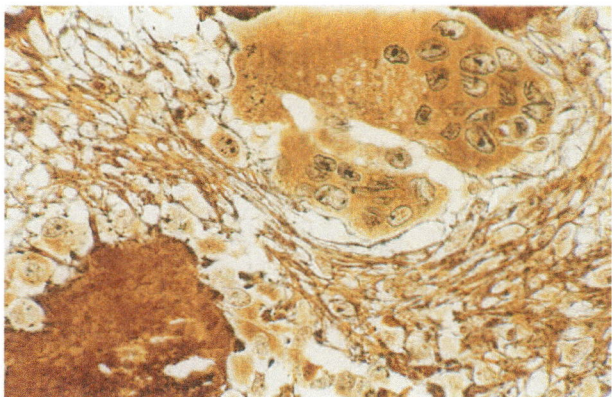

Figs. 14.1–14.6 Osteoclasts in Paget's disease of bone

Fig. 14.1 Numerous large multinucleated osteoclasts on bone inside resorption cavities or within the fibrous connective tissue stroma. Gomori

Fig. 14.2 Multinucleated osteoclast with large area of vacuolated cytoplasm as well as nuclear inclusions. Note coarse fibrosis and osteoblastic activity (lower left). Gomori

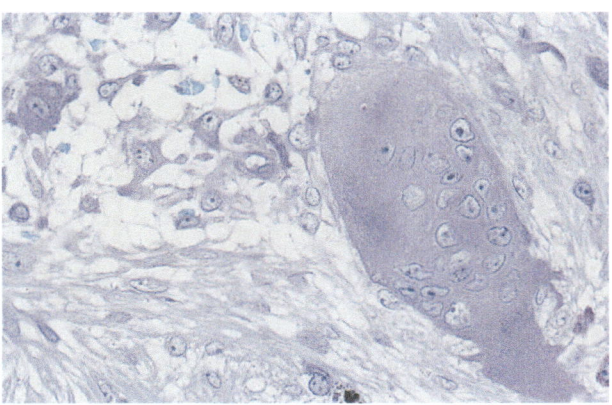

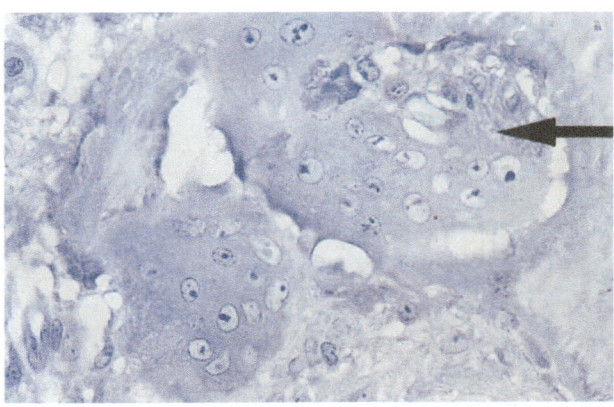

Fig. 14.3 Giant multinucleated osteoclast within loose connective tissue, but far from any osseous surface. Note small developing osteoclast (upper left). Giemsa

Fig. 14.4 Large multinucleated and nucleolated osteoclasts within erosion cavity which is lined by a layer of osteoid. Note fragment of bone (arrow) engulfed within a vacuole in the cytoplasm of the osteoclast. Giemsa. See also Fig. 14.EM1, electron microscopy of osteoclast with fragments of bone in cytoplasmic vacuoles

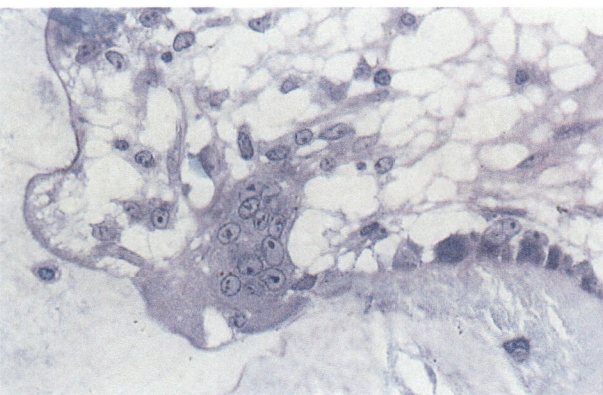

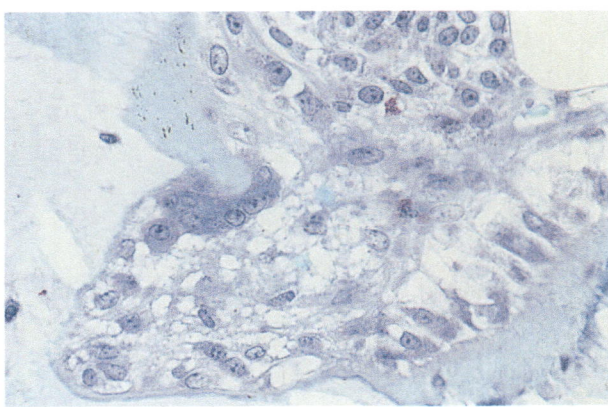

Fig. 14.5 Scalloped trabecular surface with one large osteoclast in Howship's lacuna adjacent to a layer of osteoblasts ('coupled' osseous remodelling?) and surrounded by loose connective tissue. Giemsa

Fig. 14.6 Deep excavation filled with connective tissue, with broad osteoid seam covered by layer of high-columnar osteoblasts. Note osteoclast partially surrounding protruding edge of osteoid seam (left). Giemsa

Plate 14.B

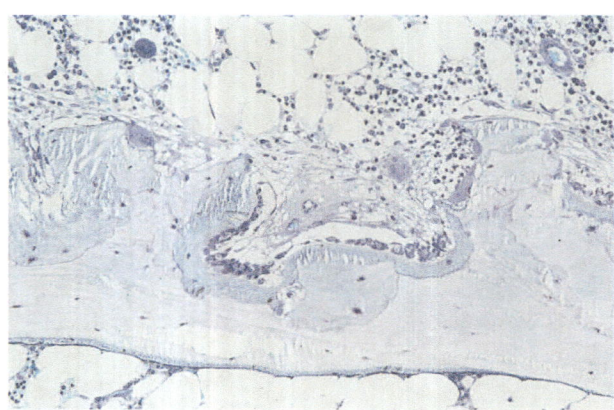

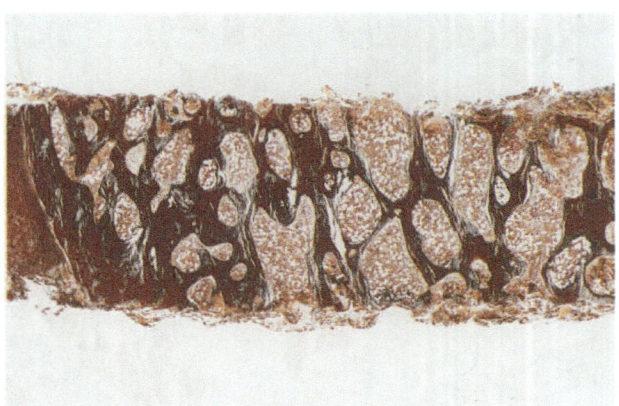

Figs. 14.7–14.12 Examples of progressive alterations of bone structure in Paget's disease

Fig. 14.7 Early case of Paget's disease of bone, with focal involvement of the upper side of an ossicle. Note unaffected lower side with smooth trabecular surface. Giemsa

Fig. 14.8 Overview of iliac crest biopsy with altered trabecular structure in the subcortical zone. Gomori

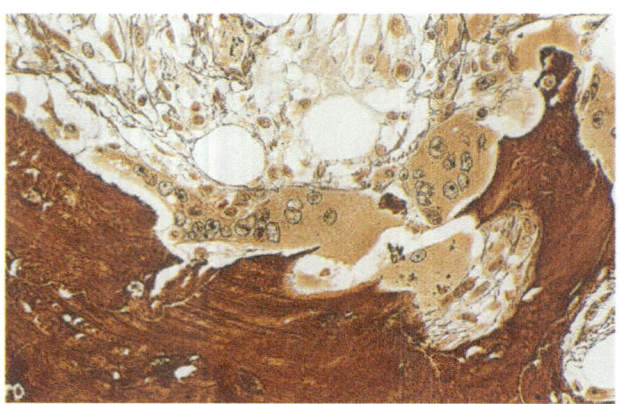

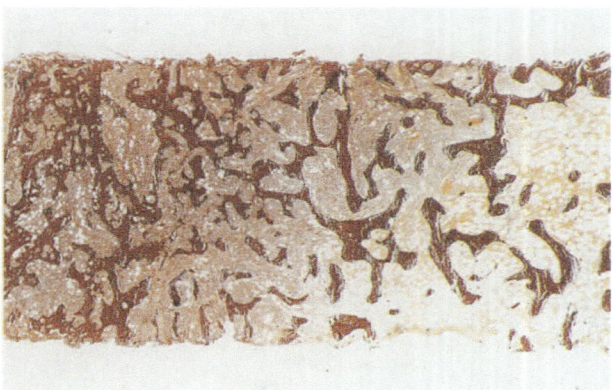

Fig. 14.9 Higher magnification of osteoclastic bone resorption from affected bone area in Fig. 14.8. Gomori

Fig. 14.10 Overview of iliac crest biopsy, two-thirds of which is clearly involved. Note porosity of the cortex and predominantly woven bone in the subcortical region. Gomori

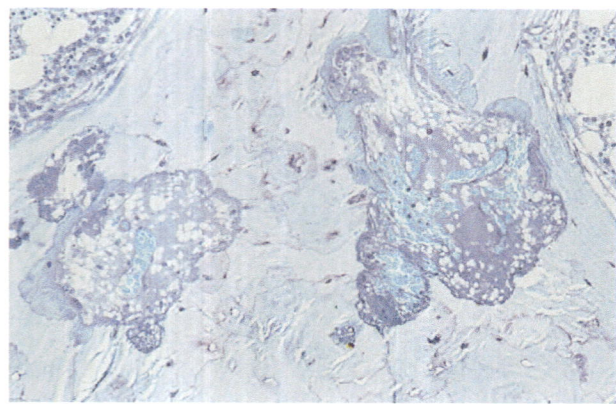

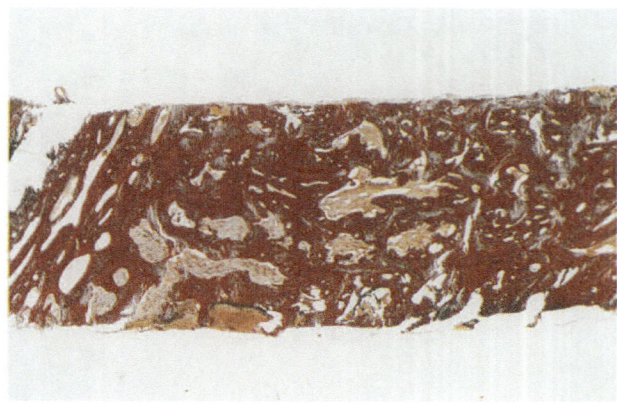

Fig. 14.11 Higher magnification to show dissecting osteoclasia and mosaic structure in cortex. Giemsa

Fig. 14.12 Overview of iliac crest biopsy taken from patient with advanced Paget's disease of the pelvis (see Figs 14.R2 and 14.R3, X-ray and bone scan, respectively). Gomori

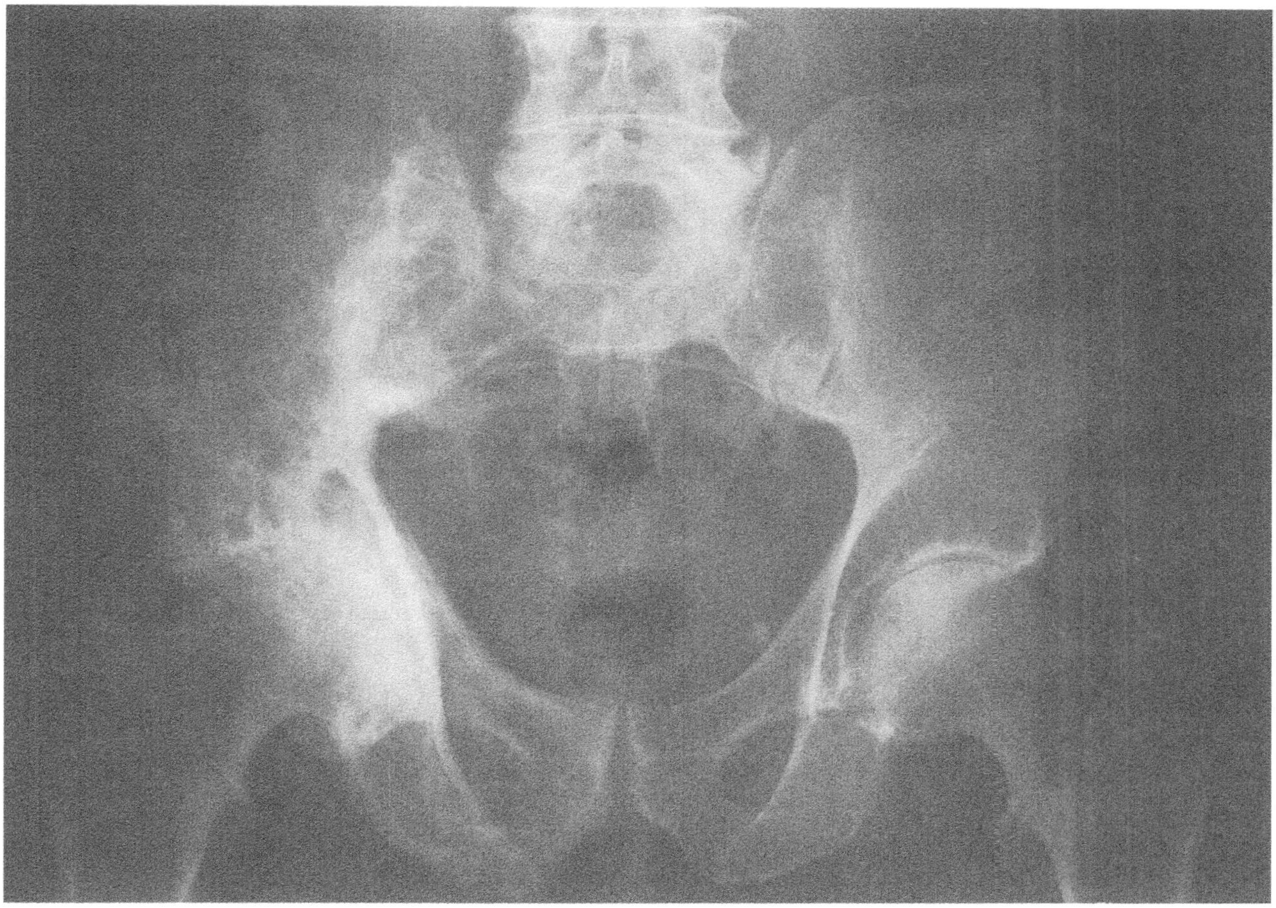

Fig. 14.R1 Active phase of Paget's disease, mixed type, of the right pelvis with coarsening of the trabecular pattern. (Kindly supplied by Prof. M. Kessler, Department of Radiology, Klinikum Großbadern, University of Munich)

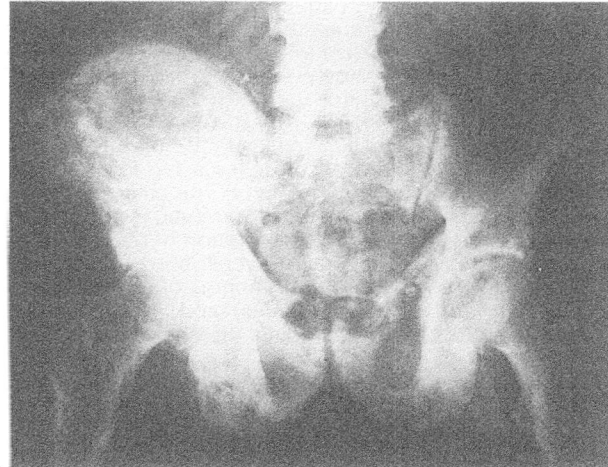

Fig. 14.R2 X-ray of patient with Paget's disease, advanced stage, showing large area of sclerotic bone in right ilium and lumbar vertebrae

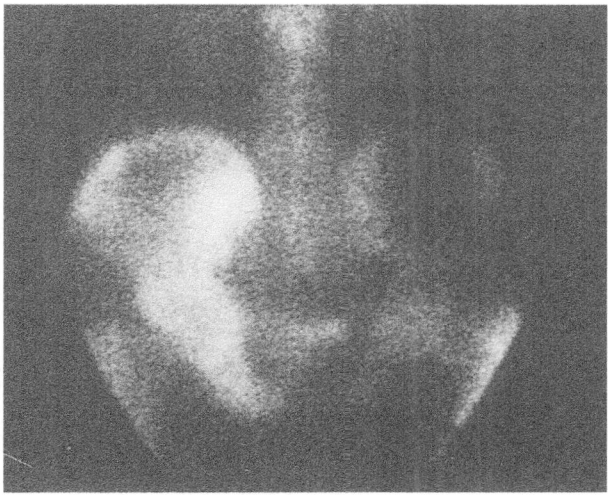

Fig. 14.R3 Bone scan of same patient as in Fig. 14.R2, illustrating increased uptake in the right ilium

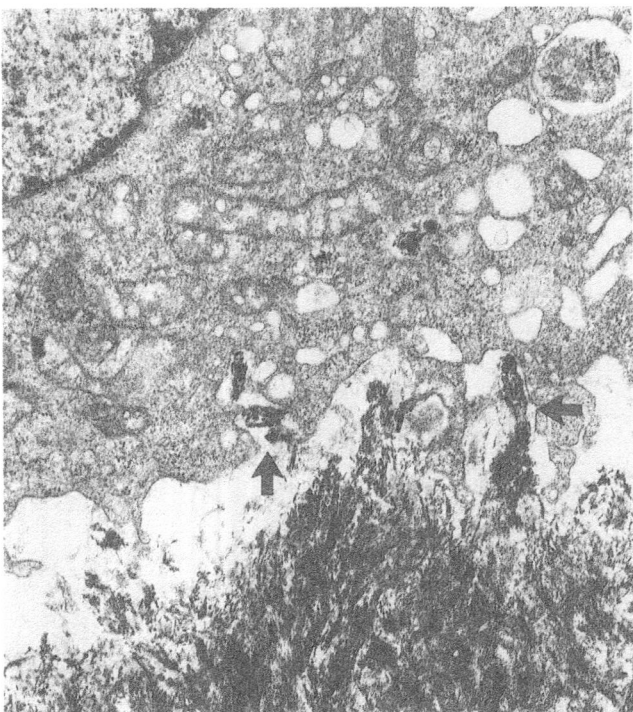

Fig. 14.EM1 Osteoclast on mineralized bone. Note fragments of electron-dense material (bone) within cytoplasmic vacuoles and in process of engulfment (arrows). EM × 32 000

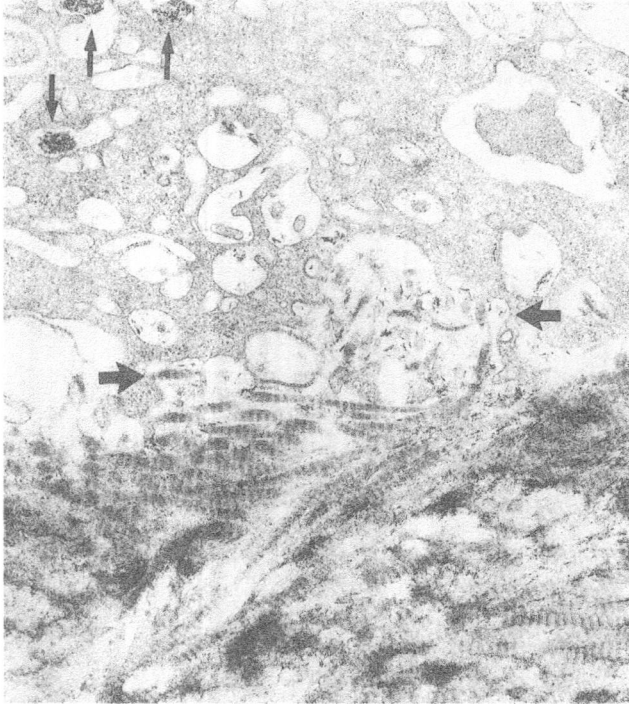

Fig. 14.EM2 Osteoclast on bone. Note both mineralized and unmineralized collagen fibres in process of phagocytosis (arrows) as well as electron-dense material (mineralized bone) within cytoplasmic vacuoles (small arrows). EM × 40 000

As in normal bone, new matrix is formed by *osteoblasts* during the formative or reparative phase: rows of osteoblasts fill the scalloped resorption cavities with osteoid[26]. It is the increased osteoblastic activity that accounts for the marked elevation of serum alkaline phosphatase and the increase in osteoid volume[22]. However, in Paget's disease some of this newly formed matrix is irregular, 'woven' rather than lamellar. This feature probably reflects the increased rate of production rather than a primary abnormality of osteoblast function. Subsequently, lamellar and woven bone mosaics are arranged in haphazard 'jigsaw' pattern, formed by the prominent cement lines. Repeated waves of resorption and formation produce this *'mosaic' pattern*, which characterizes bones involved in Paget's disease (Plate 14.C). In the chronic, or burnt-out stage, cellular activity subsides, leaving a sclerotic bone with few osteoclasts and osteoblasts, an abnormal irregular structure and high fragility. The previously prominent vasculature (Plate 14.D)[2,8] disappears, but marrow fibrosis may persist to some extent.

At a more macroscopic level the disorganized bone turnover results in effacement of the trabecular network with loss of definition between cortical and cancellous bone, leaving some areas of trabecular sclerosis and others of lysis. The rates of bone formation and resorption remain in equilibrium; however, at a particular time and site either formation or resorption may predominate, even at the microscopic level[23]. Generally an initial wave of osteoclastic activity producing rarefaction (*lytic phase*) is followed by both new bone formation and continued bone resorption, with resulting lytic and sclerotic areas (*mixed phase*) (Fig. 14.R1). Finally pagetic bone tends to become sclerotic with decrease of bone turnover (*sclerotic phase*) (Plate 14.B, Figs 14.R2 and 14.R3). The small marrow cavities are almost entirely filled with fibrous tissue, ectatic sinusoids and chronic inflammatory cells. However, this progression does not invariably occur, and the phases may differ between the various bone remodelling units involved, as demonstrable in large biopsies, and various bones may be in different phases at any one time.

The extent and activity of pagetic involvement vary considerably between individual patients, and may change either as a result of disease progression or in response to specific treatment. Changes in symptoms such as alleviation of bone pain are obviously of great clinical importance. However, radiological changes under *treatment* are not sufficiently pronounced to monitor changes in the degree of remodelling activity. The major role of bone biopsy in Paget's disease may be to monitor the effects of new therapeutic agents (such as bisphosphonates) on mineralization and turnover of the non-involved skeleton[20]. However, bone biopsy may not be the ideal way to monitor the anti-osteoclastic effects in the involved bone since site-to-site and course variations in the disease activity, rather than inhibitory effects on osteoclasts, could account for a reduction in bone resorption following treatment. Fortunately the indirect biochemical markers of bone turnover, serum alkaline phosphatase and the urinary excretion of hydroxyproline, provide reliable reflections of overall bone cell activity in Paget's disease of bone[27,39]. Inhibitors of osteoclasts (e.g. calcitonin and bisphosphonates) and, recently, gallium have been used to treat Paget's disease of bone[7,10,24].

References

1. Altman R. D. and Buschoff H. S. (1981). Correlation of pain, X-ray and bone scans in Paget's disease of the bone. *Calcif. Tissue Int.*, **33**, 327
2. Arlet J. and Mazieres B. (1975). La circulation dans l'os pagétique. Revue générale et données personelles. *Rev. Rheumatol.*, **42**, 643

Plate 14.C

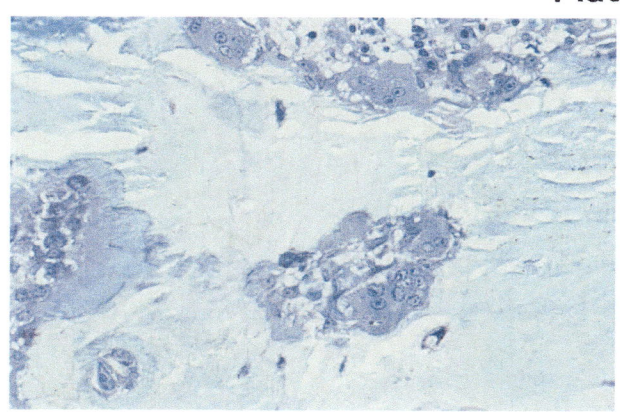

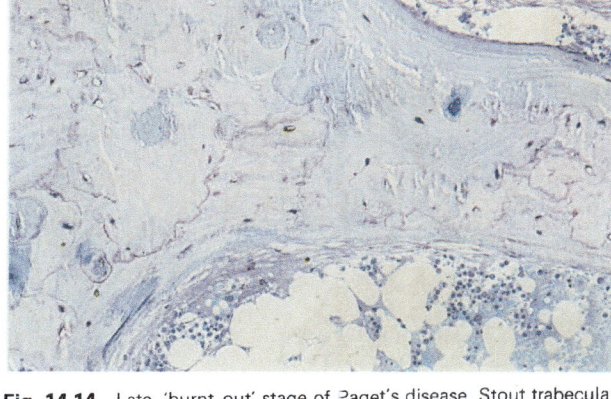

Figs. 14.13–14.18 Examples of mosaic structures of Paget's disease of bone

Fig. 14.13 Early, active stage of Paget's disease. Note superficial osteoclastic erosion, dissecting osteoclasia and reactive new bone formation with osteoid in cavity at left. Mosaic pattern has not yet been produced. Giemsa

Fig. 14.14 Late, 'burnt-out' stage of Paget's disease. Stout trabecula showing marked mosaic pattern of cement lines, absence of osteoclastic resorption but lamellar new bone formation by osteoblasts (upper right). Giemsa

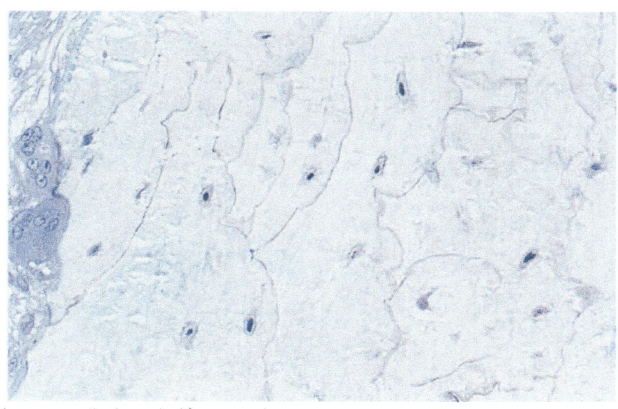

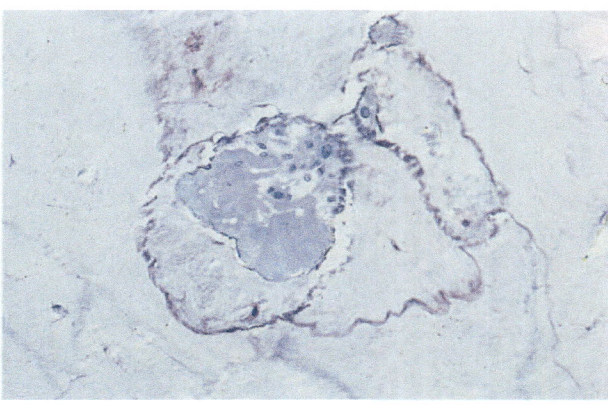

Fig. 14.15 Trabecula demonstrating numerous, closely spaced cement lines and many relatively large osteocytes. Note active osteoclastic resorption at left. Giemsa

Fig. 14.16 Dissecting osteoclasia in sclerotic bone indicating continued activity of disease. Note fairly broad cement lines (recent remodelling) as well as paler and thinner ones (earlier remodelling). Giemsa

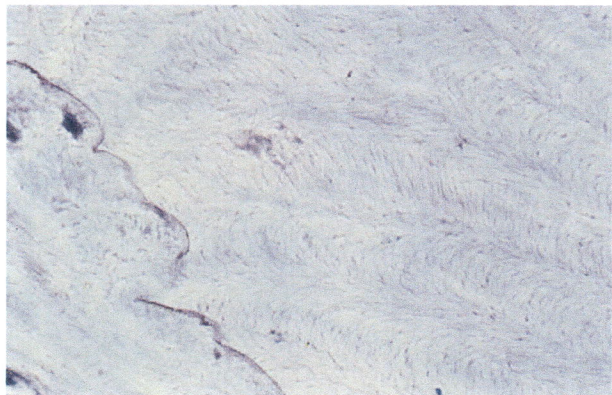

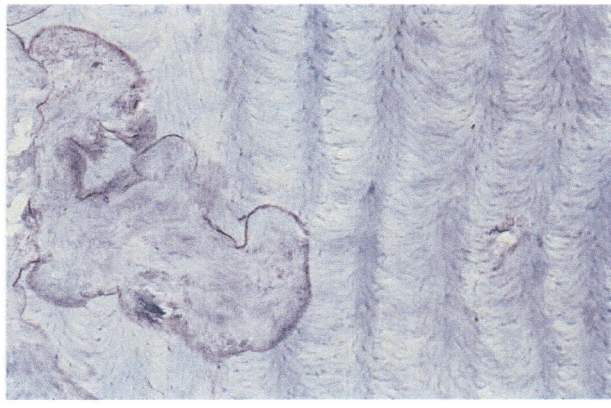

Fig. 14.17 Original lamellar structure interrupted by the disorganized remodelling (left) characteristic of Paget's disease. Giemsa

Fig. 14.18 Interruption of regular lamellar pattern by dissecting osteoclasia, now filled by woven bone. Note osteocytic canaliculi and collagen fibrils. Giemsa

Plate 14.D

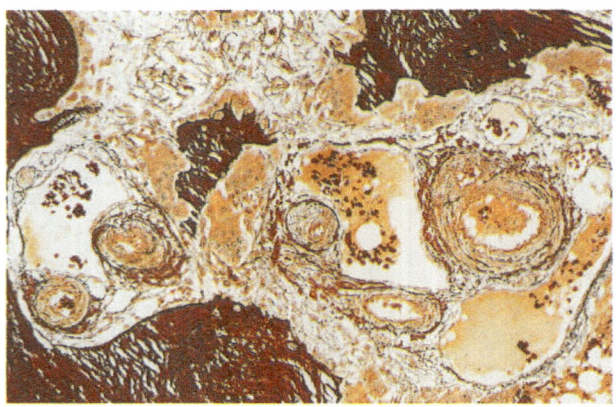

Figs. 14.19–14.23 Survey of blood vessels in iliac crest biopsy in Paget's disease of bone

Fig. 14.19 Biopsy section in which a large part of the marrow cavity is occupied by blood vessels of varying calibres. This biopsy was taken from an area of involved bone. Note active osteoclastic resorption and fibrosis. Gomori

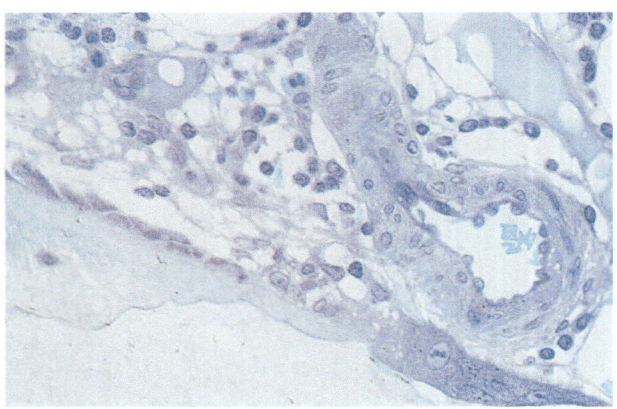

Fig. 14.20 Surface of trabecular bone with osteoblasts and osteoid at left; osteoclast (lower right) with adjacent small artery surrounded by loose connective tissue. Giemsa

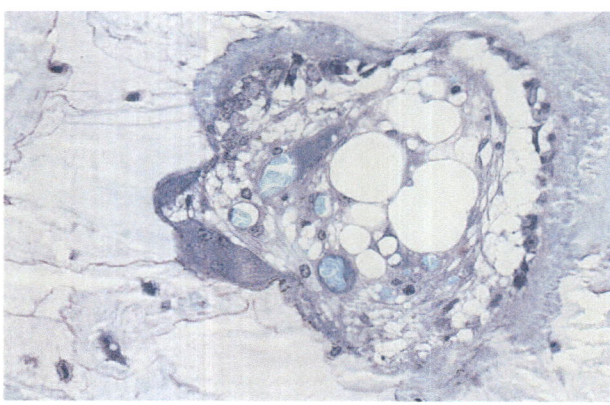

Fig. 14.21 Osteoclastic tunnel in trabecular bone. Note several small blood vessels with erythrocytes in their lumina in the loose connective tissue. Though many of the resorption lacunae are filled with osteoid and lined by osteoblasts, there is still active osteoclastosis (centre left). Giemsa

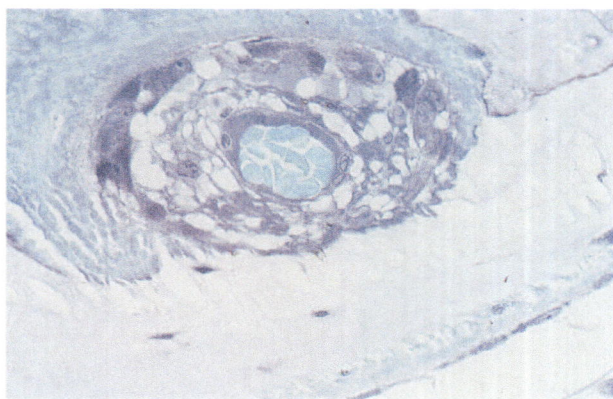

Fig. 14.22 Reparative phase as shown by broad osteoid seam (upper left) lined by osteoblasts, absence of osteoclasts and large central blood vessel. Giemsa

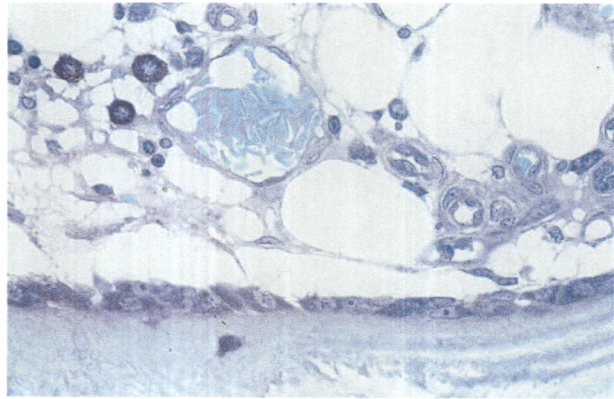

Fig. 14.23 Reparative phase with lamellar new bone formation and highly vascular loose connective tissue. Note mast cells in vicinity of capillaries and sinusoids. There is less fibrosis in the late and reparative phases of Paget's disease than in the florid, osteoclastic phase (compare Fig. 14.19 with Figs 14.20–14.23). Giemsa

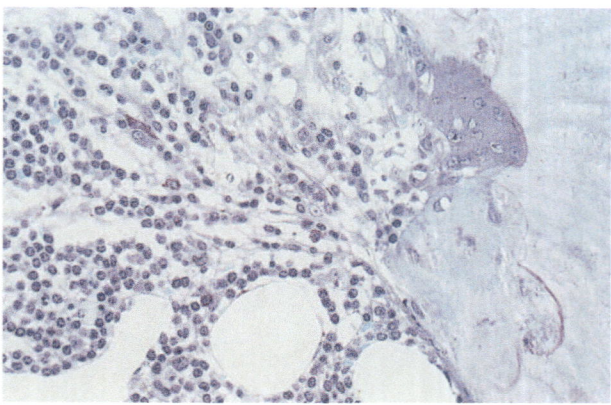

Fig. 14.24 Iliac crest biopsy of patient with Paget's disease and concomitant malignant lymphoma. Note multinucleated osteoclast and mosaic pattern at left, and lymphocytic infiltration occupying most of the intertrabecular space. Giemsa

3. Barry H. G. (1969). *Paget's Disease of Bone*. Edinburgh: Churchill Livingstone

4. Bordier P., Woodhouse N. J. Y., Joplin G. F. and TunChot S. (1972). Quantitative bone histology in Paget's disease. *J. Bone Jt Surg.*, **54B**, 553

5. Burgener F. A. and Perry P. E. (1978). Pitfalls in the radiographic diagnosis of Paget's disease of the pelvis. *Skelet. Radiol.*, **2**, 231

6. Burr D. B. and Martin R. B. (1989). Errors in bone remodeling: toward a unified theory of metabolic bone disease. *Amer. J. Anat.*, **186**, 186

7. Canfield R., Rosner W. and Skinner J. (1977). Diphosphonate therapy of Paget's disease of bone. *J. Clin. Endocrinol. Metab.*, **11**, 96

8. Demmler K. (1974). Die Vaskularisation des Pagetknochens. *Dtsch. Med. Wschr.*, **99**, 91

9. Dove J. (1980). Complete fractures of the femur in Paget's disease of bone. *J. Bone Jt Surg.*, **62B**, 12

10. Finerman G. A. M., Gonick H. C., Smith R. K. and Mayfield J. M. (1976). Diphosphonate therapy of Paget's disease. *Clin. Orthop.*, **120**, 115

11. Fogelman I. and Carr D. (1980). A comparison of scanning and radiology in the assessment of patients with symptomatic Paget's disease. *Europ. J. Nucl. Med.*, **5**, 417

12. Freydinger J., Duling J. and McDonald L. (1963). Sarcoma complicating Paget's disease of bone. *Arch. Pathol.*, **75**, 496

13. Frisch B., Lewis S. M., Burkhardt R. and Bartl R. (1985). *Biopsy Pathology of Bone and Bone Marrow*. London: Chapman & Hall

14. Grundy M. (1970). Fractures of the femur in Paget's disease of bone. *J. Bone Jt Surg.*, **52B**, 252

15. Guyer P. B. (1981). Paget's disease of bone: The anatomical distribution. *Metab. Bone Dis. Rel. Res.*, **4**, 239

16. Haibach H., Farrell C. and Dittrich F. J. (1985). Neoplasms arising in Paget's disease of bone: a study of 82 cases. *Amer. J. Clin Pathol.*, **83**, 594

17. Hamdy R. C. (1981). *Paget's Disease of Bone: Assessment and Management*. New York: Praeger

18. Howarth S. (1953). Cardiac output in osteitis deformans. *Clin. Sci.*, **12**, 271

19. Kanis J. A. (1991). *Pathophysiology and Treatment of Paget's Disease of Bone*. London: Martin Dunitz

20. Khairi M. R. A., Meunier P., Edouard C., Coupron P., Bernard J., Derosa G. P. and Johnston C. C. (1977). Quantitative bone histology in Paget's disease of bone: influence of sodium etidronate therapy. *Calc. Tissue Res.*, **22**, 355

21. Krane S. M. (1977). Paget's disease of bone. *Clin. Orthop.*, **127**, 24

22. Lee W. R. (1967). Bone formation in Paget's disease. A quantitative microscopic study using tetracycline marks. *J. Bone Jt Surg.*, **49B**, 146

23. Maldague B. and Malghem J. (1987). Dynamic radiologic patterns of Paget's disease of bone. *Clin. Orthop.*, **217**, 126

24. Matkovic V., Apseloff G., Shepard D. R. and Gerber N. (1990). Use of gallium to treat Paget's disease of bone: a pilot study. *Lancet*, **335**, 72

25. Merkow R. L. and Lane J. M. (1990). Paget's disease of bone. *Endocrinol. Metab. Clin. N. Amer.*, **19**(1), 177

26. Meunier P. J., Coindre J. M., Edouard C. M. and Arlot M. E. (1980). Bone histomorphometry in Paget's disease. Quantitative and dynamic analysis of pagetic and non pagetic bone tissue. *Arthritis Rheum.*, **23**, 1095

27. Meunier P. J., Dalson C., Mathieu L., Chapuy M. C., Delmas P., Alexandre C. and Charhon S. (1987). Skeletal distribution and biochemical parameters of Paget's disease. *Clin. Orthop. Rel. Res.*, **217**, 37

28. Mills B. G. and Singer F. R. (1976). Nuclear inclusions in Paget's disease of bone. *Science*, **194**, 201

29. Misra D. P. (1975). Crosslink in bone collagen in Paget's disease. *J. Clin. Pathol.*, **28**, 305

30. Rebel A., Malkani K., Basle M. and Bregeon C. (1987). The classic. osteoclast ultrastructure in Paget's disease. *Clin. Orthop.*, **217**, 4

31. Revell P. A. (1986). *Pathology of Bone*. Berlin: Springer

32. Riffat M. G. (1968). Myelome plasmocytaire et maladie osseuse de Paget. *Lyon Med.*, **219**, 1035

33. Russell R. G. G. (1984). Paget's disease. Nordin B. E. C., *Metabolic Bone and Stone Disease* (p. 190). Edinburgh: Churchill Livingstone

34. Schmorl G. (1932). Über Ostitis deformans Paget. *Virch. Arch. Pathol. Anat. Physiol.*, **283**, 694

35. Singer F. R. (1980). Paget's disease of bone: a slow virus infection? *Calcif. Tissue Int.*, **31**, 185

36. Singer F. R. and Krane S. M. (1990). Paget's disease of bone. Avioli L. V. and Krane S. M., *Metabolic Bone Disease* (p. 546). Philadelphia: Saunders

37. Singer F. R. and Mills B. G. (1989). Primary bone cell dysfunction I – Paget's disease of bone. Tam C. S., Heersche J. N. M. and Murray T. M., *Metabolic Bone Disease: Cellular and Tissue Mechanisms* (p. 33). Boca Raton: CRC Press

38. Wick M. R., Siegal G. P. and Urni G. P. (1981). Sarcomas of bone complicating osteitis deformans (Paget's disease): fifty years' experience. *Amer. J. Surg. Pathol.*, **5**, 47

39. Woodard H. Q. (1959). Long-term studies of the blood chemistry in Paget's disease of bone. *Cancer*, **12**, 1226

40. Yates A. J. P. (1988). Paget's disease of bone. *Clin. Endocrinol. Metab.*, **2**(1), 267

41. Ziegler R., Holz G., Rotzler B. and Minne H. (1985). Paget's disease of bone in West Germany. Prevalence and distribution. *Clin. Orthop. Rel. Res.*, **194**, 199

Miscellaneous bone diseases

15

The osseous disorders described in this chapter are relatively rare, but are included because of their pathophysiology and because they may affect the ilium and therefore may be encountered in a bone biopsy.

CONGENITAL HAEMOLYTIC ANAEMIAS

Chronic haemolysis by virtue of continuous excessive red cell production leads to extreme marrow hyperplasia. There is extension of haematopoietic marrow into the long bones, marrow fat cells are totally replaced and even skeletal changes are demonstrable. These disorders are mainly congenital, and extension of haematopoiesis into the shafts of the long bones may occur. Iron overload by frequent transfusions may further influence the activity and number of osteoblasts, and thus induce the development of osteopenia (see also Chapter 8). However, to what extent iron affects osteoblast function has not yet been conclusively determined[19]. Some studies have shown accelerated bone turnover associated with chronic erythroid hyperplasia[77].

In *β-thalassaemia* the bone marrow expansion may lead to deformities of the skull, giving rise to the classical mongoloid facies. The extreme augmentation of erythropoiesis is possible only at cost of the other cell lines and of the trabecular bone, reflected in striking radiological changes which include a typical 'hair on end' appearance of the skull (Fig. 15.R1). The main skeletal changes in β-thalassaemia are

1. disproportionate widening of the marrow cavities in the diaphysis, giving long bones a characteristic 'squared' appearance,
2. cortical thinning caused by an unbalanced endosteal resorption and periostal bone formation,
3. coarsening of the trabecular architecture with loss of the less weight-bearing trabeculae, and
4. retarded skeletal maturation[42,57].

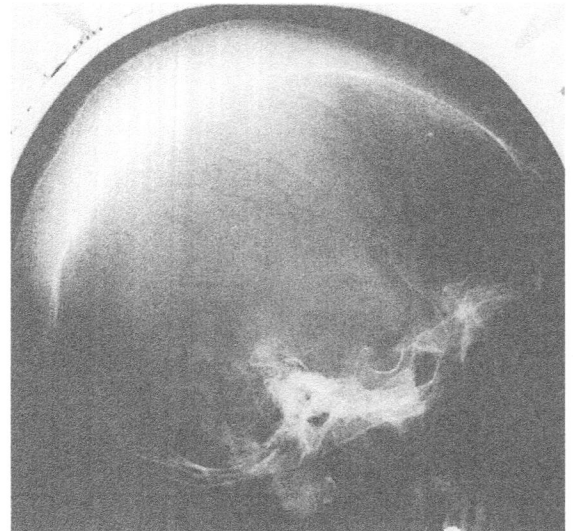

Fig. 15.R1 X-ray of skull of child with thalassaemia major illustrating 'hair on end' appearance of the skull

Sickle cell disease, a congenital disorder of haemoglobin synthesis, affects the musculoskeletal system in a similar way, and in combination with vaso-occlusive crises, a variety of skeletal lesions have been described: localized osteolyses with or without marginal sclerosis, bone necrosis, osteoporosis, osteomyelitis and widening of the shafts of long bones, even 'vanishing' of vertebrae (see also Chapters 6 and 7)[9,12,30,59,64].

A bone biopsy reveals wide bone marrow cavities filled with erythropoietic precursors and the trabeculae are thin and far apart. Similar osteopenic lesions occur with hyperplasia of haematopoiesis due to other causes, reactive as well as neoplastic.

STORAGE DISEASES

Storage diseases are due to inborn errors of metabolism in the form of enzyme deficiencies. Some of these disorders are classified together as the lysosomal storage diseases, comprising Gaucher's disease, Fabry's disease, the mucopolysaccharidoses and others[58]. Because of the defective enzymes, lysosomes become engorged, thereby inhibiting the activities of other enzymes, so that a variety of macromolecules are 'stored'. The skeletal manifestations are secondary to the expansion of the marrow cavities by ever greater numbers of storage cells, causing osteopenia, osteolytic lesions and even bone infarcts, due to interference with the blood supply.

GAUCHER'S DISEASE

Gaucher's disease is characterized by the presence of glucocerebroside-containing cells ('Gaucher cells') in the bone marrow, spleen and liver, due to a deficiency of glucocerebrosidase[11]. Three clinical types are now recognized[55]:

Type 1 (chronic, *adult*), by far the most common (more than 99% of cases) and defined by the absence of neurological involvement.
Type 2 (acute, *infantile*), a fulminant disorder with severe neurological manifestations and causing death usually within the first 18 months of life.
Type 3 (subchronic, *juvenile*), characterized by a later onset of neurological symptoms.

All patients may have hepatosplenomegaly, myelophthisic bone marrow involvement and severe and extensive bone complications[55,72]. Episodes of 'bone crisis', also called 'pseudo-osteomyelitis' or 'aseptic osteomyelitis'[80], are one of the most painful manifestations of Gaucher's disease. The crisis may occur in all long bones, but the ilium and spine are also affected. Bone marrow transplantation has been tried in patients with bone marrow failure due to replacement. Enzyme replacement is now available[7].

Skeletal X-ray shows two different types of abnormalities[4,8,34,66,73]:

1. *generalized osteopenia* and cortical thinning due to expansion of the infiltrated marrow spaces, and
2. *focal osteonecrosis* due to loss of local blood supply[5]. Infarcts can be massive in size and multiple, or they may be subtle with patchy osteosclerosis[79]. Flaring of the distal femur (Erlenmeyer-flask deformity) is the most typical finding, together with marrow infarctions

and subchrondral bony collapse resulting from osteonecrosis.

The *Gaucher cell* is large and has the appearance of crumpled silk or tissue paper (Plate 15.A)[51,55,63]. Histochemical and immunohistological studies have demonstrated its monocytic–macrophage origin. Paratrabecular aggregates of Gaucher cells cause rarefaction of the trabecular bone, though direct bone destruction by Gaucher cells has not been documented. Gaucher bone biopsies, analysed by Stowens and co-workers had evidence of accelerated bone remodelling, with a relative increase of resorption as compared to formation, leading to osteopenia[72]. Bilateral and multifocal corticomedullary osteonecrotic lesions resulting from 'Gaucher's crisis' have been reported, and osteosclerotic areas may present the reparative end-stage of medullary infarction[34,72]. Histopathology of necrotic bone may be complex due to the cycles of bone necrosis, revascularization and repair, and recurrent necrosis which can affect the bone in this disease. A detailed review of Gaucher's disease has recently been published[10].

Cells similar in appearance to Gaucher cells have been observed in the bone marrow in CML, after intensive therapy of haematological malignancies and in other bone marrow disorders with a high cellular turnover rate. They are called *'pseudo-Gaucher cells'* and they may be indistinguishable from those in Gaucher's disease (Figs 15.7 and 15.8).

NIEMANN-PICK DISEASE

This lipid storage disease is due to sphingomyelinase deficiency, with accumulation of abnormal amounts of lipids in the spleen, liver, lymph nodes and bone marrow[63]. The 'Niemann-Pick cell' is large with a clear cytoplasm in histological section. Most cases run a rapidly fatal course, and only rare patients survive as long as a year after diagnosis has been made. Because of the rapid course few osseous abnormalities such as cortical expansion of long bones have been reported.

FABRY'S DISEASE

This is also called *angiokeratoma corporis diffusum* and is inherited in an X-linked recessive manner. The clinical manifestations are mainly due to intralysosomal deposits of trihexoside in cells of the RES, in endothelial cells of vessels, and in the glomeruli. Recent reports that a grafted kidney supplied a therapeutically useful amount of the missing enzyme as well as relieving uraemia have not been confirmed.

The storage cells have a foamy appearance, and in the bone marrow they may induce a marked perivascular and paratrabecular fibrosis with osteoclastic bone resorption (Figs. 15.13 and 15.14).

MUCOPOLYSACCHARIDOSES AND MUCOLIPIDOSES

These are a group of seven inborn errors of metabolism in which the activity of one of the exoglycosidases is deficient[63]. The primary storage products are carbohydrate polymers, producing secondary changes in lysosomal function..The clinical entities are characterized by variable degrees of skeletal dysplasia, and the most common variants are *Hurler's syndrome, Hunter's syndrome, Morquio disease* and *Scheie disease.*

The term *mucolipidoses* was introduced to encompass a group of patients with clinical features which were a mixture of those encountered in the sphingolipidoses and the mucopolysaccharidoses, but did not have abnormal mucopolysacchariduria. All six conditions of the mucolipidoses (variants I–IV) are inherited in an autosomal recessive manner and usually develop severe dysostosis multiplex.

LANGERHANS CELL HISTIOCYTOSIS

Synonyms: histiocytosis X, Langerhans cell (eosinophilic) granulomatosis.

This term describes a pathological process with numerous clinical manifestations but a fairly uniform histopathological picture: proliferation and infiltration of tissue by histiocytes and secondarily by eosinophils[18,25,65]. The syndrome runs a gamut from the most benign form called eosinophilic granuloma to the more chronic variant of Hand–Schüller–Christian disease on to the most malignant type known as Letterer–Siwe disease[52]. The aetiology is unknown, but clinical course and histological features virtually rule out a neoplastic process[35]. It seems likely that the underlying abnormality is one of faulty intercellular communication (abnormalities in suppressor T lymphocytes or their lymphokines)[24]. Other features suggest an inflammatory cause, possibly due to a virus[24].

The degree of bone marrow infiltration varies from small eosinophilic granulomas to total replacement by 'histiocytosis X' cells[50]. The common sites of skeletal involvement are the pelvic bones, skull, thorax, spine and major long bones. The usual solitary lesion of eosinophilic granuloma is a relatively small, well-circumscribed lytic area, while the skeletal lesions in Hand–Schüller–Christian disease are multiple, usually lytic and widely disseminated. Transformations between these variants have been described. The occurrence of Langerhans cell histiocytosis has also been described in association with Hodgkin's disease[46].

Solitary eosinophilic granulomas in the skeleton occur as circumscribed lytic lesions varying in size from 1 to 5 mm^2 (Fig. 15.R2)[54,67]. The inner and outer tables of flat bones are eroded, often with a central sequestra thus simulating pyogenic osteomyelitis. Reactive marginal sclerosis is uncommon. A bone biopsy from an involved site shows eosinophils, plasma cells, lymphocytes, fibroblasts and storage cells[22]. Marked osteoclastic resorption occurs within areas with dense infiltration, possibly due to osteoclast-activating factors released by 'histiocytosis X' cells. The foci may heal with a margin of sclerosis[62].

Hand–Schüller–Christian disease (Figs 15.9–15.12), a more extensive and more serious variant, comprises about

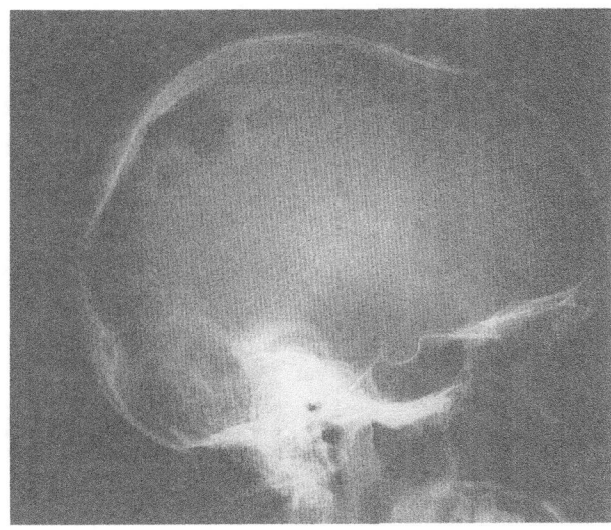

Fig. 15.R2 Multiple eosinophilic granulomas in the skull

[continued on p. 168]

Plate 15.A

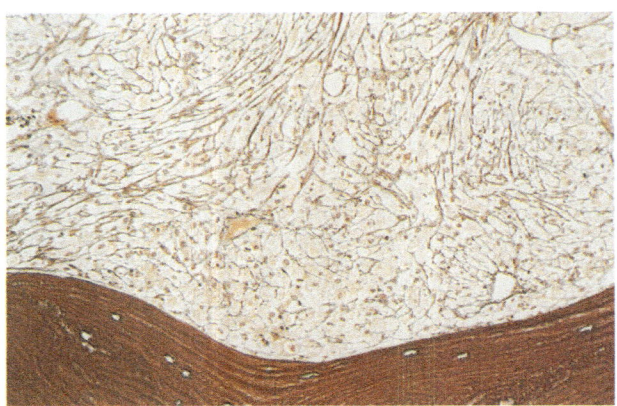

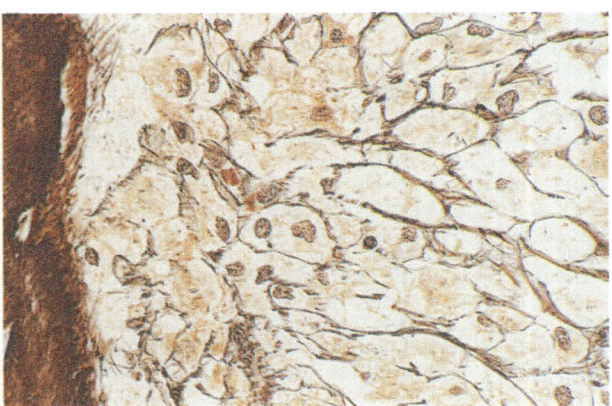

Figs. 15.1–15.4 Iliac crest biopsy of patient with Gaucher's disease, acute type

Fig. 15.1 The normal marrow has been completely replaced by the typical storage cells. Gomori

Fig. 15.2 Higher magnification from section of Fig. 15.1 demonstrating 'Gaucher cells' adjacent to the trabecular surface, with marked reactive fibrosis. Gomori

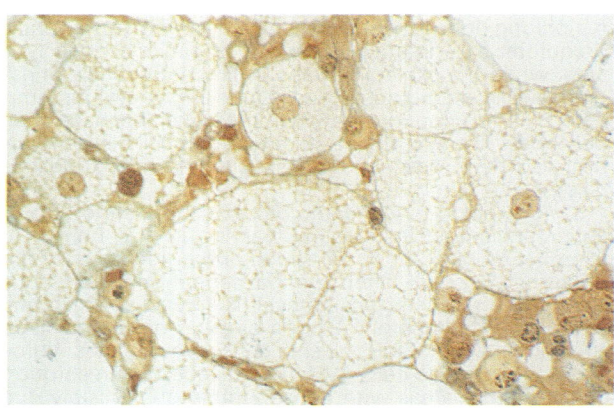

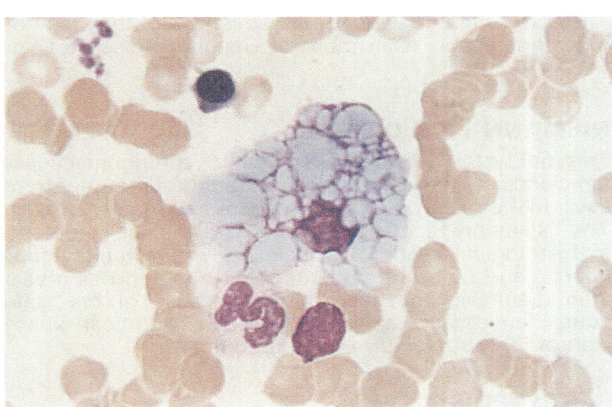

Fig. 15.3 Higher magnification showing typical 'Gaucher cells' of variable size, with characteristic 'wrinkled tissue-paper' appearance of cytoplasm. Gomori

Fig. 15.4 'Gaucher cell' in smear of bone marrow aspirate. Pappenheim

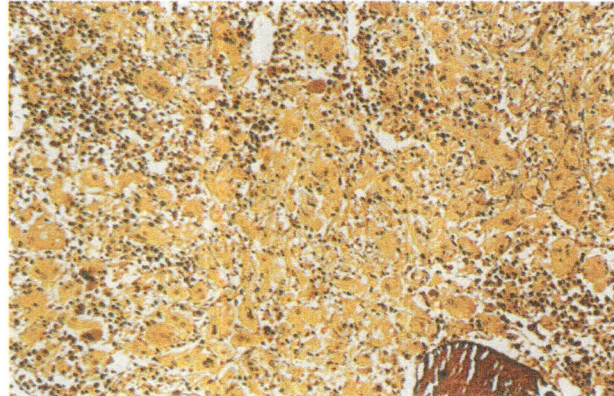

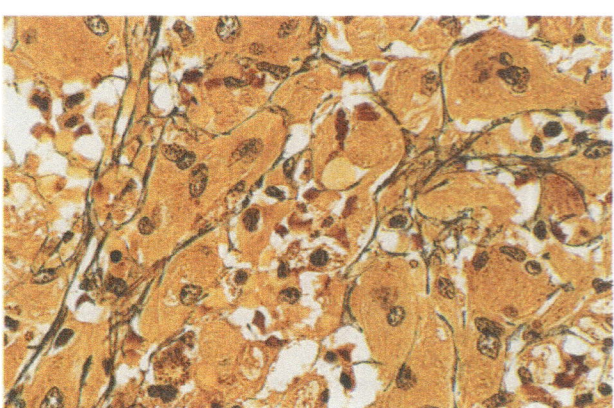

Figs. 15.5 and **15.6** Iliac crest biopsy of patient with storage disease. In spite of intensive investigation, a definite diagnosis was not made in this case

Fig. 15.5 Patchy infiltration of the marrow spaces by storage cells, with residual haematopoiesis between (upper left and lower right). Gomori

Fig. 15.6 Higher magnification of Fig. 15.5 showing macrophages of variable size and with one or several nuclei, and reactive fibrosis. Gomori

Plate 15.B

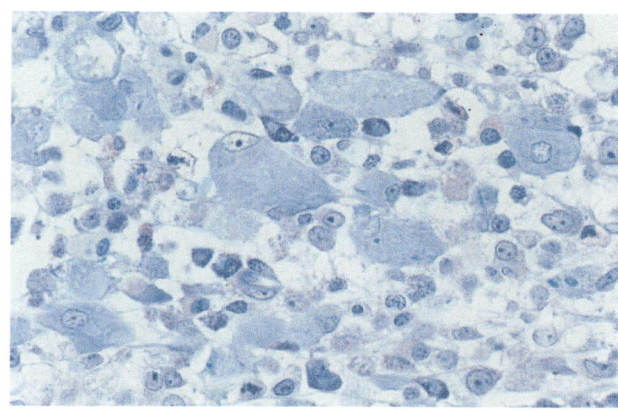

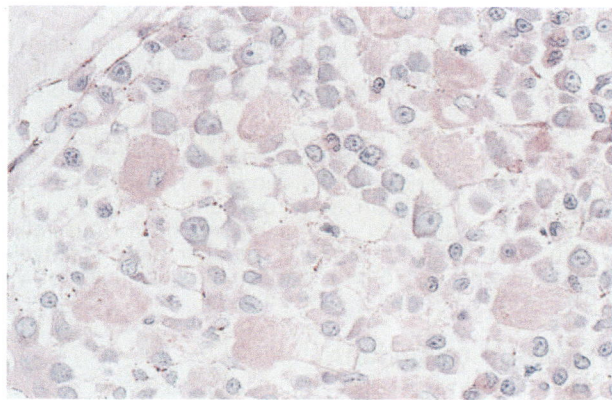

Figs. 15.7 and **15.8** 'Pseudo-Gaucher cells' in chronic myeloid leukaemia

Fig. 15.7 Multiple large macrophages between neutro- and eosinophilic granulocytes. Giemsa

Fig. 15.8 Macrophages with PAS-positive cytoplasm. PAS

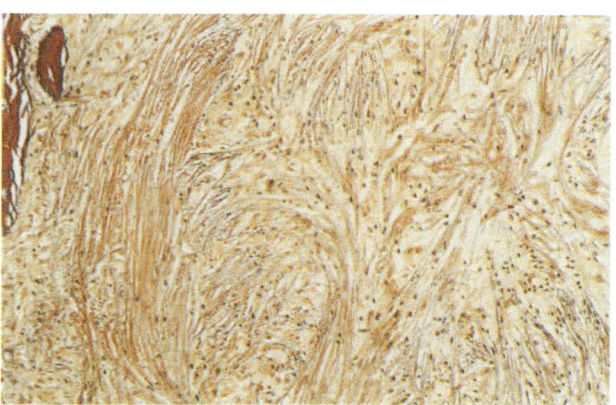

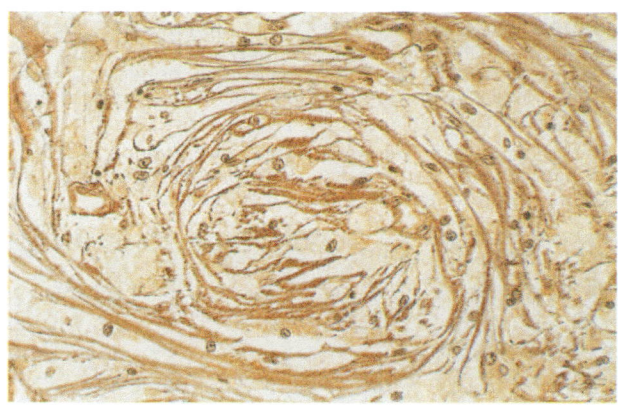

Figs. 15.9–15.12 Iliac crest biopsy of 10-year-old patient with Hand–Schüller–Christian disease

Fig. 15.9 Complete replacement of the bone marrow by storage cells and coarse reactive fibrosis. Gomori

Fig. 15.10 Higher magnification of section from Fig. 15.9 showing a whorl-like arrangement of storage cells and fibres. Gomori

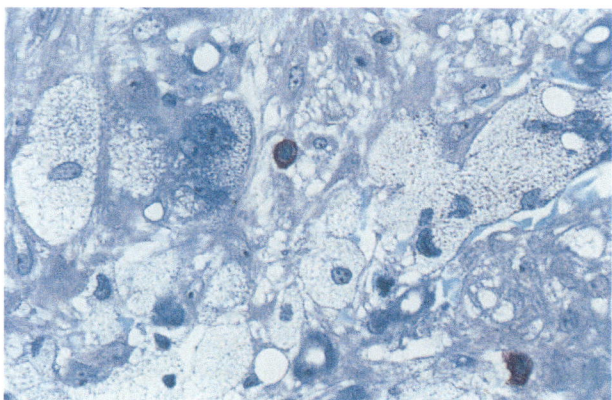

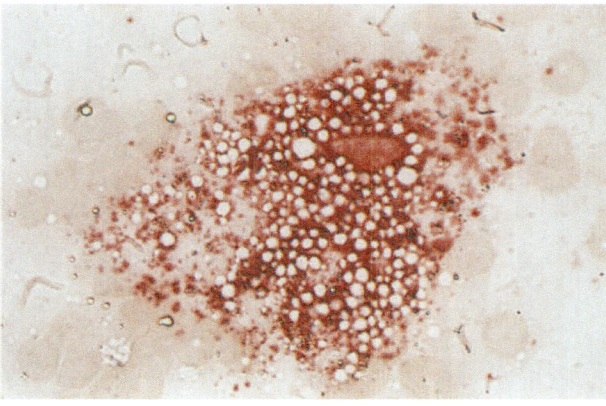

Fig. 15.11 Higher magnification of the storage cells revealing abundant cytoplasm and fine vacuolization; presence of mast cells and connective tissue. Giemsa

Fig. 15.12 Large, vacuolated storage cell in imprint of the bone marrow biopsy. Acid phosphatase

10% of all cases of histiocytosis X. It is classically known as a syndrome consisting of osteolytic lesions in the skull, exophthalmus and diabetes insipidus. The osteolytic lesions are scattered throughout the skeleton with an affinity to the skull ('the geographical skull') and to other flat bones.

Letterer–Siwe disease is a disseminated variant with a very poor prognosis, occurring in less than 2% of the entire group. Multiple destructive lesions in the haematopoietic areas of the skeleton are prominent. In bone biopsy, extensive aggregates of proliferating histiocytes mixed with eosinophils and fibrosis are characteristic. Myelosclerosis and myelofibrosis may occur in children with histiocytosis X.

FIBROUS DYSPLASIA

This is a fibro-osseous aberration of the skeleton, probably a developmental disorder of the mesenchyme of bone tissue[21,33]. The aetiology remains unclear, but the disease does not appear to be heritable. The common period of clinical presentation is in the first two decades of life, and both sexes are affected[17]. The fundamental abnormality is replacement of bone and marrow by masses of fibrous tissue, within which bone may develop later. Clinically the main features of fibrous dysplasia are bone pain, deformities, and fractures[39]. The commonest sites of skeletal involvement are the pelvis (Figs 15.R3 and 15.R4), the major long bones, the facial bones and ribs[29].

The disease may be divided into three main clinical categories[70]:

1. the *monostotic* variant is relatively common in orthopaedic practice, and the diagnosis is made from the radiographic and histological findings;

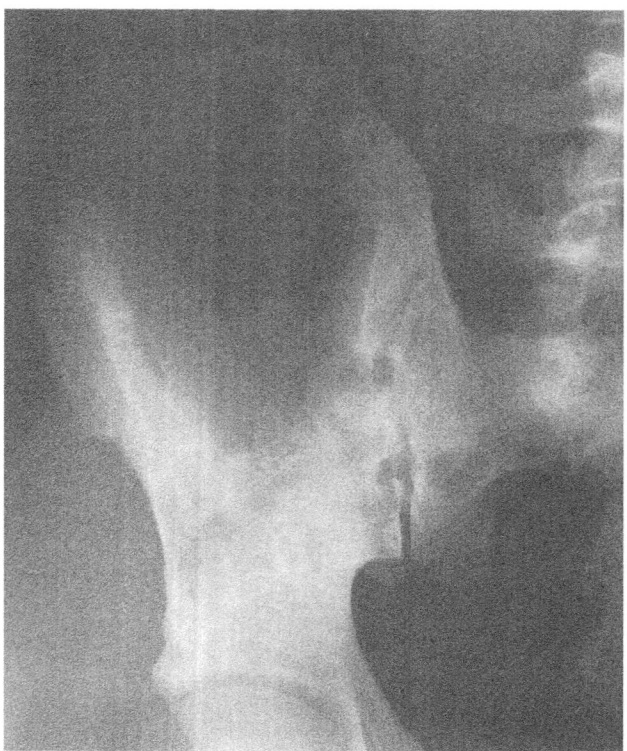

Figs. 15.R3 and **15.R4** Monostotic fibrous dysplasia of the pelvis

Fig. 15.R3 This localized focus in the right os ilium was discovered accidentally on X-ray. The translucent zone is surrounded by dense reactive sclerosis ('rind' sign)

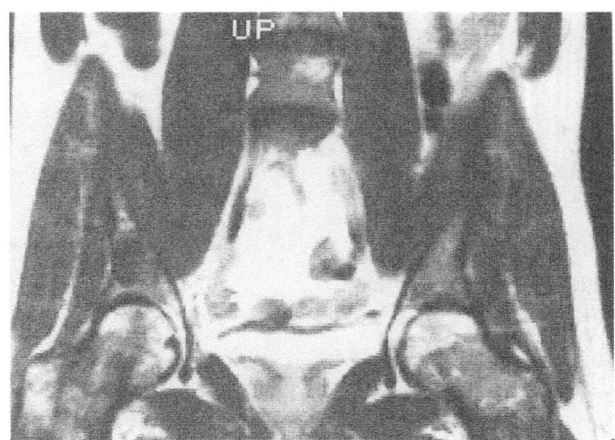

Fig. 15.R4 The lesion in the ilium is also shown in MNR

2. the *polyostotic* type tended to be unilateral, and the lesions may be distributed segmentally[53], and
3. the '*McCune–Albright syndrome*', in which multiple bone lesions occur with skin pigmentations and endocrine abnormalities[23].

The differential diagnosis includes bone cysts, Paget's disease and pHPT[37,56].

Microscopically, varying mixtures of fibrous connective tissue and new bone are seen[63]. Fibrous dysplasia appears to commence in the marrow space, the defects then encroaching on both cortical and trabecular bone, causing fragility and distortion of the normal bone contours (Figs 15.15–15.18). The fibrous tissue is composed of spindle cells arranged in whorls interspersed with islands of woven bone, osteoblasts and some osteoclasts. Cysts, if present, vary in size and are often accompanied by multinuclear osteoclast-type giant cells and foam cells[70]. Rapid progression of bone lesions during pregnancy has been described and related to the presence of both oestrogen and progesterone receptors in osteogenic cells – a finding relevant to a possible direct action of oestrogen on human bone cells[45]. In approximately 10% of cases, islands of hyaline cartilage are present. Malignant transformation has been observed in less than 1% both of the monostotic and polyostotic forms[70].

AMYLOIDOSIS

Amyloidosis is characterized by an accumulation of a protein–polysaccharide complex in various tissues[16,49]. The primary type is distinguished from the secondary by immunohistological stainings, absence of chronic disease and a predilection for specific sites. Amyloid represents linear fibrils composed of polypeptide chains, and *four main amyloid fibril proteins* have been recognized[61,69]:

1. AL, immunoglobulin light chains (myeloma-associated amyloidosis);
2. AA, acute phase reactant serum amyloid A (secondary amyloidosis);
3. AF, prealbumin (heredofamilial amyloidosis), and
4. β_2-M, β_2-microglobulin (haemodialysis-associated amyloidosis).

Amyloid is readily recognized in Giemsa-stained sections of bone biopsies (Plates 15.D and 15.E). It appears as homogeneous dark blue deposits usually located within the vessel walls or, more diffusely distributed, in the interstitium. Congo red and immunohistological stainings are applied for further confirmation and classification

[continued on p. 172]

Plate 15.C

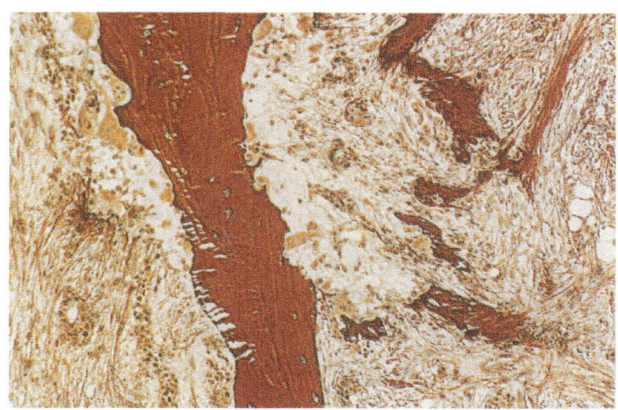

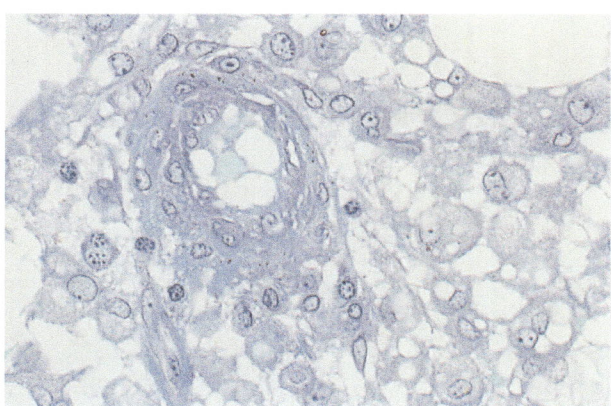

Figs. 15.13 and **15.14**   Iliac crest biopsy of patient with Morbus Fabry

Fig. 15.13   Complete replacement of the bone marrow by storage cells and fibrosis. Note marked osseous remodelling: osteoclastic bone resorption with Howship lacunae (centre) and multiple foci of newly formed woven bone (right). Gomori

Fig. 15.14   Higher magnification showing perivascular infiltration by relatively small storage cells. Homogeneous dark-blue deposits in the adventitia of the small artery. Giemsa

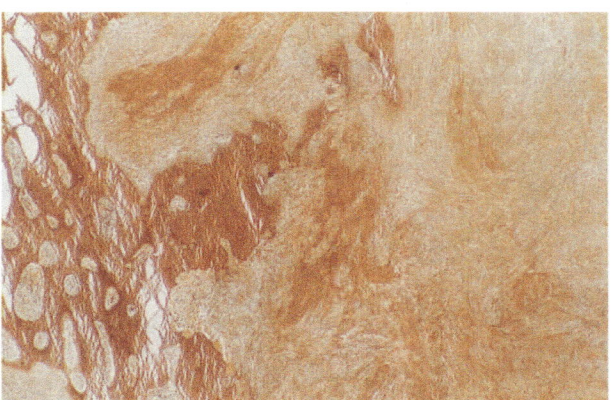

Figs. 15.15–15.18   Fibrous dysplasia in iliac crest biopsy

Fig. 15.15   Overview of biopsy section demonstrating complete transformation of trabecular bone and bone marrow into a mass of fibrous tissue. Note cortical bone at left. Giemsa

Fig. 15.16   Higher magnification of cortical and subcortical area illustrating marked porosity of cortex and subcortical residue of trabecular bone. Note substitution of ossicles by primitive, poorly mineralized woven bone. Gomori

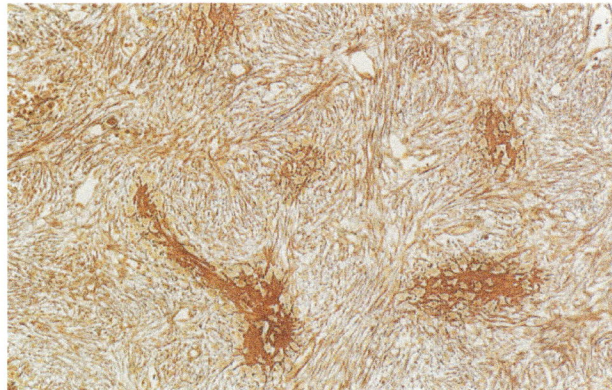

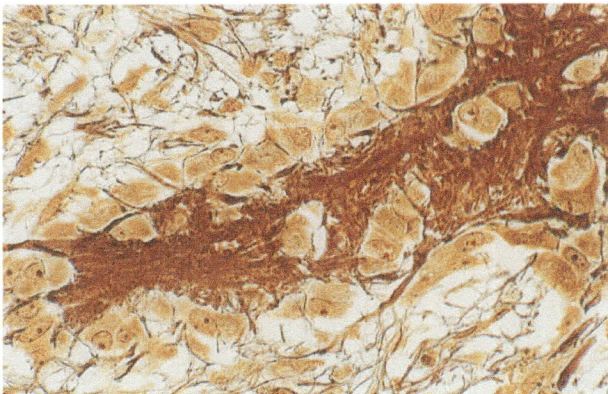

Fig. 15.17   Area from deeper part of biopsy shown in Fig. 15.15 illustrating the dense fibrosis and several foci of osteoblastic new bone formation. Gomori

Fig. 15.18   Higher magnification of focus of osteoblastic bone formation. Note entrapment of large osteoblasts within the woven bone. Gomori

Plate 15.D

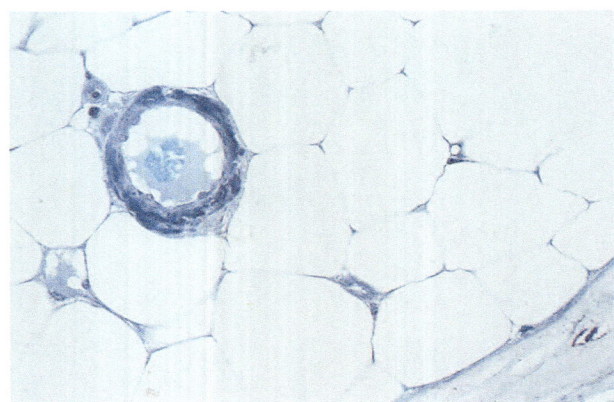

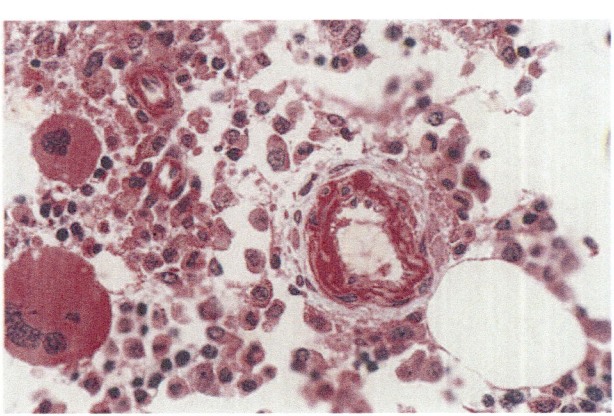

Figs. 15.19–15.21 Iliac crest biopsies in haemodialysis-associated amyloidosis

Fig. 15.19 Deposits of amyloid (dark blue) in small artery; aplastic marrow. Giemsa

Fig. 15.20 Patchy deposits of amyloid (dark red) in small artery and perivascular inflammatory reaction; normocellular marrow. Ladewig

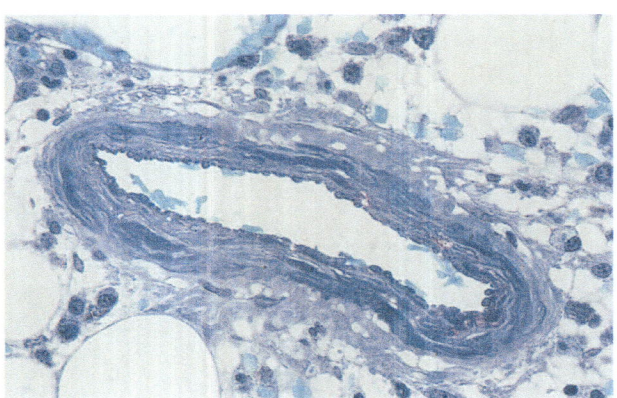

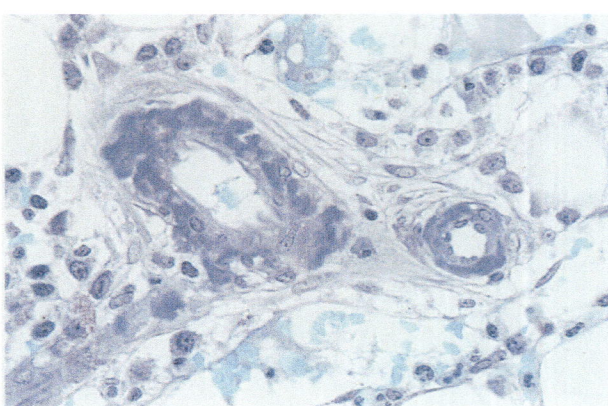

Fig. 15.21 Layers of amyloid in the media of an artery, with perivascular plasmacytosis. Giemsa. Evidence of AB amyloidosis (β_2-microglobulin) by immunohistology performed on sections of the same biopsy

Figs. 15.22–15.24 Iliac crest biopsy in primary amyloidosis

Fig. 15.22 Small artery (left) and arteriole (right) showing amyloid deposition in their walls. Giemsa

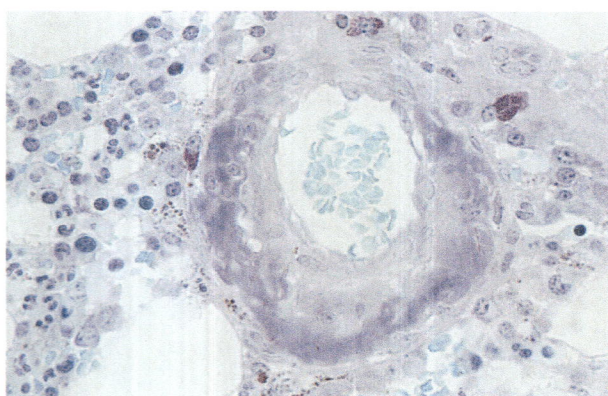

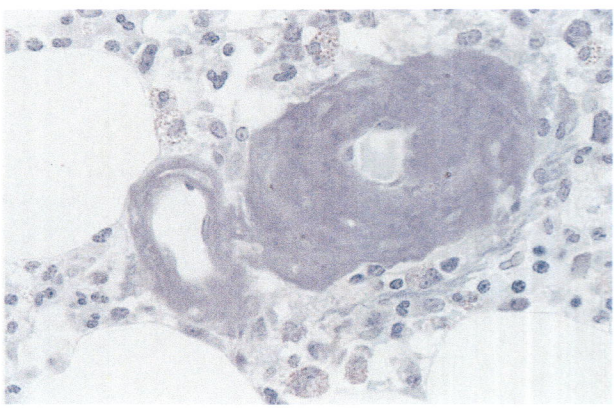

Fig. 15.23 Thickened wall of an artery with patchy deposits of amyloid, surrounded by mast cells, plasma cells and macrophages with haemosiderin (dark brown). Giemsa

Fig. 15.24 Thick homogeneous deposits of amyloid in the vessel wall with consequent narrow lumen. Giemsa

Plate 15.E

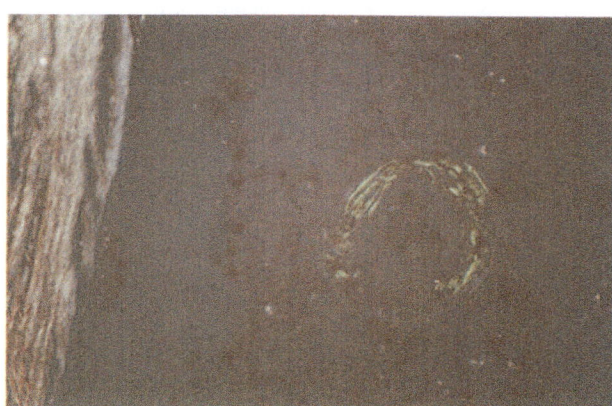

Figs. 15.25–15.30 Aspects of amyloidosis in iliac crest biopsies

Fig. 15.25 Biopsy section stained with Congo red and viewed in polarized light: amyloid in arterial wall shows characteristic green fluorescence

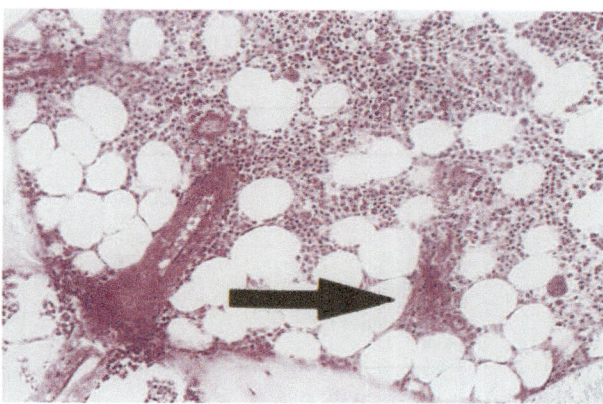

Fig. 15.26 Low-power view of iliac crest biopsy section illustrating both vascular and interstitial amyloidosis. Note amorphous interstitial deposits (arrow) and intramural deposits in artery, capillary and sinusoid. Methyl violet

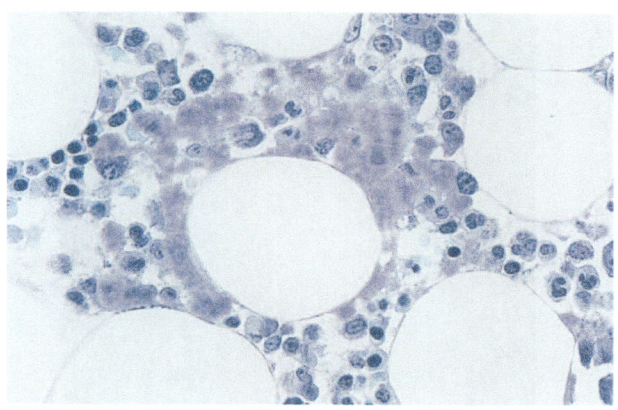

Fig. 15.27 Interstitial deposits of amyloid around a fat cell (centre). Giemsa

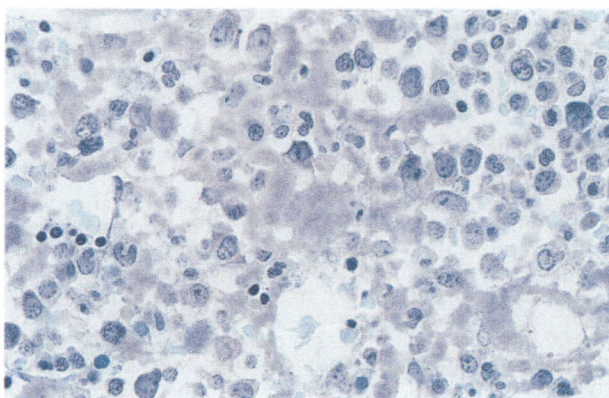

Fig. 15.28 Interstitial deposits of amyloid between haematopoietic cells. Giemsa

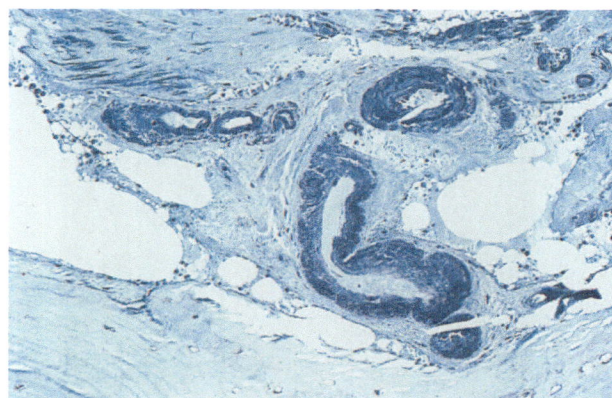

Fig. 15.29 Vascular amyloidosis in the periosteum of the iliac crest biopsy. Giemsa

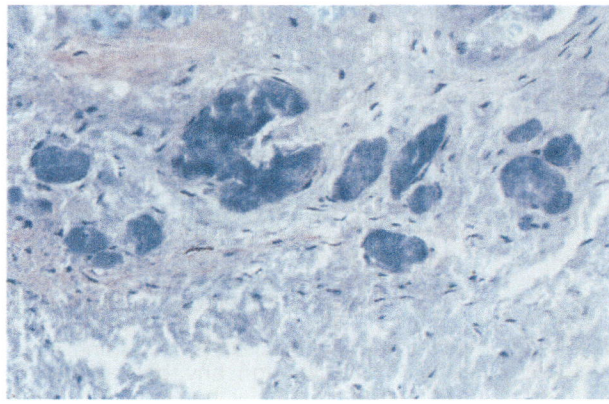

Fig. 15.30 Multiple periosteal deposits of AB amyloid (β_2-microglobulin) in a patient with haemodialysis-associated amyloidosis (as shown by immunohistology). Giemsa

Table 15.1 Frequency of organ involvement by amyloidosis according to results of biopsies. Note high rate of involvement in iliac crest biopsies (85 patients investigated in our series)

Biopsy	Frequency (%)
Kidney	87–100
Liver	50–96
Spleen	100
Rectum	64–96
Bone	**78**
Muscle	75–80
Gingiva	27–100
Subcutaneous fat	42–75
Skin	77–87

(Fig. 15.25). In our series, iliac crest biopsy was positive in 78% of the patients with proven amyloidosis, detected as readily as in biopsies of the rectum or the kidney (Table 15.1)[48]. Lytic bone lesions[6,28,36,76] appear in combination with dense amyloid deposits in the marrow cavities, and have been especially observed in patients on long-term haemodialysis (Figs 15.21 and 15.30)[15,68]. Systemic vascular amyloidosis usually leads to haematopoietic hypoplasia (Fig. 15.19) and generalized low-turnover osteopenia. In about 10% of patients with multiple myeloma, secondary amyloidosis aggravates rarefaction of trabecular bone structure[49,74].

OXALOSIS

Synonym: primary hyperoxaluria.

This rare metabolic disorder is characterized by increased urinary excretion of oxalic acid. Hyperoxalaemia and hyperoxaluria cause recurrent kidney stones and progressive renal failure. Bone biopsy reveals the generalized depositions of calcium oxalate crystals in the periosteum and in the marrow cavities (Plate 15.F)[63]. Cystic rarefaction with marginal sclerosis may be present in the trabecular bone[3,78]. Osseous changes due to secondary hyperparathyroidism may also be evident in cases of renal insufficiency[13].

GORHAM'S DISEASE

Synonyms: massive osteolysis, vanishing bone disease, disappearing bone disease, phantom bone.

Jackson (1838) was the first to report a case of spontaneous absorption of bone ('a boneless arm') (see ref. 14). In 1955 Gorham and Stout reviewed 24 cases with disappearing bones, and they emphasized the angiogenic component of the osteolytic lesions[31]. A review of the literature, based on 46 patients with Gorham's disease[1,2,14,26,27,32,38,40,41,43,44,60,71,75], revealed the following characteristics:

1. The disorder affects mainly young adults, with a mean age of 26 years. The sex incidence is equal. No genetic, metabolic or endocrine abnormalities were identified. The disease was monostotic in eight cases and polyostotic in 38 patients.
2. Initially the disease affects a single bone, with involvement of adjacent bones as the process spreads (Figs 15.R5 and 15.R6). The most commonly affected regions were the pelvis (13 cases), thorax, spine, major long bones and skull; though any bone could be affected, even the short tubular bones of the hands and feet (four cases) (Fig. 15.S1).
3. The rate of progression was unpredictable. In some instances the disorder stabilized after a number of years; alternatively involvement of critical areas such

as thorax and spine led to severe complications. One of our patients had massive pulmonary complications due to disappearance of the ribs.
4. The aetiology of the disorder is still unclear; the following pathomechanisms have been suggested:

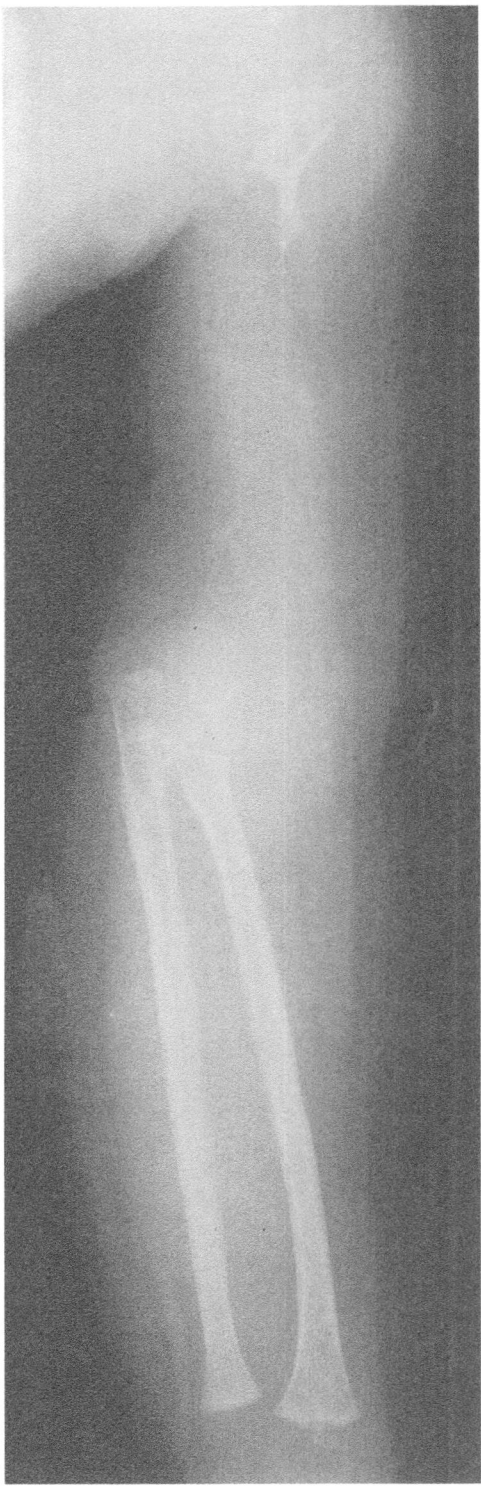

Fig. 15.R5 Gorham's disease in a child with 'vanishing' of the humerus

Plate 15.F

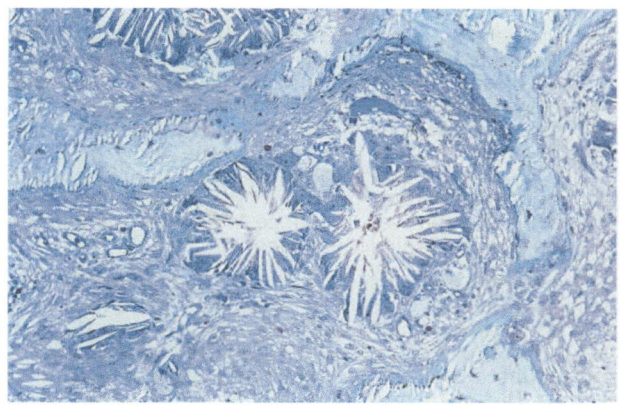

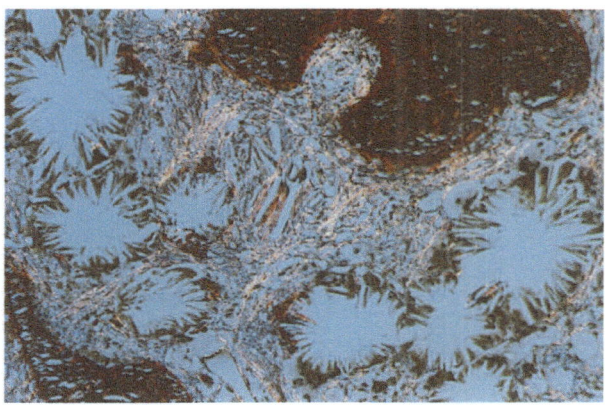

Figs. 15.31–15.36 Iliac crest biopsy of young patient with hereditary oxalosis complicated by chronic renal failure, aluminium intoxication under haemodialysis and pancytopenia

Fig. 15.31 Variably sized rosettes of calcium oxalate needles in bone marrow space with complete replacement of haematopoiesis by connective tissue. Note marked osseous remodelling of the trabeculae with broad osteoid seams. Giemsa

Fig. 15.32 Multiple rosettes of calcium oxalate crystals in the intertrabecular marrow spaces, surrounded by coarse fibrosis and newly formed woven bone (above). There is no residual haematopoiesis. Gomori, polar.

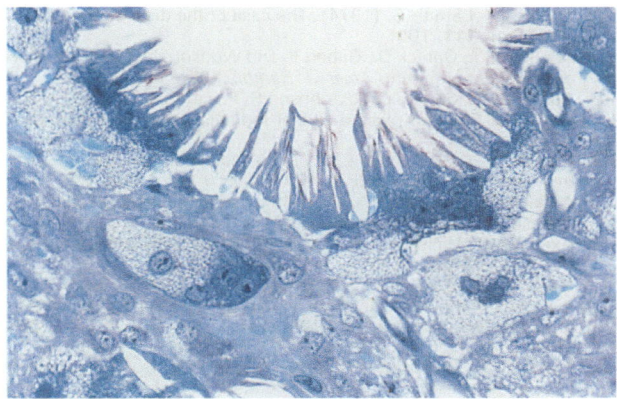

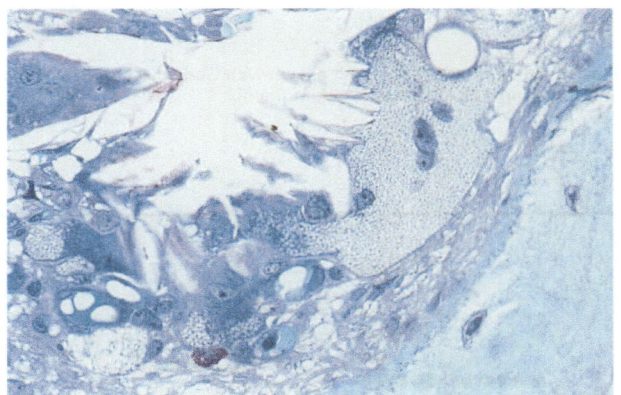

Fig. 15.33 Rosette with radiating bundles of calcium oxalate needles surrounded by large macrophages with vacuolated cytoplasm. Note nucleolated osteoclast-like cell with partly vacuolated cytoplasm (left). Giemsa

Fig. 15.34 Rosette with giant macrophage adjacent to an ossicle (right). Note broad seam of osteoid and two osteocytes. Giemsa

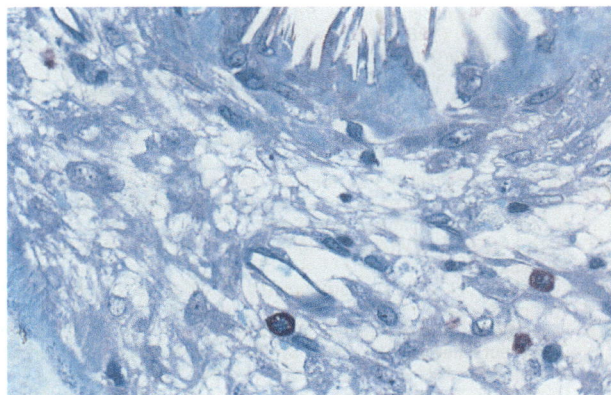

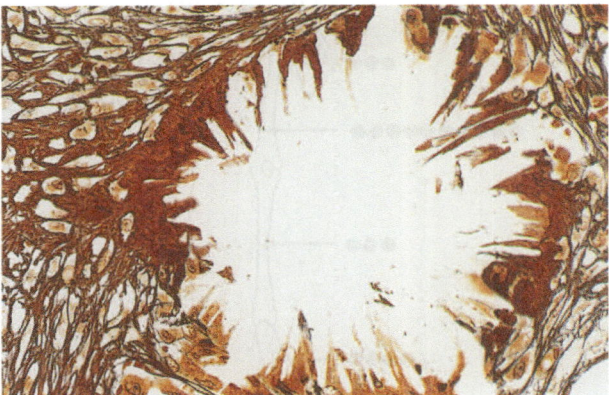

Fig. 15.35 Part of rosette with marginal zone of newly formed osteoid between the oxalate needles. Broad rim of connective tissue, vessels and plasma cells. Ossicle covered by osteoid lower left. Giemsa

Fig. 15.36 Rosette with needles partly composed of osteoid (dark brown) and surrounded by coarse, partly calcified fibrosis (left). Gomori

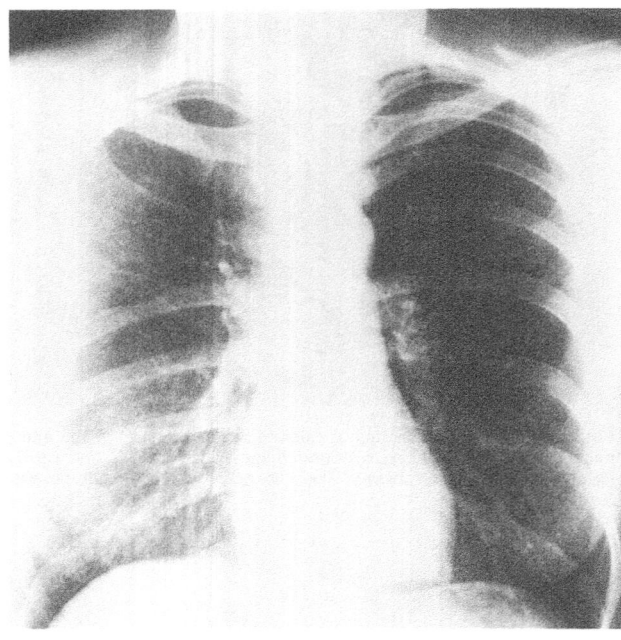

Fig. 15.R6   Chest X-ray of adult patient with Gorham's disease showing 'vanishing' bone disease affecting the ribs

trauma, haemangiomatous proliferation[27,38], reactive hyperaemia, vegetative and neural disturbances, inflammations, circulatory defects, congenital dysplasia of vasculature[40,47] and finally osteoclastic activating factors secreted by lymphoid cells in the vicinity.

5. Treatment usually consists of extensive local resection and insertion of a free vascularized bone graft, but recurrence is not infrequent. Spontaneous remission has been reported. Therapy with bisphosphonates or with calcitonin was not successful in our patient with extensive thoracic involvement.

Histological examination of involved skeletal sites revealed marked osteoclastic bone resorption; the osteoclasts appeared morphologically normal (Plate 15.G). In other cases, osteoclasts were not numerous, and atypical ultrastructure was detected in osteoblasts and endothelial cells[20]. The resorption lacunae were filled with fibrous, oedematous and highly vascularized connective tissue, in which plasma cells, mast cells and lymphocytes were dispersed. Osteoid seams with or without lining osteoblasts covered the bone adjacent to the lytic lesions.

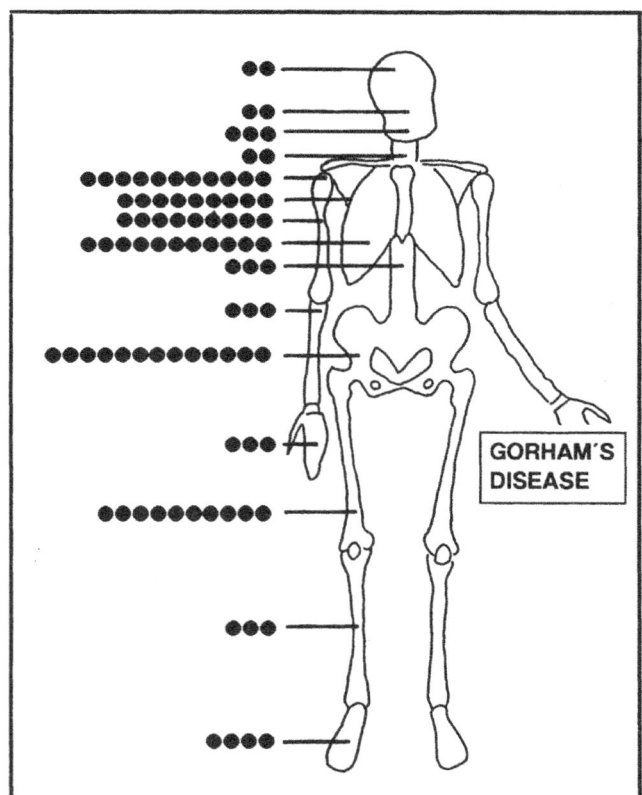

GORHAM'S DISEASE

Fig. 15.S1   Involvement of skeletal sites in Gorham's vanishing bone disease. Data compiled from review of the literature, each dot represents one involved site reported

References

1. Abel M. and Smith G. (1974). The case of the disappearing pelvis. *Radiology*, **111**, 105
2. Abrahams J., Ganick D., Gilbert E. and Wolfson J. (1980). Massive osteolysis in an infant. *Amer. J. Radiol.*, **135**, 1084
3. Adams N. D., Carrera G. F., Johnson R. P., Latorraca R. and Lemann J. (1982). Calcium-oxalate-crystal-induced bone disease. *Amer. J. Kidney*, **1**, 294
4. Amstutz H. C. and Carey E. J. (1966). Skeletal manifestations and treatment of Gaucher's disease. *J. Bone Jt Surg.*, **48A**, 670
5. Arkin A. M. and Schein A. J. (1948). Aseptic necrosis in Gaucher's disease. *J. Bone Jt Surg.*, **30A**, 631
6. Axelsson U., Hallén A. and Rausig A. (1970). Amyloidosis of bone. Report of 2 cases. *J. Bone Jt Surg.*, **528**, 717
7. Barton N. W., Brady R. O. and Dambrosia J. M. (1991). Replacement therapy for inherited enzyme deficiency – macrophage-targeted glucocerebrosidase for Gaucher's disease. *N. Engl. J. Med.*, **324**, 1464
8. Beighton P., Goldblatt J. and Sacks S. (1982). Bone involvement in Gaucher's disease: a century of delineation and research. Desnick R. J. and Grabowski G. A., *Progress in Clinical and Biological Research*, vol. 95. (p. 107). New York: Alan R. Liss
9. Bennett O. M. and Namnyak S. S. (1990). Bone and joint manifestations of sickle cell anaemia. *J. Bone Jt Surg.*, **72B**, 494
10. Beutler E. (1991). Gaucher's disease. *N. Engl. J. Med.*, **325**, 1354
11. Blandet A. (1987). Gaucher's disease. *N. Engl. J. Med.*, **316**, 619
12. Bohrer S. P. (1970). Acute long bone diaphyseal infarcts in sickle cell disease. *Brit. J. Radiol.*, **43**, 685
13. Brancaccio D., Poggi A. and Ciccarelli C. (1981). Bone changes in end-stage oxalosis. *Amer. J. Roentgenol.*, **136**, 935
14. Cannon S. R. (1986). Massive osteolysis: a review of seven cases. *J. Bone Jt Surg.*, **68B**, 24
15. Casey T. T., Stone W. J., DiRaimondo C. R., Brantley B. D., DiRaimondo C. V., Gorevic P. D. and Page D. L. (1986). Tumoral amyloidosis of bone of beta-2-microglobulin origin in association with long-term hemodialysis: a new type of amyloid disease. *Hum. Pathol.*, **17**, 731
16. Cohen A. S. (1985). Amyloidosis. McCarthy D. J., *Arthritis and Allied Conditions: a Textbook of Rheumatology*, 10th edn (p. 1108). Philadelphia: Lea & Febiger
17. DeGeorge A. M. (1975). Albright's syndrome: is it coming of age? *J. Pediatr.*, **87**, 1018
18. Dehner L. P. (1991). Morphologic findings in the histiocytic syndromes. *Semin. Oncol.*, **18**, 8
19. Diamond T., Pojer R., Steil D., Alfrey A. and Posen S. (1991). Does iron affect osteoblast function? Studies in vitro and in patients with chronic liver disease. *Calcif. Tissue Int.*, **48**, 373
20. Dickson G. R., Hamilton A., Hayes D., Carr K. E., Davis R. and Mollan R. A. B. (1990). An investigation of vanishing bone disease. *Bone*, **11**, 205
21. Editorial. (1971). Fibrous dysplasia of bone. *Brit. Med. J.*, **1**, 685
22. Elema J. D. and Atmosoerodjo-Briggs J. E. (1984). Langerhans' cells and macrophages in eosinophilic granuloma: an enzyme-

Plate 15.G

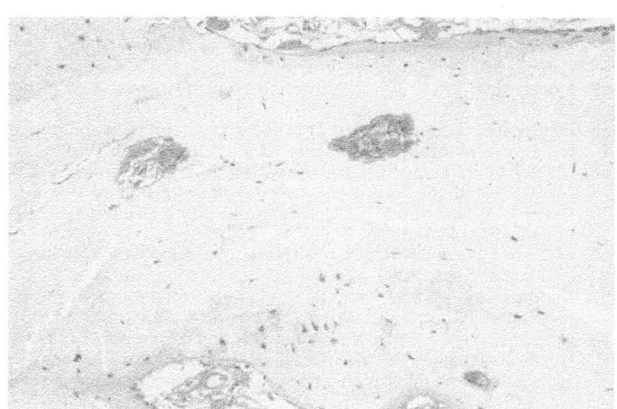

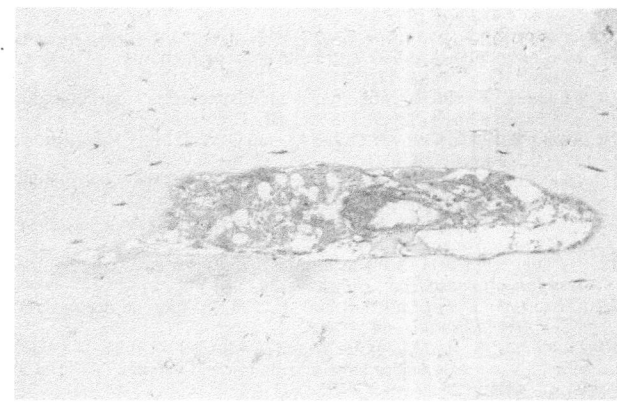

Figs. 15.37–15.42 Gorham's disease in surgical biopsy of rib, taken from margin of osteolytic lesion (see chest X-ray in Fig. 15.R6)

Fig. 15.37 Overview of the cortex near the osteolytic lesion revealing two foci of dissecting osteoclasia (centre). Giemsa

Fig. 15.38 Larger lacuna filled with connective tissue cells, some osteoclasts (left), endosteal sinusoid (below) and small artery (centre). Giemsa

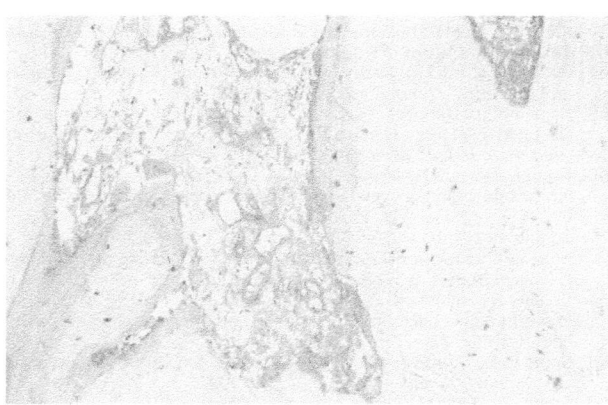

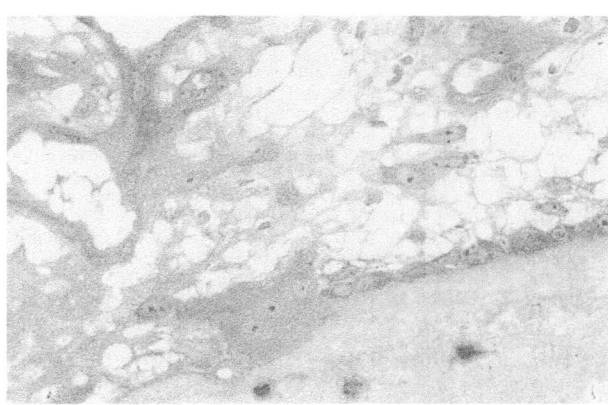

Fig. 15.39 Increased osseous remodelling with deep resorption cavity and adjacent new bone formation with seams of osteoid covered by osteoblasts. Giemsa

Fig. 15.40 Higher magnification of Fig. 15.39, with nucleolated osteoclast, osteocytes and osteoblastic formation of appositional bone (left). Note atypical vessels with wide lumira and connective tissue cells. Giemsa

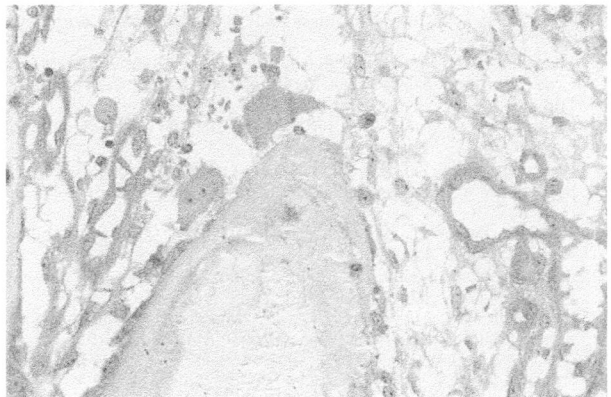

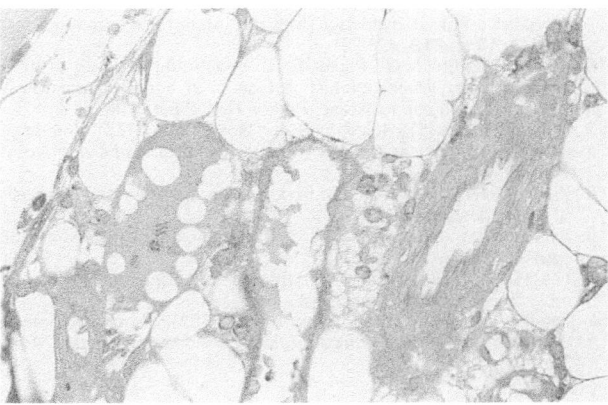

Fig. 15.41 Higher magnification of Fig. 15.39 showing active osteoclasts within the lumen of an endosteal sinusoid; ossicle completely covered by osteoid. Atypical vessels in the marrow space. Giemsa

Fig. 15.42 Inflammatory reaction in small artery (left) with mast cells and plasma cells in the adventitia. Note variations of atypical sinusoids (right). Giemsa

histochemical, enzyme-cytochemical, and ultrastructural study. *Cancer*, **54**, 2174

23. Falconer M. A. and Cope C. L. (1942). Fibrous dysplasia of bone with endocrine disorders and cutaneous pigmentation (Albright's disease). *Q. J. Med.*, **11**, 121

24. Favara B. E. (1991). Langerhans' cell histiocytosis – pathobiology and pathogenesis. *Semin. Oncol.*, **18**, 3

25. Favara B. E., McCarthy R. C. and Mierau G. W. (1983). Histiocytosis X. *Hum. Pathol.*, **14**, 663

26. Geigl D., Seidel L. and Marmor A. (1981). Gorham's disease of the clavicle with bilateral pleural effusions. *Chest*, **79**, 242

27. Fornasier V. L. (1970). Haemangiomatosis with massive osteolysis. *J. Bone Jt Surg.*, **52B**, 444

28. Gardner H. (1961). Bone lesions in primary systemic amyloidosis. A report of a case. *Brit. J. Radiol.*, **34**, 778

29. Gibson M. J. and Middlemiss J. H. (1971). Fibrous dysplasia of bone. *Brit. J. Radiol.*, **44**, 1

30. Golding J. S. R., MacIver J. E. and Went L. N. (1959). The bone changes in sickle cell anemia and its genetic variants. *J. Bone Jt Surg.*, **41B**, 711

31. Gorham L. W. and Stout A. P. (1955). Massive osteolysis (acute spontaneous absorption of bone, phantom bone, disappearing bone): its relation to hemangiomatosis. *J. Bone Jt Surg.*, **37A**, 985

32. Gorham L. W., Wright, A. W., Schultz H. H. and Maxon F. C. (1954). Disappearing bones: a rare form of massive osteolysis: report of 2 cases, 1 with autopsy findings. *Amer. J. Med.*, **17**, 674

33. Grabias S. L. and Campbell C. J. (1977). Fibrous dysplasia. *Orthop. Clin. N. Amer.*, **8**, 771

34. Greenfield G. B. (1970). Bone changes in chronic adult Gaucher's disease. *Amer. J. Roentgenol.*, **110**, 800

35. Groopman J. E. and Golde D. W. (1981). The histiocytic disorder: a pathophysiologic analysis. *Ann. Intern. Med.*, **94**, 95

36. Grossman R. E. and Hensley G. T. (1967). Bone lesions in primary amyloidosis. *Amer. J. Roentgenol.*, **10**, 872

37. Hahn S.-B., Lee S. B. and Kim D. H. (1991). Albright's syndrome with hypophosphatemic rickets and hyperthryoidism: a case report. *Yonsei Med. J.*, **32**, 179

38. Hambach R., Pujman J. and Maly V. (1958). Massive osteolysis due to haemangiomatosis. *Radiology*, **71**, 43

39. Harris W. H., Dudley H. R. and Parry R. J. (1962). The natural history of fibrous dysplasia. An orthopaedic, pathological and roentgenographic study. *J. Bone Jt Surg.*, **44A**, 207

40. Hemingway A., Leuny A. and Lavender J. (1983). Familial vanishing limbs: four generations of idiopathic multicentric osteolysis. *Clin. Radiol.*, **34**, 585

41. Heyden G., Kindblom L. G. and Nielsen J. M. (1977). Disappearing bone disease: a clinical and histological study. *J. Bone Jt Surg.*, **59A**, 57

42. Johnson N. A. (1990). Musculoskeletal problems in hemoglobinopathy. *Orthop. Clin. N. Amer.*, **21**(1), 191

43. Johnson P. M. and McClure J. G. (1958). Observations on massive osteolysis: a review of the literature and report of a case. *Radiology*, **71**, 28

44. Jones G. B., Smith G. S. and Midgley R. L. (1970). Massive osteolysis – disappearing bone. *J. Bone Jt Surg.*, **52B**, 452

45. Kaplan F. S., Fallon M. D., Boden S. D., Schmidt R., Senior M. and Haddad J. G. (1988). Estrogen receptors in bone in a patient with polyostotic fibrous dysplasia (McCune-Albright Syndrome). *New Engl. J. Med.*, **319**, 421

46. Keen C. E., Philip G., Parker B. C. and Souhami R. L. (1990). Unusual bony lesions of histiocytosis X in a patient previously treated for Hodgkin's disease. *Pathol. Res. Pract.*, **186**, 519

47. Kohler E. Babbitt D., Huizenga B. and Good T. A. (1973). Hereditary osteolysis. A clinical, radiological and chemical study. *Radiology*, **108**, 99

48. Krause J. R. (1977). Value of bone marrow biopsy in the diagnosis of amyloidosis. *South. Med. J.*, **70**, 1072

49. Kyle R. A. and Bayrd E. D. (1975). Amyloidosis: review of 236 cases. *Medicine*, **54**, 271

50. Lee R. E. (1988). Histiocytic diseases of bone marrow. *Hematol./Oncol. Clin. N. Amer.*, **2**(4), 657

51. Lee R. E., Peters S. P. and Glew R. H. (1982). Gaucher's disease: clinical, morphological and pathogenic considerations. *Pathol. Ann.*, **12**, 309

52. Lichtenstein L. (1953). Histiocytosis X: integration of eosinophilic granuloma of bone, 'Letterer–Siwe disease' and 'Schüller–Christian disease' as related manifestations of a single nosologic entity. *Arch. Pathol.*, **56**, 84

53. Lichtenstein L. (1938). Polyostotic fibrous dysplasia. *Arch. Surg.*, **36**, 874

54. Lichtenstein L. and Jaffe H. L. (1940). Eosinophilic granuloma of bone, with report of a case. *Amer. J. Pathol.*, **16**, 595

55. Mankin H. J., Doppelt S. H., Rosenberg A. E. and Barranger J. A. (1990). Metabolic bone disease in patients with Gaucher's disease. Avioli L. V. and Krane S. M., *Metabolic Bone Disease* (p. 730). Philadelphia: Saunders

56. McCune D. J. and Bruch H. (1937). Osteodystrophia fibrosa. *Amer. J. Dis. Child*, **54**, 806

57. Middlemiss J. H. and Raper A. B. (1966). Skeletal changes in the haemoglobinopathies. *J. Bone Jt Surg.*, **48A**, 693

58. Mogilner B. M., Barak Y., Amitay M. and Zlotogora J. (1990). Hyperphosphatasemia in infantile GMI gangliosidosis: possible association with microscopic bone marrow osteoblastosis. *J. Pediatr.*, **117**(5), 758

59. Ozoh J. O., Onuigbo M. A. C., Nwankwo N., Ukabam S. O., Umerah B. C. and Emewruwa C. C. (1990). 'Vanishing' of vertebra in a patient with sickle cell hemoglobinopathy. *Brit. Med. J.*, **301**, 1368

60. Pedicelli G., Mattia P., Zorzoli A., Sorrone A. and deMartino F. (1984). Gorham-syndrome. *Amer. J. Med.*, **252**, 1449

61. Pepys M. B. (1987). Amyloidosis. Weatherall D. J., Ledingham J. G. G. and Warrell D. A., *Oxford Textbook of Medicine* (p. 9.145). Oxford: Oxford Medical Publications

62. Pinckney L. and Parker B. R. (1977). Myelosclerosis and myelofibrosis in treated histiocytosis X. *Amer. J. Roentgenol.*, **129**, 521

63. Revell P. A. (1986). *Pathology of Bone*. Berlin: Springer

64. Reynolds J. (1977). Radiologic manifestations of sickle cell hemoglobinopathy. *J. Amer. Med. Assoc.*, **238**, 247

65. Risdall R. J., Dehner L. P., Duray P., Krobinsky N., Robinson L. and Nesbit M. E. (1983). Histiocytosis X (Langerhans' cell histiocytosis). *Arch. Pathol. Lab. Med.*, **107**, 59

66. Rourke J. A. and Heslin D. J. (1965). Gaucher's disease: roentgenologic bone changes over 20 year interval. *Amer. J. Roentgenol.*, **94**, 621

67. Schajowicz A. R. and Slullitel J. (1973). Eosinophil granuloma of bone and its relationship to Hand-Schüller–Christian and Letterer–Siwe syndromes. *J. Bone Jt Surg.*, **55B**, 545

68. Schiller B., Hillebrand G., Bartl R. and Linke R. P. (1992). Chronische Arthralgien bei einem 46-jährigen Patienten mit Niereninsuffizienz. *Internist*, **33**, 117

69. Scott P. P., Scott W. W. and Siegelman S. S. (1986). Amyloidosis: an overview. *Semin. Roentgenol.*, **21**, 103

70. Smith R. (1987). Fibrous dysplasia. Weatherall D. J., Ledingham J. G. G. and Warrell D. A., *Oxford Textbook of Medicine* (p. 17.33). Oxford: Oxford University Press

71. Stout A. P. (1959). Massive osteolysis. *Radiology*, **73**, 435

72. Stowens D. W., Teitelbaum S. L., Kahn A. J. and Barranger J. A. (1985). Skeletal complications of Gaucher's disease. *Medicine*, **64**, 310

73. Strickland B. (1958). Skeletal manifestations of Gaucher's disease with some unusual findings. *Brit. J. Radiol.*, **30**, 246

74. Subbarao K. and Jacobson H. G. (1986). Amyloidosis and plasma cell dyscrasias of the musculoskeletal system. *Semin. Roentgenol.*, **21**, 139

75. Thompson J. S. and Schurman D. J. (1974). Massive osteolysis. Case report and review of the literature. *Clin. Orthop. Rel. Res.*, **103**, 206

76. Weinfeld A., Stern M. H. and Marx L. H. (1970). Amyloid lesion of bone. *Amer. J. Roentgenol.*, **108**, 799

77. Weinstein R. S. and Lutcher C. L. (1983). Chronic erythroid hyperplasia and accelerated bone turnover. *Metab. Bone Dis. Rel. Res.*, **5**, 7

78. Wiggelinkhuizen J. and Fisher R. M. (1982). Oxalosis of bone. *Pediatr. Radiol.*, **12**, 307

79. Windholz F. and Foster S. E. (1948). Sclerosis of bones in Gaucher's disease. *Amer. J. Roentgenol.*, **60**, 246

80. Yossipovitch Z. H., Herman G. and Makin M. (1965). Aseptic osteomyelitis in Gaucher's disease. *Isr. J. Med. Sci.*, **1**, 531

Systemic mastocytosis

16

Mast cells are connective tissue elements containing cytoplasmic granules that stain metachromatically. They are a storehouse for many chemical mediators including histamine, serotonin, heparin, prostaglandins and proteoglycans (Fig. 16.S1)[21,35]. The mature mast cell has a variable contour, round, oval or spindle-shaped, and the morphological variations may reflect diverse functional states[30,47,56]. In the bone marrow, mast cells are primarily located adjacent to blood vessels or in close proximity to the trabecular surface (Figs 16.1–16.2)[4,19,31]. Tables 3.3 and 5.1 show the density of mast cells in the bone marrow according to age and skeletal site, with higher average values in the elderly and in females.

An *increase in marrow mast cells* together with plasma cells and lymphocytes has been observed in a variety of conditions: inflammations, wound and fracture healing, oedema and fibrosis (Fig. 16.S2)[1,35]. Immunocytic and lymphocytic marrow infiltrations often have a high content of mast cells. The connective tissue of certain tumours may contain numerous mast cells, possibly participating in local tissue resistance against tumour growth or, in contrast, in angioneogenesis[41,26]. Mast cell proliferation at osseous surfaces is also a consequence of secondary HPT. The close association between mast cells and HPT, both primary and secondary, has been established by many workers[1,14,38]. In 1968 Frame and Nixon focused attention on the relation between mast cells and postmenopausal osteoporosis, suggesting that mast cells accelerate trabecular bone loss by increasing the bone turnover rate[18]. In 1983, Fallon *et al.* confirmed the association between osteoporosis and increased bone

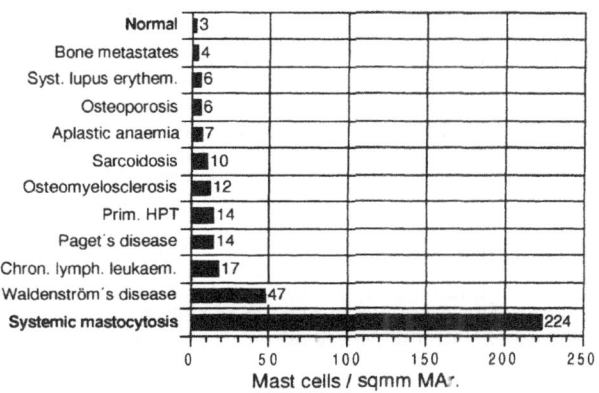

	Mast cells / sqmm MAr.
Normal	3
Bone metastates	4
Syst. lupus erythem.	6
Osteoporosis	6
Aplastic anaemia	7
Sarcoidosis	10
Osteomyelosclerosis	12
Prim. HPT	14
Paget's disease	14
Chron. lymph. leukaem.	17
Waldenström's disease	47
Systemic mastocytosis	224

Fig. 16.S2 Mast cells in iliac crest biopsy in increasing order of frequency in various pathological conditions

marrow mast cell counts[16]. However, the impact of the mast cell on normal bone metabolism remains controversial, and clinical observations have revealed their presence in osteosclerosis as well as osteoporosis. For instance, certain mast cell products, such as heparin or prostaglandin, could cause osteopenia, whereas osteosclerosis could be the result of prostaglandin-stimulated bone formation.

We assessed the frequency of reactive bone marrow mastocytosis in 850 patients with chronic myeloproliferative disorders (CMPD), and there were striking differences in the various clinical entities: OMS 35%, MF 25%, IT 14%, PV 9% and CML only 1%[8]. Characteristic mast cell granulomas were found in only 0.3% of the patients with CMPD. The very low mast cell numbers in CML, as well as the observation of mastocytosis in patients with severe neutropenia, suggest that the granulocyte macrophage-colony stimulating factor (GM-CSF) may inhibit mast cell growth, and therefore one strategy of therapy in patients with systemic mastocytosis might be to administer GM-CSF consecutively[7]. Reactive mastocytosis has been reported in myeloproliferative disorders, myelofibrosis, myelodysplastic syndrome, lymphoproliferative disorders and aplastic anaemia[13,17,24,36,51,52,54,58,59].

Mastocytosis (mast cell disease) is characterized by a proliferation of mast cells in various organs and tissues[30,40,49,50,53]. The hyperplasia of mast cells that defines systemic mastocytosis in most cases is neither clonal or neoplastic[20]. It is *localized* to the skin (cutaneous mastocytosis, urticaria pigmentosa)[39], *systemic* in distribution (systemic mastocytosis)[22,25,27,42], *sarcomatous* (mast cell sarcoma)[30], or even *leukaemic* (mast cell leukaemia) (Fig. 16.36)[11,12,33,48].

Several classifications of mastocytosis have been published, and a recent *consensus classification of systemic mastocytosis* describes four variants[2,32]:

1. an indolent type, which constitutes the majority of patients and without major influence or life expectancy;

2. a haematological type, which is associated with basic myeloproliferative or myelodysplastic disorders;

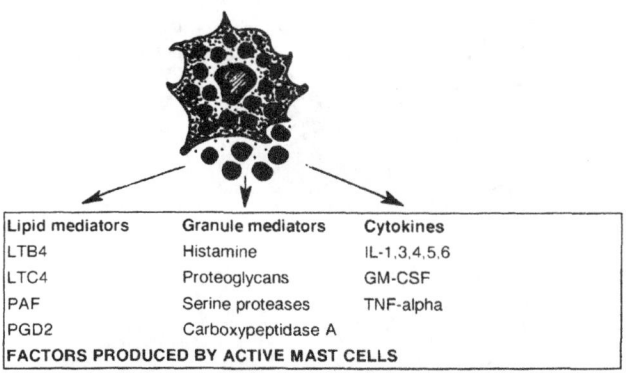

Lipid mediators	Granule mediators	Cytokines
LTB4	Histamine	IL-1,3,4,5,6
LTC4	Proteoglycans	GM-CSF
PAF	Serine proteases	TNF-alpha
PGD2	Carboxypeptidase A	
FACTORS PRODUCED BY ACTIVE MAST CELLS		

Leukocyte responses	Fibroblast responses	Microvascular reponses
Adherance	Proliferation	Augmented vascular permeability
Chemotaxis	Collagen production	Leukocyte adherence
Phagocytosis	Substrate responses	Constriction
IgE production	Protein degradation	Dilatation
Mast cell proliferation	Coagulation activation	
Eosinophil activation		
RESPONSES TO THE MAST CELL FACTORS		

Fig. 16.S1 Diagram of the various factors known to be produced by mast cells as well as the responses that may be evoked by them. Modified from Stevens R. L. and Austen K. F. (1989). Recent advances in the cellular and molecular biology of mast cells. *Immunology Today*, **10**, 381

3. an aggressive type, in which the extent of mast cell proliferation in parenchymal organs determines the prognosis; and
4. mast cell leukaemia, a rare and fatal disease.

In 1982, Webb *et al.* reported that the systemic variant constitutes approximately 10% of all mastocytoses[55].

We investigated bone biopsies of 85 adult patients with established systemic mastocytosis[4,19], and bone marrow involvement was present in 80% of the cases. Histomorphometric data are given in Fig. 16.S3. Survival statistics documented a favourable life expectancy: within a follow-up period of 5 years only six of 45 patients with systemic mastocytosis died. Malignant (immature, leukaemic) types of systemic mastocytosis were observed in only four cases. Eight patients had bone marrow involvement and very short survivals, but additional malignancies (malignant lymphomas, multiple myeloma, bronchial carcinoma) were detected during follow-up (see also refs 6 and 9).

The characteristic histological lesion is the presence of *mast cell granulomas* (Plates 16.A–D)[4,5,19,42,43]. These are located predominantly in the endosteal and perivascular regions. The granulomas consist of spindle-shaped mast cells variably granulated, lymphocytes, plasma cells, eosinophils and sea-blue histiocytes, all within a network of fibres and capillaries. Mast cells are also loosely dispersed among fat and haematopoietic cells and on the trabecular surface. In advanced cases (10%) the granulomas have coalesced and occupy large areas of the marrow or even completely replace haematopoiesis in the biopsy sections[4,19,29,34,53,55].

Patients were assigned to one of *three stages*, depending on the amount and pattern of mast cell infiltration in bone biopsy:

1. a small solitary mast cell granuloma;
2. multiple mast cell granulomas, together with an interstitial, perivascular and paratrabecular mast cell infiltration; and
3. extensive granulomatous infiltration of the marrow cavities with marked fibrosis, replacement of normal haematopoiesis and increased bone remodelling.

Skeletal changes are noted in approximately 70% with systemic mastocytosis[23,43,44,46,53,60], and they may be osteolytic[37], osteoporotic[10,16] or osteosclerotic[45,48], circumscribed[22] and/or diffuse[57]. They are more frequent in skull, vertebrae and pelvis than in long bones. Systemic mastocytosis may be the underlying cause of spinal osteopenia more frequently than is generally realized, and the osseous lesions may resemble metastatic malignant bone disease (Fig. 16.R1)[3,57].

Paratrabecular granulomas invariably induce a local *osseous reaction* (Plates 16.E and F): osteoblastic bone formation with thickening of the trabeculae in 22%, while in 33% of the biopsies osteoclastic bone resorption caused osteoporotic and osteolytic bone lesions. Normal trabecular bone volumes were present in only half of the patients: 26% had osteopenia (less than 16 vol% bone) and 17% osteosclerosis (more than 30 vol% bone). Biopsies of six patients were characterized by concomitant lytic and sclerotic lesions. The frequency and degree of bone reactions correlated with the degree of bone marrow involvement. Skeletal lesions on X-rays were observed in 70% of the patients: osteopenia 44%, multiple osteolyses 27%, osteosclerotic lesions 17%. Serum alkaline phosphatase was increased in 40% of the patients.

The indolent course, as well as the granulomatous features, in systemic mastocytosis suggest an immunological, non-neoplastic pathogenesis favouring the designation of *mast cell granulomatosis* (Fig. 16.S4).

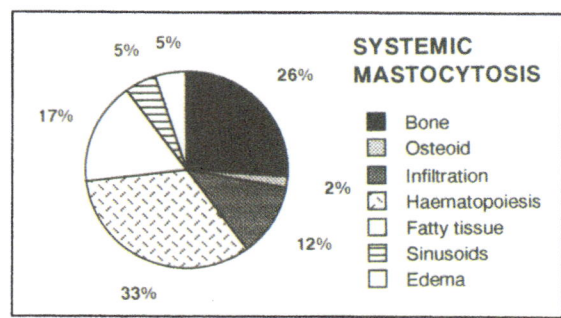

Fig. 16.S3 Histomorphometry of iliac crest biopsies in systemic mastocytosis

Malignant, usually leukaemic or sarcomatous, variants are very rare. However, there is an increased risk of haematological malignancy in patients with systemic mastocytosis[33,52,55].

Antiproliferative drugs and radiotherapy have been used in systemic mastocytosis, but without success. Low doses of prednisone may be useful. Recently response to interferon-α_{2b} was very encouraging. Indeed, *in vitro* studies with atypical bone marrow mast cells revealed that interferon-α_{2b} reduced spontaneous and induced degranulation, and it is quite possible that cytokines regulate the activity of the mast cell in systemic mastocytosis[2,28].

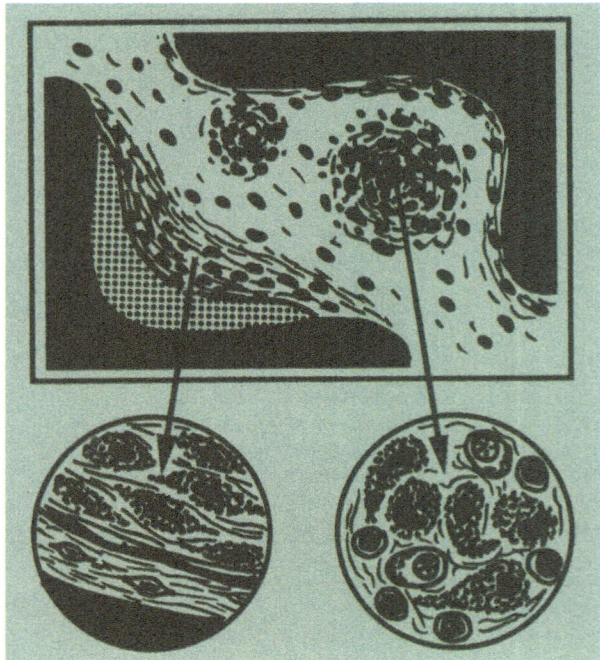

Fig. 16.S4 Systemic mastocytosis in the bone marrow. There is a patchy involvement with paratrabecular (left circle), intertrabecular (right circle) and perivascular granulomas consisting of a heterogeneous cell population though the majority are mast cells, plasma cells and lymphocytes ('mast cell granulomatosis'). Mast cells, both round and spindle-shaped, are also scattered among the fat cells and haematopoietic elements. Production of woven bone (left) in apposition to paratrabecular mast cell granulomata

Plate 16.A

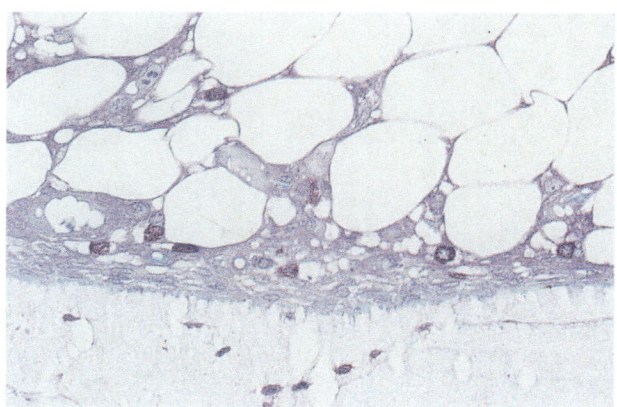

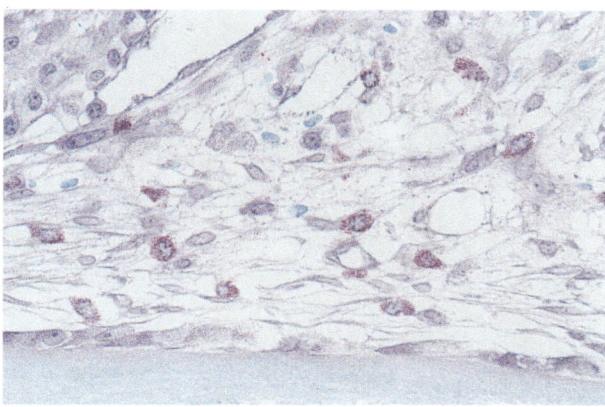

Figs. 16.1 and **16.2**   Reactive mastocytosis in iliac crest biopsies

Fig. 16.1   Small, round mast cells diffusely distributed between fat cells in a patient with aplastic anaemia. Giemsa

Fig. 16.2   Round mast cells scattered between connective tissue cells in patient with sclerosing myelitis. Note broad osteoid seam covered by osteoblasts. Giemsa

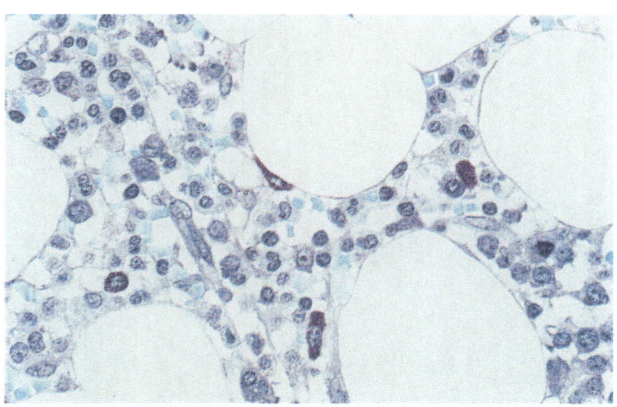

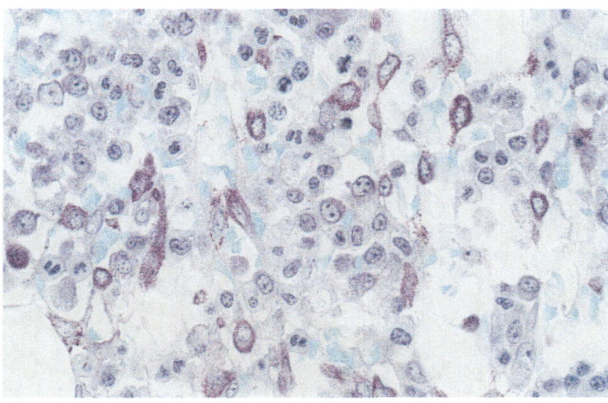

Figs. 16.3–16.6   Iliac crest biopsies with interstitial and perivascular involvement in systemic mastocytosis

Fig. 16.3   Minimal interstitial infiltration of the bone marrow by mast cells. Note characteristic fibroblast-like mast cell on the surface of a fat cell (centre). Giemsa

Fig. 16.4   Dense interstitial infiltration of the bone marrow by variably shaped mast cells. Giemsa

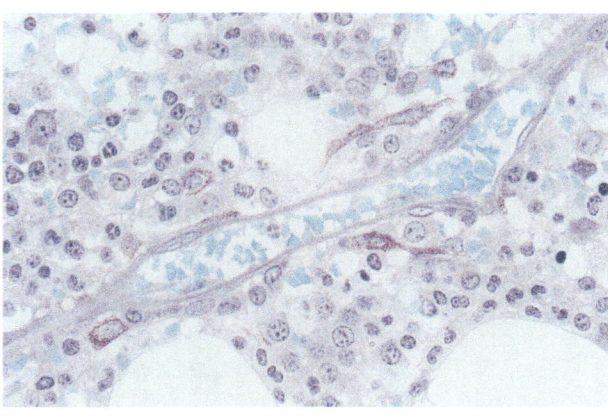

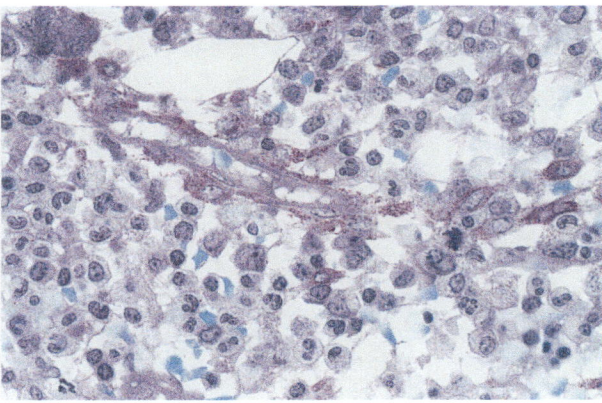

Fig. 16.5   Elongated, fibroblast-like mast cells located around a central sinusoid. Giemsa

Fig. 16.6   Arteriole with mast cell infiltration. Giemsa

Plate 16.B

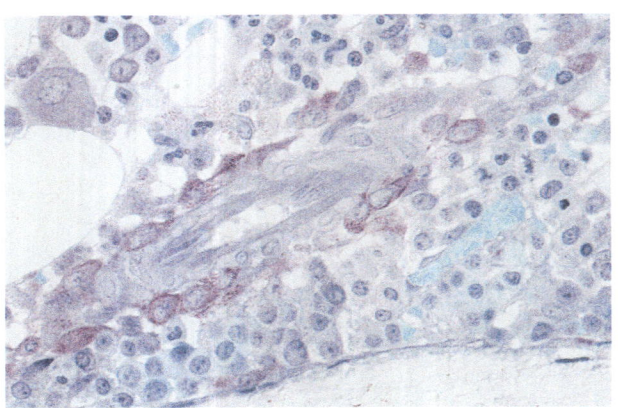

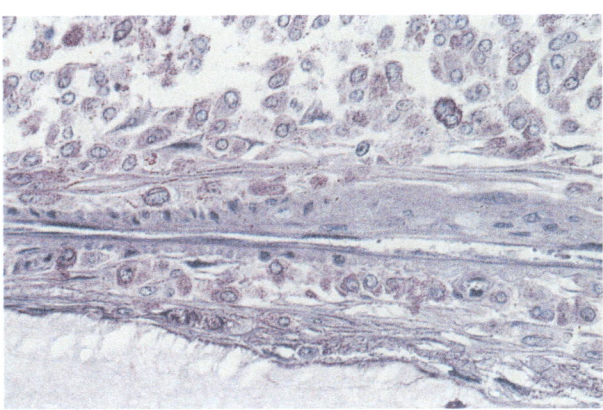

Figs. 16.7–16.12 Iliac crest biopsies with perivascular and granulomatous involvement in systemic mastocytosis

Fig. 16.7 Small artery surrounded by a layer of mast cells. Giemsa

Fig. 16.8 Dense mast cell infiltration around a longitudinally cut artery, near an ossicle. Giemsa

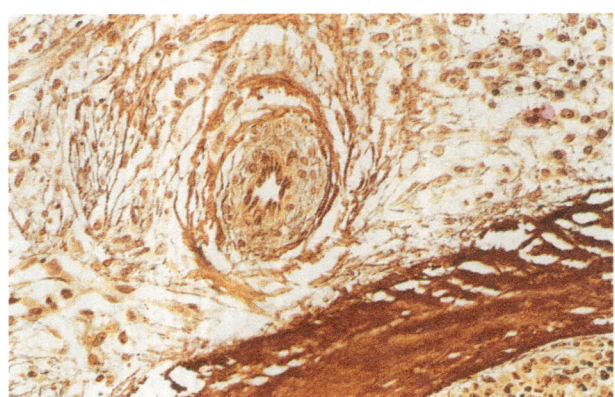

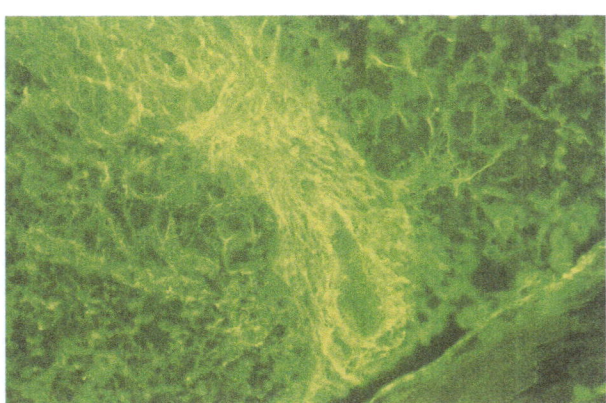

Fig. 16.9 Characteristic perivascular mast cell granuloma with coarse fibrosis. Gomori

Fig. 16.10 Perivascular fibrosis due to mast cell infiltration. Section incubated for demonstration of collagen type III. The fibres show green fluorescence while the trabecular bone (lower right) is negative. Cryostat section, immunofluorescence

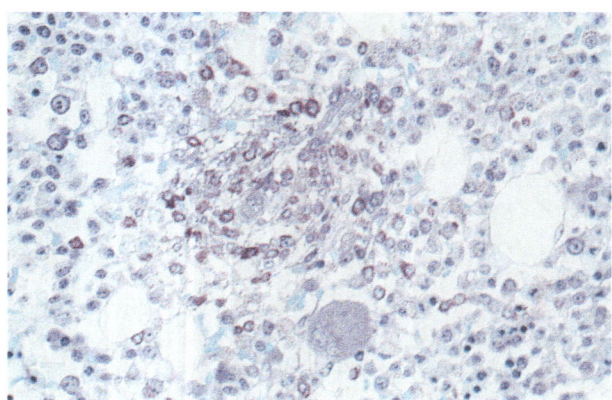

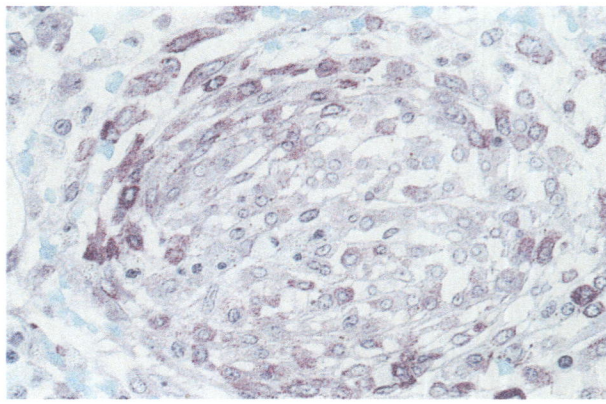

Fig. 16.11 Small mast cell nodule in the bone marrow between haematopoietic tissue. Giemsa

Fig. 16.12 Larger mast cell nodule (granuloma) with lymphoid cells in the centre. Giemsa

Plate 16.C

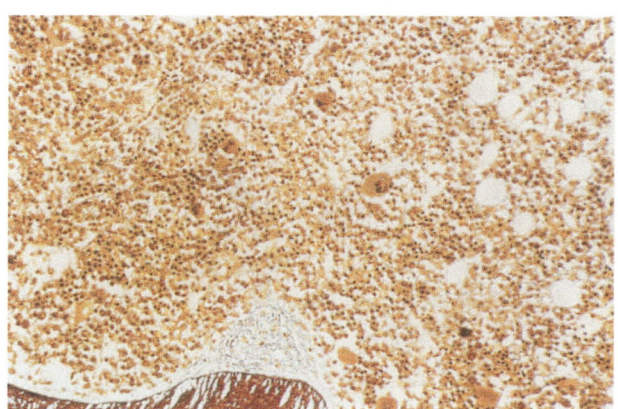

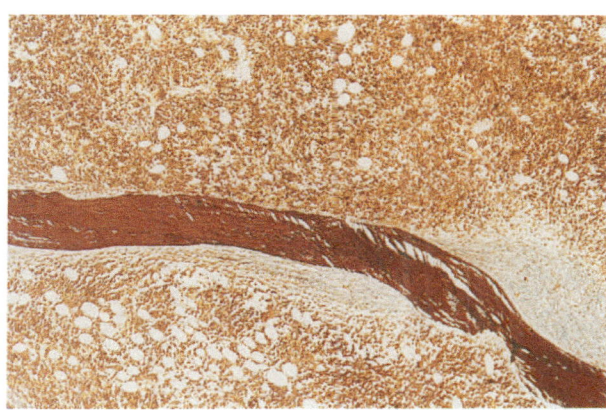

Figs. 16.13–16.18 Variations of paratrabecular mast cell granulomas and osseous reactions in systemic mastocytosis

Fig. 16.13 Small mast cell granuloma on the surface of an ossicle. Gomori

Fig. 16.14 Attenuation of trabecula by typical mast cell granuloma (right) and extensive superficial erosion with paratrabecular fibrosis at the lower part of the trabecular surface. Gomori

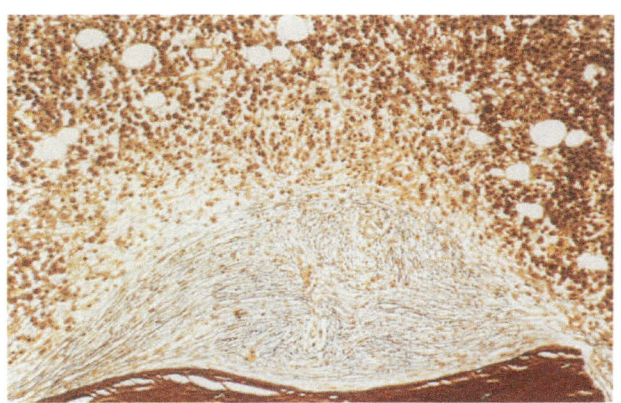

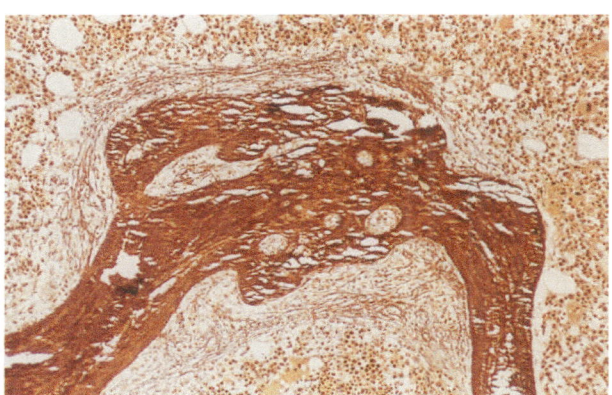

Fig. 16.15 Large mast cell granuloma on the surface of an ossicle, without osseous reaction. Gomori

Fig. 16.16 Thickened ossicles encased in mast cell granuloma. Gomori

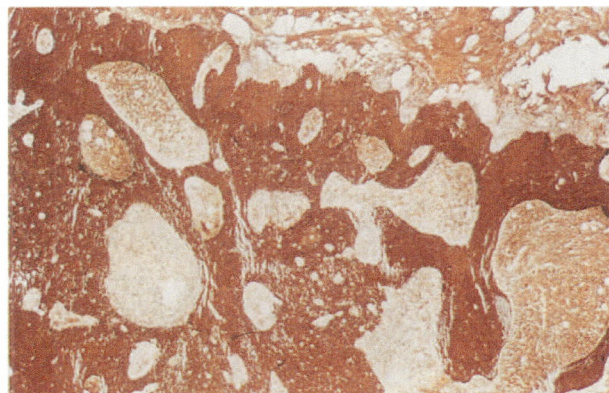

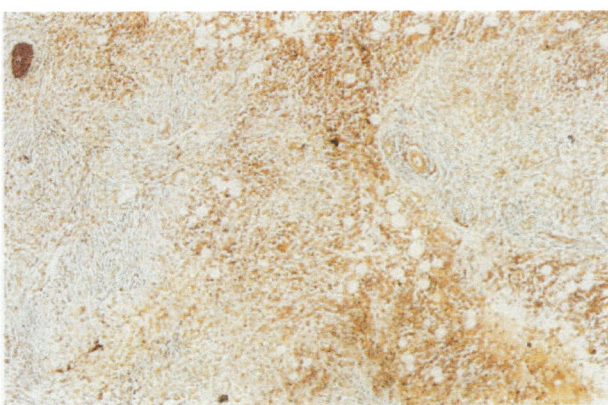

Fig. 16.17 Osteosclerotic variant of systemic mastocytosis. Note disorganized trabecular structure. Gomori

Fig. 16.18 Confluent granulomas in iliac crest biopsy of patient with advanced systemic mastocytosis and osteolytic lesions. Note residual small island of cancellous bone (upper left); 'button phenomenon'. Gomori

Plate 16.D

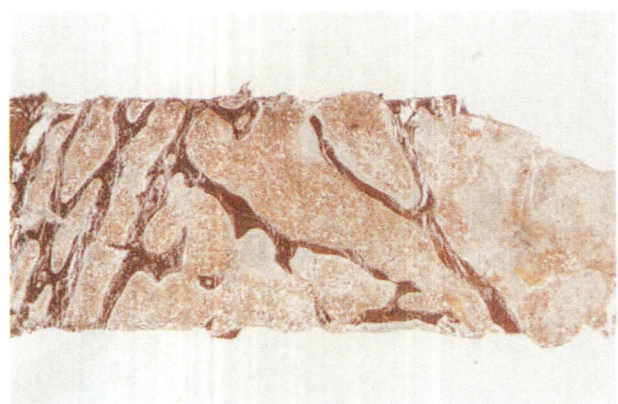

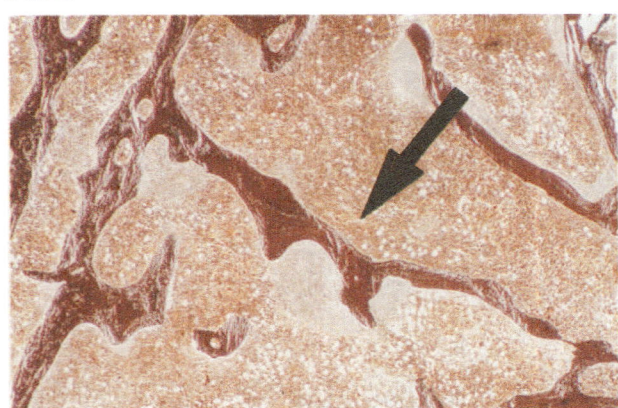

Figs. 16.19–16.24 Iliac crest biopsy of a patient with systemic mastocytosis

Fig. 16.19 Overview of bone biopsy. Note focal infiltration, mainly paratrabecular, incipient osteopenia and osteolysis (right) (see Fig. 16.R1 showing X-ray of vertebrae of same patient)

Fig. 16.20 Higher magnification of subcortical region in Fig. 16.19. Note several paratrabecular granulomas. Gomori

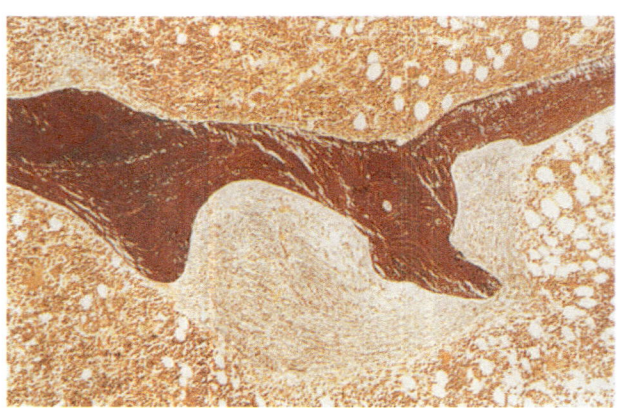

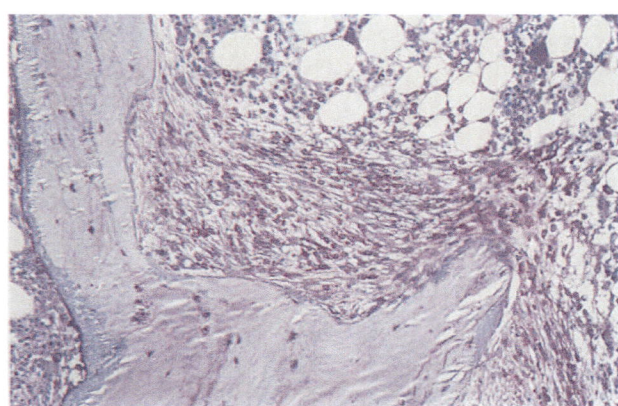

Fig. 16.21 Higher magnification of area indicated by arrow in Fig. 16.20 with dense fibrosis enclosing part of the trabecula and the granuloma (lower centre), and a very small granuloma on the trabecular surface (upper left). Gomori

Fig. 16.22 Higher magnification of round and spindle-shaped mast cells with variable granulation in a mast cell granuloma. Giemsa

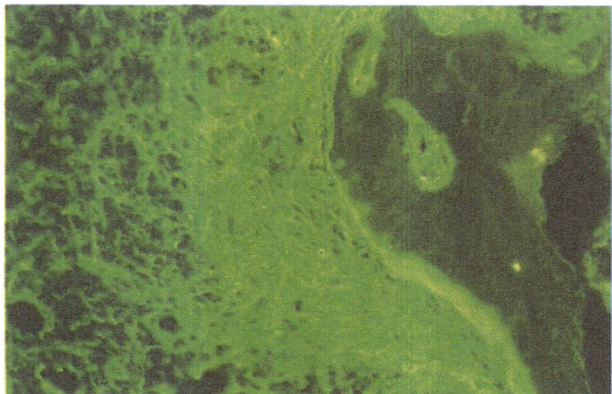

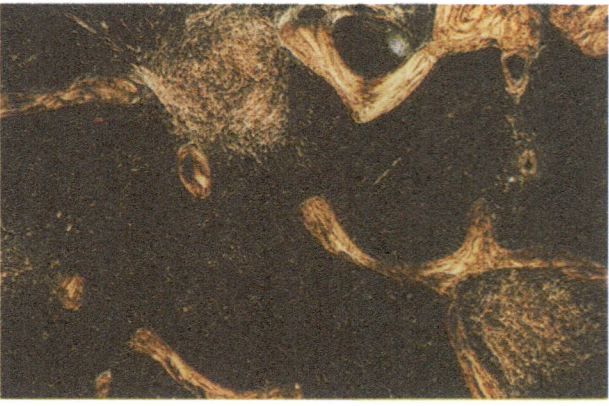

Fig. 16.23 Paratrabecular mast cell granuloma. Section incubated for demonstration of collagen type III. The fibres of the granuloma show green fluorescence, while the trabecular bone (right) is negative. Cryostat section, immunofluorescence

Fig. 16.24 Granulomas highlighted by their framework of fibres viewed in polarized light. Gomori, polar.

Plate 16.E

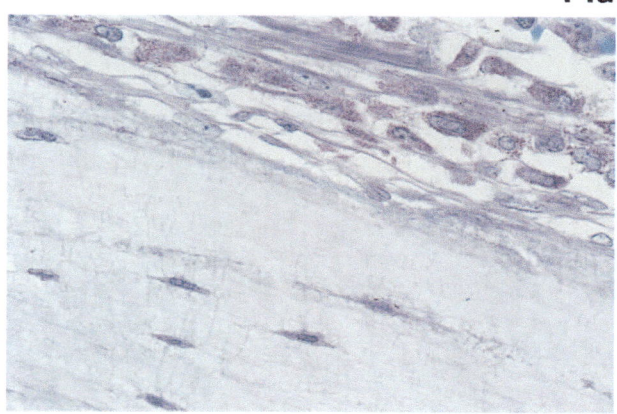

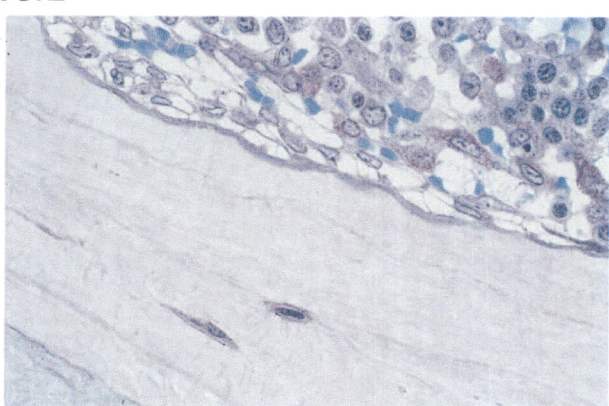

Figs. 16.25–16.30 Variations of osseous reaction in systemic masto-cytosis I

Fig. 16.25 Paratrabecular mast cell infiltration but unaffected bone. Note smooth trabecular surface, normal osteocytes and absence of osteoid. Giemsa

Fig. 16.26 Paratrabecular mast cell infiltration with scalloped trabecular surface, but absence of osteoclasts. Giemsa

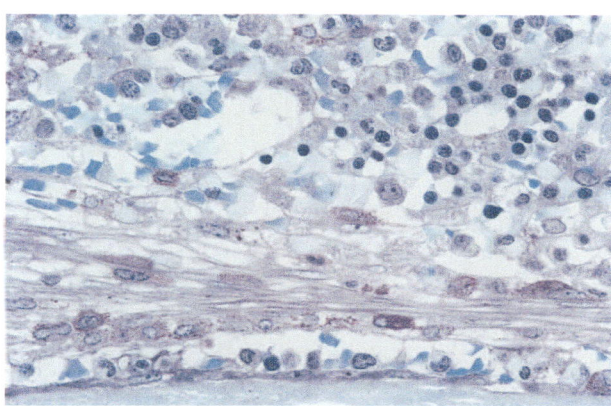

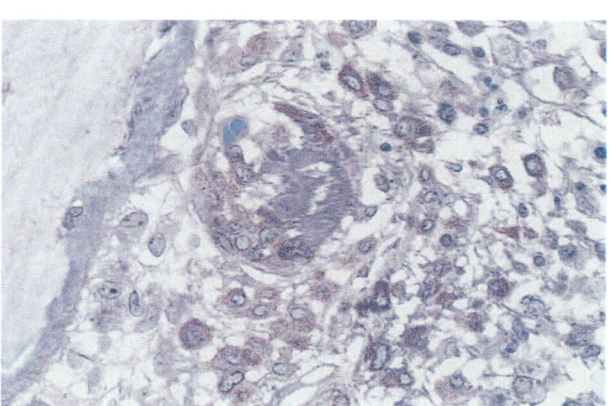

Fig. 16.27 Paratrabecular mast cell infiltration, broad endosteal sinusoid and seam of osteoid covered by osteoblasts. Giemsa

Fig. 16.28 Mast cell granuloma with broad seam of osteoid and island of newly formed woven bone (centre). Giemsa

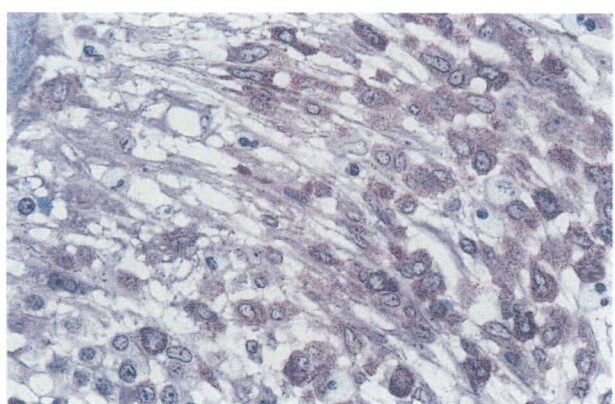

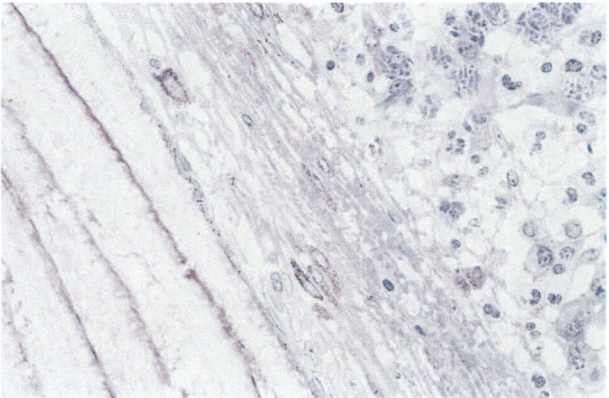

Fig. 16.29 Fibres radiating from focus of woven bone (upper left), together with dense mast cell infiltration. Giemsa

Fig. 16.30 Part of a trabecula showing lamellae separated by cement lines, parallel in the lower left hand corner indicating successive waves of osteoblastic bone formation. Giemsa

Plate 16.F

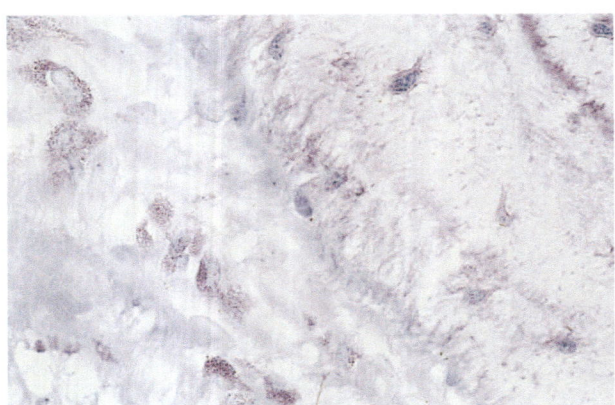

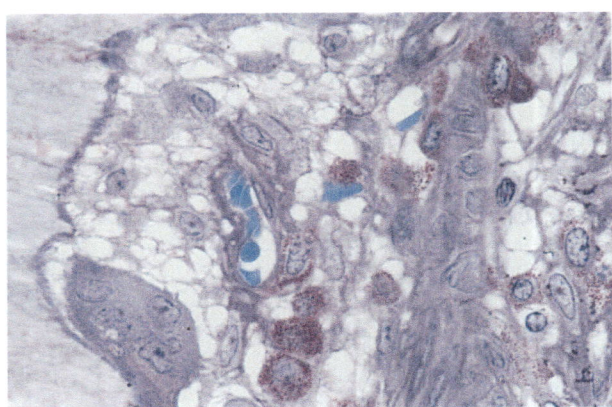

Figs. 16.31–16.34 Variations of osseous reaction in systemic masto-cytosis II

Fig. 16.31 Higher magnification of large, fibrocyte-like mast cells in close apposition to the surface of an ossicle. Note distinct cement line (upper right). Giemsa

Fig. 16.32 Resorption cavity with multinucleated osteoclast, close to mast cells, fibrocytes and vessels. Giemsa

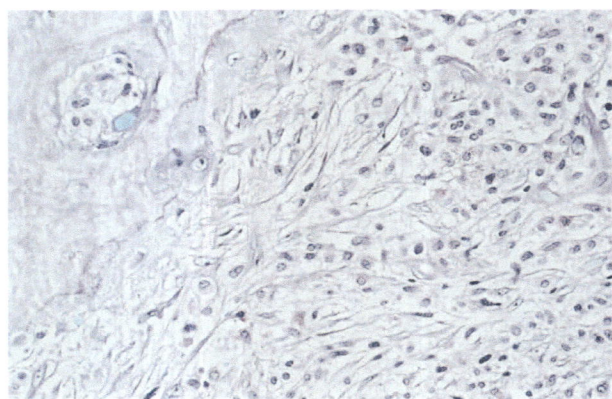

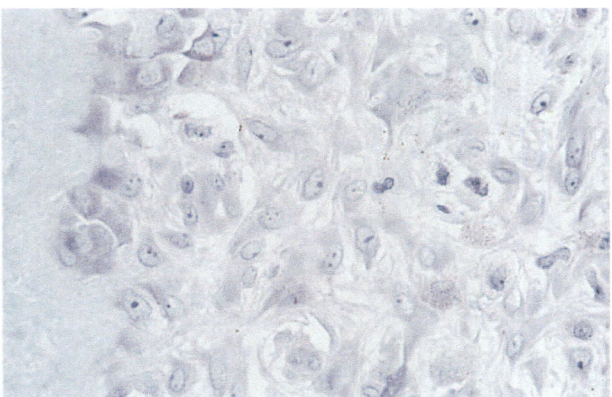

Fig. 16.33 Increased bone remodelling with cement lines resembling 'mosaic structure' in area of dense mast cell infiltration. Note almost complete absence of mast cell granulation. Giemsa

Fig. 16.34 Higher magnification of section in Fig. 16.33 revealing spindle-shaped, almost degranulated mast cells and large, partly nucleo-lated mast cells. Note osteoid seam covered by cuboidal osteoblasts (left). Giemsa

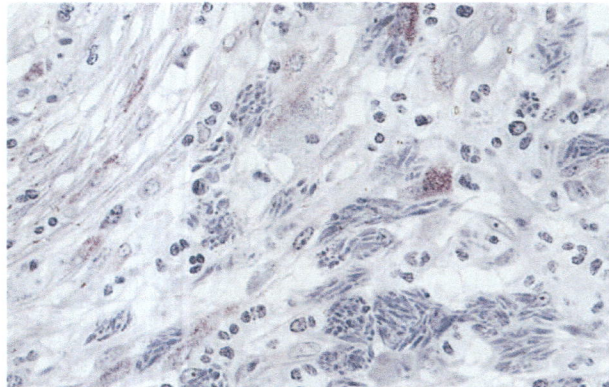

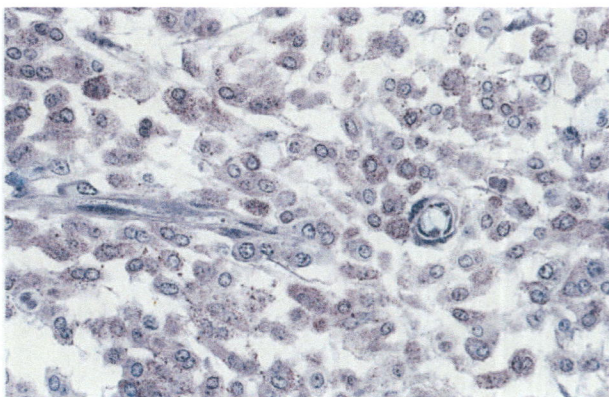

Fig. 16.35 Aggregate of crystal-containing macrophages in mast cell granuloma consisting mainly of spindle-shaped mast cells with variable granulation, and granulocytes. Giemsa

Fig. 16.36 Iliac crest biopsy of patient with systemic mastocytosis who developed acute leukaemia. Giemsa

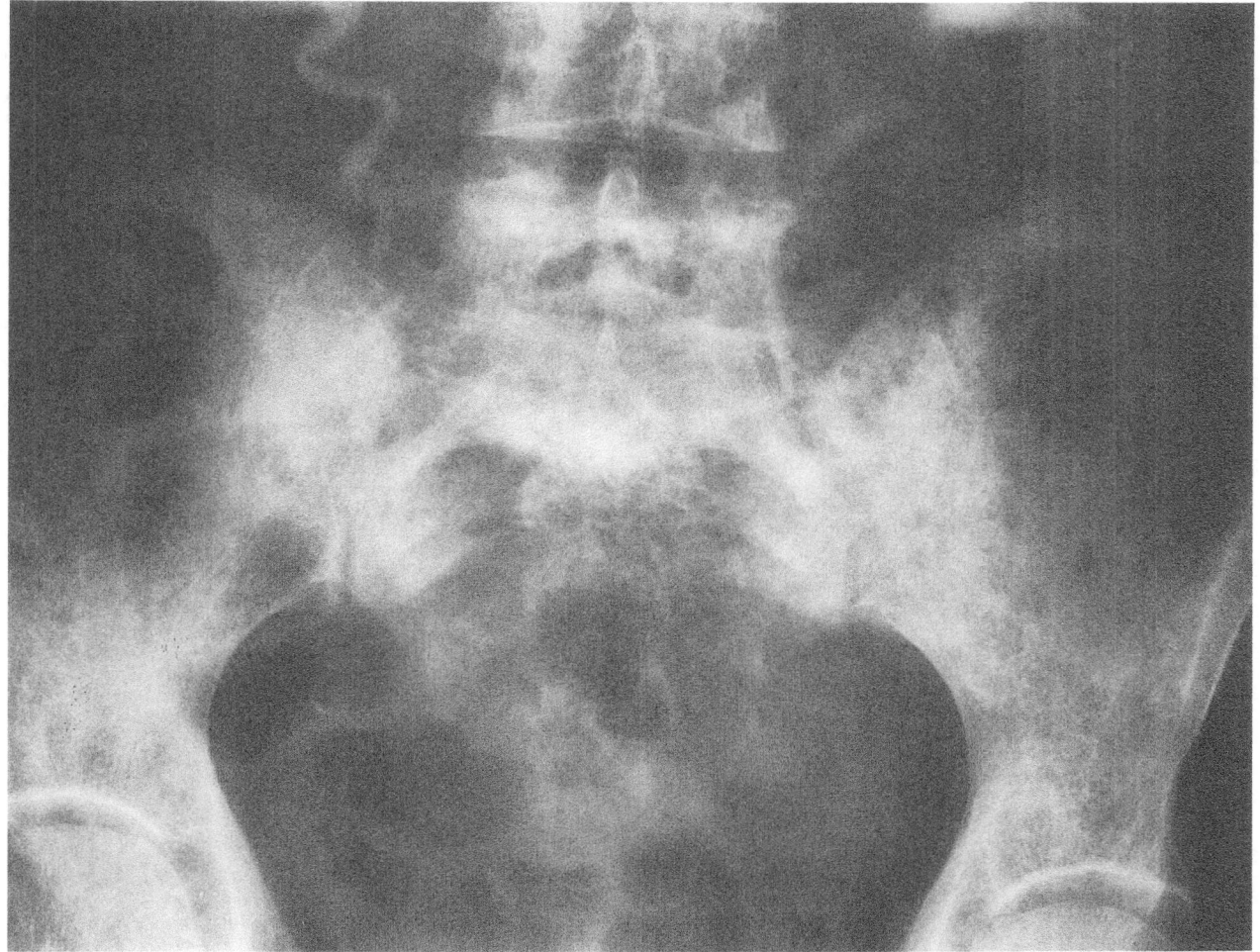

Fig. 16.R1 Systemic mastocytosis, with diffuse involvement of the spine and pelvis showing a mixed pattern of osteosclerosis and osteopenia. X-ray kindly supplied by Dr F. Weigert

References

1. Asboe-Hansen G. (1973). The mast cell in health and disease. *Acta Dermatol. (Stockholm)*, **73S**, 139
2. Austen K. F. (1992). Systemic mastocytosis. *N. Engl. J. Med.*, **326**, 639
3. Barer M., Peterson L. F. A., Dahlin D. C., Winkelmann R. K. and Stewart J. R. (1968). Mastocytosis with osseous lesions resembling metastatic malignant lesions in bone. *J. Bone Jt Surg.*, **50A**, 142
4. Bartl R., Frisch B. and Burkhardt R. (1985). *Bone Marrow Biopsies Revisited: a New Dimension for Haematologic Malignancies*. Basel: Karger
5. Bartl R., Jäger H. G. and Burkhardt R. (1982). Mastocytosis – a disease with frequent bone marrow involvement. *Blut*, **45**, 230
6. Bowdler A. J. and Tullett G. L. (1960). Urticaria pigmentosa and polycythaemia vera, a case report. *Brit. Med. J.*, **1**, 396
7. Bressler R. B., Thompson H. L., Keffer J. M. and Metcalfe D. D. (1989). Inhibition of the growth of interleukin-3-dependent mast cells from murine bone marrow by recombinant granulocyte-macrophage colony stimulating factor. *J. Immunol.*, **143**, 135
8. Burkhardt R. Jäger K., Bartl R., Kettner G. and Sund M. (1984). Mastozytose im Knochenmark bei myeloproliferativen Krankheiten. *Verh. Dtsch. Ges. Pathol.*, **68**, 456
9. Cohen A. H. and Vogel J. M. (1972). Systemic mastocytosis and multiple carcinoma. *Mt Sinai J. Med.*, **39**, 365
10. Colver G. B., Dawber R. P. R., Smith R., Ryan T. J. and Wojnarowska F. (1985). Osteoporosis and mastocytosis with late appearance of urticaria pigmentosa. *J. Roy. Soc. Med.*, **78**, 866

11. Coser P., Quaglino D., DePasquale A. and Colombetti W. (1980). Cytobiological and clinical aspects of tissue mast cell leukaemia. *Brit. J. Haematol.*, **45**, 5
12. Dalton R., Chan L., Batten E. and Eridani S. (1986). Mast cell leukaemia: evidence for bone marrow origin of the pathological clone. *Brit. J. Haematol.*, **64**, 397
13. Dash S., Rao N. R., Deodhar S. D. and Varma N. (1991). Malignant mastocytosis and myelodysplastic syndrome. *Brit. J. Haematol.*, **79**, 530
14. Ellis H. A. and Peart K. M. (1976). Iliac bone marrow mast cells in relation to the renal osteodystrophy of patients treated by haemodialysis. *J. Clin. Pathol.*, **29**, 502
15. Fallon M. D., Whyte M. P., Craig R. B. and Teitelbaun S. L. (1983). Mast-cell proliferation in postmenopausal osteoporosis. *Calcif. Tissue Int.*, **35**, 29
16. Fallon M. D., Whyte M. P. and Teitelbaum S. L. (1981). Systemic mastocytosis associated with generalized osteopenia. *Hum. Pathol.*, **12**, 813
17. Fohlmeister I., Reber T. and Fischer R. (1985). Bone marrow mast cell reaction in preleukaemic myelodysplasia and in aplastic anaemia. *Virchows Arch. (Pathol. Anat.)*, **405**, 503
18. Frame B. and Nixon R. K. (1968). Bone marrow mast cells in osteoporosis and aging. *N. Engl. J. Med.*, **279**, 626
19. Frisch B. and Bartl R. (1990). *Atlas of Bone Marrow Pathology*. Dordrecht: Kluwer
20. Galli S. J. (1990). Biology of disease. New insights into 'The riddle of the mast cells': microenvironmental regulation of mast cell

development and phenotypic heterogeneity. *Lab. Invest.,* **62**, 5

21. Gordon J. R., Burd P. R. and Galli S. J. (1990). Mast cells as a source of multifunctional cytokines. *Immunol. Today,* **11**, 458

22. Harvard C. W. H. and Scott R. B. (1956). Urticaria pigmentosa with visceral and skeletal lesions. *Q. J. Med.,* **28**, 459

23. Hills E., Dunstan C. R. and Evans R. A. (1981). Bone metabolism in systemic mastocytosis. *J. Bone Jt Surg.,* **63A**, 665

24. Horny H. P., Ruck M., Wehrmann M. and Kaiserling A. (1990). Blood findings in generalized mastocytosis: evidence of frequent simultaneous occurrence of myeloproliferative disorders. *Brit. J. Haematol.,* **76**, 186

25. Katsuda S., Okada Y., Oda Y., Tanimoto K. and Takabatake S. (1987). Systemic mastocytosis without cutaneous involvement. *Acta Pathol. Jpn.,* **37**, 167

26. Kessler D. A., Langer R. S., Pless N. A. and Folkman J. (1976). Mast cells and tumor angiogenesis. *Int. J. Cancer,* **18**, 703

27. Kettelhut B. V. and Metcalfe D. D. (1991). Pediatric mastocytosis. *J. Invest. Dermatol.,* **96**, 15S

28. Kluin-Nelemans H. C., Jansen J. H., Breukelman H., Wolthers B. G., Kliun P. M., Kroon H. M. and Willemze R. (1992). Response to interferon alfa-2b in a patient with systemic mastocytosis. *N. Engl. J. Med.,* **326**, 619

29. Lawrence J. B., Friedman B. S., Travis W. D., Chinchilli V. M., Metcalfe D. D. and Gralnick H. R. (1991). Hematologic manifestations of systemic mast cell disease: a prospective study of laboratory and morphologic features and their relation to prognosis. *Amer. J. Med.,* **91**, 612

30. Lennert K. and Parwaresch R. (1979). Mast cells and mast cell neoplasia: a review. *Histopathology,* **3**, 349

31. McKenna M. J. and Frame B. (1985). The mast cell and bone. *Clin. Orthop. Rel. Res.,* **200**, 226

32. Metcalfe D. D. (1991). Classification and diagnosis of mastocytosis: current status. *J. Invest. Dermatol.,* **96**, 2S

33. Mezger J., Permanetter W., Gerhartz H., Bartl R., Bauchinger M., Schmetzer H. and Sauer H. (1990). Philadelphia chromosome-negative acute hematopoetic malignancy: ultrastructural, cytochemical and immunocytochemical evidence of mast cell and basophil differentiation. *Leukemia Res.,* **14**, 169

34. Parker R. I. (1991). Hematologic aspects of mastocytosis: II: Management of hematologic disorders in association with systemic mast cell disease. *J. Invest. Dermatol.,* **96**, 52S

35. Parwaresch M. R., Horny H. P. and Lennert K. (1985). Tissue mast cells in health and disease. *Pathol. Res. Pract.,* **179**, 439

36. Prococimer M. and Polliack A. (1981). Increased bone marrow mast cells in preleukemic syndromes, acute leukemia, and lymphoproliferative disorders. *Amer. J. Clin. Pathol.,* **75**, 34

37. Raffi M., Firooznia H., Golimbu C. and Balthazar E. (1983). Pathologic fracture in systemic mastocytosis. Radiographic spectrum and review of the literature. *Clin. Orthop.,* **180**, 260

38. Rebel A. and Malkani K. (1974). Fine structure of mast cells in iliac crest biopsies during renal osteodystrophy. *Pathol. Biol.,* **22**, 221

39. Ridell B., Olafsson J. H., Roupe G., Swolin B., Granerus G., Rödjer S. and Enerbäck L. (1986). The bone marrow in urticaria pigmentosa and systemic mastocytosis. *Arch. Dermatol.,* **122**, 422

40. Roberts L. J. and Oates J. A. (1991). Biochemical diagnosis of systemic mast cell disorders. *J. Invest. Dermatol.,* **96**, 19S

41. Roche W. R. (1986). The nature and significance of tumour-associated mast cells. *J. Pathol.,* **148**, 175

42. Rohner H. G., Bartl R., Klingmüller G., Kreysel H. W. and Geisler L. S. (1980). Die Mastozytose – eine Krankheit mit häufiger Systemisierung. *Therapiewoche,* **30**, 6773

43. Rohner H. G., Bartl R., Koischwitz D. and Rodermund O. E. (1982). Haut- und Knochenbefunde bei der Mastozytose. *Radiologe,* **22**, 545

44. Rosenbaum R. C., Frieri M. and Metcalfe D. D. (1984). Patterns of skeletal scintigraphy and their relationship to plasma and urinary histamine levels in systemic mastocytosis. *J. Nucl. Med.,* **25**, 859

45. Rosinus V. (1980). Spongiosasklerose bei systemischer Mastozytose. *Schweiz. Med. Wschr.,* **110**, 1980

46. Sagher F., Cohen C. and Schorr S. (1952). Concomitant bone changes in urticaria pigmentosa. *J. Invest. Dermatol.,* **18**, 425

47. Sagher F. and Even-Paz Z. (1967). *Mastocytosis and the Mast Cell.* Chicago: Year Book Medical Publishers

48. Sagher F., Liban E., Ungar H. and Schorr S. (1956). Urticaria pigmentosa with bone involvement. Mast cell aggregates in bones and myelosclerosis found at autopsy in a case dying of monocytic leukemia. *J. Invest. Dermatol.,* **27**, 355

49. Tharp M. D. (1985). The spectrum of mastocytosis. *Amer. J. Med. Sci.,* **289**, 119

50. Travis W. D., Li C.-Y. and Su W. P. D. (1985). Adult-onset urticaria pigmentosa and systemic mast cell disease. *Amer. J. Clin. Pathol.,* **84**, 710

51. Travis W. D., Li C. Y., Yam L. T., Bergsralh E. J. and Swee R. G. (1988). Significance of systemic mast cell disease with associated hematologic disorders. *Cancer,* **62**, 965

52. Travis W. D., Li C.-Y. and Bergstralh E. J. (1989). Solid and hematologic malignancies in 60 patients with systemic mast cell disease. *Arch. Pathol. Lab. Med.,* **113**, 365

53. Travis W. D., Li C.-Y., Bergstralh E. J., Yam L. T. and Swee R. G. (1988). Systemic mast cell disease: analysis of 58 cases and literature review. *Medicine,* **67**, 345

54. Udoji W. C. and Razavi S. A. (1975). Mast cells and myelofibrosis. *Amer. J. Clin. Pathol.,* **63**, 203

55. Webb T. A., Li C.-Y. and Yam L. T. (1982). Systemic mast cell disease: a clinical and hematopathologic study of 26 cases. *Cancer,* **49**, 927

56. Weidner N. and Austen K. F. (1991). Ultrastructural and immunohistochemical characterization of normal mast cells at multiple body sites. *J. Invest. Dermatol.,* **96**, 26S

57. Weigert F. and Bartl R. (1984). Diffuse Stammskelettveränderungen bei systemischer Mastozytose. *Fortschr. Röntgenstr.,* **3**, 353

58. Yoo D., Lessin L. S. and Jensen W. N. (1978). Bone marrow mast cells in lymphoproliferative disorders. *Ann. Intern. Med.,* **88**, 753

59. Yoo D. and Lessin L. S. (1982). Bone marrow mast cell content in preleukemic syndrome. *Amer. J. Med.,* **73**, 539

60. Zak F. G., Covey J. A. and Snodgrass J. J. (1957). Osseous lesions in urticaria pigmentosa. *N. Engl. J. Med.,* **256**, 56

Osteomyelosclerosis

17

The normal bone marrow has few fibres and these are found mainly in association with trabecular bone surfaces and blood vessels. *Fibrosis of the bone marrow* takes place in response to many different toxic, inflammatory, osteolytic and malignant processes and is always of collagen type III[1,18]. The basic disorders associated with bone marrow fibrosis are given in Table 17.1[27,45]. Fibrosis may occur in varying degrees of severity[7] and has been roughly divided into three grades[27] (Fig. 17.S1):

Table 17.1 Bone marrow fibrosis (grades II/III) and its basic disorders

Basic disorders	Patients
Haematological neoplasias	
Myeloproliferative disorders	1255
Acute/subacute leukaemias	80
Multiple myeloma	250
Non-Hodgkin's lymphomas	797
Hodgkin's disease	69
Metastatic cancer	
Breast	156
Prostate	51
Lung	32
Others	27
Unknown primaries	90
Inflammatory reactions	
Toxic	38
Infectious	8
Unknown	42
Osteopathies	
Paget's disease	102
Primary hyperparathyroidism	112
Myelodysplastic syndrome	43
Total	3152

Grade I: a diffuse increase in reticular fibres in the marrow parenchyma.
Grade II: both fine and patchy coarse fibrosis around megakaryocytes and vessels.
Grade III: widespread coarse fibrosis with replacement of haematopoiesis.

The median survivals of patients in the different groups were 54, 47 and 39 months, respectively; however, with no significant differences[3,4].

Morphological signs of chronic inflammation such as lymphocytes, lymphoid nodules, plasma cells, mast cells and oedema are always present. The ectatic sinusoids

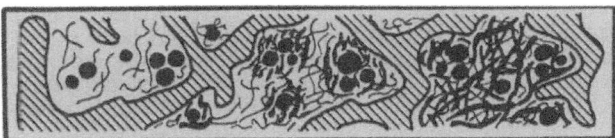

GRADE I GRADE II GRADE III

Fig. 17.S1 Degree of bone marrow fibrosis in MF/OMS. Grade I: Diffuse increase in fine fibres near megakaryocytic clusters. Grade II: Both fine and coarse fibrosis around megakaryocytes and vessels. Grade III: Widespread coarse fibrosis

show sclerotic walls, constituting a rigid blood–marrow barrier[4,24,27].

Reactive fibrosis[32] on the basis of a *myeloproliferative disorder* (MPD) is called *myelofibrosis* (MF) or, when primitive bone is present, *osteomyelosclerosis* (OMS)[5,10,11,28–30,53]. Variable amounts of this poorly mineralized bone (collagen type I) are randomly interwoven with the fibrous tissue (collagen type III) which occupies the intertrabecular cavities. The extent of overall osseous increase is variable even in the same biopsy, and *three grades* of bone sclerosis in OMS are distinguishable[27] (Fig. 17.S2):

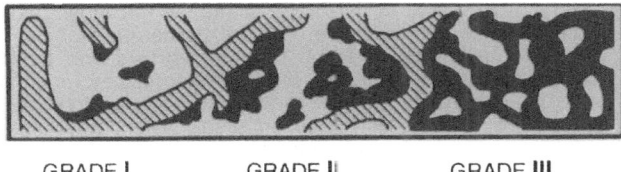

GRADE I GRADE II GRADE III

Fig. 17.S2 Degree of new bone formation in OMS. Grade I: Small foci of woven bone at site of increased trabecular appositional bone. Grade II: Increased appositional and woven bone in approximately equal proportions. Grade III: Almost complete replacement of normal trabecular architecture by a network of primitive bone

Grade I: small foci of primitive bone and slightly increased trabecular bone apposition.
Grade II: increased appositional and woven bone in approximately equal proportions.
Grade III: almost complete replacement of normal trabecular architecture by a network of poorly mineralized primitive bone.

There are usually more residual fat cells in OMS than in MF, though the latter has less remaining haematopoiesis[27]. OMS occurs more frequently in young patients and in females. There are differences in the clinical course and prognosis (more favourable in OMS, with median survivals of 59 and 56 months, respectively), in spite of the close pathogenic relationship between them[4]. MF and OMS represent qualitatively and quantitatively different modes of stromal reactions. On the basis of follow-up studies we were able to show that OMS is not necessarily an advanced state of MF[4,27].

Transformation to MF and OMS was observed in about half of the patients with MPD[28]. The basic myeloproliferative disorder was known in 70% of the patients with MF/OMS, but it could not be identified in the remaining 30%. The frequencies of the main underlying MPD in OMS patients were, with the frequencies in MF cases in parentheses: chronic myeloid leukaemia 39% (38%), polycythaemia vera 28% (35%) and idiopathic thrombocythaemia 8% (8%) (Fig. 17.S3). When still recognizable, the underlying myeloproliferative process, at least the basic clinical diagnosis, should be defined, e.g. 'OMS secondary to PV'[24,25,27]. The term 'idiopathic' OMS should be used only when the patients present the full-blown picture of OMS and no cause can be identified. Cases in the MPD with proliferation of megakaryocytes have a particular tendency to develop MF/OMS[25]. Generally the

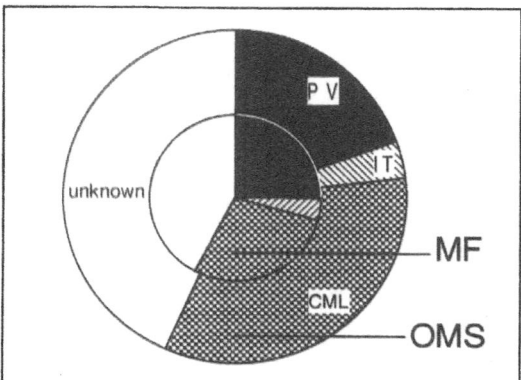

Fig. 17.S3 Underlying myeloproliferative disorders in MF and OMS in 2860 untreated patients at initial diagnosis

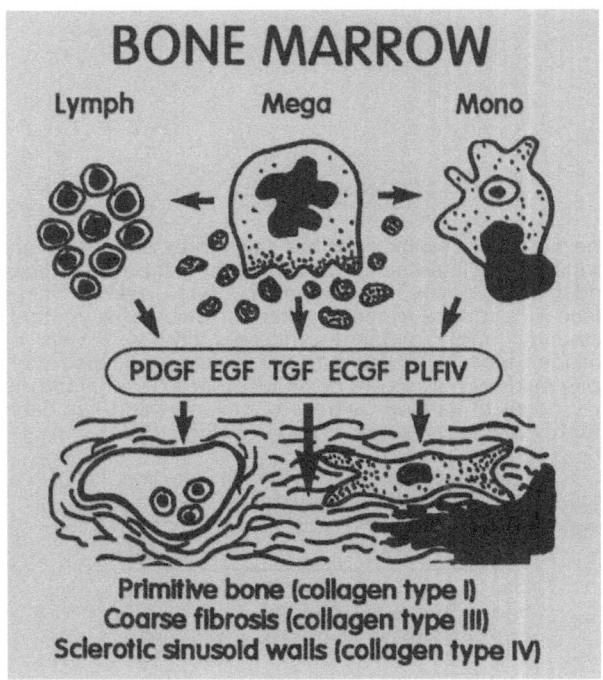

Fig. 17.S4 Illustration of the pathogenic mechanisms in MF/OMS: Interactions between heterotopic megakaryocytes, interstitially deposited platelets, monocytes and lymphoid nodules induce the production of various growth factors: e.g. platelet derived growth factor (PDGF), epidermal growth factor (EGF), transforming growth factor β (TGF), endothelial cell growth factor (ECGF) and platelet factor IV (PLF IV). All these growth factors induce fibroblast proliferation and fibrillogenesis: production of collagen type I (woven bone), type III (coarse fibres in the marrow spaces) and type IV (basement membrane material, sclerotic walls of the sinusoids)

development of fibrosis and of primitive bone runs a slowly progressive course over years[4]. A terminal blast crisis has been observed in a small percentage of both MF and OMS cases[4]. Bone marrow fibrosis and bone sclerosis, being dependent on the neoplastic clone, is potentially reversible if the clone is eradicated. However, the presence of fibrosis may adversely affect haematopoietic recovery after chemotherapy and bone marrow transplantation[44]. Apparently, sufficient time must elapse before resolution of the fibrosis (sclerosis) is accomplished, or the presence of the fibrous tissue prevents complete eradication of the neoplastic clone.

Acute (malignant) myelofibrosis (AMF) shows a rapidly progressive and fatal course, but it is only one extreme in the spectrum of 'idiopathic' myelofibrosis[9,42,43,55,58]. Three different histopathological forms were found in the bone biopsies of the 16 patients with clinical AMF: myelodysplastic (eight cases), blastic (six cases) and atrophic (two cases) types[43]. All biopsies investigated were characterized by infiltration of immature myeloid cells, though distributed in variable numbers and in variable topographic arrangement. We have also observed metamorphosis of a *myelodysplastic syndrome* (MDS), usually the MDS fibrotic type, directly to MF/OMS in 12 cases[6].

Three *pathogenic mechanisms* of bone marrow fibrosis (Figure 17.S4, Plates 17.A and B) have been proposed[27,33,34,37,38,58]:

1. A chronic inflammatory reaction mediated by circulating immune complexes[2,14,35], and evidenced by the presence of plasma cells, monocytes, mast cells and lymphocytes – all cells known to have the capacity to produce and secrete growth factors[31,50,56,59].
2. The production and release of the fibroblast-stimulating growth factor derived from megakaryocytes and platelets (platelet-derived growth factor, PDGF)[8,13,40,51] and of the collagenase inhibiting growth factor (platelet factor 4, PF4)[16].
3. The production of the transforming growth factor β (TGF-β), an important regulator of mesenchymal cell proliferation, differentiation, and synthesis of extracellular matrix[15,23,39,49,52].

In support of the second mechanism, deposition of platelets into the interstitium instead of into the sinusoids in areas of incipient fibrosis has been observed[4,11,12,17,19,20]. These mechanisms induce fibroblast proliferation and fibrillogenesis composed of collagen type III[21]. Follow-up studies including sequential biopsies emphasize the importance of megakaryocytes in MPD: the significance

of their number and maturity as well as their topographic arrangement[4,25,27].

The *histological picture of OMS* (Fig. 17.S5) is characterized by a diffuse network of coarse fibrosis accompanied by an increase of bone: appositional osteoblastic bone formation onto the pre-existing trabeculae and woven bone within the marrow spaces[4,14,27,29]. The main histomorphometric values (vol%) are given in Fig. 17.S6. In advanced stages of OMS the lamellar bone may be totally replaced by woven bone (Plate 17.C). Clusters of polymorphic megakaryocytes surrounded by fibres are located close to the sclerotic walls of ectatic sinusoids, or even in their lumina. Morphological signs of inflammation as described above are always present. Focal osteolytic lesions have also been observed, possibly due to local factors released by clusters of neoplastic myeloid cells in adjacent marrow spaces[36,41]. In some cases of OMS there were thick seams of unmineralized osteoid covered by mainly flat osteoblasts (osteomalacic variant). Indeed, an imbalance of vitamin D metabolites causing abnormal osseous remodelling in OMS has been postulated[22,46,47]. When osteoclasts are present they are more frequently observed on calcified bone[54]. Clusters of atypical megakaryocytes may be located at the bone surface, and possibly these also interfere with bone resorption.

The *radiological findings* reflect the pathological changes, and the pelvis, ribs, spine and proximal ends of femora and humeri are the most frequently affected skeletal sites (Fig. 17.R1). Diffuse osteoporosis may be the initial finding in the early stages, though zones of

[continued on p. 192]

Plate 17.A

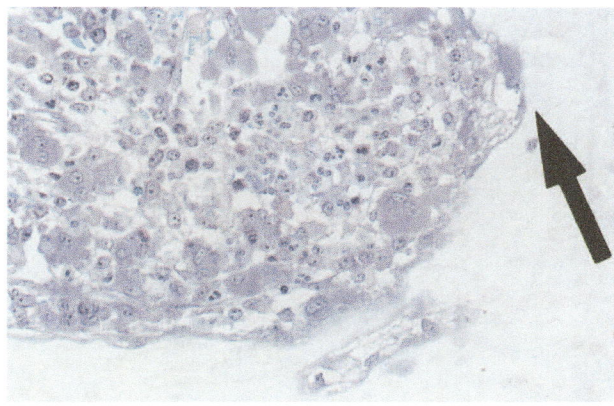

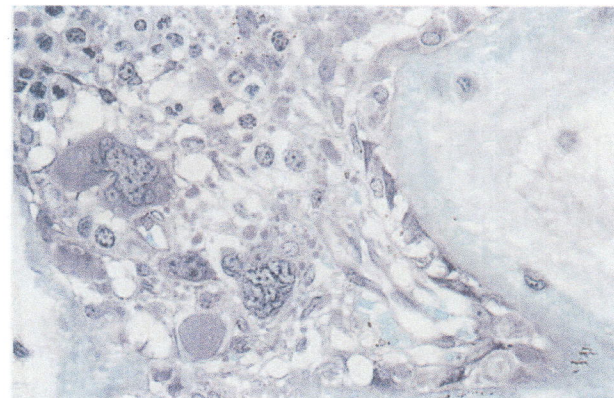

Figs. 17.1–17.6 Aspects of pathogenic mechanisms in osteomyelo-sclerosis (OMS)

Fig. 17.1 Uneven trabecular surface due to osteoclastic erosion (arrow). Note the neoplastic megakaryocytic proliferation, which is thought to be at least partly responsible for the reactive fibrosis and osteosclerosis in OMS. Giemsa

Fig. 17.2 Part of biopsy section showing loose connective tissue with atypical, polymorphous megakaryocytes, interstitial platelets and fibroblasts. Note osteoblastic appositional new bone formation (right). Giemsa

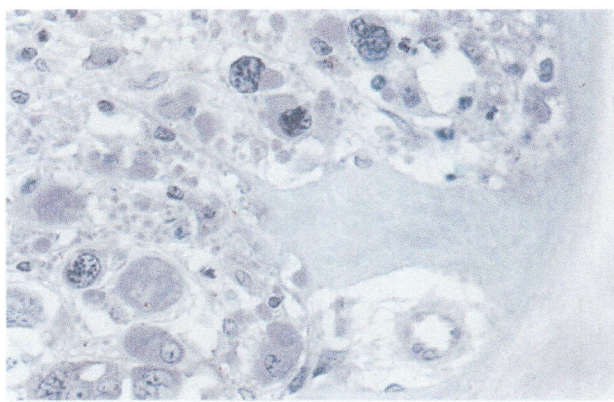

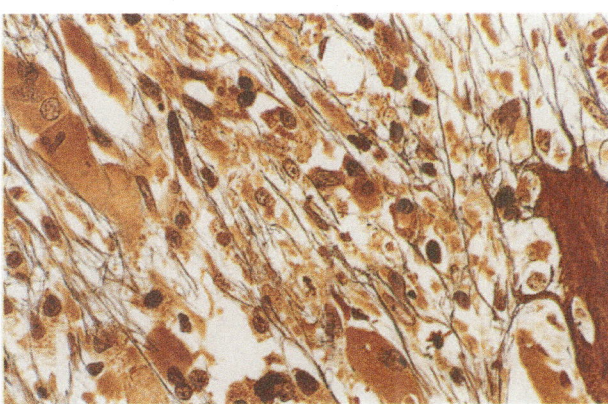

Fig. 17.3 Another part of section shown in Fig. 17.2. Note sprout of osteoid continuous with coarse collagenous fibres – example of development of woven bone in absence of osteoblasts. Atypical mega-karyocytes, fragments of megakaryocytic cytoplasm and platelets in the surrounding marrow. Giemsa

Fig. 17.4 Section of iliac crest biopsy in more advanced stage of OMS: hypercellular bone marrow with megakaryocytic hyperplasia and spicule of woven bone (right). Gomori

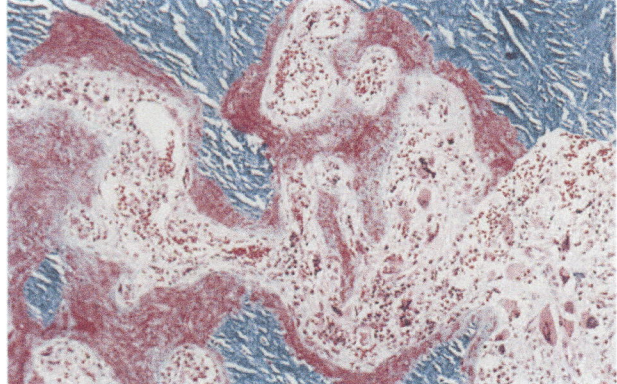

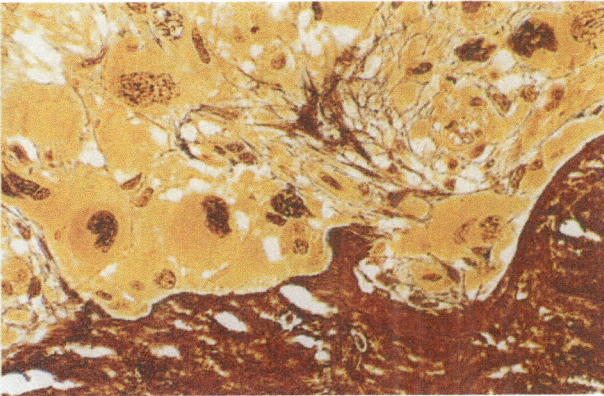

Fig. 17.5 Lower magnification of section shown in Fig. 17.4 demon-strating relatively large amount of unmineralized bone (red). Note decrease in marrow cellularity. Ladewig

Fig. 17.6 Large cluster of megakaryocytes at trabecular surface with ossifying coarse collagen fibres in the centre. Gomori

Plate 17.B

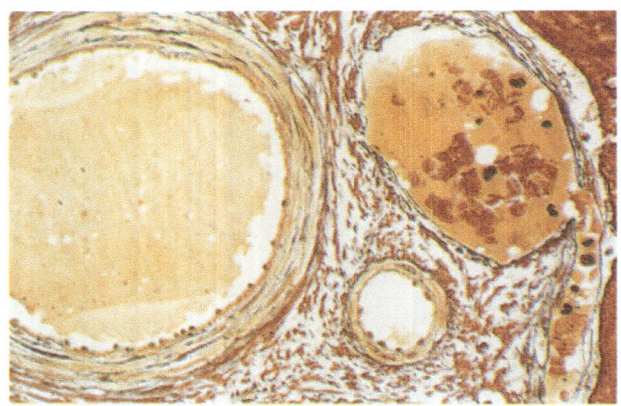

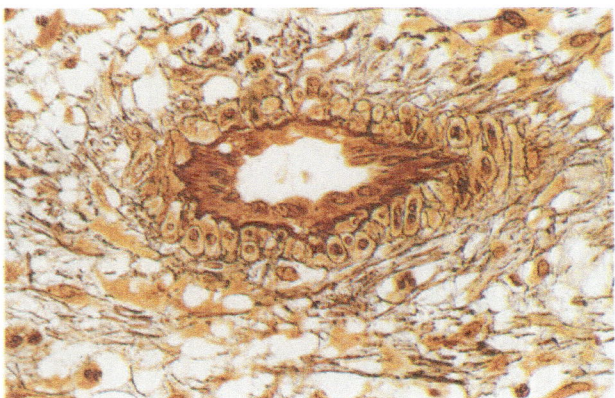

Figs. 17.7–17.12 Aspects of blood vessels in OMS

Fig. 17.7 Section of iliac crest biopsy showing unusually large artery in intertrabecular space, together with a smaller one and an endosteal sinusoid (upper right) and vein (upper right). Gomori

Fig. 17.8 Intertrabecular small artery with marked adventitial fibrosis and surrounding inflammatory reaction. Gomori

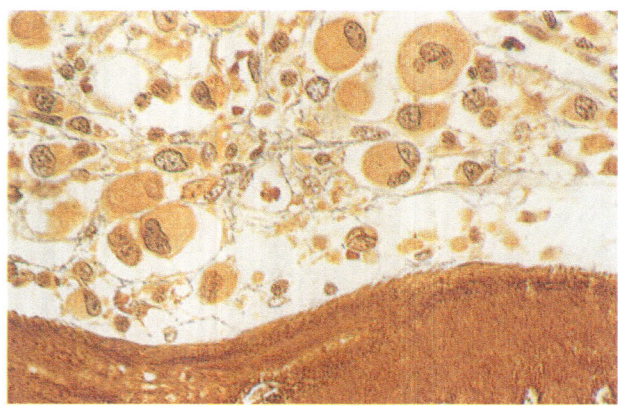

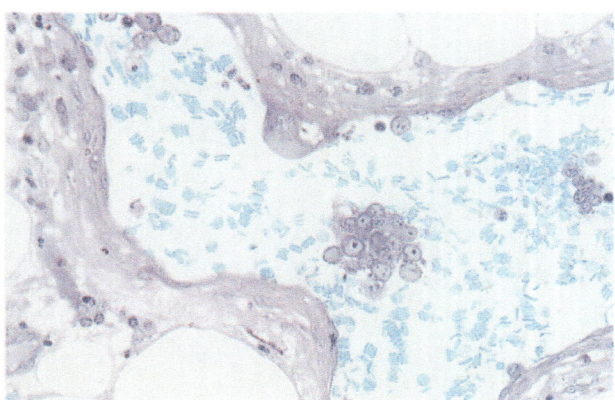

Fig. 17.9 Paratrabecular sinus with haematopoietic precursors in the lumen. Note numerous megakaryocytes at different maturation stages in the interstitium. Gomori

Fig. 17.10 High magnification of intertrabecular sinusoid with markedly sclerotic wall, and an erythron (=island of immature erythroid precursors) in the lumen. One megakaryocyte attached to the endothelium (upper centre). Intravascular haematopoiesis is a characteristic feature of OMS. Giemsa

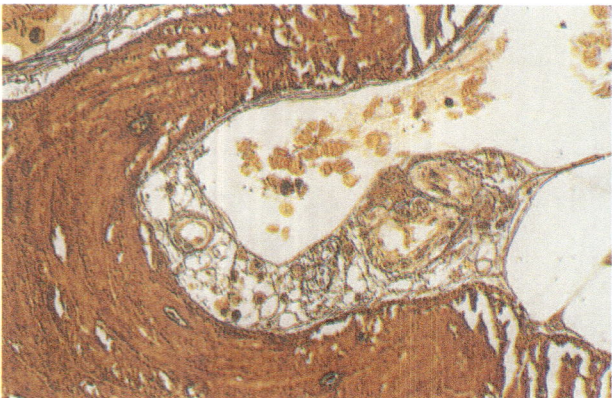

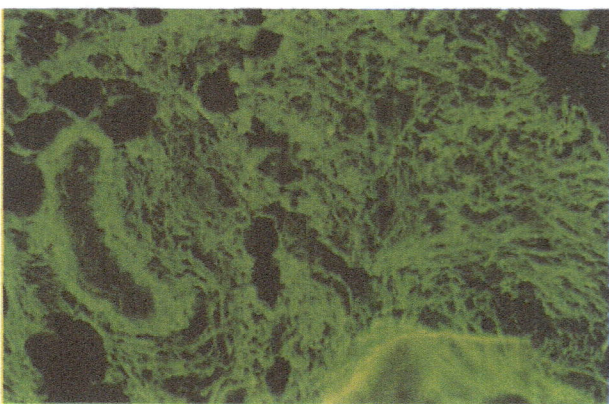

Fig. 17.11 The paratrabecular space is occupied almost entirely by variably sized blood vessels, reflecting the greatly increased bone marrow vascularity in OMS. Gomori

Fig. 17.12 Interstitial and vascular fibrosis composed of collagen type III. Cryostat section, immunofluorescence

Plate 17.C

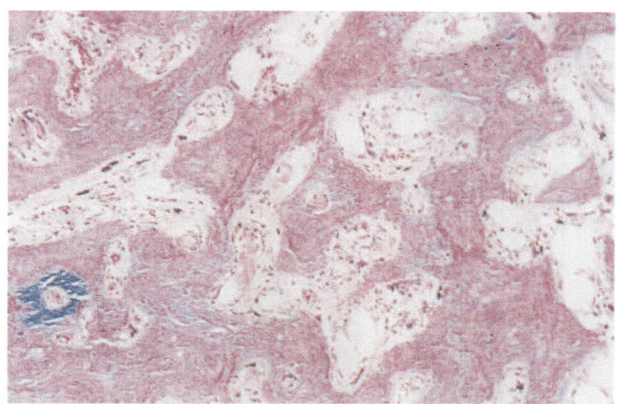

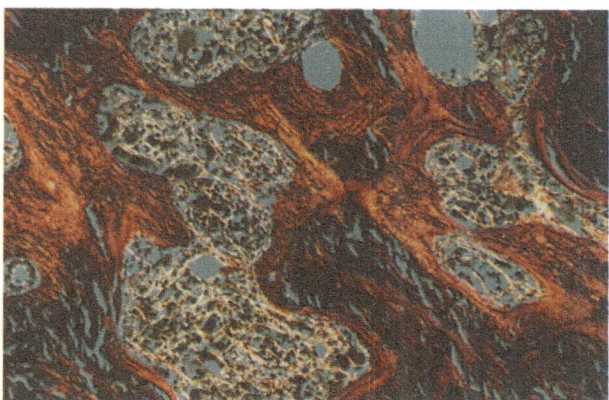

Figs. 17.13–17.18 Sections of iliac crest biopsies illustrating later stages of OMS

Fig. 17.13 Sclerotic area consisting entirely of osteoid, except for a small island of mineralized bone (blue) at left. Ladewig

Fig. 17.14 Another section of the biopsy in Fig. 17.13. Sclerosis of intertrabecular cavities with residual haematopoiesis, especially mega-karyocytes. Gomori, polar.

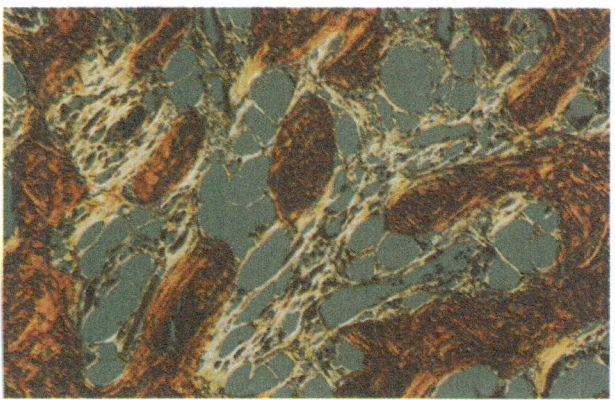

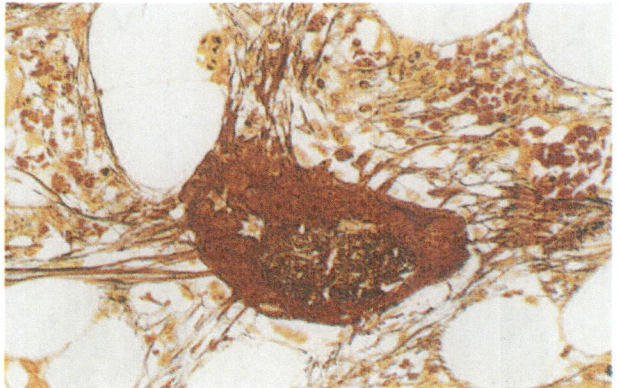

Figs. 17.15 and **17.16** Examples of 'burnt-out' OMS

Fig. 17.15 A network of fibres spans the empty marrow between the spicules of woven bone. Gomori, polar.

Fig. 17.16 Higher magnification of section in Fig. 17.15 demonstrating coarse collagen fibres radiating out from the island of woven bone which is surrounded by fat cells and blood vessels (atrophic arrow). Gomori

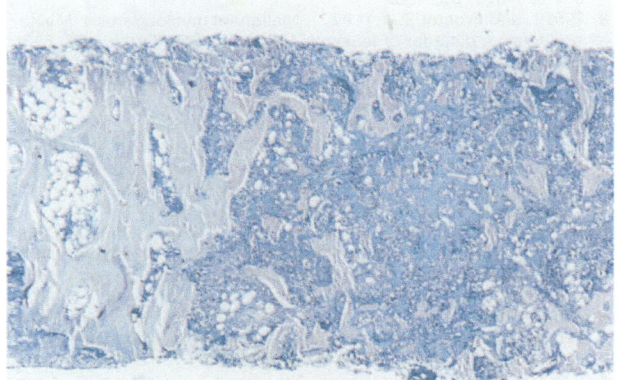

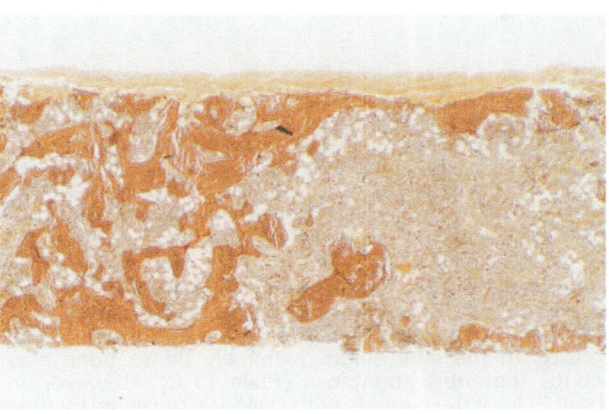

Fig. 17.17 Overview of iliac crest biopsy showing OMS with central focus exclusively consisting of newly formed woven bone (dark blue). Gomori

Fig. 17.18 Overview of iliac crest biopsy in OMS, an example of the extreme variability in bone density and architecture that may be encountered even in a single biopsy: osteosclerosis at left and osteolytic lesion at right. Gomori

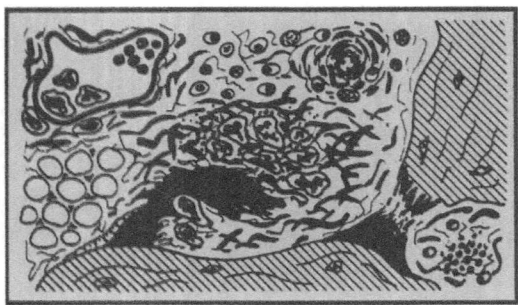

Fig. 17.S5 Histological criteria in OMS: (1) and (2) appositional and woven bone formation; periosseous clusters of megakaryocytes and interstitial platelets (centre); (3) ectatic sinusoids with sclerotic walls and intravascular haematopoiesis; (4) perivascular inflammatory infiltration and fibrosis; (5) inflammatory infiltrates of plasma cells, mast cells and lymphoid cells; (6) benign lymphoid nodules; and (7) variable increase in fat cells

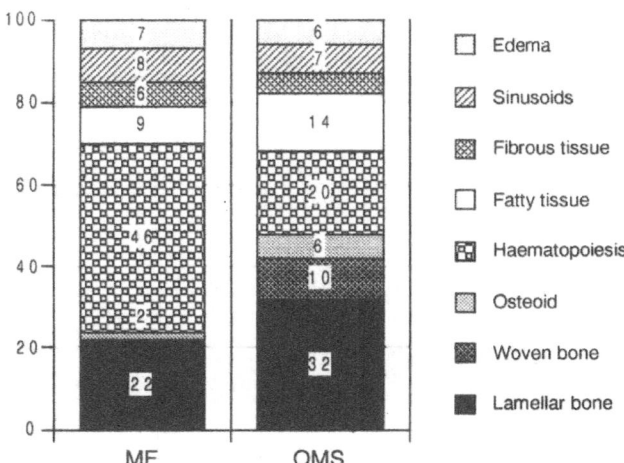

Fig. 17.S6 Histomorphometry of iliac crest biopsies in MF ($n = 100$) and OMS ($n = 100$)

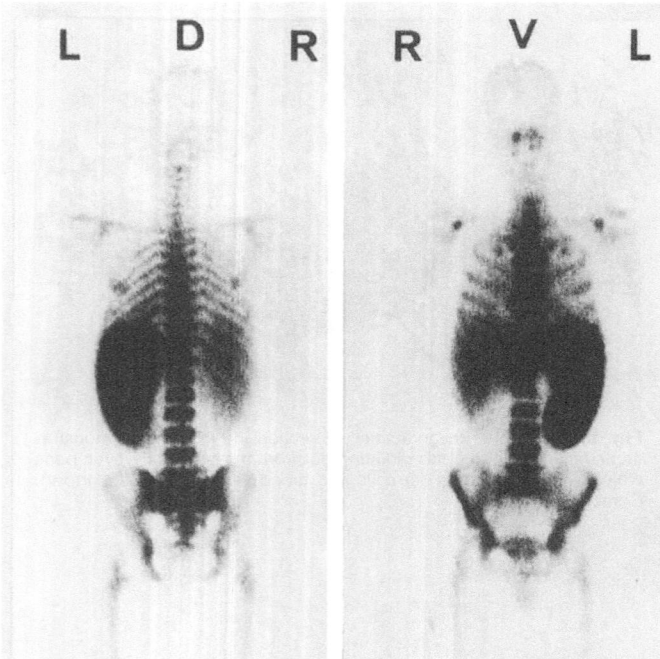

Fig. 17.R1 Bone marrow scintigraphy using ^{99m}Tc-labelled monoclonal antibodies against NCA 95 in a patient with 'post CML-myelofibrosis'. Note massively enlarged spleen and expansion of haematopoiesis to the proximal extremities. D = dorsal, V = ventral, R = right, L = left. (Kindly supplied by Dr C.-M. Kirsch, Division of Nuclear Medicine, Department of Radiology, Klinikum Großhadern, University of Munich)

radiolucent mottling corresponding to marrow fibrosis may also be observed. As new bone is deposited in the marrow cavities the radiographs show islands of increased density. In the later stages extremely dense bone may occupy the entire spongiosa (Plate 17.C). However, in about 30% of the patients with OMS we observed marked discrepancies between the considerable increase of poorly mineralized woven bone in the biopsy and the osseous changes on X-rays, i.e. histology not reflected in the radiographs.

References

1. Apaja-Sarkkinen M., Autio-Harmainen H., Alavaikko M., Risteli J. and Risteli L. (1986). Immunohistochemical study of basement membrane proteins and type III procollagen in myelofibrosis. *Brit. J. Haematol.*, **63**, 571
2. Baglin T. P., Simpson A. W., Price S. M. and Boughton B. J. (1987). Composition of immune complexes and their relation to plasma fibronectin in chronic myeloproliferative disorders. *J. Clin. Pathol.*, **49**, 1468
3. Bartl R., Burkhardt R., Frisch B. and Schlag R. (1982). Prognosis of bone marrow fibrosis in haematologic malignancies. Levy E., *Advances in Pathology*, vol. 1 (p. 425). Oxford: Pergamon Press
4. Bartl R., Frisch B. and Burkhardt R. (1985). *Bone Marrow Biopsies Revisited. A New Dimension for Haematologic Malignancies*. Basel: Karger
5. Bartl R., Frisch B. and Burkhardt R. (1991). Bone marrow histology. Catovsky D., *Methods in Hematology: The Leukemic Cell*, 2nd edn. (p. 47). Edinburgh: Churchill Livingstone
6. Bartl R., Frisch B. and Baumgart R. (1992). Morphologic classification of the myelodysplastic syndromes (MDS): combined utilisation of bone marrow aspirates and trephine biopsies. *Leukemia Res.*, **16**(1), 15
7. Bentley S. A. and Herman C. J. (1979). Bone marrow fiber production in myelofibrosis: a quantitative study. *Brit. J. Haematol.*, **42**, 51
8. Bernabei P. A., Arcangeli A., Casini M., Grossi A., Padovani R. and Rossi-Ferreni P. (1986). Platelet-derived growth factor(s) mitogenic activity in patients with myeloproliferative disease. *Brit. J. Haematol.*, **63**, 483
9. Bird T. and Proctor S. J. (1977). Malignant myelosclerosis. Myeloproliferative disorder of leukemia? *Amer. J. Clin. Pathol.*, **67**, 512
10. Burkhardt R., Bartl R., Jäger K., Frisch B., Kettner G., Mahl G. and Sund M. (1984). Chronic myeloproliferative disorders (CMPD). *Pathol. Res. Pract.*, **179**, 131
11. Burkhardt R., Bartl R., Beil E., Demmler K., Hoffmann E., Kronseder A., Langegger H., Saar U., Ulrich M. and Wiemann H. (1975). Myelofibrosis-osteosclerosis syndrome. Review of literature and histomorphometry. *Advances in the Biosciences*, vol. 16 (p. 9). Oxford/Braunschweig: Pergamon Press/Vieweg
12. Burkhardt R., Bartl R., Jäger K., Frisch B., Kettner G., Mahl G. and Sund M. (1986). Working classification of chronic myeloproliferative disorders based on histological, haematological, and clinical findings. *J. Clin. Pathol.*, **39**, 237
13. Burstein S. A., Malpass T. W. and Yee E. (1984). Platelet factor-4 excretion in myeloproliferative disease: implications for the aetiology of myelofibrosis. *Brit. J. Haematol.*, **57**, 383
14. Caligaris-Cappio F., Vigliani R., Novariono A., Camussi G., Campana D. and Gavosto F. (1981). Idiopathic myelofibrosis: a possible role for immune-complexes in the pathogenesis of bone marrow fibrosis. *Brit. J. Haematol.*, **49**, 17
15. Canalis E., McCarthy T. and Centrella M. (1988). Growth factors and the regulation of bone remodeling. *J. Clin. Invest.*, **81**, 277

16. Castro-Malaspina H. (1984). Pathogenesis of myelofibrosis: role of ineffective megakaryopoiesis and megakaryocyte components. Berk P. D., Castro-Malaspina H. and Wasserman L. R., *Myelofibrosis and the Biology of the Connective Tissue* (p. 427). New York: Alan R. Liss

17. Castro-Malaspina H. and Moore M. A. S. (1982). Pathophysiological mechanisms operating in the development of myelofibrosis: role of the megakaryocytes. *Nouv. Rev. Franc. Haematol.*, **24**, 221

18. Charron D., Robert L., Couty M. C. and Binet J. L. (1979). Biochemical and histological analysis of bone marrow collagen in myelofibrosis. *Brit. J. Haematol.*, **41**, 151

19. Chauvet M., Hollard D., Cousin F. and Leger J. (1987). Myelofibrosis. Pathology of the microenvironment. *Nouv. Rev. Franc. Haematol.*, **29**, 119

20. Deschamps J. F. and Caen J. P. (1984). Abnormal megakaryocyte release and myelofibrosis. *Lancet*, **1**, 567

21. Ellis J. T. and Peterson P. (1984). Myelofibrosis in the myeloproliferative disorders. Berk R. D., Castro-Malaspina H., Wasserman L. R., *Myelofibrosis and the Biology of Connective Tissue* (p. 19). New York: Alan R. Liss

22. Eugster C., BrunDelRe G. P. and Bucher U. (1987). The role of 1,25-di-hydroxyvitamin D3 (1,25 (OH)2D3) in the treatment of idiopathic myelofibrosis, **65**, 381

23. Fava R. A., Casey T. T., Wicox J., Pelton R. W., Moses H. L. and Nanney L. B. (1990). Synthesis of transforming growth factor-β1 by megakaryocytes and its localization to megakaryocyte and platelet alpha-granules. *Blood*, **76**, 1946

24. Frisch B. and Bartl R. (1990). *Atlas of Bone Marrow Pathology*. Dordrecht: Kluwer

25. Frisch B., Bartl R., Burkhardt R., Jäger K., Mahl G. and Kettner G. (1984). Classification of myeloproliferative disorders by bone marrow histology. Frisch B. and Bartl R., *Bone Marrow Biopsies Updated. New Prospects for Clinical Diagnostics*. Basel: Karger

26. Frisch B., Bartl R., Burkhardt R. and Jäger K. (1984). Histologic criteria for classification and differential diagnosis of chronic myeloproliferative disorders. *Haematologia*, **17**, 209

27. Frisch B. and Bartl R. (1985). Histology of myelofibrosis and osteomyelosclerosis. Lewis S. M., *Myelofibrosis* (p. 51). New York: Marcel Dekker

28. Frisch B., Bartl R. and Jäger K. (1989). Histologic diagnosis of chronic myeloproliferative disorders. *Hematol. Rev.*, **3**, 131

29. Frisch B., Lewis S. M., Burkhardt R. and Bartl R. (1985). *Biopsy Pathology of Bone and Bone Marrow*. London: Chapman & Hall

30. Georgii A., Vykoupil K. F. and Thiele J. (1984). Classification of chronic myeloproliferative diseases by bone marrow biopsies. Hematological and cytogenetic findings and clinical course. Frisch B. and Bartl R., *Bone Marrow Biopsies Updated. New Prospects for Clinical Diagnostics* (p. 41). Basel: Karger

31. Gordon B. R., Coleman M., Kohen P. and Day N. K. (1981). Immunologic abnormalities in myelofibrosis with activation of the complement system. *Blood*, **58**, 904

32. Greenberg B. R., Woo L. and Veomett I. C. (1987). Cytogenetics of bone marrow fibroblastic cells in idiopathic chronic myelofibrosis. *Brit. J. Haematol.*, **66**, 487

33. Groopman J. E. (1980). The pathogenesis of myelofibrosis in myeloproliferative disorders. *Ann. Intern. Med.*, **92**, 857

34. Hasselbalch H. (1990). Idiopathic myelofibrosis: a review. *Europ. J. Haematol.*, **45**, 65

35. Hasselbalch H., Nielsen H., Berild D. and Kappelgaard E. (1985). Circulating immune complexes in myelofibrosis. *Scand. J. Haematol.*, **34**, 177

36. Herrera A., Urbanitz D., Rossner A., Lingg G. and Grundmann E. (1986). Case report 402: megakaryocytic myelosis with disseminated osteolysis and osteomyelosclerosis. *Skeletal Radiol.*, **15**, 672

37. Hunstein W. (1975). Experimental myelofibrosis. *Clin. Haematol.*, **11**, 457

38. Jacobson R. J., Salo A. and Fialkow P. J. (1978). Agnogenic myeloid metaplasia: a clonal proliferation of hematopoietic stem cells with secondary myelofibrosis. *Blood*, **51**, 189

39. Joyce M. E., Jingushi S. and Bolander M. E. (1990). Transforming growth factor-β in the regulation of fracture repair. *Orthop. Clin. N. Amer.*, **21** (1), 199

40. Kimura A., Katoh O. and Kuramoto A. (1988). Effects of platelet derived growth factor, epidermal growth factor and transforming growth factor-β on the growth of human marrow fibroblasts. *Brit. J. Haematol.*, **69**, 1

41. Kosmidis P. A., Palacas C. G. and Axelrod A. R. (1980). Diffuse purely osteolytic lesions in myelofibrosis. *Cancer*, **46**, 2263

42. Lohman T. P. and Beckman E. N. (1983). Progressive myelofibrosis in agnogenic myeloid metaplasia. *Arch. Pathol. Lab. Med.*, **107**, 593

43. Mahl G., Frisch B., Bartl R., Jäger K., Pappenberger R., Schlag R. and Burkhardt R. (1984). Acute myelofibrosis: only one extreme in the spectrum of 'idiopathic' myelofibrosis. Lennert K. and Hübner K., *Pathology of the Bone Marrow* (p. 206). Stuttgart: G. Fischer

44. McGlave P. B., Brunning R. D., Hurdand D. D. and Kim T. H. (1982). Reversal of severe bone marrow fibrosis and osteosclerosis following allogeneic bone marrow transplantation for chronic granulocytic leukaemia. *Brit. J. Haematol.*, **52**, 189

45. McCarthy D. M. (1985). Fibrosis of the bone marrow: content and causes (Annotation). *Brit. J. Haematol.*, **59**, 1

46. McCarthy D. M., Hibbin J. A. and Goldman J. M. (1984). A role for 1,25-dihydroxyvitamin D3 in control of bone-marrow collagen deposition? *Lancet*, **1**, 78

47. McKinley R., Kwan Y. L., Ford D. Lam-Po-Yang P. R., Mason R. S. and Manoharan A. (1987). Clinical and laboratory studies of 1,25-dihydroxycholecalciferol in myelofibrosis. *Brit. J. Haematol.*, **65**, 245

48. Moore M. A. S. (1982). Pathogenesis of myelofibrosis. Hoffbrand A. V., *Recent Advances in Haematology* (p. 136). Edinburgh: Churchill Livingstone

49. Roberts A. B., Sporn M. B. and Assoian R. K. (1986). Transforming growth factor-β: rapid induction of fibrosis and angiogenesis in vivo and stimulation of collagen formation in vitro. *Proc. Natl. Acad. Sci. USA*, **83**, 4167

50. Rondeau E., Solal-Celigny P. and Dhermy D. (1983). Immune disorders in agnogenic myeloid metaplasia: relations to myelofibrosis. *Brit. J. Haematol.*, **53**, 467

51. Ross R. and Vogel A. (1978). The platelet-derived growth factor. *Cell*, **14**, 203

52. Seyer J. M. (1985). Mediators of increased collagen synthesis in fibrosing organs. *Fund. Appl. Toxicol.*, **5**, 228

53. Smith R. E., Chelmowski M. K. and Szabo E. J. (1988). Myelofibrosis: a concise review of clinical and pathologic features and treatment. *Amer. J. Hematol.*, **29**, 74

54. Thiele J., Hoeppner B., Wienhold S., Schneider G., Fischer R. and Zankovich R. (1989). Osteoclasts and bone remodeling in chronic myeloproliferative disorders. *Pathol. Res. Pract.*, **184**, 591

55. Thiele J., Krech R., Vykoupil K. F. and Georgii A. (1984). Malignant (acute) myelosclerosis – a clinical and pathological study in 6 patients. *Scand. J. Haematol.*, **33**, 95

56. Thiele J., Rompcik V., Wagner S. and Fischer R. (1992). Vascular architecture and collagen type IV in primary myelofibrosis and polycythaemia vera: an immunomorphometric study on trephine biopsies of the bone marrow. *Brit. J. Haematol.*, **80**, 227

57. Thiele J., Simon K. G., Fischer R. and Zankowich R. (1988). Follow-up studies with sequential bone marrow biopsies in chronic myeloid leukaemia and so-called (idiopathic) osteomyelofibrosis. Evolution of histopathological lesions and clinical course in 40 patients. *Pathol. Res. Pract.*, **183**, 434

58. Truong L. D., Saleem A. and Schwartz M. R. (1984). Acute myelofibrosis. A report of four cases and review of the literature. *Medicine*, **63**, 182

59. Udoji W. C. and AliRazavi S. (1975). Mast cells and myelofibrosis. *Amer. J. Clin. Pathol.*, **63**, 203

Multiple myeloma

18

The spectrum of plasma cell dyscrasias varies in severity and prognosis from benign (stable) to malignant (progressive). The benign type is best described as *'monoclonal gammopathy of unknown significance'* (MGUS), which denotes the presence of a stable monoclonal protein (M-protein) in the absence of bone lesions, anaemia and hypercalcaemia[41,44]. The term 'benign monoclonal gammopathy' (BMG) is inappropriate because at initial diagnosis it is not known whether the M-protein will remain stable or will develop to a lymphoproliferative disease. Bone biopsy reveals no characteristic features in MGUS patients. The number of plasma cells may be increased, but only in patients with underlying inflammatory disorders. Histomorphometrically bone mass, trabecular structure, mineralization and osseous remodelling are all within normal ranges[4,5]. The incidence of MGUS increases with advancing age; it is present in about 4% of individuals over 80 years[2,44]. Furthermore, patients with connective tissue diseases, chronic inflammatory disorders, Paget's disease and Gaucher's disease have a higher risk of developing MGUS. Approximately 15–30% of patients with MGUS develop multiple myeloma or related diseases after approximately 10 years of follow-up, indicating a premyelomatous rather than a 'benign' condition[41,44].

Multiple myeloma (MM) is a malignant neoplasm of plasma cells with a broad spectrum of initial presentations (Fig. 18.S1)[3,7,9,22,23,43,46,53]. Solitary extramedullary plasmacytomas tend to remain localized and some cases are healed by local treatment. In contrast, many of the so-called solitary plasmacytomas of bone appear to represent early stages of generalized MM – thus a bone biopsy is indicated for early recognition of dissemination[1,4,9,10,33]. Although a few patients with osteolyses had no involvement in the iliac crest biopsy at initial investigation, follow-up bone biopsies revealed a nodular growth pattern (multifocal MM)[9,10]. However, most MM patients show widespread dissemination in the skeleton from the start (myelomatosis), evidenced by the interstitial growth

pattern[9]. It has been proposed that MM is disseminated by circulating clonogenic cells that home to the bone marrow, and that bone marrow stromal cells are involved in supporting the growth of B lymphocytes, plasma cells and osteoclasts, and the spread of MM[18].

It is astonishing that the *morphological diagnosis of MM*, the most frequent primary malignancy of bone, is still based on arbitrarily defined percentages of aspirated plasma cells[4,29,43,46], in spite of the fact that equal or even much higher numbers of plasma cells may be present in non-malignant conditions (reactive plasmacytosis). In bone biopsies topographic characteristics in particular proved to be more reliable in differential diagnosis. The main histological criteria for distinguishing minimal neoplastic plasma cell infiltration from *reactive plasmacytosis* are given in Fig. 18.S2)[7]. Moreover, a *morphological classification of MM* has not yet been widely adopted, though many authors have described plasmacytomas with different features and prognoses[6,9,17,32,43,46]. MM may be divided into six histological types (Fig. 18.S3):

1. Marschalko type (59% of the cases, median survival of 38 months);
2. small cell type (11%, 44 months);
3. cleaved type (8%, 18 months);
4. polymorphous type (9%, 20 months);
5. asynchronous type (10%, 19 months); and
6. blastic type (2%, 8 months).

These types may be combined into *three prognostic grades*, comparable to the malignant lymphomas: MM of low (71%, 40 months), intermediate (28%, 20 months) and high grade malignancy (2%, 8 months)[9,28]. Bone biopsy also provides information on *tumour cell burden*, i.e. quantity of infiltration in the bone marrow biopsy corresponding to the histological stage of MM (Figs 18.S4 and 5), and *tumour growth* (Fig. 18.S6), which proved to be important and independent prognostic parameters[4–10]. Furthermore it permits early identification of patients with smouldering MM, which should not be treated[9,10,42].

A characteristic feature of MM is *skeletal destruction*[43,46], which also accounts for many of its troublesome complications such as bone pain, pathological fractures, hypercalcaemia and renal damage[22,43,46]. Seventy per cent

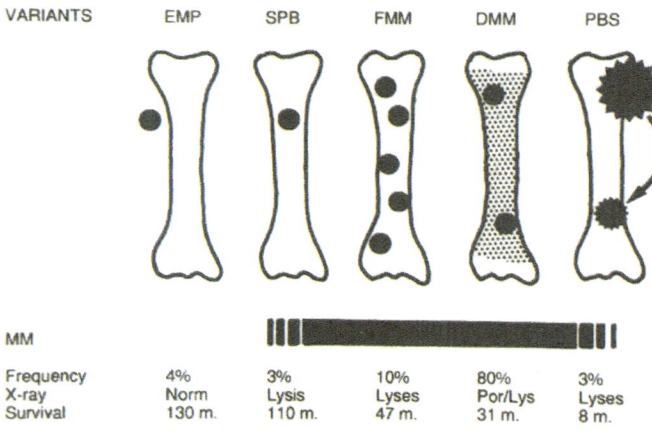

VARIANTS	EMP	SPB	FMM	DMM	PBS
MM					
Frequency	4%	3%	10%	80%	3%
X-ray	Norm	Lysis	Lyses	Por/Lys	Lyses
Survival	130 m.	110 m.	47 m.	31 m.	8 m.

Fig. 18.S1 Types of plasmacellular neoplasias and their skeletal manifestations[20]. EMP = extramedullary plasmocytoma; SPB = solitary plasmocytoma of bone; FMM = multifocal myelomatosis; DMM = diffuse myelomatosis; PBS = plasmablastic sarcoma

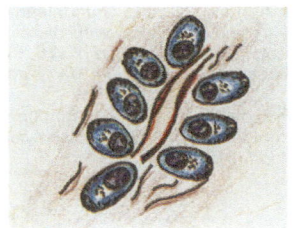

Reactive plasmacytosis

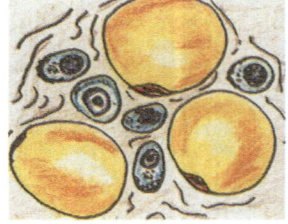

Neoplastic plasmacytosis

Fig. 18.S2 Diagram depicting topographic significance of reactive and neoplastic plasmacytosis as well as illustrating the cytological differences between the two groups of plasma cells

TYPE   GRADE

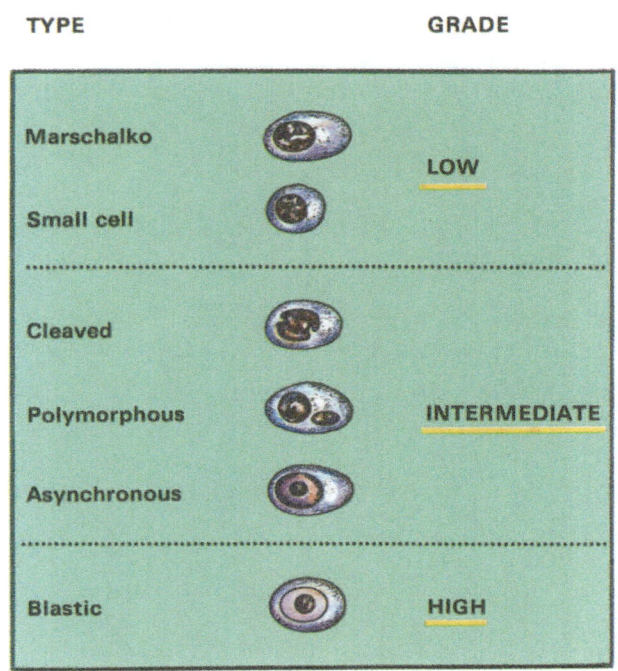

Fig. 18.S3 Histological classification of MM grouped into three grades of malignancy, analogous to the malignant lymphomas

of patients with MM present with bone pain as their major complaint, which is also the most persistent symptom most patients suffer from. Abnormal skeletal radiographs are found in 80% or more of patients at diagnosis[25]. In fact, if skeletal lesions are not present the diagnosis of MM may be difficult to establish. Characteristically, skeletal surveys show multiple *punched-out osteolytic lesions* involving sites of red marrow (e.g. ribs, sternum, vertebrae, skull, pelvic girdle)[25]. The lesions vary in size from a diameter of 1–2 mm to areas as large as 10 cm, with no radiological evidence of osteoblastic bone formation at the margins (Figs 18.R1–3). Ultimately, the small lesions

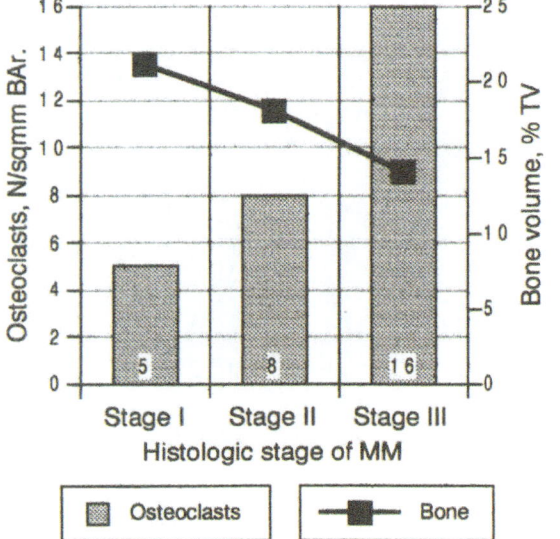

Fig. 18.S4 Correlation of histological stage of MM with osteoclastic resorption. Stage I: <20 vol% plasma cells in the biopsy; stage II: 20–50 vol%; stage III: >50 vol%

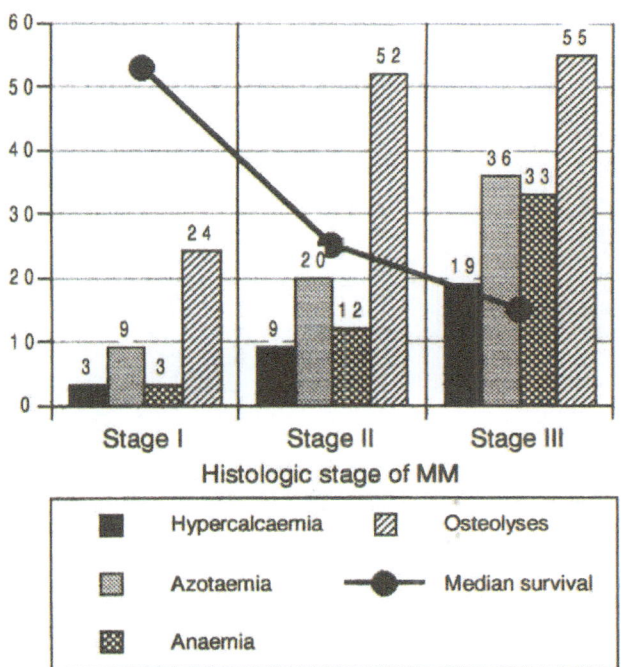

Fig. 18.S5 Correlation of histological stage of MM with clinical and prognosis parameters (% and months, respectively)

extend and coalesce until both cortical and trabecular bone in the whole area is destroyed. *Generalized osteopenia* with or without lytic lesions is seen in 60% of patients at diagnosis, and represents the sole skeletal abnormality found in up to 20% of patients. In smouldering MM osteoporosis without any lytic lesions was present in 40% of the cases. Osteopenia in MM is similar to that seen in senile or postmenopausal osteoporosis, and in both types pathological fractures of the vertebral bodies are common. *Osteosclerotic MM* occurs in less than 1% of patients with MM[21]. It is often associated with peripheral neuropathy, organomegaly, endocrinopathy, *M protein* and skin changes (POEMS syndrome). In two patients with sclerotic MM and thrombocytosis bone biopsy revealed the coexistence of a megakaryocytic myelosis accompanied by an osteomyelosclerotic reaction. Sclerosis sometimes occurs after chemotherapy, radiation, and also when MM is complicated by amyloidosis, Paget's disease, Gaucher's disease, metastatic bone disease or chronic MPD.

Standard radiographic skeletal survey is still the best diagnostic way to evaluate the presence and distribution of bone lesions in patients with MM[25]. Magnetic resonance imaging (MRI) and computed tomography (CT)

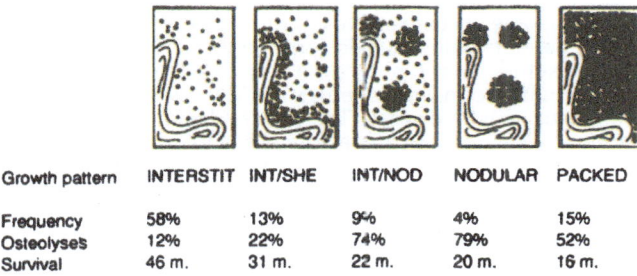

Growth pattern	INTERSTIT	INT/SHE	INT/NOD	NODULAR	PACKED
Frequency	58%	13%	9%	4%	15%
Osteolyses	12%	22%	74%	79%	52%
Survival	46 m.	31 m.	22 m.	20 m.	16 m.

Fig. 18.S6 Growth patterns of MM in iliac crest biopsies, their frequencies, X-ray manifestations and associated median survivals

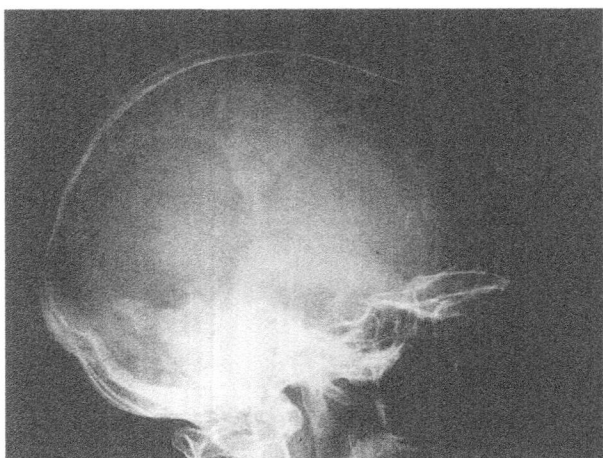

Fig. 18.R1 X-ray of skull showing large, well-circumscribed osteolytic lesions in a patient with MM

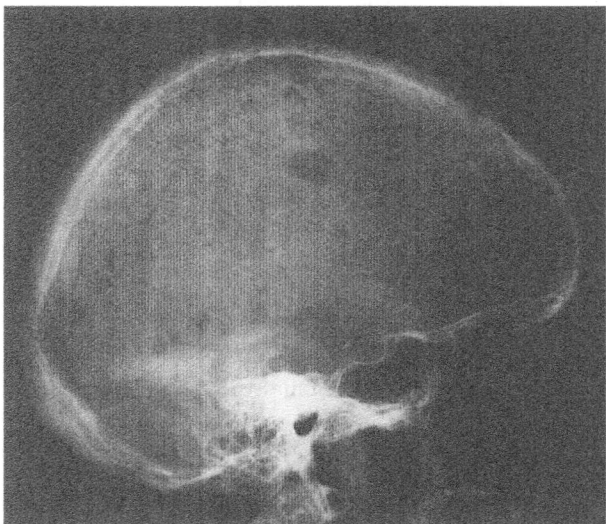

Fig. 18.R2 X-ray of skull illustrating typical punched-out lesions in a patient with MM

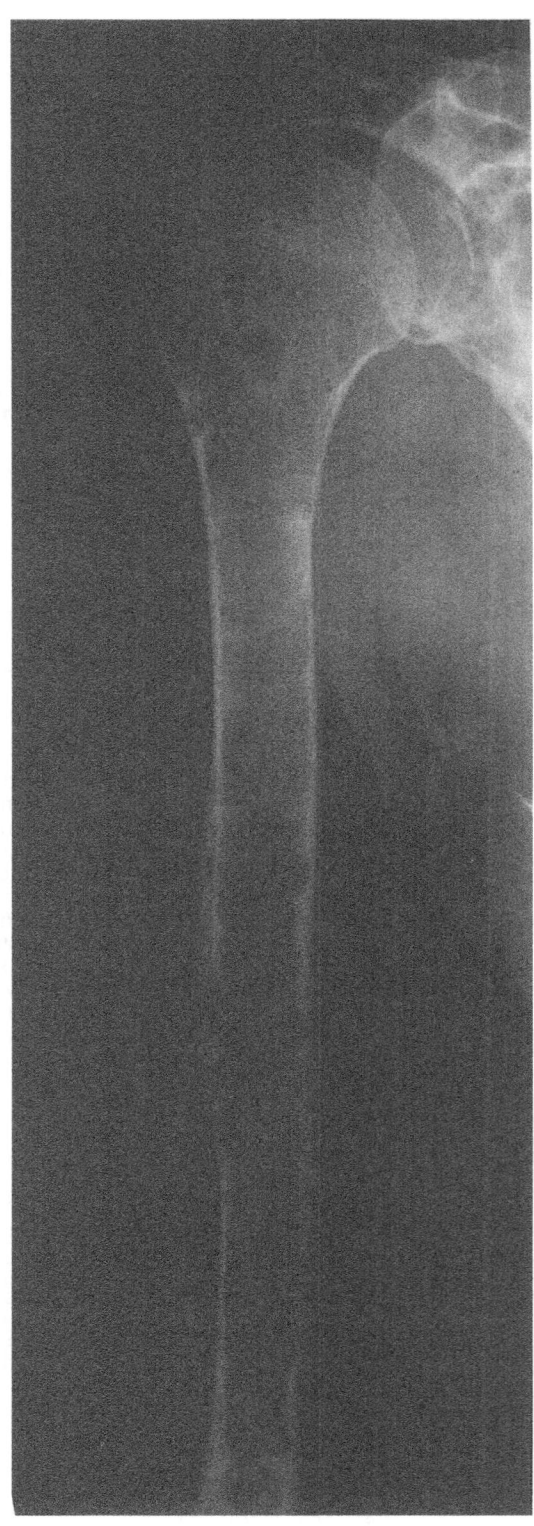

Fig. 18.R3 Dense, multiple punched-out lesions in the humerus and scapula eroding the cortex. Same patient as in Fig. 18.R2

are also useful for evaluating focal bone problems (Fig. 18.R4). Radionuclide scans are less sensitive than conventional roentgenograms for detection of osteolytic lesions in patients with MM, in contrast to their effectiveness in patients with other malignant tumours[45,47,48]. Bone scans often underestimate the size of osteolytic lesions and in some instances these are missed altogether. In some patients with costal lesions a bone scan has proved to be useful. The serum alkaline phosphatase level generally remains normal in patients with MM, even in the face of extensive lytic disease. The punched-out lytic lesions, normal alkaline phosphatase levels and negative bone scans all reflect the lack – or at least a very low level – of local osteoblastic activity around myeloma lesions. This has given rise to speculations that myeloma cells secrete an osteoblast inhibiting factor, as documented in *in-vitro* studies[26].

A major mediator of skeletal destruction in MM is the cytokine family *'osteoclast activating factor'* (OAF)[3,19,22–24,49,51,52,59]. There is histological evidence of increased

[continued on p. 201]

Plate 18.A

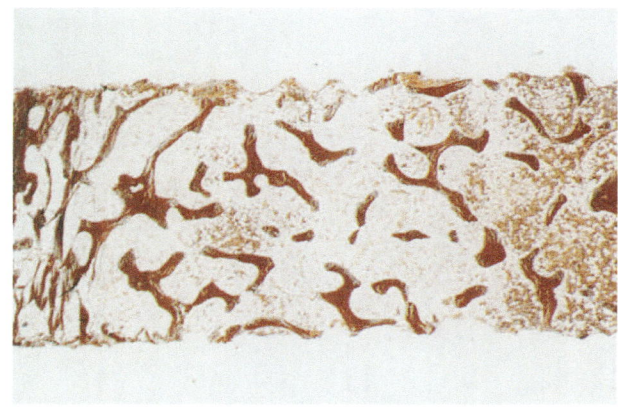

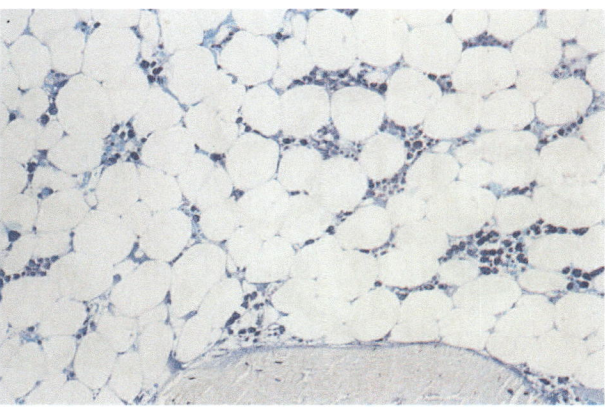

Figs. 18.1–18.6 Examples of minimal infiltration in multiple myeloma (MM) and the effect on bone

Fig. 18.1 Overview of bone biopsy with minimal patchy interstitial infiltration (centre and right) in a patient with smouldering MM. Gomori

Fig. 18.2 Minimal interstitial infiltration and marked hypocellular marrow. Note absence of bone remodelling. Giemsa

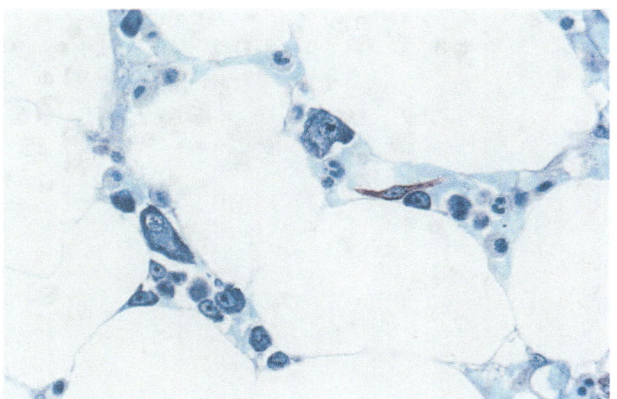

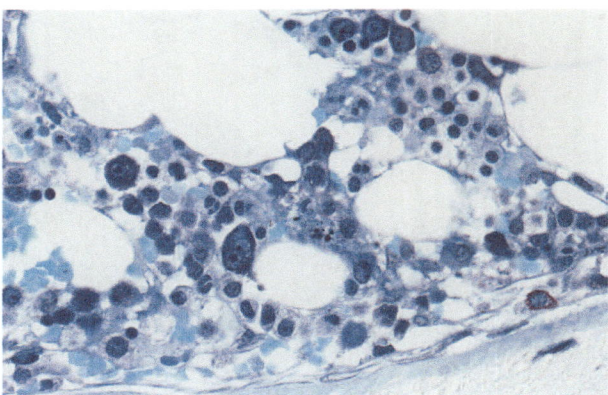

Fig. 18.3 Higher magnification of section from Fig. 18.2 showing some nucleolated plasma cells between fat cells: characteristic finding in smouldering MM. Giemsa

Fig. 18.4 Minimal interstitial infiltration with one large, nucleolated plasma cell in the centre. Note small seam of osteoid, but absence of osteoblasts. Giemsa. Myeloma patient in the plateau phase under chemotherapy

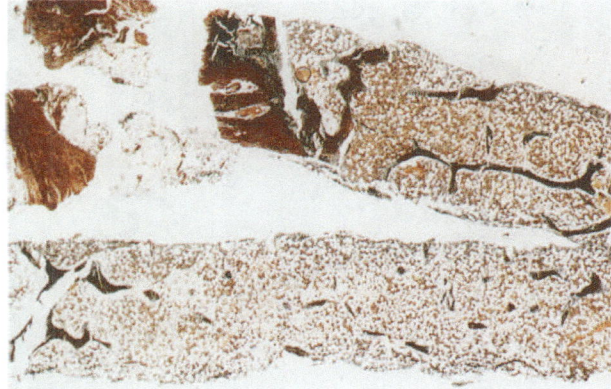

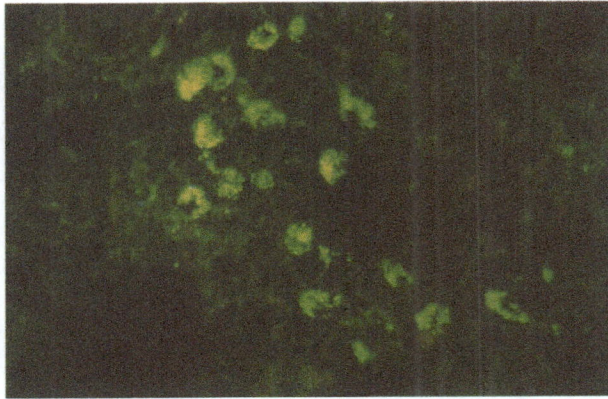

Fig. 18.5 Overview of bone biopsy with minimal interstitial myelomatous infiltration in hypocellular bone marrow. Massive reduction in trabecular bone. Gomori

Fig. 18.6 Immunohistology demonstrating monoclonality of plasma cells in case of non-secretory MM. FITC conjugated antibodies, frozen sections

Plate 18.B

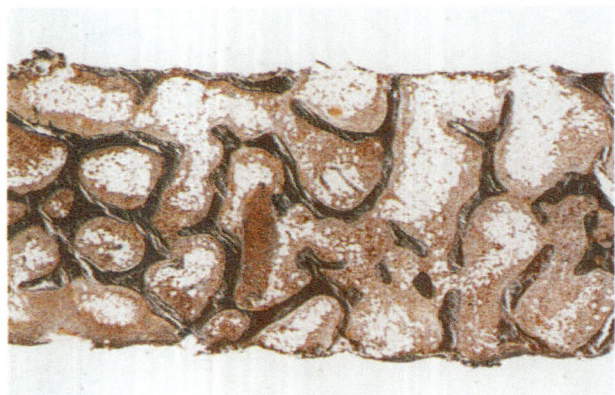

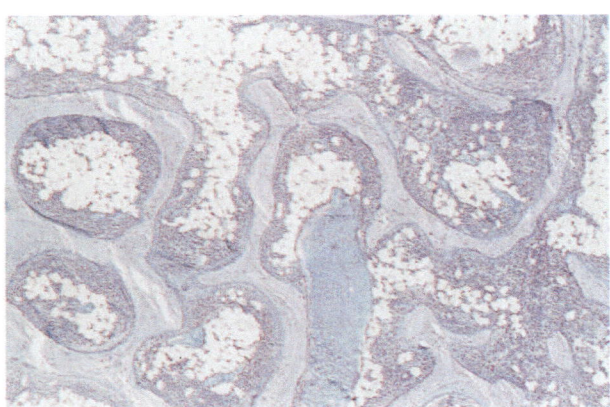

Figs. 18.7–18.12 Examples of paratrabecular infiltration in MM and the effect on bone

Fig. 18.7 Almost the whole trabecular network is surrounded by cuff of myeloma cells. Note hypocellular bone marrow in the central areas. Gomori

Fig. 18.8 Higher magnification of part of Fig. 18.7. Note large ectatic sinusoid (centre). In spite of the close apposition of the myeloma cells to the ossicles there is no reduction in trabecular bone. Giemsa

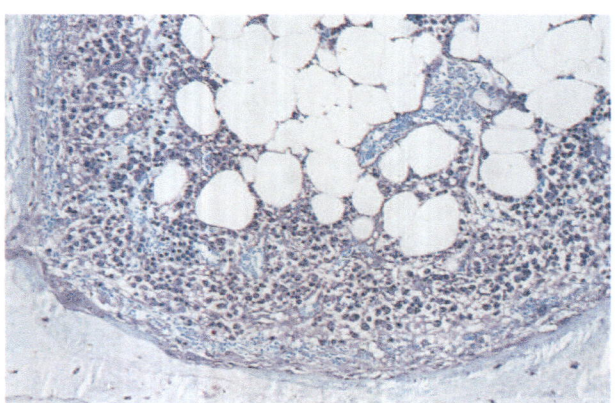

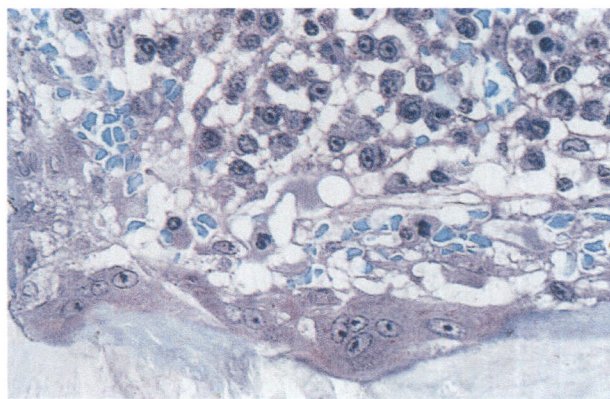

Fig. 18.9 Higher magnification of part of Fig. 18.8 showing that the paratrabecular layer of cells consists almost entirely of plasma cells except for a small erythroid island (left) and a few isolated myeloid precursors. Giemsa

Fig. 18.10 Higher magnification of the trabecular surface in Fig. 18.9 (extreme left). Note that the trabecular surface and the osteoclasts are separated from the plasma cells by slight paratrabecular fibrosis and sinusoids. Gomori

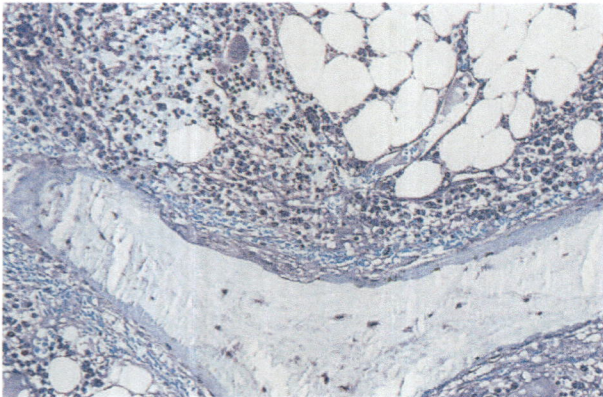

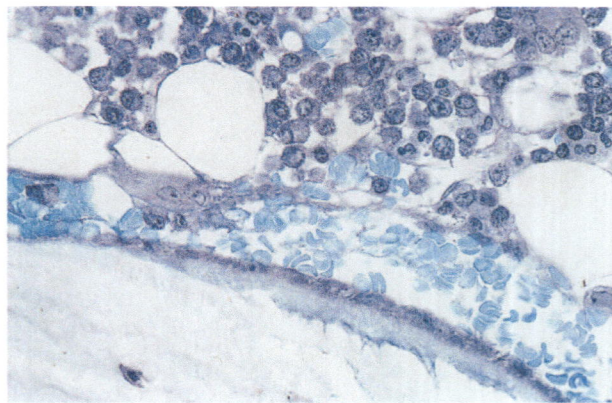

Fig. 18.11 Higher magnification of an area from another part of the same biopsy. Note trabecular surface with scalloped edge lined by layer of osteoclasts and separated from the plasma cells by a distinct band of connective tissue fibres. Gomori

Fig. 18.12 Another part of an area from the same biopsy with paratrabecular sinusoid and layer of osteoblasts on an osteoid seam. The balanced osseous remodelling in this biopsy most probably accounts for the well-preserved trabecular network as seen in Figs 18.7 and 18.8. Giemsa

Plate 18.C

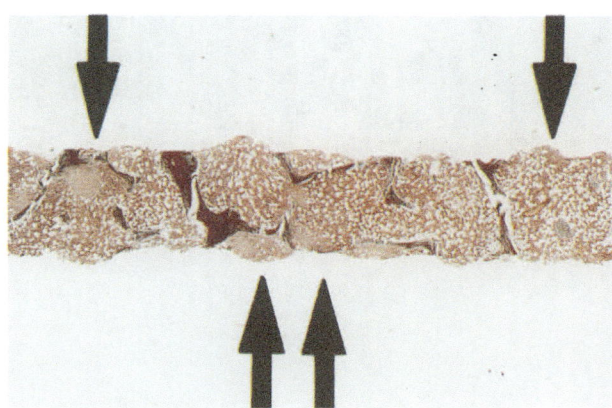

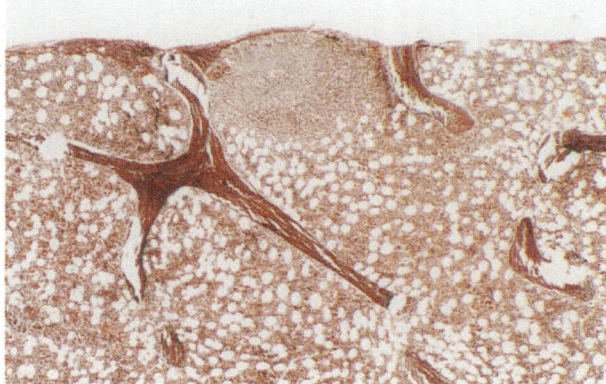

Figs. 18.13–18.18 Examples of nodular involvement in iliac crest biopsies in patients with multiple myeloma (MM)

Fig. 18.13 Overview showing multiple small nodules (arrows). The trabecular bone shows patchy osteopenia not associated with the nodules. Gomori

Fig. 18.14 Bone biopsy showing only a single nodule. The trabecular bone is osteopenic and the bone marrow shows a slight increase in fat cells. Gomori

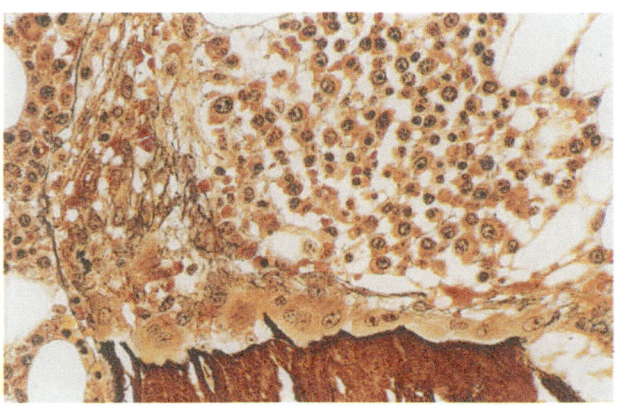

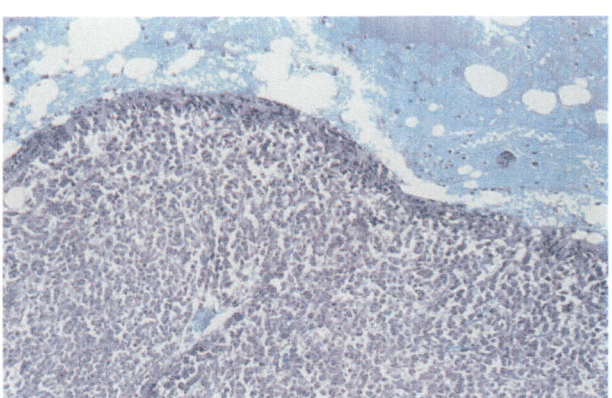

Fig. 18.15 Well-defined edge of large myeloma nodule sharply delineated from surrounding normocellular bone marrow. Giemsa

Fig. 18.16 Small myeloma nodule encapsulated by fibres separated from trabecular surface by a layer of active osteoclasts. Gomori

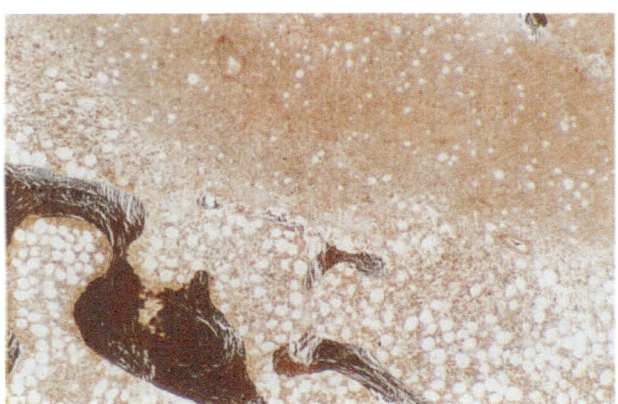

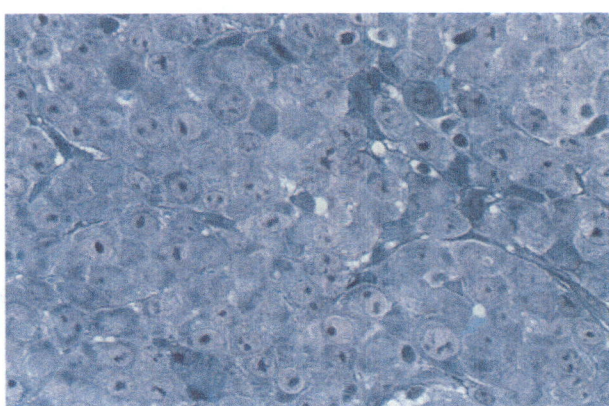

Fig. 18.17 Part of large myeloma nodule within osteolytic lesion. Note marked osteoclastic bone resorption on trabecular surface below the nodule. Gomori

Fig. 18.18 High magnification of typical immature plasma cells (plasmablasts) from nodule in Fig. 18.17. Giemsa

Plate 18.D

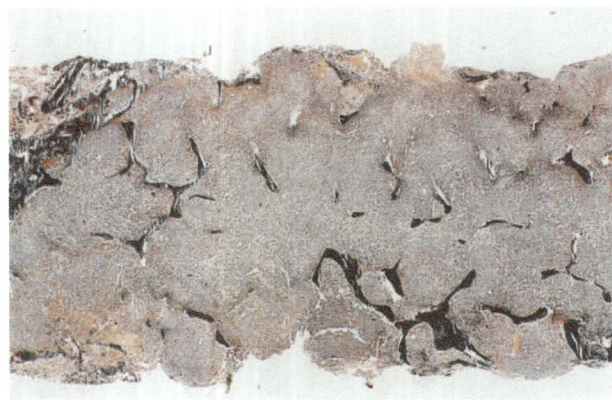

Figs. 18.19–18.24 Examples of iliac crest biopsies with 'packed marrow' pattern in MM and variable osseous reactions

Fig. 18.19 Overview of iliac crest biopsy showing complete occupation of the marrow cavities by myeloma ('packed marrow' pattern). Note variable trabecular bone structure, osteolytic region in centre and fairly stout ossicles (below). Gomori

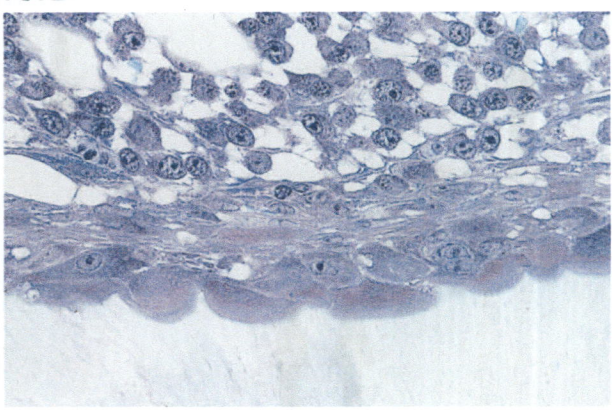

Fig. 18.20 Massive osteolytic bone resorption in vicinity of dense infiltration in a biopsy of another patient with osteolytic lesions and hypercalcaemia. Giemsa

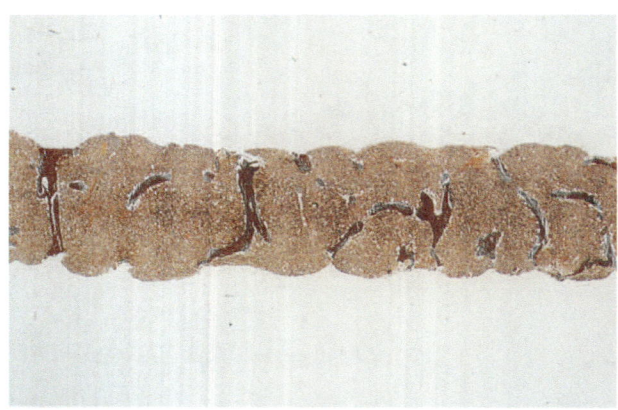

Fig. 18.21 'Packed marrow' type of MM, with reduction in trabecular bone volume, osteoporosis, histological type B (see Chapter 8). Gomori

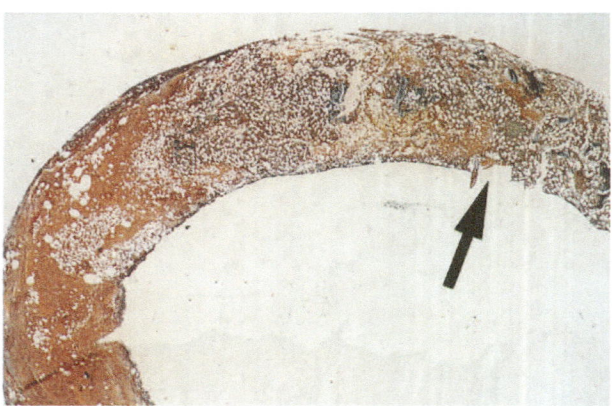

Fig. 18.22 Iliac crest biopsy with minimal interstitial involvement by MM and almost no residual trabecular bone. The curvature of the biopsy is probably due to complete loss of rigidity because of absence of trabecular network. Note haemorrhage (brown area lower left) and lymphoid nodule beneath an isolated trabecula (arrow). Gomori

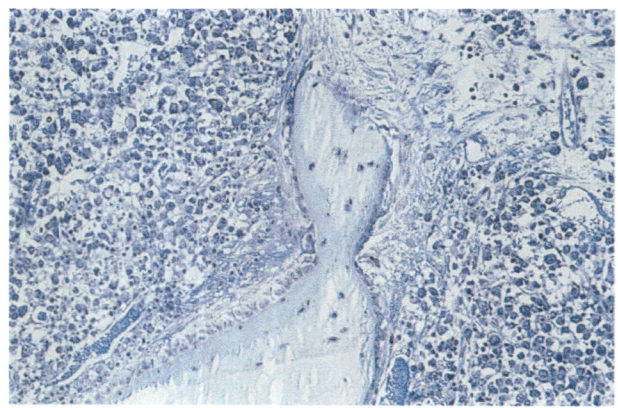

Fig. 18.23 Example of both resorption and formation of bone in MM. Giemsa

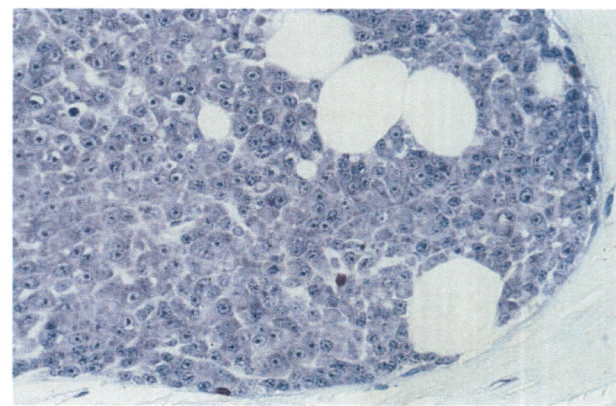

Fig. 18.24 Asynchronous plasma cell type in packed marrow, but with normal trabecular bone volume and minimal osseous remodelling. Giemsa

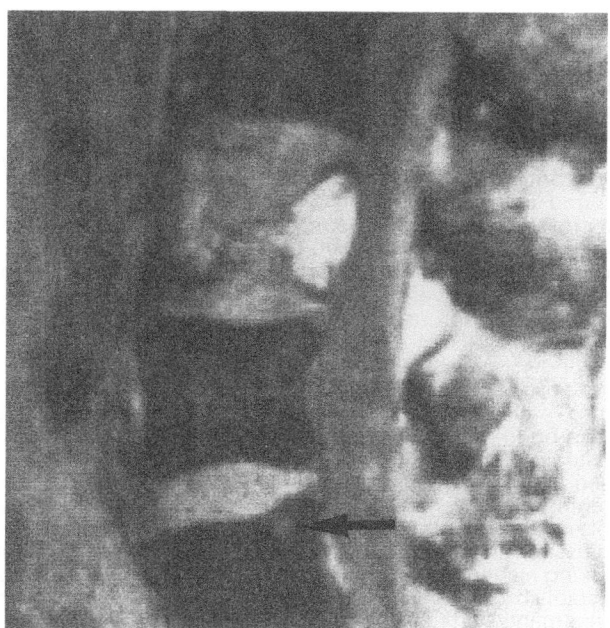

Fig.18.R4 Opposed GE-image (TR 500, TE 17, α 90°) of the lower lumbar spine of a patient with multiple myeloma: isolated destruction of the 3rd lumbar vertebra. Note a small myeloma nodule at arrow, not visible on the X-ray performed at the same time. (Kindly supplied by Dr A. Stäbler, Department of Radiology, Klinikum Großhadern, University of Munich)

numbers of active osteoclasts at bone surfaces adjacent to myeloma cell infiltrations, and this is consistent with the proposal that myeloma cells produce a locally active agent capable of stimulating osteoclasts[5,7,12,57]. This conclusion is also supported by the efficacy of primarily anti-osteoclastic agents such as bisphosphonates, mithramycin and corticosteroids[34] in lowering the serum calcium levels in patients with MM. Cultures of myeloma cells produce osteoclast activating factor(s) that can be clearly distinguished from PTH, prostaglandins of the E-type and vitamin D metabolites[30,35,54]. Moreover, studies have shown that several cytokines (lymphokines and monokines) can function as OAFs, including agents such as interleukin-1 (IL-1), lymphotoxin and tumour necrosis factors (TNF-α and TNF-β)[13,30,55,56]. Bataille and co-workers reported a significant enhancement of osteoblast recruitment in the early stage of MM, and these stimulated osteoblasts produce high amounts of IL-6[16,27,37,39,40], IL-3[11] and the granulocyte macrophage colony stimulating factor (GM-CSF)[38], all potent myeloma growth factors and involved in the formation of new osteoclasts and osteolytic bone resorption[14,15]. According to Mundy it is possible that OAF represents a family of bone resorbing factors with identical biological effect, and they may be subdivided into three subgroups according to their cell origin: T-cell, B-cell and monocyte OAFs[49,51,52]. Bone marrow plasma cells of patients with MM produce IL-1 and/or TNF[55]; consequently IL-1 released *in vivo* by malignant plasma cells is thought to have a major role in pathogenesis of lytic bone lesions[31,36]. OAFs are more likely local rather than systemic factors, since when myeloma cell OAF is injected systemically it fails to cause hypercalcaemia, unlike PTH. However we found that myeloma patients without involvement in the biopsy also had increased numbers of osteoclasts, suggesting the existence of a systemic PTH-like factor in MM. Osteoblastic activity and bone collagen synthesis is inhibited in

MM, though some coupling of osteoclastic resorption with osteoblastic new bone formation was always demonstrable in biopsies in MM.

Hypercalcaemia is a frequent complication of MM[43,50], occurring in 20–40% of patients, and it is also associated with malignant lymphomas and acute leukaemias[49]. It is influenced in part by tumour burden, OAF activity and presence of Bence-Jones protein, but it does not commonly occur unless the patient has impaired glomerular filtration. PTH, PTH-like factors, prostaglandins and TGFs may also be responsible for hypercalcaemia and increased bone resorption in special situations. Hypercalcaemia is exacerbated by immobilization or prolonged bed rest, which also increase bone resorption. Since most older people have some degree of decrease in renal function, hypercalcaemia occurs more frequently in the older age group.

In order to evaluate bone changes in MM, *bone biopsies* from 700 patients with MM were analysed by semiquantitative and histomorphometric methods[7,9]. *Osteoclastic resorption* surfaces were markedly increased compared with controls (Plate 18.E). Increased osseous remodelling was found in most biopsies and both the numbers of osteoclasts and osteoblasts correlated with the quantity of plasma cell infiltration (Figs 18.S7–10). However, the type of skeletal lesion (osteolysis versus osteopenia) depended mainly on the type of *tumour growth*: patients with interstitial and packed marrow patterns usually had diffuse rarefaction of trabecular bone (generalized osteoporosis), while patients with nodules were characterized by local osteoclastic resorption (osteolytic lesions). Therefore osteolytic lesions are a reflection of the tumour growth pattern (nodularity) rather than the tumour load[9]. This histotopographic correlation provides confirmation of myeloma-induced OAF effects on osteoclasts. OAF appears to have a very local action, stimulating osteoclasts mainly adjacent to myeloma cell infiltrations. Thus the pattern of bone loss – diffuse (osteoporosis) versus focal (lytic bone lesions) – represents bony expressions of the underlying growth patterns of MM. Nodular myeloma growth correlated predominantly with osteolytic lesions, while interstitial growth showed diffuse, generalized osteopenia. In the packed marrow pattern the advanced stage of myeloma growth, both osteolyses and osteopenia, were prominent in bone biopsies and on roentgenograms. The type of M-component

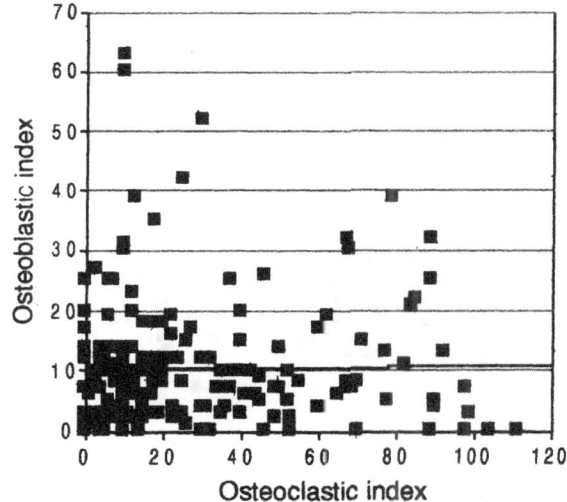

Fig.18.S7 Correlation of numbers of osteoclasts and osteoblasts in iliac crest biopsies in MM. Note complete lack of correlation indicating 'uncoupling' of resorption and formation

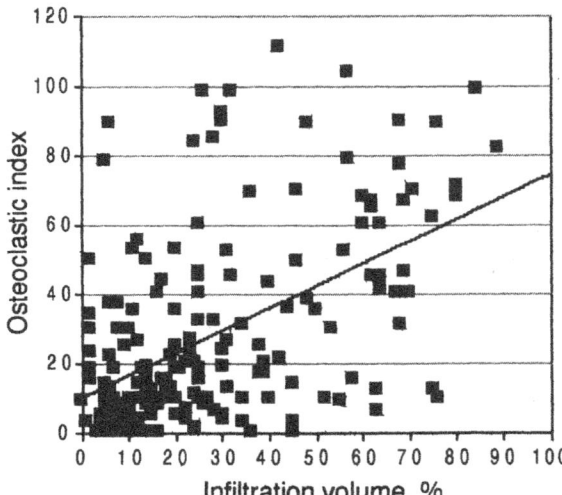

Fig. 18.S8 Correlation of infiltration volumes and numbers of osteoclasts in iliac crest biopsies in MM

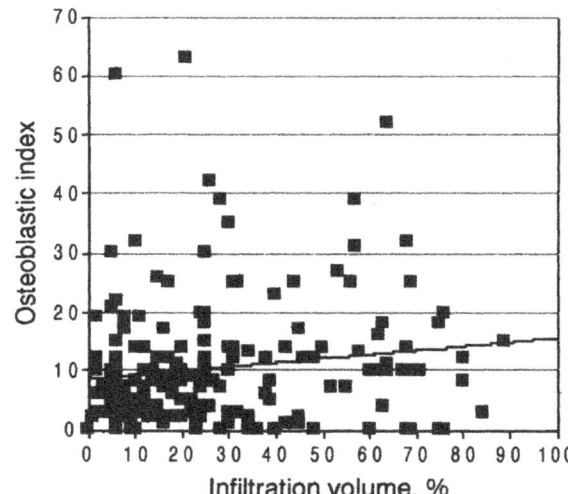

Fig. 18.S9 Correlation of infiltration volumes and numbers of osteoblasts in iliac crest biopsies in MM

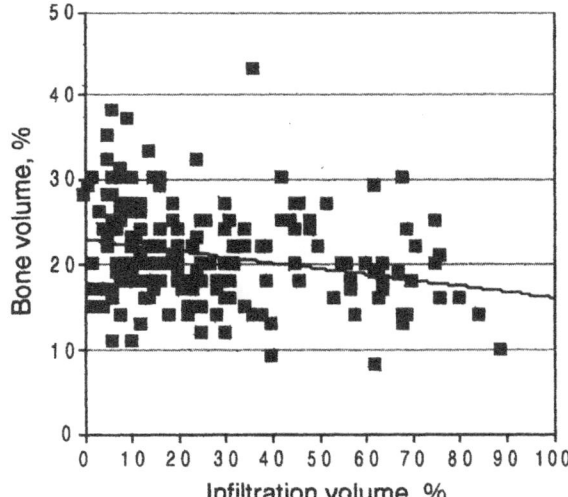

Fig. 18.S10 Correlation of infiltration volumes and bone volumes in iliac crest biopsies in MM

did not influence osteoclastic activity, in contrast to the conclusions of Bataille *et al.*, that Ig A and pure Bence-Jones MM appeared more osteoclastic than Ig G cases[12]. Direct bone resorption by myeloma cells was observed in only two patients who had plasma cell sarcoma[9].

MM is generally characterized by osteoclastic resorption together with *inhibited bone formation* (Plate 18.F). In contrast to the radiological findings, however, we found increased numbers of osteoblasts and a slightly increased volume of osteoid in the bone biopsies, both in areas completely invaded by plasma cells and in non-involved regions. A decoupling effect between resorption and formation was only evident adjacent to dense myeloma infiltrations, usually consisting of nucleolated plasma cells.

Under successful *chemotherapy*, especially together with use of anti-osteoclastic therapy such as bisphosphonates[48], we observed a marked reduction of osteoclastic resorption coupled with an increase in osteoblasts, osteoid seams and trabecular bone volume. Furthermore, sequential biopsies may characterize variations in tumour regression under therapy, or may herald imminent relapse, often before other clinical evidence of disease progression[10]. Refractory cytopenia is also an indication for taking sequential biopsy specimens, to exclude or to establish other causes of a refractory tendency towards treatment, such as aplasia, myelodysplasia, fibrosis, amyloidosis, leukaemia or other secondary neoplasms (Plate 18.D). Interferon-α and interleukin-6 suggest some benefit with respect to relapse rate and survival in myeloma patients, and allogeneic bone marrow transplantation appears to be a promising new method of treatment for some patients with MM[3,23,42].

References

1. Apitz K. (1940). Die neuen Anschauungen vom Plasmozytom des Knochenmarks, dem sog. multiplen Myelom. *Klin. Wschr.*, **40**, 1025
2. Axelsson U. (1986). A 20-year follow-up study of 64 subjects with M-components. *Acta Med. Scand.*, **219**, 519
3. Barlogie B., Epstein J., Selvanayagam P. and Alexanian R. (1989). Plasma cell myeloma – new biological insights and advances in therapy. *Blood*, **73**, 865
4. Bartl R. (1988). Histologic classification and staging of multiple myeloma. *Hematol. Oncol.*, **6**, 107
5. Bartl R., Frisch B., Burkhardt R., Fateh-Moghadam A., Mahl G., Gierster P., Sund M. and Kettner G. (1982). Bone marrow histology in myeloma: its importance in diagnosis, prognosis, classification and staging. *Brit. J. Haematol.*, **51**, 361
6. Bartl R., Frisch B. and Burkhardt R. (1985). *Bone Marrow Biopsies Revisited: a New Dimension of Haematologic Malignancies – Multiple Myeloma*. Basel: Karger
7. Bartl R. and Frisch B. (1989). Bone marrow histology in multiple myeloma: prognostic relevance of histologic characteristics. *Hematol. Rev.*, **3**, 87
8. Bartl R., Frisch B., Diem H., Mündel M. and Fateh-Moghadam A. (1989). Bone marrow histology and serum beta 2 microglobulin in multiple myeloma – a new prognostic strategy. *Europ. J. Haematol.*, **51**, Suppl., 88
9. Bartl R., Frisch B., Fateh-Moghadam A., Kettner G., Jäger K. and Sommerfeld W. (1987). Histological classification and staging of multiple myeloma. Retrospective and prospective study of 674 cases. *Amer. J. Clin. Pathol.*, **87**, 342
10. Bartl R., Frisch B., Diem H., Mündel M., Nagel D., Lamerz R. and Fateh-Moghadam A. (1991). Histologic, biochemical and clinical parameters for monitoring multiple myeloma. *Cancer*, **68**, 2241
11. Barton B. E. and Mayer R. (1989). IL-3 induces differentiation of bone marrow precursor cells to osteoclast-like cells. *J. Immunol.*, **143**, 3211
12. Bataille R., Chappard D., Alexandre C. and Sany J. (1986). Importance of quantitative histology of bone changes in monoclonal gammapathy. *Brit. J. Cancer*, **53**, 805
13. Bataille R., Chappard D., Marcelli C., Dessauw P., Sany J., Baldet P. and Alexandre C. (1989). Mechanisms of bone destruction in multiple myeloma. The importance of an unbalanced process in

Plate 18.E

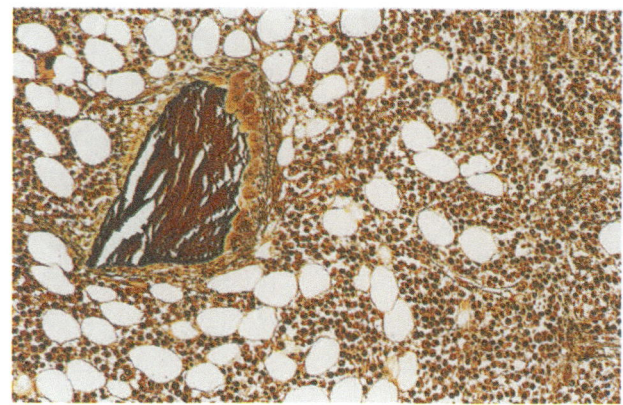

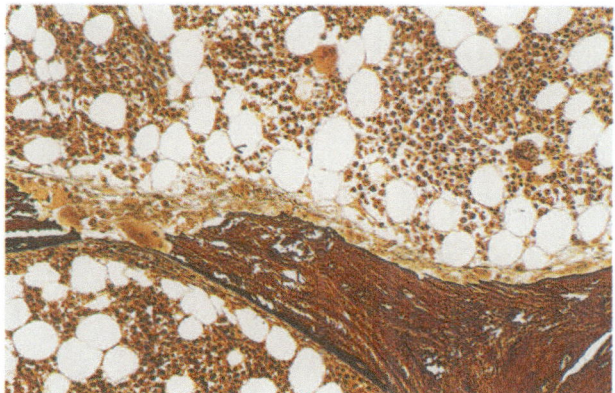

Figs. 18.25–18.30 Osteoclastic bone resorption in MM

Fig. 18.25 Band of osteoclasts on scalloped surface of an ossicle. Note dense plasma cell infiltration at right. Giemsa

Fig. 18.26 Transecting osteoclasia (left) of a longitudinally cut trabecula, and osteoblastic repair (upper right). Interstitial plasma cell infiltration in normocellular haematopoietic tissue. Gomori

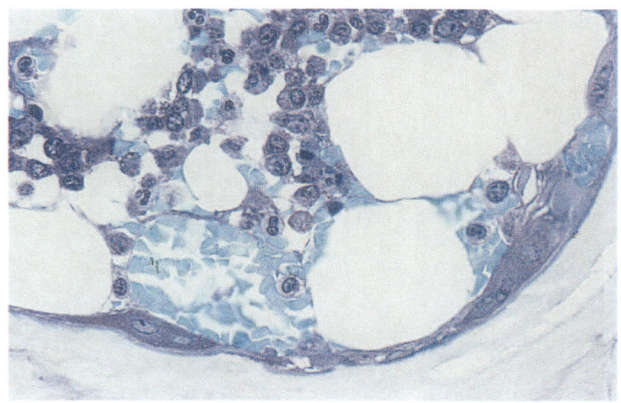

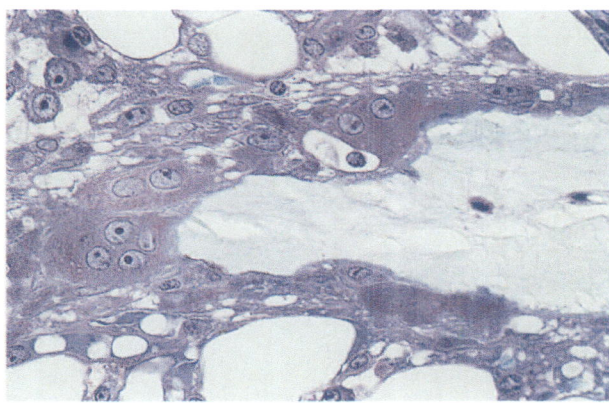

Fig. 18.27 Higher magnification of part of a 'mini-aggregate' to illustrate the atypical and small plasma cells. Note flat osteoclasts on trabecular surface. Giemsa

Fig. 18.28 Multiple nucleolated osteoclasts resorbing a small trabecula. Two nucleolated plasma cells upper left. Giemsa

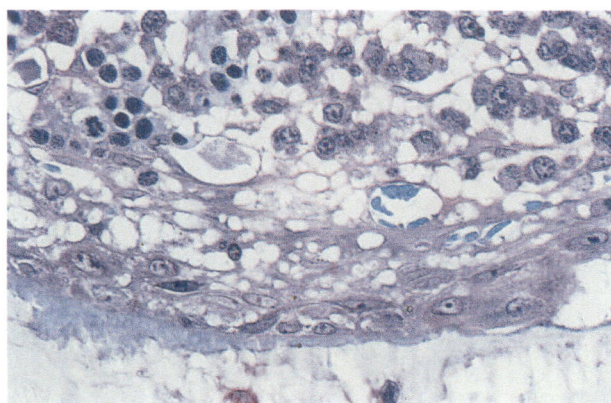

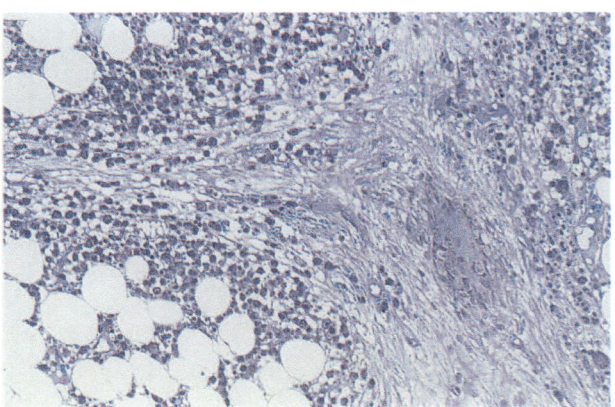

Fig. 18.29 Coupled osteoclastic bone resorption (right) and osteoblastic bone formation (left) on surface of an ossicle. The plasma cell infiltration above is separated by a broad zone of connective tissue from the bone cells. Giemsa

Fig. 18.30 Total resorption of a trabecula and replacement by fibrous connective tissue and an island of woven bone, surrounded by a zone of plasma cells. Giemsa

Plate 18.F

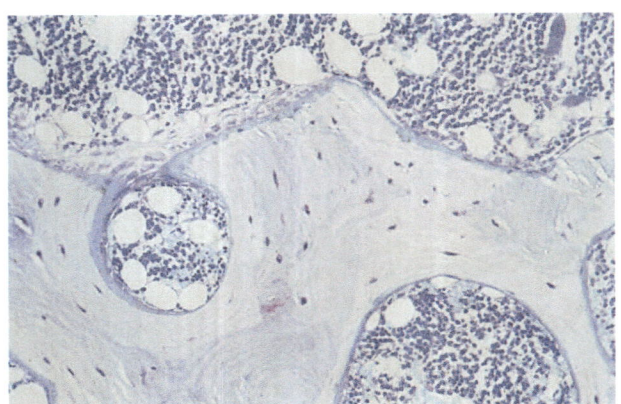

Figs. 18.31–18.36 Osteoblastic bone formation in MM

Fig. 18.31 Thick trabecular network partly covered by small osteoid seams. Note diffuse plasma cell infiltration in the surrounding bone marrow. Giemsa

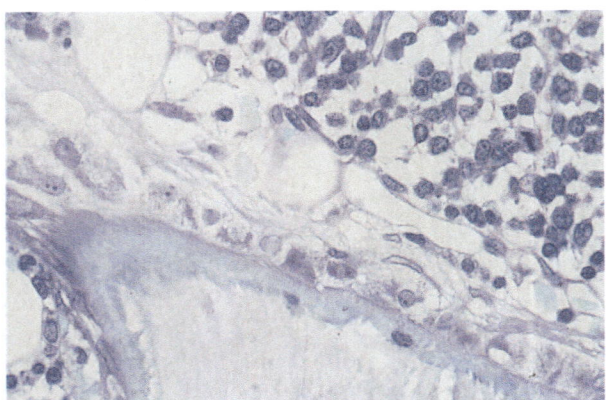

Fig. 18.32 Higher magnification from Fig. 18.31 showing repair of previous bone resorption, with broad seam of osteoid and lined by osteoblasts. Giemsa

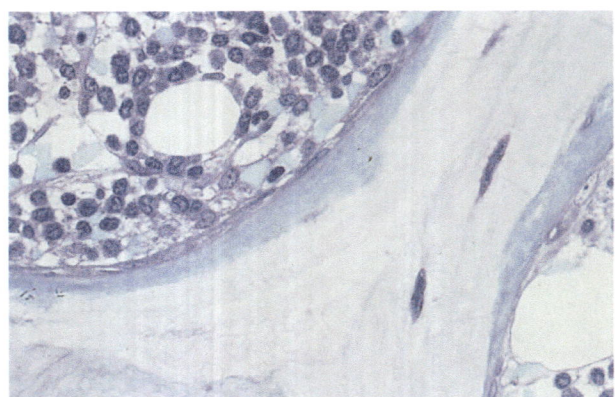

Fig. 18.33 Trabecula with broad osteoid seam on both sides and lined by flat endosteal lining cells. Plasma cell infiltration upper left. Giemsa

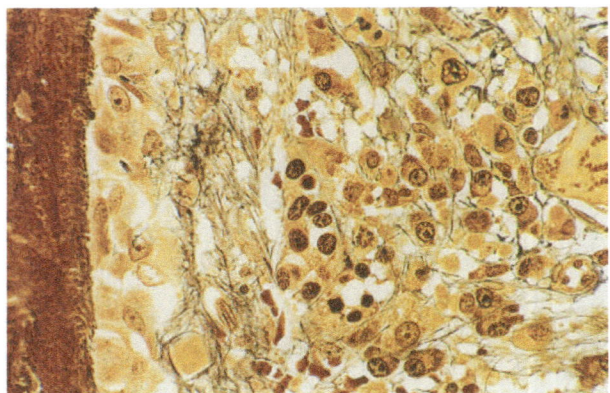

Fig. 18.34 Trabecular surface showing band of large osteoblasts separated from the myeloma cells by a distinct band of connective tissue. Gomori

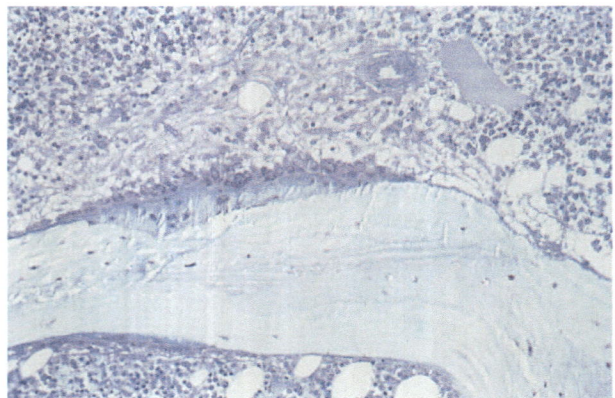

Fig. 18.35 Layer of osteoblasts on osteoid seam separated from the plasma cells by band of fibrous connective tissue on one side of the trabecula while there is minimal osseous remodelling, no paratrabecular fibrosis and some residual haematopoiesis on the other side (left). Giemsa

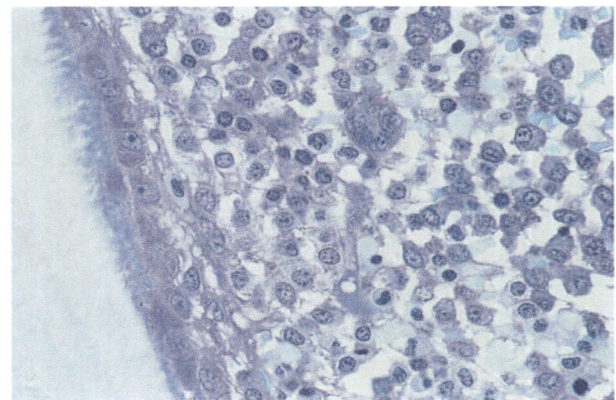

Fig. 18.36 Osteoid lined by cuboidal osteoblasts. Plasma cells diffusely scattered within hypercellular marrow. Giemsa

Plate 18.G

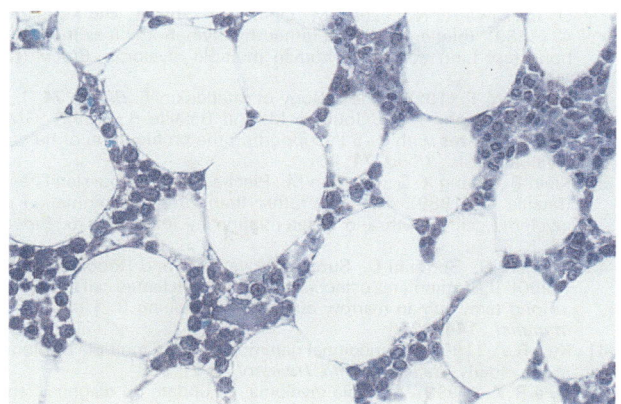

Figs. 18.37–18.42 Complications in MM

Fig. 18.37 Atrophic marrow, with plasma cells between fat cells (evidence of myelopoiesis depressing factor produced by myeloma cells?). Giemsa

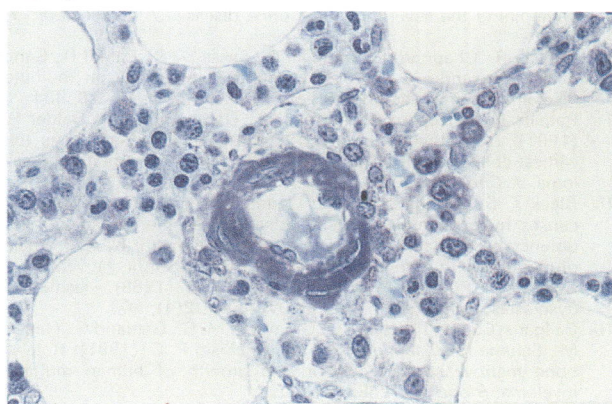

Fig. 18.38 Unexpected finding of secondary amyloidosis in refractory MM. Note minimal plasma cell infiltration in the perivascular region. Giemsa

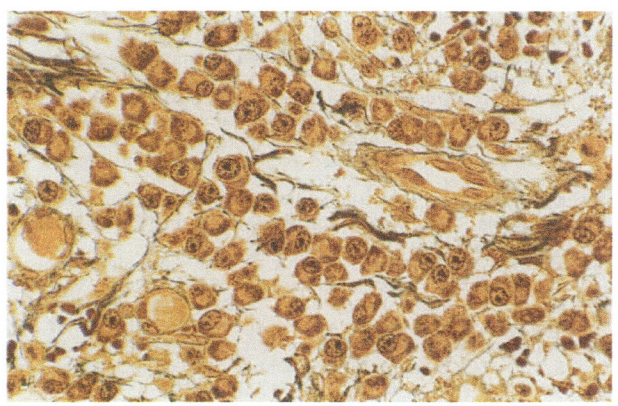

Fig. 18.39 Dense plasma cell infiltration with coarse fibrosis in refractory MM. Gomori

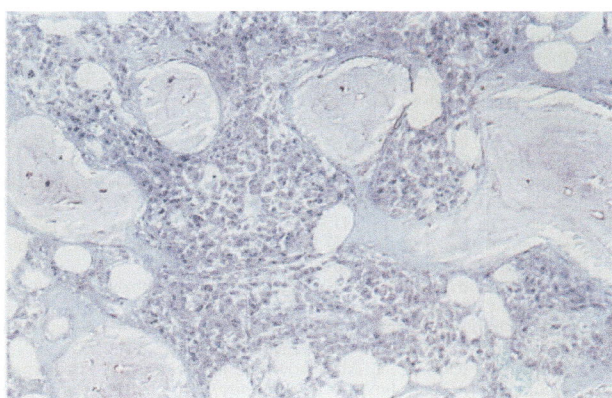

Fig. 18.40 Biopsy showing extensions of the trabecular network formed by fibrous tissue and unmineralized primitive bone in area of myelomatous infiltration. Part of biopsy showing osteosclerotic variant of MM. Giemsa

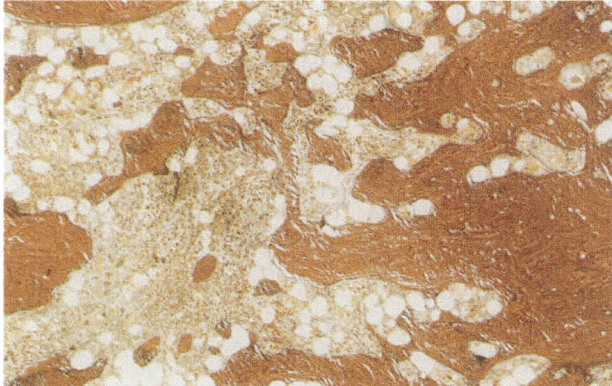

Figs. 18.41 and **18.42** Iliac crest biopsy of another patient with osteosclerotic MM

Fig. 18.41 Increased bone volume (osteosclerosis) at left, plasma cell infiltration within fibrous area and clusters of megakaryocytes (upper and lower right). Gomori

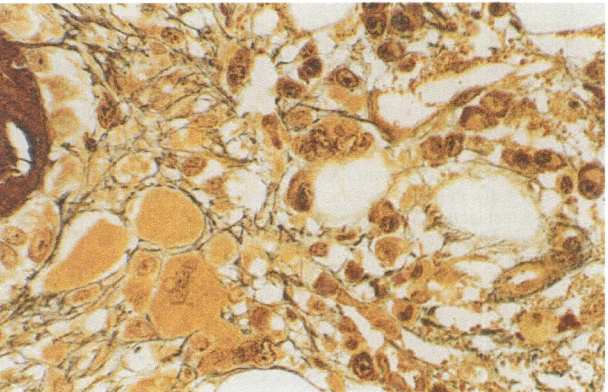

Fig. 18.42 Higher magnification of biopsy shown in Fig. 18.5 revealing cluster of polymorphic and atypical megakaryocytes. Marked fibrosis of the bone marrow and plasma cell infiltration (centre and right). The osteomyelosclerosis in this case (in contrast to that illustrated in Fig. 18.40) is most probably due to the concomitant myeloproliferative disorder. Gomori

determining the severity of lytic bone disease. *J. Clin. Oncol.*, **7**, 1009

14. Bataille R., Chappard D., Marcelli C., Sessauw P., Baldet P., Sany J. and Alexandre C. (1990). Osteoblast stimulation in multiple myeloma lacking lytic bone lesions. *Brit. J. Haematol.*, **76**, 484

15. Bataille R., Chappard D., Marcelli C., Dessauw P. and Baldet P. (1991). Recruitment of new osteoblasts and osteoclasts is the earliest critical event in the pathogenesis of human multiple myeloma. *J. Clin. Invest.*, **88**, 62

16. Black K. S., Mundy G. R. and Garrett I. R. (1990). Interleukin-6 causes hypercalcemia *in vivo* and enhances the bone resorbing potency of interleukin-1 and tumor necrosis factor by two orders of magnitude *in vitro*. *J. Bone Miner. Res.*, **5**(Suppl. 2), 787

17. Buss D. H., Prichard R. W. and Cooper M. R. (1988). Plasma cell dyscrasias. *Hematol./Oncol. Clin. N. Amer.*, **2**(4), 603

18. Caligaris-Cappio F., Bergui L., Gregoretti M. G., Gaidano G., Gaboli M., Schena M., Zallone A. Z. and Marchisio P. C. (1991). Role of bone marrow stromal cells in the growth of human multiple myeloma. *Blood*, **77**, 2688

19. Canalis E., McCarthy T. and Centrella M. (1988). Growth factors and regulation of bone remodeling. *J. Clin. Invest.*, **81**, 277

20. Dixon W. J. and Brown M. B. (1987). *BMDP-87: Biomedical Computer Programs P-Series: System Program and Statistical Development*. Berkeley: University of California Press

21. Driedger M. and Prizanski W. (1979). Plasma cell neoplasia with osteosclerotic lesions. A study of five cases and a review of the literature. *Arch. Intern. Med.*, **139**, 892

22. Durie B. G. M. (1988). The biology of multiple myeloma. *Hematol. Oncol.*, **6**, 77

23. Durie B. G. M. (1991). Multiple myeloma: biology and treatment. *Oncol. Today*, **3**, 15

24. Durie B. G. M., Salmon S. E. and Mundy G. R. (1981). Relation of osteoclast activating factor production to extent of bone disease in multiple myeloma. *Brit. J. Haematol.*, **47**, 21

25. Edeiken J., Dalinka M. and Karasick D. (1990). *Edeiken's Roentgen Diagnosis of Diseases of Bone*. Baltimore: Williams & Wilkins

26. Evans C. E., Galasko C. S. B. and Ward C. (1989). Does myeloma secrete an osteoblast inhibiting factor? *J. Bone Jt Surg.*, **71B**, 288

27. Feyen J. H. M., Elford P., DiPadova F. E. and Trechsel U. (1989). Interleukin 6 is produced by bone and modulated by parathyroid hormone. *J. Bone Miner. Res.*, **4**, 633

28. Frisch B. and Bartl R. (1990). *Atlas of Bone Marrow Pathology*. Dordrecht: Kluwer

29. Fritz E., Ludwig H. and Kundi M. (1984). Prognostic relevance of cellular morphology in multiple myeloma. *Blood*, **63**, 1072

30. Garrett I. R., Durie B. G. M., Nedwin G. E., Gillespie A., Bringman T., Sabatini M., Bertolini D. R. and Mundy G. R. (1987). Production of lymphotoxin, a bone resorbing cytokine, by cultured human myeloma cells. *N. Engl. J. Med.*, **317**, 526

31. Gozzolino F., Torcia M., Aldinucci D., Rubartelli A., Miliani A., Shaw R., Lansdorp A. R. and DiGuglielmo R. (1989). Production of interleukin 1 by bone marrow myeloma cells. *Blood*, **74**, 380

32. Greipp P. R., Raymond N. M., Kyle R. A. and O'Fallon W. M. (1985). Multiple myeloma: significance of plasmablastic subtype in morphologic classification. *Blood*, **65**, 305

33. Huvos A. G. (1991). Multiple myeloma, including solitary osseous myeloma. Huvos A. G., *Bone Tumors: Diagnosis, Treatment and Prognosis* (p. 653). Philadelphia: Saunders

34. Ishikawa H., Tanaka H., Iwato K., Tanabe O., Asaouku H., Nobuyoshi M., Yamamoto I., Kawano M. and Kuramoto A. (1990). Effect of glucocorticoids on the biologic activities of myeloma cells: inhibition of interleukin-1β osteoclast activating factor-induced bone resorption. *Blood*, **75**, 715

35. Josse R. G., Murray T. M., Mundy G. R., Jez D. and Heersche J. N. M. (1981). Observations on the mechanism of bone resorption induced by multiple myeloma marrow culture fluids and purified osteoclast-activating factor. *J. Clin. Invest.*, **67**, 1472

36. Kawano M., Yamamoto I., Iwato K., Tanaka H., Asaoku H., Tanabe

O., Ishikawa H., Nobuyoshi M., Ohmoto Y., Hirai Y. and Kuramoto A. (1989). Interleukin 1 beta rather than lymphotoxin as the major bone resorbing activity in human multiple myeloma. *Blood*, **73**, 1646

37. Kishimoto T. (1989). The biology of interleukin-6. *Blood*, **74**, 1

38. Klein B., Zhang K. G., Jourdan M. and Bataille R. (1989). GM-CSF synergizes with IL-6 in supporting the proliferation of human myeloma cells. *Blood*, **74**, 201

39. Klein B., Zhang X. G., Jourdan M., Piechaczyk M., Houssiau F. and Bataille R. (1989). Paracrine rather than autocrine regulation of myeloma cell growth and differentiation by interleukin-6. *Blood*, **73**, 517

40. Kurihara N., Bertolini D., Suda T, Akiyama Y. and Roodman G. D. (1990). IL-6 stimulates osteoclast-like multinucleated cell formation in long term human marrow cultrues by inducing IL-1 release. *J. Immunol.*, **144**, 4226

41. Kyle R. A. (1987). Monoclonal gammopathy and multiple myeloma in the elderly. *Bailliére's Clin. Hematol.*, **1**(2), 533

42. Kyle R. A. (1990). Multiple myeloma: an update on diagnosis and management. *Acta Oncol.*, **29**, 1

43. Kyle R. A. and Bayrd E. D. (1976). *The Monoclonal Gammopathies: Multiple Myeloma and Related Plasma-Cell Disorders*. Springfield: Charles C. Thomas

44. Kyle R. A. and Lust J. A. (1989). Monoclonal gammopathies of undetermined significance. *Semin. Hematol.*, **26**, 176

45. Leonard R. C. F., Owen J. P., Proctor S. J. and Hamilton P. J. (1981). Multiple myeloma: radiology or bone scanning. *Clin. Radiol.*, **32**, 2917

46. Ludwig H. (1982). *Multiples Myelom*. Berlin: Springer

47. Ludwig H., Kampen W. and Sinzinger H. (1982). Radiography and bone scintigraphy in multiple myeloma, a comparative analysis. *Brit. J. Radiol.*, **55**, 1737

48. Merlini G., Parrinello G. A., Piccinini L., Crema F., Fiorentini M., Riccardi A., Pavesi F., Novazzi F., Silingardi V. and Ascari E. (1990). Long-term effects of parenteral dichloromethylene biphosphonate (Cl2MBP) on bone disease of myeloma patients treated with chemotherapy. *Haematol. Oncol.*, **8**, 23

49. Mundy G. R. (1990). Hypercalcemia of malignancy. Avioli L. V. and Krane S. M., *Metabolic Bone Disease* (p. 793). Philadelphia: Saunders

50. Mundy G. R. and Bertolini D. R. (1986). Bone destruction and hypercalcemia in plasma cell myeloma. *Semin. Oncol.*, **13**, 291

51. Mundy G. R. and Martin T. J. (1982). The hypercalcemia of malignancy: pathogenesis and management. *Metabolism*, **31**, 1247

52. Mundy G. R., Raisz L. G., Cooper R. A., Schechter G. P. and Salmon S. E. (1974). Evidence for the secretion of an osteoclast stimulating factor in myeloma. *N. Engl. J. Med.*, **291**, 1041

53. Oken M. M. (1984). Multiple myeloma. *Med. Clin. N. Amer.*, **68**, 757

54. Rossi J. F. and Bataille R. (1984). In vitro osteolytic activity of human myeloma plasma cells and the clinical evaluation of myeloma osteoclastic bone lesions. *Brit. J. Cancer*, **50**, 119

55. Stashenko P., Dewhirst F. E., Peros W. J. and Kent R. I. (1987). Synergistic interactions between interleukin-1, tumor necrosis factor and lymphotoxin in bone resorption. *J. Immunol.*, **138**, 1464

56. Thomson B. M., Mundy G. R. and Chambers T. J. (1987). Tumor necrosis factors alpha and beta induce osteoblastic cells to stimulate osteoclastic bone resorption. *J. Immunol.*, **138**, 775

57. Valentin-Opran A., Charhon S. A., Meunier P. J., Edouard G. M. and Arlot M. E. (1982). Quantitative histology of myeloma-induced bone changes. *Brit. J. Haematol.*, **52**, 601

58. Woolfenden J. M., Pitt M. J., Durie B. G. M. and Moon T. E. (1980). Comparison of bone scintigraphy and radiography in multiple myeloma. *Radiology*, **134**, 7237

59. Yoneda T. and Mundy G. R. (1979). Prostaglandins are necessary for osteoclast activating factor production by activated peripheral leucocytes. *J. Exp. Med.*, **149**, 279

Leukaemias and lymphomas in bone

19

Acute leukaemia (AL) (Plate 19.A) is the most common malignant disease *of childhood*, and the lymphoblastic subtype (ALL) accounts for about 80% of the cases. In half of the children with ALL bone pain occurs during the course of disease[51]. The pain is typically migratory and located in para-articular regions, simulating juvenile rheumatoid arthritis. Radiologically the skeleton is affected in approximately half the cases, but the true incidence of bone lesions at autopsy may be significantly higher[12,25,31,40,43,64]. Simmons reviewed skeletal roentgenograms of 172 young patients with AL and found the following forms of osseous lesions[54]:

1. osteolytic lesions 30%,
2. diffuse osteopenia 16%,
3. periosteal reaction 20%,
4. metaphyseal bands 17%, and
5. mixed lesions 18%.

The first roentgenological abnormalities may be horizontal radiolucent bands in the metaphyses of long bones[25,40]. Periosteal reactions of long bones often reflect the infiltration of the cortex by leukaemic cells. With increasing tumour load and expansion in the rigid marrow cavities, generalized thinning of the cortex and the trabeculae cause systemic osteopenia. Multiple, small, clearly defined radiolucent defects may assume a 'raindrop' pattern similar to that in multiple myeloma. In the terminal phase, massively destructive confluent lesions may be observed, and pathological fractures are then common[51]. The increase in bone resorption may be attributed either to resorptive activity of the leukaemic cells themselves or to a circulating factor secreted by them that activates osteoclastic bone resorption. Osteoblast activating factors, prostaglandins, vitamin D metabolites, ectopically produced PTH and various PTH-like substances have all been implicated as mediators – local and/or systemic – of osteoclast recruitment and activation[16,20,24,32,49,65]. Furthermore leukaemia-induced changes of the bone marrow (vascularization, stromal microenvironment, haematopoietic stem cell pool) may also contribute to osseous rarefaction[27,30]. Some degree of osteosclerosis – diffuse or local – may occur, but is very rare and usually observed during the treatment phase or in patients with underlying osteopetrosis.

Adults with acute leukaemia rarely show bone abnormalities (less than 10% of cases)[8,9,20,27,33,34,41,47,53,57]. The main histomorphometric parameters in adult acute leukaemia at initial diagnosis are shown in Table 19.1. The median trabecular bone volume was within the normal range. The osteoid volume and the bone remodelling parameters, however, were decreased, indicating an inactive bone surface. There were no notable differences of bone histomorphometry between the different cellular subtypes of AL. During the course of treatment, generalized osteopenia, lytic lesions[59] and osteosclerotic reactions due to extensive marrow necrosis[60] have been observed (Fig. 19.R1). Demineralization may improve during remission, especially as a consequence of physical activity.

In *chronic myeloid leukaemia* (CML, CGL), skeletal abnormalities are considered uncommon, although radiologically demonstrable lesions have been reported in up to 29% of patients[8,9,19,25,27,30,33,36,40,48,58]. Osteolytic lesions

have also been reported in chronic myelomonocytic leukaemia[18,45]. As may be expected, the red marrow-containing segments of the skeleton are mainly affected. Generalized demineralization is by far the commonest abnormality in bone. In bone biopsy osteopenia is characteristically of histological type B (thick, but short trabeculae with disruption of the trabecular network and large, confluent marrow cavities). In contrast, osteopenia in polycythaemia vera (PV) shows attenuated trabeculae, but with preservation of the network (histological type A)[8,9,27] (see also Chapter 4). Destructive lesions, poorly outlined, may also occur in CML and the sites most commonly involved are the ends of long bones, the spine and the pelvis[17]. Osteolytic lesions and/or hypercalcaemia are most frequently observed in the accelerated and blastic phase[46,61], or due to complications such as infection, infarction or response to injury[38]. Osteosclerotic and mixed lesions in CML and PV are usually signs of transformation to MF/OMS[28,56].

Although the individual *malignant lymphomas* (ML) are histologically distinct and present with different clinical manifestations and radiological features, they have enough in common to be considered together, emphasizing where necessary their distinguishing characteristics[15,37,52,55,63].

Destruction of bone and hypercalcaemia are relatively infrequent in lymphomas of bone, except for Hodgkin's disease, chronic lymphocytic leukaemia, Burkitt's lymphoma and some T-cell lymphomas[13,24,32,35,44]. Recently, the lymphokine *lymphotoxin* has been shown to be a potent bone-resorbing agent *in vitro*. It is secreted by both T- and B-cells. Lymphomas of T-cell origin with

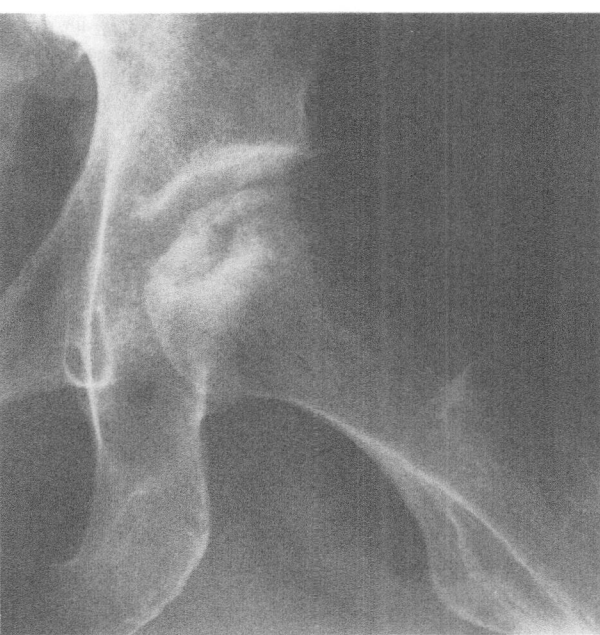

Fig. 19.R1 Osteolytic lesion (bone necrosis) with a rim of reactive sclerosis in the femoral head, during the course of aggressive chemotherapy in a patient with AL

Plate 19.A

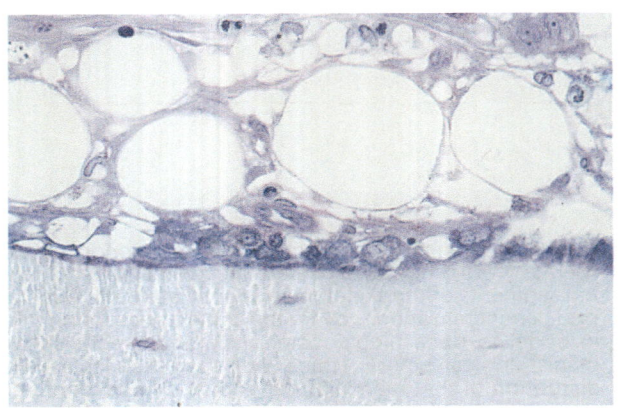

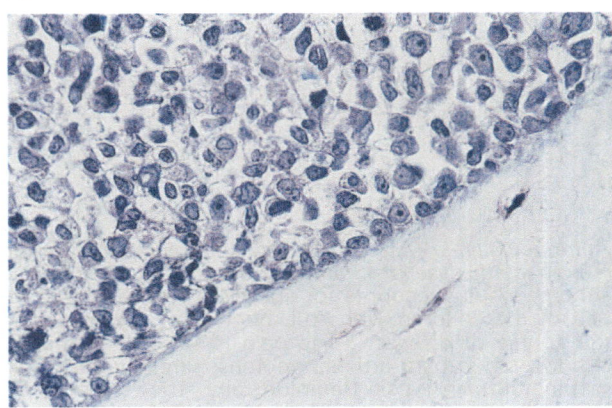

Figs. 19.1–19.6 Aspects of trabecular bone in acute leukaemia (AL)

Fig. 19.1 Case of hypocellular AL showing oedematous stroma and flat endosteal surface without remodelling. Giemsa

Fig. 19.2 Case of hypercellular AL. Sheet of monomorphic leukaemic blasts in apposition to inactive, flat trabecular surface as in Fig. 19.1. Giemsa

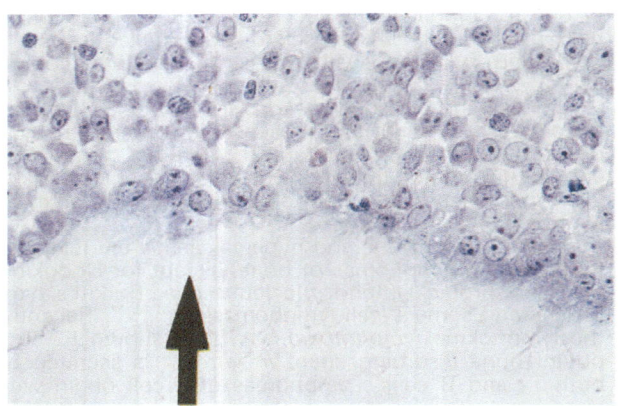

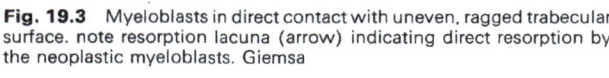

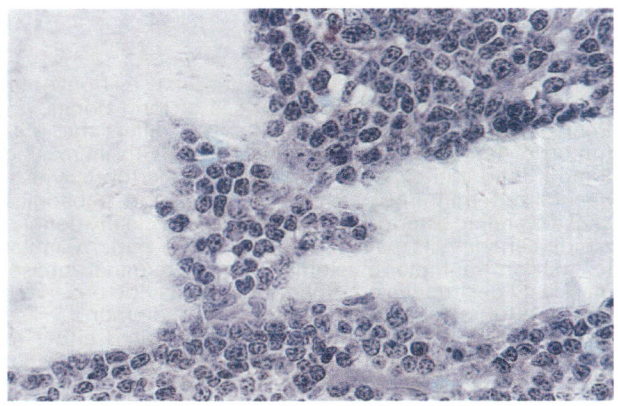

Figs. 19.3 and **19.4** Trabecular bone in two cases of AL with 'packed marrow' and reduction in trabecular bone volume

Fig. 19.3 Myeloblasts in direct contact with uneven, ragged trabecular surface. note resorption lacuna (arrow) indicating direct resorption by the neoplastic myeloblasts. Giemsa

Fig. 19.4 Example of more advanced direct trabecular resorption in AL, not mediated by osteoclasts. Giemsa

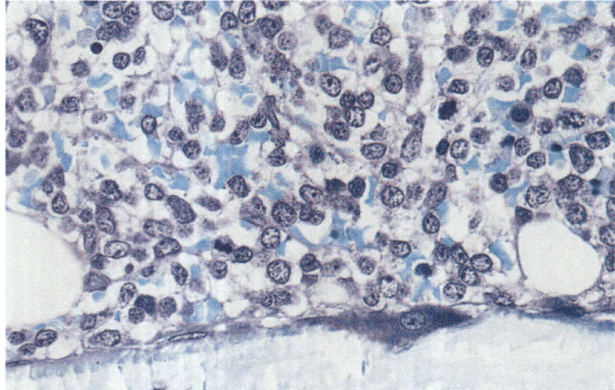

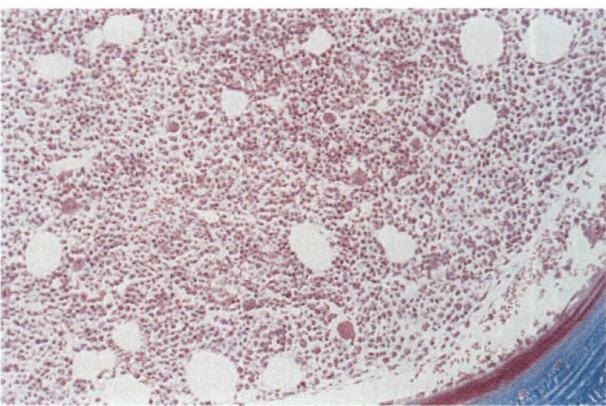

Fig. 19.5 Iliac crest biopsy of another case of AL illustrating osteoclastic resorption. Giemsa

Fig. 19.6 'Oncogenic osteomalacia' in AL, with broad seam of osteoid. Ladewig

characteristics of mature helper–inducer cells produce osteoclast activating factors with consequent destructive bone lesions and hypercalcaemia[13,39]. Interleukin-1, a monocyte product, is probably responsible for a series of other biological phenomena such as fibroblast proliferation and release of prostaglandins, and may play an important role in stromal and osseous reactions, for example in Hodgkin's disease. Hypercalcaemia associated with certain lymphomas may be caused by the increased synthesis of calcitriol by lymphoma cells[16].

Tables 19.1–3 and Plates 19.B–D summarize our histological, clinical and prognostic findings on bone changes in various *non-Hodgkin's lymphomas* (NHL) involving the skeleton[5,8–11].

In patients with *chronic lymphocytic leukaemia* (CLL)[37,42] and *Waldenström's disease* (WM)[7], trabecular osteopenia occurred in about 15%, and osteosclerosis was found in 7% of patients[3,7,35]. Hypercalcaemia has also been reported in the literature[35,44,62]. However, active remodelling, as indicated by the presence of osteoblasts and osteoclasts, was minimal and rare, though a mosaic trabecular structure with prominent cement lines reminiscent of that seen in Paget's disease of bone was observed in 5% of the biopsies. Osteolytic lesions have been reported especially in elderly patients[29].

Most cases with *ML centrocytic* (cleaved FCC lymphoma) showed a characteristic paratrabecular infiltration accompanied by coarse fibres radiating into the bone marrow. The histological parameters of bone remodelling were most prominent in this type of ML[5,8,10,11,27,30]. In contrast, cases with *ML centroblastic/centrocytic*, which had a nodular, mainly intertrabecular infiltration pattern, did not show any unusual activity of bone cells[8]. Following chemo- and/or radiation therapy the bone marrow may show remission but without complete restitution of haematopoiesis. In some cases the presence of minimal paratrabecular infiltration may raise the question of residual ML or reactive (benign) lymphocytosis.

In *hairy cell leukaemia* (HCL)[1,6,23,50] the volume percentages of the trabecular bone showed a marked negative correlation with those of the HC infiltration (correlation factor: −0.4). Cases of HCL of the convoluted and indented types (indicating an unfavourable prognosis) may exhibit solitary or multiple osteolytic lesions on skeletal X-rays (Fig. 19.R2)[6].

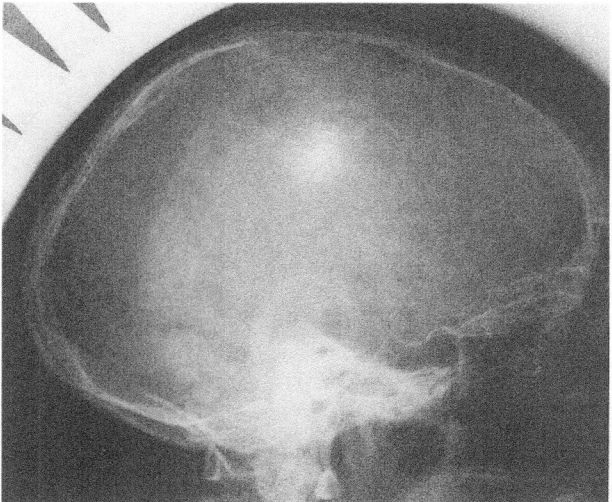

Fig. 19.R2 Multiple small osteolytic lesions in cranial bones in a patient with hairy cell leukaemia

Table 19.1 Bone changes in skeletal X-rays and in iliac crest biopsies in haematological malignancies

Parameters	Units	PV	CML	AL	NHL	HD	MM
Patients	n	210	190	200	510	85	300
Skeletal X-ray							
Normal	%	72	69	89	72	84	32
Porotic	%	22	27	3	23	10	24
Lytic	%	2	4	6	4	4	44
Sclerotic	%	4	0	2	1	2	2
Bone biopsy							
Bone structure							
Normal	%	69	60	63	65	72	52
Porotic	%	27	37	23	28	19	44
Sclerotic	%	4	3	4	7	9	4
Bone remodelling							
Increased	%	15	8	3	4	53	80

Table 19.2 Frequency and bone involvement in iliac crest biopsies in ML

Malignant lymphomas	Frequency (percentage of all cases)	Bone involvement (percentage in each group)
Lymphocytic (LC)	16	99
Lymphoblastic (LB)	2	45
Hairy cell leukaemia (HCL)	8	95
Centrocytic (CC)	4	71
Centroblastic/cytic (CB/CC)	3	20
Centroblastic (CB)	1	25
Immunocytic (IC)	15	85
Immunoblastic (IB)	1	29
Plasmacytic (PC)	30	94
Plasmablastic (PB)	12	79
Hodgkin's disease (HD)	5	8
Angioimmunoblastic (AILD)	2	70
Unclassifiable (UCL)	2	–

Table 19.3 Frequency of patterns of bone involvement and their prognostic relevance in different types of ML (percentage in each histological class; median survival time (months) in parentheses)

ML	Nodular	Nodular/Interstitial	Interstitial	Para-trabecular	Focal	Packed
LC	–	32 (107)	42 (36)	–	–	26 (25)
IC	41 (74)	33 (56)	6 (34)	–	–	20 (17)
PC	4 (20)	9 (22)	58 (46)	13 (31)	–	15 (16)
CC	–	–	–	60 (29)	–	40 (19)
CB/CC	80 (50)	–	–	–	–	20 (12)
Blastic	–	–	–	–	–	100 (6)
HCL	–	–	–	–	75 (28)	25 (18)
HD	–	–	–	–	65 (35)	35 (29)
AILD	–	–	–	–	76 (34)	24 (12)

In *ML of high-grade malignancy*, excluding ALL, osteolytic lesions have been found in about one-third of patients[8–11,27]. Osteoclast-activating factors, prostaglandin E as well as immunoreactive PTH have been implicated in the pathogenesis of bone destruction[24,32].

The overall incidence of *Hodgkin's disease* (HD) in the bone marrow of patients at initial presentation was 6% in our recent bone biopsy evaluation[2,4,9,11,27]. Radiographic bone involvement occurs in 20% of HD patients and in 4% at the initial presentation[2,4,14,21,26]. Based on autopsy

[continued on p. 213]

Plate 19.B

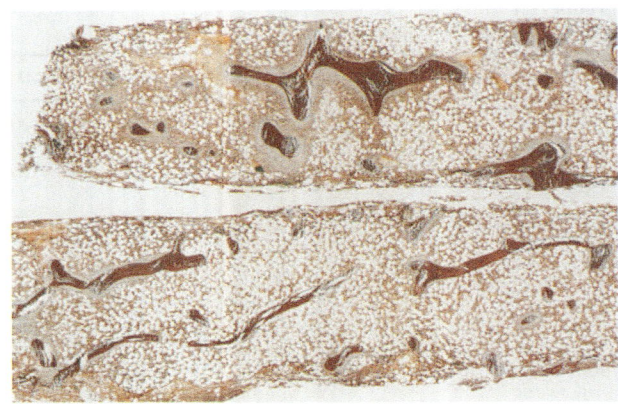

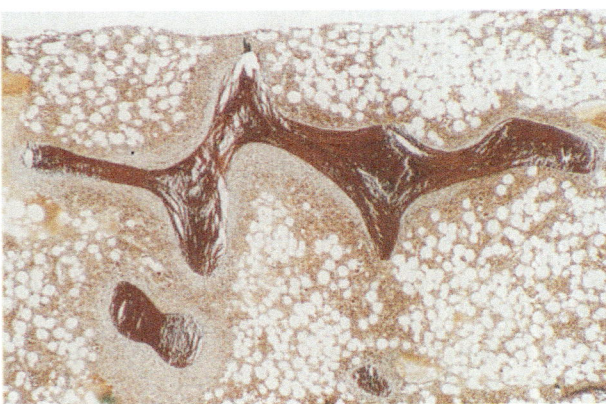

Figs. 19.7–19.12 Cancellous network in malignant lymphoma (ML) with paratrabecular involvement

Fig. 19.7 Overview of iliac crest biopsy demonstrating partly paratrabecular infiltration, hypocellular bone marrow and overall reduction in trabecular bone volume. It is of interest that the affected trabeculae are not attenuated. Gomori

Fig. 19.8 Higher magnification of biopsy shown in Fig. 19.7 illustrating dense infiltration in direct apposition to trabecular surface. Gomori

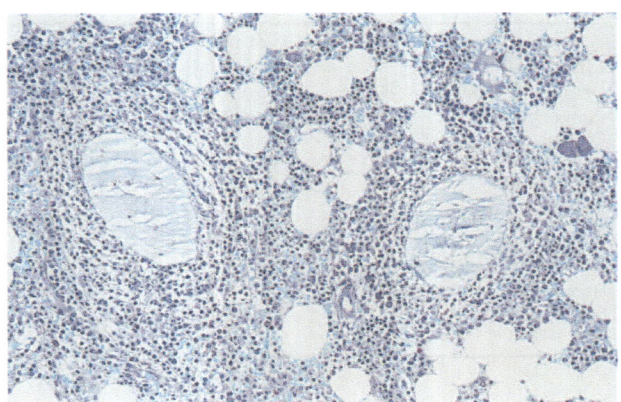

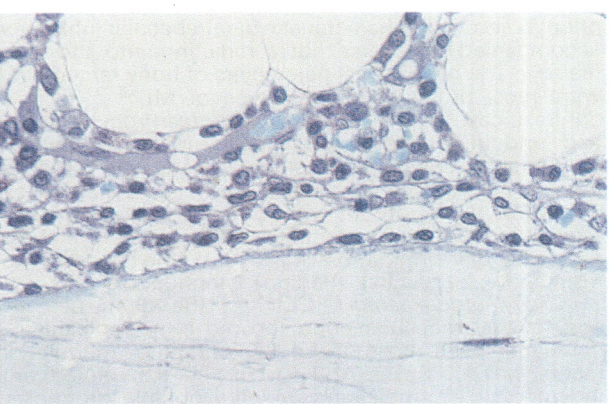

Fig. 19.9 Cross-sections of trabeculae with smooth surfaces, minimal osseous remodelling surrounded by broad band of infiltrating cells; example of the characteristic pattern in centrocytic lymphoma. Giemsa

Fig. 19.10 Higher magnification of section from Fig. 19.9 showing paratrabecular seam of small lymphoid cells and some fibres in ML centrocytic. Note smooth trabecular surface and absence of bone remodelling. Giemsa

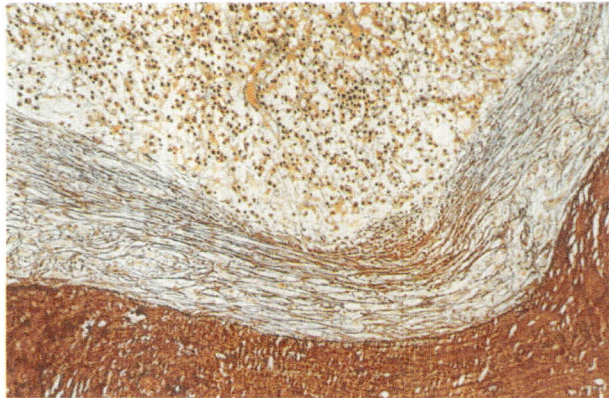

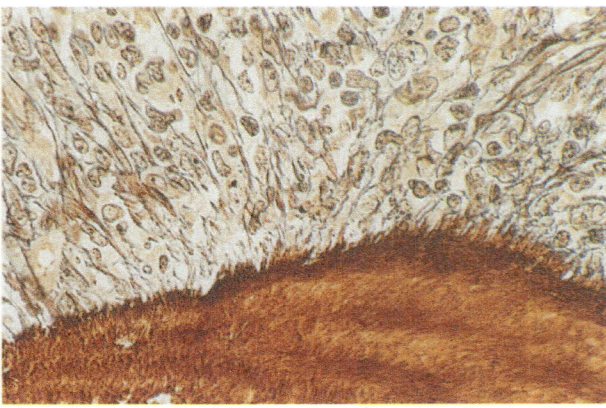

Fig. 19.11 Another case of centrocytic lymphoma which; in contrast to that illustrated in the previous figures, shows massive paratrabecular fibrosis (longitudinal section). Gomori

Fig. 19.12 High magnification showing attachment of coarse fibres to trabecular surface (simulating appearance of 'hair on end' skull). Gomori

Plate 19.C

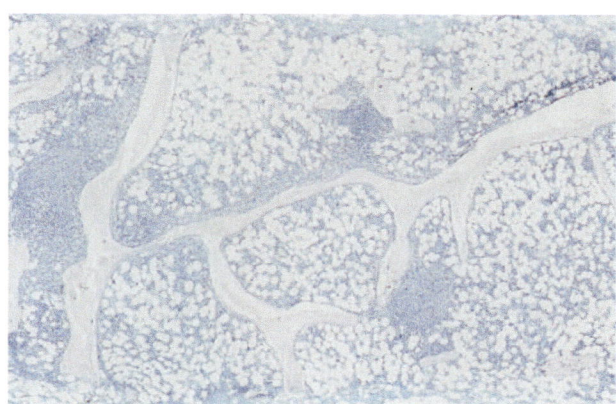

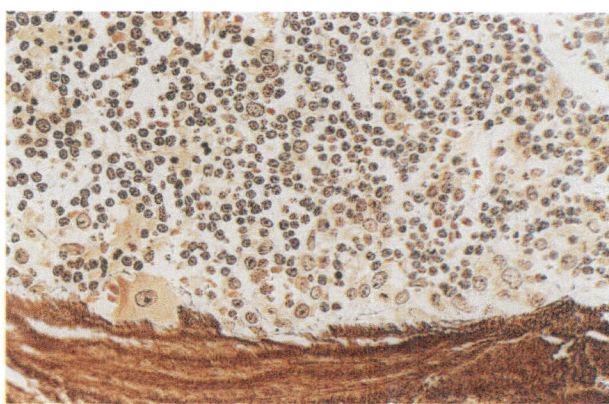

Figs. 19.13–19.18 Aspects of nodular bone involvement in iliac crest biopsies in ML

Fig. 19.13 Low magnification showing both paratrabecular and nodular involvement. Giemsa

Fig. 19.14 Higher magnification of biopsy from Fig. 19.13 showing nodular infiltration and adjacent osteoclastic bone resorption. Gomori

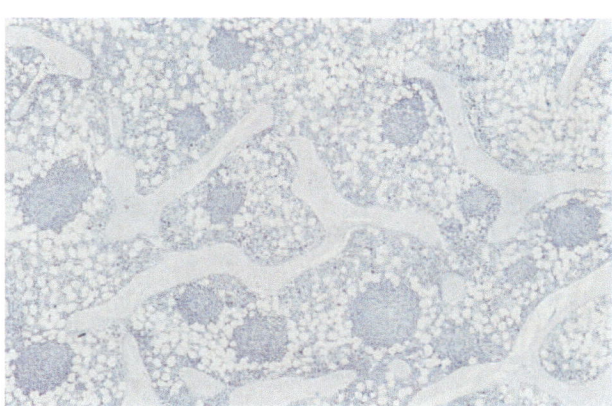

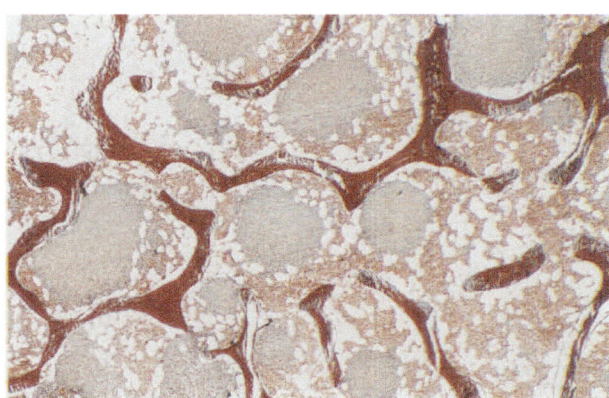

Fig. 19.15 Another case with multiple small intertrabecular nodules. Note preservation of trabecular structure. Giemsa

Fig. 19.16 Bone biopsy showing increasing involvement but with residual fat cells and haematopoietic tissue. Gomori. Patients with ML and nodular bone marrow involvement rarely develop bone marrow failure

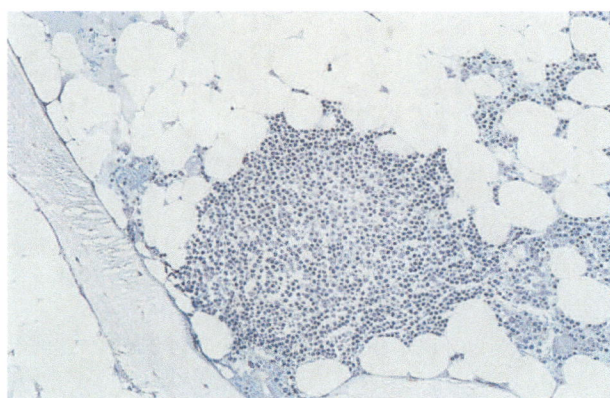

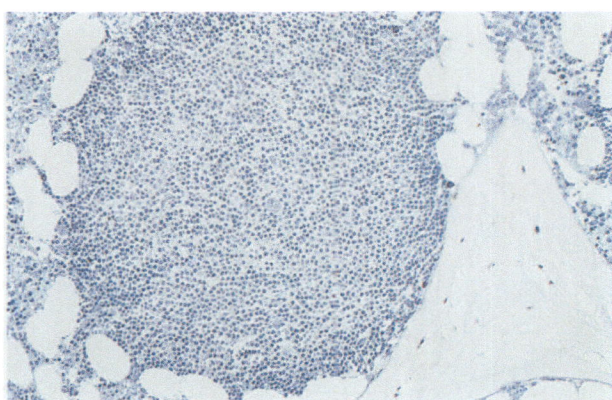

Fig. 19.17 Another aspect of same biopsy illustrating separation of the lymphomatous nodules by a layer of fat cells from a thin trabecula. Giemsa

Fig. 19.18 A larger lymphomatous nodule attached to the trabecular surface (right). Giemsa

Plate 19.D

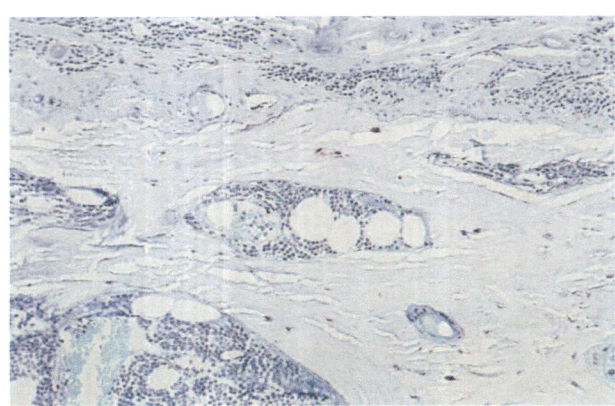

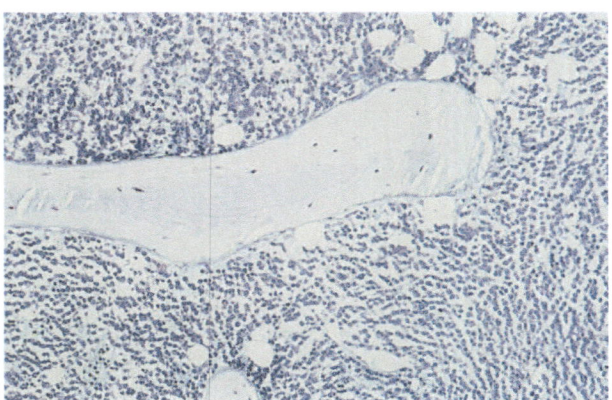

Figs. 19.19–19.21 Aspects of 'packed marrow' pattern in iliac crest biopsies in ML

Fig. 19.19 Cortical bone showing extension of the infiltration into the cavities of the cortical bone as well as the periosteum (upper part). Giemsa

Fig. 19.20 Attenuated trabecular bone from same biopsy with minimal remodelling. Giemsa

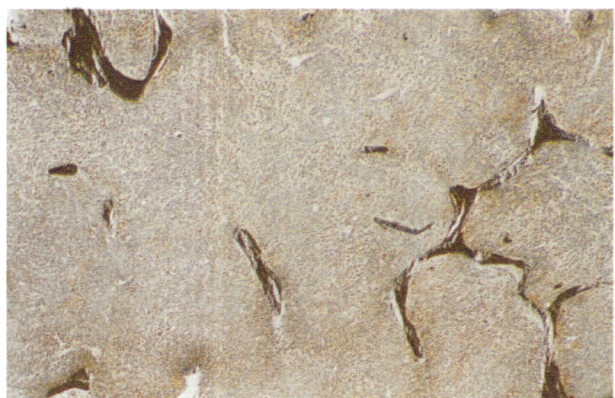

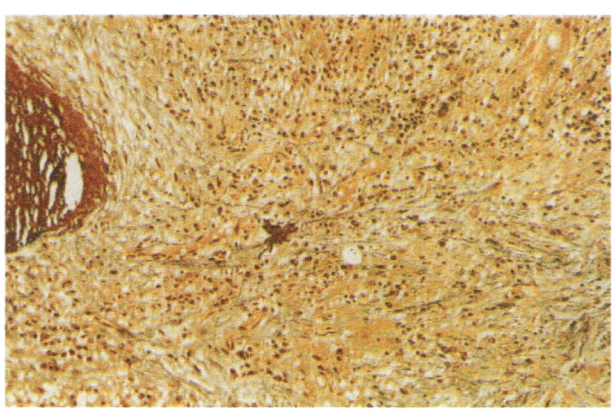

Fig. 19.21 Terminal stage of involvement with marked reduction in trabecular bone volume leading to osteolytic lesions. Gomori

Figs. 19.22–19.24 Effects of cytotoxic therapy in AL and ML

Fig. 19.22 Biopsy taken shortly after first course of therapy for AL showing partial degeneration, haemorrhage, fibrosis and incipient reconstitution of haematopoiesis. Note osteoblastic bone remodelling, osteoid seam and remodelling-related paratrabecular fibrosis. Gomori

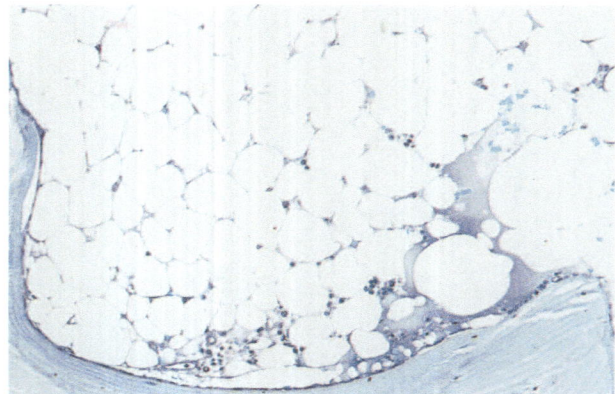

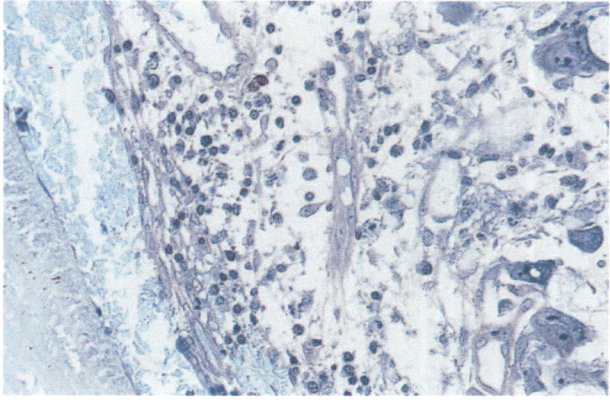

Fig. 19.23 Post-chemotherapy bone marrow in lymphoma patient with moderate pancytopenia and question of residual involvement, or chemotherapy-induced hypoplasia/dysplasia of haematopoiesis. The biopsy showed replacement by fat cells with minimal residual lymphocytic infiltration. Note seam of osteoid. Giemsa

Fig. 19.24 Post-therapy iliac crest biopsy of patient with ML highgrade malignancy showing residual involvement. Giemsa

findings the frequency of bone involvement is much higher, and varies between 34% and 78%. HD arising primarily in bone is a very rare occurrence[4,22]. Bone involvement signifies stage IV lymphoma. Hodgkin lymphoma is radiographically indistinguishable from non-Hodgkin lymphomas in the individual patient. The axial skeleton is more frequently involved (77%) than the appendicular skeleton (23%). Osteolytic lesions – often marked by a sclerotic margin – may be solitary (33%) or polyostotic (66%), varying in size from a few millimetres to large areas. Osteolysis is the rule in HD, but patchy sclerosis, 'ivory vertebra' and mixed lesions are also found.

The lesions in involved biopsies (Plate 19.E) were usually focal and ranged from small paratrabecular foci to large, confluent patches of 'lymphogranulomatous tissue'. For initial diagnosis identification of Reed–Sternberg cells within granulomatous tissue is required, but when HD has already been documented elsewhere atypical mononuclear cells within a suitable background are taken as evidence of involvement. Bone biopsies with epithelioid-cell granulomas or with foci of fibrosis and/or lymphocytic nodules are designated as negative. Bone lesions were predominantly lytic in about 50% of cases, with marked osteoclastic activity and surrounded by a lymphogranulomatous tissue with low content of lymphocytes but with a large number of Reed–Sternberg and Hodgkin cells. Osteosclerotic reactions were observed in 20% of the biopsies involved, especially in areas with a high content of lymphocytes and with inflammatory reactions, and culminating in the appearance of an 'ivory' vertebra. In 12% of the positive biopsies areas of osteoclastic resorption and osteoblastic formation were found, mimicking metastatic carcinoma on skeletal X-rays.

Post-therapy biopsies are indicated in patients who had bone involvement before treatment, to check for incomplete remission[4].

References

1. Arkel Y. S., Lake-Lewin D., Savopoulos A. A. and Berman E. (1984). Bone lesions in hairy cell leukemia. A case report and response of bone pains to steroids. *Cancer*, **53**, 2401
2. Bartl R., Burkhardt R., Lengsfeld H. and Huhn D. (1976). Die Bedeutung der histologischen Knochenmarksbeurteilung bei Morbus Hodgkin. *Klin. Wschr.*, **54**, 1061
3. Bartl R., Frisch B., Burkhardt R., Hoffmann-Fezer G., Demmler K. and Sund M. (1982). Assessment of marrow trephine in relation to staging in chronic lymphocytic leukaemia. *Brit. J. Haematol.*, **51**, 1
4. Bartl R., Frisch B., Burkhardt R., Huhn D. and Pappenberger R. (1982). Assessment of bone marrow histology in Hodgkin's disease: correlation with clinical factors. *Brit. J. Haematol.*, **51**, 345
5. Bartl R., Frisch B., Burkhardt R., Kettner G., Mahl G., Fateh-Moghadam A. and Sund M. (1982). Assessment of bone marrow histology in the malignant lymphomas (non-Hodgkin's): correlation with clinical factors for diagnosis, prognosis, classification and staging. *Brit. J. Haematol.*, **51**, 511
6. Bartl R., Frisch B., Hill W., Burkhardt R., Sommerfeld W. and Sund M. (1983). Bone marrow histology in hairy cell leukemia: identification of subtypes and their prognostic significance. *Amer. J. Clin. Pathol.*, **79**, 531
7. Bartl R., Frisch B., Mahl G., Burkhardt R., Fateh-Moghadam A., Pappenberger R., Sommerfeld W. and Hoffmann-Fezer G. (1983). Bone marrow histology in Waldenstroem's macroglobulinaemia. Clinical relevance of subtype recognition. *Scand. J. Haematol.*, **31**, 359
8. Bartl R., Frisch B. and Burkhardt R. (1985). *Bone Marrow Biopsies Revisited: A New Dimension for Haematologic Malignancies*. Basel: Karger
9. Bartl R., Frisch B. and Burkhardt R. (1991). Bone marrow histology. Catovsky D., *Methods in Hematology: The Leukemic Cell*, 2nd edn. (p. 47). Edinburgh: Churchill Livingstone
10. Bartl R., Frisch B., Kettner G., Hill W., Hoffmann-Fezer G., Sund M. and Burkhardt R. (1984). Histologic classification of lymphoproliferative disorders in the bone marrow. Frisch B. and Bartl R., *Bone Marrow Biopsies Updated: New Prospects for Clinical Diagnostics* (p. 98). Basel: Karger
11. Bartl R., Frisch B., Burkhardt R., Jaeger K., Pappenberger R. and Hoffmann-Fezer G. (1984). Lymphoproliferations in the bone marrow: identification and evolution, classification and staging. *J. Clin. Pathol.*, **37**, 233
12. Baty J. M. and Vogt E. C. (1935). Bone changes of leukemia in children. *Amer. J. Roentgenol.*, **34**, 310
13. Blayney D. W., Jaffe E. S. and Fisher R. I. (1983). The human T-cell lymphoma virus, lymphoma, lytic bone lesions and hypercalcemia. *Ann. Intern. Med.*, **98**, 144
14. Braunstein E. M. (1980). Hodgkin disease of bone; radiographic correlation with the histological classification. *Radiology*, **137**, 643
15. Braunstein E. M. and White S. J. (1980). Non-Hodgkin lymphoma of bone. *Radiology*, **135**, 59
16. Breslau N. A., McGuire J. L., Zerwekh J. E., Frenkel E. P. and Pak C. Y. C. (1984). Hypercalcemia associated with increased serum calcitriol levels in three patients with lymphoma. *Ann. Intern. Med.*, **100**, 1
17. Campbell E., Maldonado W. and Suhrland G. (1975). Painful lytic bone lesion in an adult with chronic myelogenous leukemia. *Cancer*, **33**, 1354
18. Chabner B. A., Haskell C. M. and Canellos G. P. (1969). Destructive bone lesions in chronic granulocytic leukemia. *Medicine*, **48**, 401
19. Clements D. G. and Kalmon E. H. (1956). Chronic myelogenous leukemia. Unusual bone changes in an adult. *Radiology*, **67**, 339
20. Cohn S. L., Morgan E. R. and Mallette L. E. (1987). The spectrum of metabolic bone disease in lymphoblastic leukemia. *Cancer*, **59**, 346
21. Coles W. C. and Schultz M. D. (1948). Bone involvement in malignant lymphoma. *Radiology*, **50**, 458
22. Cowie F., Benghiat A. and Holgate C. (1991). Primary Hodgkin's disease of bone. *Clin. Oncol.*, **3**, 233
23. Demanes D. J., Lane N. and Beckstead J. H. (1982). Bone involvement in hairy cell leukemia. *Cancer*, **49**, 697
24. Demers L. M., Allegra J. C. and Harvey H. A. (1977). Plasma prostaglandins in hypercalcemic patients with neoplastic disease. *Cancer*, **39**, 1559
25. Edeiken J., Dalinka M. and Karasick D. (1990). *Edeiken's Roentgen Diagnosis of Diseases of Bone*. Baltimore: Williams & Wilkins
26. Ferrant A., Rodhain J. and Michaux J. L. (1975). Detection of skeletal involvement in Hodgkin's disease: a comparison of radiography, bone scanning, and bone marrow biopsy in 38 patients. *Cancer*, **35**, 1346
27. Frisch B. and Bartl R. (1990). *Atlas of Bone Marrow Pathology*. Dordrecht: Kluwer
28. Frisch B., Bartl R., Burkhardt R., Jäger K., Mahl G. and Kettner G. (1984). Classification of myeloproliferative disorders by bone marrow histology. Frisch B. and Bartl R., *Bone Marrow Biopsies Updated: New Prospects for Clinical Diagnostics* (p. 57). Basel: Karger
29. Frisch B. and Bartl R. (1988). Histologic classification and staging of chronic lymphocytic leukaemia. A retrospective and prospective study of 503 cases. *Acta Haematol.*, **79**, 140
30. Frisch B., Lewis S. M., Burkhardt R. and Bartl R. (1985). *Biopsy Pathology of Bone and Bone Marrow*. London: Chapman & Hall
31. Gallagher D., Heinrich S. D., Craver R., Ward K. and Warrier R. (1991). Skeletal manifestations of acute leukemia in childhood. *Orthopedics*, **14**, 485
32. Goltzman D., Stewart A. F. and Broaders A. E. (1981). Malignancy-associated hypercalcemia evaluation with a cytochemical bioassay for parathyroid hormone. *J. Clin. Endocrinol. Metab.*, **53**, 899
33. Huvos A. G. (1991). Skeletal manifestations of malignant lymphomas and leukemias. Huvos A. G., *Bone Tumors: Diagnosis, Treatment and Prognosis* (p. 625). Philadelphia: Saunders
34. Lands R. and Karnad A. (1991). Non T-cell lymphoblastic lymphoma with extensive osteolytic lesions and hypercalcemia. *South. Med. J.*, **84**, 1405
35. Littlewood T. J., Lydon A. P. M. and Barton C. J. (1990). Hypercalcaemia and osteolytic lesions associated with chronic lymphatic leukaemia (CLL). *Brit. Med. J.*, **43**, 877
36. Martell R. W., Myers H. S. and Jacobs P. (1986). Bone lesions in chronic granulocytic leukaemia. *Brit. J. Haematol.*, **62**, 31
37. McKenna R. W. and Hernandez J. A. (1988). Bone marrow in malignant lymphoma. *Hematol./Oncol. Clin. N. Amer.*, **2**(4), 617
38. Mora J. J., Heron J. F., L'Hirondel J. L. and Loyan G. (1979). Lesion osteolytique au cours de la leukemic myeloid chronique. *Nouv. Presse Med.*, **8**, 3171
39. Mundy G. R., Luben R. A., Raisz L. G., Oppenheim J. J. and Buell D. N. (1974). Bone-resorbing activity in supernatants from lymphoid cell line. *N. Engl. J. Med.*, **290**, 867
40. Murray R. O., Jacobson H. G. and Stoker D. J. (1990). *The*

Plate 19.E

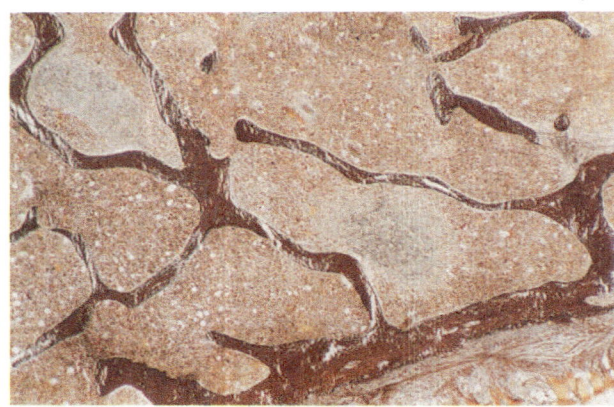

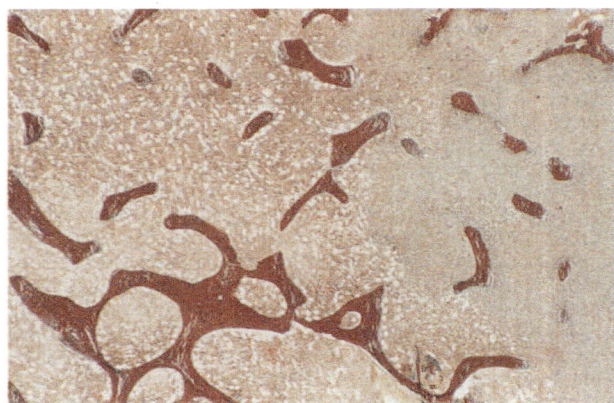

Figs. 19.25–19.30 Aspects of bone involvement in Hodgkin's disease (HD)

Fig. 19.25 Part of iliac crest biopsy showing mainly nodular subcortical involvement with no effect on the trabecular network. No changes found on skeletal X-ray or bone scan. Gomori

Fig. 19.26 Bone biopsy with large area of involvement and osteolytic lesions, also seen on skeletal X-ray. Gomori

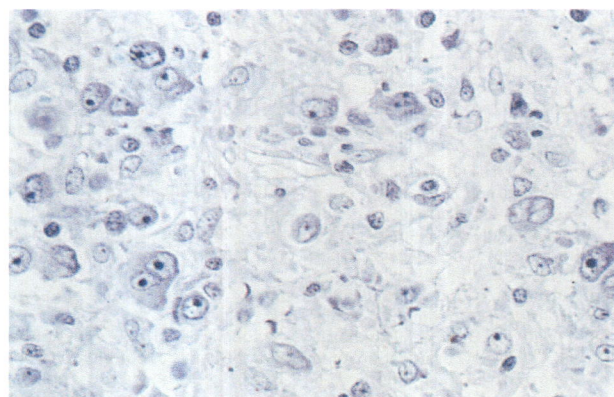

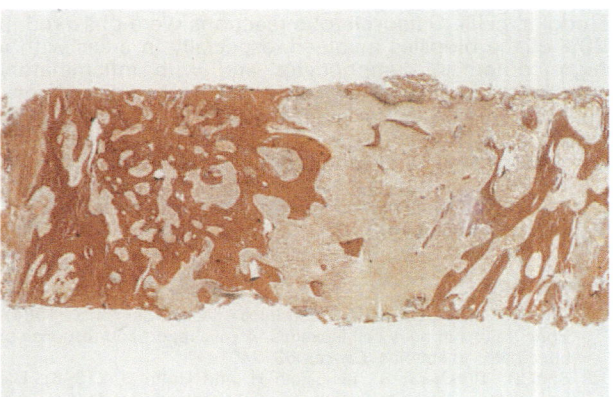

Fig. 19.27 High-power view of cellular area from Fig. 19.26 showing lymphocyte depletion HD. Note typical Reed–Sternberg cell left. Giemsa

Fig. 19.28 Overview of iliac crest biopsy demonstrating mixed osteolytic/osteosclerotic lesions. Gomori

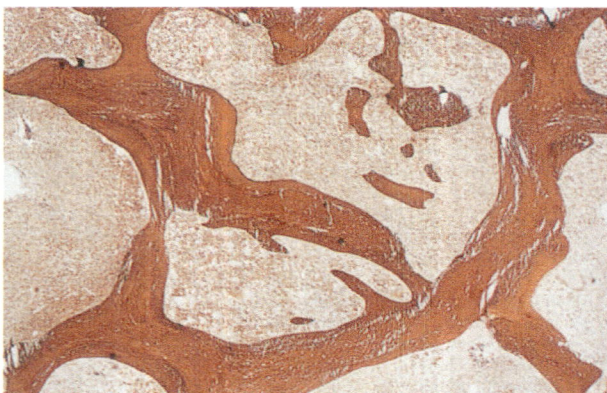

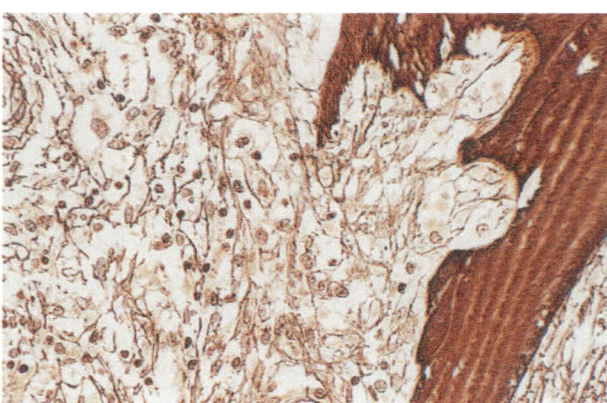

Fig. 19.29 Osteoblastic appositional and woven bone formation from sclerotic area. Gomori

Fig. 19.30 Bone resorption from edge of osteolytic area. Note absence of osteoclasts in deep resorption cavities. Gomori

Radiology of Skeletal Disorders. Edinburgh: Churchill Livingstone
41. Ngan H., James K. W., McCready V. R. and MacDonald J. S. (1966). Bone changes in adult acute leukaemia. *Brit. J. Radiol.,* **41**, 66
42. Ngan H. and Preston B. J. (1975). Non-Hodgkin's lymphoma presenting with osseous lesions. *Clin. Radiol.,* **26**, 351
43. Nixon G. W. and Gwinn J. L. (1973). The roentgen manifestations of leukemia in infancy. *Radiology,* **107**, 603
44. Norby K. and Vikrot O. (1975). Hypercalcaemia in chronic lymphatic leukemia. *Scand. J. Haematol.,* **15**, 132
45. Ohri S. K., Sharp D. J. and Coutts G. B. (1990). Osteolytic lesions in chronic myelomonocytic leukaemia. *Brit. J. Clin. Pract.,* **44**, 672
46. Opperman H. C., Ludwig R. and Georgi P. (1979). Osteolytic lesion in chronic myelogenous leukemia (CML). Initial manifestation of blastic crisis? *Pediatr. Radiol.,* **8**, 254
47. Parker B. R., Marglin S. and Castellino R. A. (1980). Skeletal manifestations of leukemia, Hodgkin disease, and non-Hodgkin lymphoma. *Semin. Roentgenol.,* **15**, 302
48. Pear B. L. (1974). Skeletal manifestations of the lymphomas and leukemias. *Semin. Roentgenol.,* **9**, 229
49. Ramsey N. K., Brown D. M., Nesbit M. E., Coccia P. F., Krivit W. and Krutzik S. (1979). Autonomous production of parathyroid hormone by lymphoblastic leukemia cells in culture. *J. Pediatr.,* **94**, 623
50. Rhyner K., Streuli R. and Kistler S. (1977). Haarzell-Leukämie (hairy cell leukemia) mit osteolytischen Knochenveränderungen. *Schweiz. Med. Wschr.,* **107**, 863
51. Rogalsky R. J., Black G. B. and Reed M. H. (1986). Orthopaedic manifestations of leukaemia in children. *J. Bone Jt Surg.,* **68A**, 494
52. Schajowicz F. (1981). *Tumors and Tumor-like Lesions of Bone and Joints.* New York: Springer
53. Silverman F. N. (1948). The skeletal lesion in leukemia. *Amer. J. Roentgenol.,* **59**, 819
54. Simmons C. R., Harle T. S. and Singleton E. B. (1986). The osseous manifestations of leukemia in children. *Radiol. Clin. N. Amer.,* **6**, 115
55. Spagnoli I., Gattoni F. and Viganotti G. (1982). Roentgenographic aspects of non-Hodgkin's lymphomas presenting with osseous lesions. *Skeletal Radiol.,* **8**, 39
56. Thiele J., Hoeppner B., Wienhold S., Schneider G., Fischer R. and Zankowich R. (1989). Osteoclasts and bone remodeling in chronic myeloproliferative disorders. A histochemical and morphometric study on trephine biopsies in 165 patients. *Pathol. Res. Pract.,* **184**, 591
57. Thomas L. B., Forkner C. E. and Frei E. (1961). The skeletal lesions of acute leukemia. *Cancer,* **14**, 608
58. Valimaki M., Vuopio P. and Liewendahl K. (1981). Bone lesions in chronic myelogenous leukaemia. *Acta Med. Scand.,* **210**, 403
59. Vassilopoulou-Sellin R. and Ramirez I. (1992). Severe osteopenia and vertebral compression fractures after complete remission in an adolescent with acute leukemia. *Amer. J. Hematol.,* **39**, 142
60. Vesterby A. and Jensen O. M. (1985). Aseptic bone/bone marrow necrosis in leukaemia. *Scand. J. Haematol.,* **35**, 365
61. Walter R. M. and Greenberg B. R. (1980). Hypercalcemia in the accelerated phase of chronic myelogenous leukemia. *Cancer,* **46**, 1174
62. Wang J. C., Steiner W., Aung M. K. and Tobin M. S. (1978). Primary hyperparathyroidism and chronic lymphatic leukaemia. *Cancer,* **42**, 1964
63. Wilner D. (1982). *Radiology of Bone Tumors and Allied Disorders.* Philadelphia: Saunders
64. Wilson J. K. V. (1959). The bone lesions of childhood leukemia: survey of 140 cases. *Radiology,* **72**, 672
65. Zidar B. L., Shadduck R. K., Winkelstein A., Zeigler Z. and Hawker C. D. (1976). Acute myelogenous leukemia and hypercalcemia: a case of probable ectopic parathyroid hormone production. *N. Engl. J. Med.,* **295**, 692

Metastatic bone disease

20

Bone metastases are common, especially in advanced cancer, and constitute one of the fundamental problems in clinical oncology[18,23,62,76,80]. In recent years, increasingly aggressive attempts have been made to arrest the growth of metastatic cancer involving bone[18,62]. Prevention of osseous metastases is not yet possible as multiple micrometastases may already be present at the time of initial presentation, diagnosis and therapy[35,62]. As shown by immunocytological studies, it is almost certain that dissemination has occurred by the time cancer is first detectable clinically at any site, but the extent of the threat posed thereby has not yet been estimated. A statistical evaluation of the fifth report on the End Results Group Program showed that at least 9% of breast cancer patients carry metastasis for more than 10 years[91]. At least four mechanisms have been proposed to account for this phenomenon of *tumour dormancy*:

1. lack of vascularization,
2. microenvironmental effects,
3. supply of growth factors and hormones, and
4. presence of defence cells (immune surveillance).

Only under the influence of further stimuli – hormonal, immunological and other as yet unknown factors – do these foci grow and become clinically apparent[10,62].

Bone scintigraphy for the detection of bone metastases has changed the management and monitoring of carcinoma patients (Fig. 20.R1)[18,32,50,62,69,82]. Because of their greater sensitivity bone scans may detect bone metastases up to 18 months before their appearance on roentgenograms. Scintigraphy may detect lesions as small as 2 mm, but due to low specificity, abnormal findings need to be confirmed by roentgenograms. The false-negative rate for bone scans is reported to be 8%, whereas the false-

positive rate may be as high as 50%. Although metastases most commonly present as 'hot' lesions, 'cold' areas are also possible and caused by obliterations of supplying blood vessels. The *roentgenographic diagnosis* is usually not difficult[21], but the absence of bone alterations does not exclude bone metastases (Plate 20.A). For example in patients with oat cell carcinoma of the lung the entire skeleton may be infiltrated by tumour tissue, but the roentgenogram shows only non-specific osteopenia or no change at all. According to Adams *et al*. up to 50% of the trabecular bone must be destroyed before radiological demonstration is possible, and even lesions with a diameter of 10 mm may be undetectable[3]. *Computed tomography* (CT)[36,62] or *magnetic resonance imaging* (MRI)[62] are more sensitive techniques in these cases, but they are not applicable as routine investigations for assessment of the skeleton. Osteolytic metastases may be solitary or multiple, sometimes with sclerotic marginal reactions. Osteoblastic metastases are usually seen in well-differentiated, slow-growing tumours. They are frequently observed in prostatic carcinoma, where they often increase in density after successful therapy. With disease progression, mixed lesions develop in previously stable sclerotic or progressive osteolytic lesions.

Metastases to the skeleton clearly outnumber primary bone tumours. The *frequency* of bone metastases in carcinoma patients reported in the literature varies from 28% to 85%, the wide range presumably reflecting the method of investigation, the stage of disease and the thoroughness of search[2,4,14,19,24,35,49,56,62,74,88,89]. Jaffe has stated that when careful post-mortem examinations are performed on all patients dying of malignancy, over 90% show osseous metastases[40]. They are especially common from carcinomas arising in breast, prostate, lung and kidney (Table 20.1), accounting for more than 80% of metastatic bone lesions[15,88–90]. Radiological ante-mortem studies have established the diagnosis of bone metastases in about 50% of patients with metastatic cancer originating from breast, prostate and lung cancer[52,55,66,68]. Metastases of these cancers demonstrate *osteotropism*[53], i.e. they possess a unique affinity for bone[18]. In breast cancer this correlates with positive steroid receptors, and in prostate cancer with histological grade[31]. Of the bronchial cancers, oat cell carcinoma metastasizes to bone more frequently than other histological types[16]. Further possible

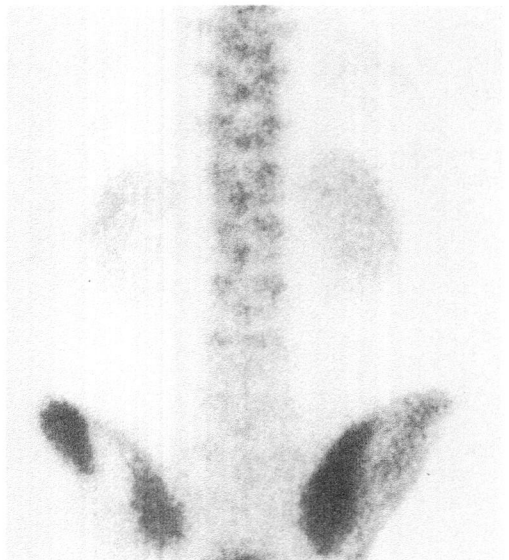

Fig. 20.R1 Bone scan of a patient with metastatic breast cancer with increased uptake in both posterior iliac crests. Infiltration documented by iliac crest biopsies taken from these areas

Table 20.1 Frequency of positive bone biopsies in carcinoma patients[27]

	Patients	Positive biopsies	Percentage
Primary tumour			
Breast	504	211	42
Prostate	255	80	32
Lung	389	56	14
Others	294	48	19
Unknown	283	205	72
Biopsy size			
< 60 mm²	1230	357	29
≥ 60 mm²	495	243	49
Total	1725	600	35

Plate 20.A

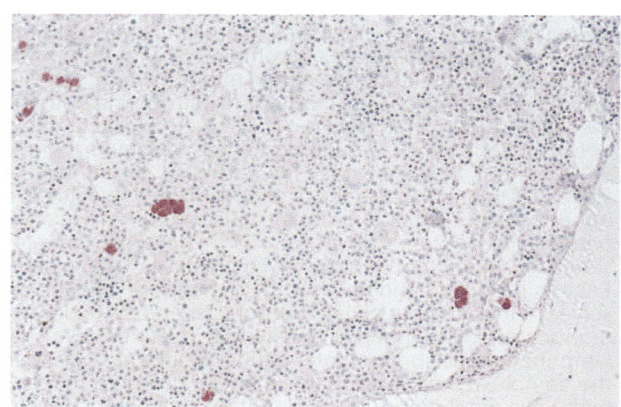

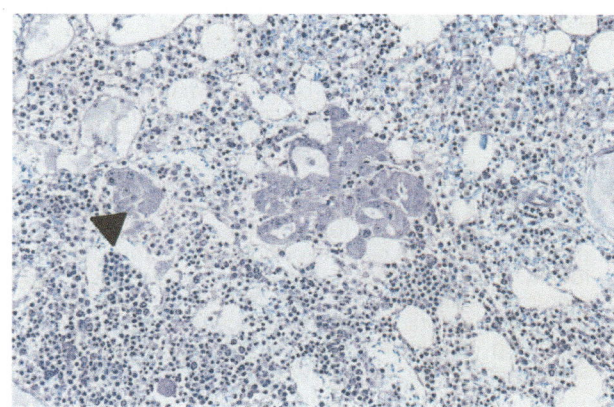

Figs. 20.1–20.6 Metastatic involvement in iliac crest biopsies without an osseous reaction

Fig. 20.1 Isolated tumour cells dispersed in cellular bone marrow. PAS

Fig. 20.2 Small and large interstitial metastases with minimal stromal reaction. Giemsa

Figs. 20.3 and **20.4** Bone biopsy of patient with breast cancer, no abnormalities on skeletal X-ray or bone scan

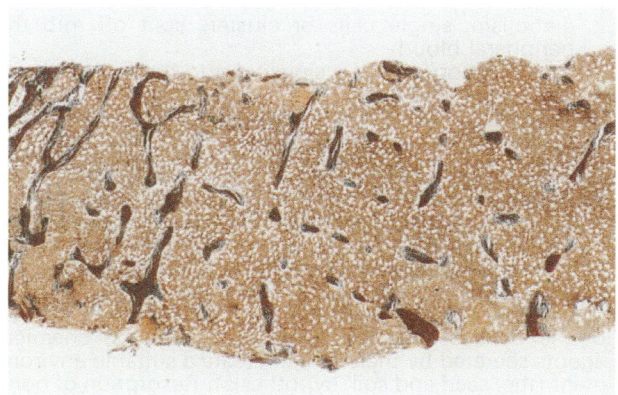

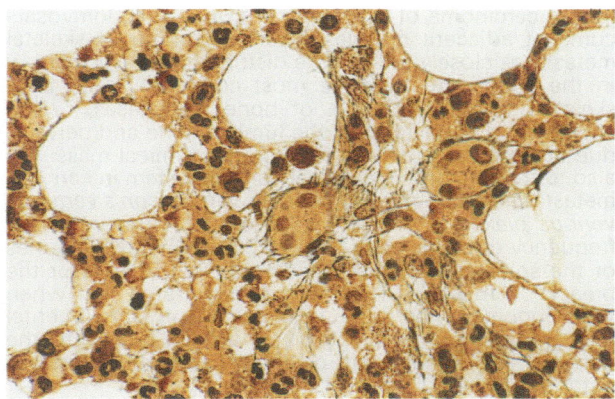

Fig. 20.3 Focal metastatic involvement in the subcortical (left) and deeper (lower right) zones. Gomori

Fig. 20.4 Higher magnification of section in Fig. 20.3, to show two very small interstitial metastases surrounded by fine fibrosis. Gomori

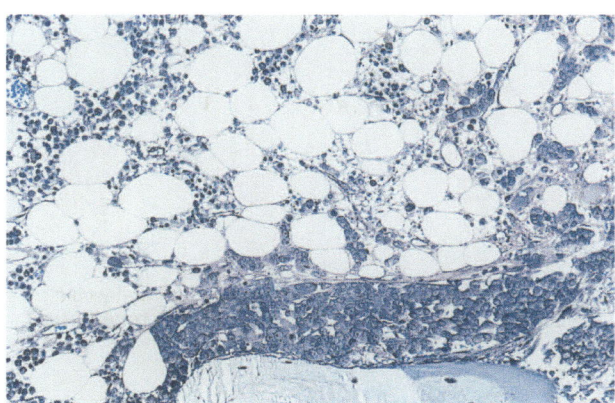

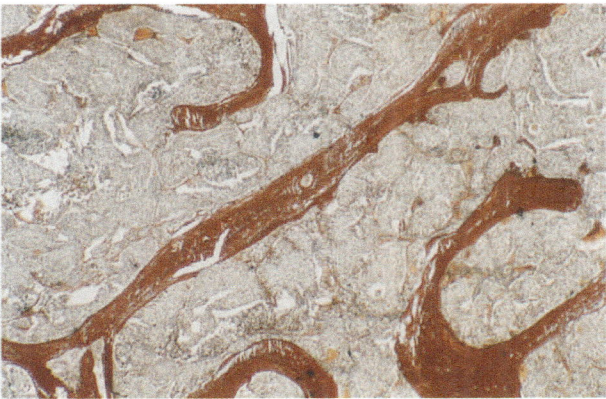

Fig. 20.5 Endosteal sinusoid engorged with tumour cells and many small groups of tumour cells scattered in the bone marrow, accompanied by reactive fibrosis. The trabecular surface underlying the sinusoid shows osteoblastic new bone formation. Giemsa

Fig. 20.6 Bone biopsy of patient with bronchial cancer and pancyto-penia, but normal skeletal X-rays and bone scan. Solid masses of tumour cells (oat cell carcinoma) separated by septa containing blood vessels. Normal trabecular bone structure. Gomori

mechanisms for predilection of bone invasion may be[7,13,22,24,25,54,62]:

1. stimulation of tumour growth by local growth factors and hormones present in bone and marrow;
2. large gaps and lack of basement membrane in the marrow sinusoids, with low endothelial cell resistance to tumour cell penetration;
3. partially very low blood flow in the sinusoidal system of the bone marrow, enabling intravascular 'dormant' tumour emboli over a long period of time;
4. circulating tumour cells responding to factors diffusing locally out of the bone – for example collagen fragments and minerals derived from normal bone resorption are chemotactic for tumour cells *in vitro*; and
5. shedding of platelets into the marrow sinusoids and subsequent release of growth factors.

Metastatic disease involves the skeleton mainly through the vascular system[56]. Therefore bone metastases are usually widespread by the time of their first clinical manifestation. Lymphatic vessels apparently are absent in the bone marrow and therefore they cannot contribute to transporting tumour cell emboli to the skeleton[26]. Direct invasion of bone may rarely occur from a tumour of an adjacent organ, for example direct invasion of the ilium from a carcinoma of the cervix or from a rhabdomyosarcoma of adjacent muscles. The distribution of skeletal metastases closely reflects the distribution of red marrow in the adult, and they are most common in the axial skeleton (more than 80% of bone metastases)[62]. The incidence of metastases in the lumbar spine and pelvis is due not only to their considerable anatomical mass, but also to the role of the vertebral venous system in carrying metastases to bone. Retrograde flow in *Batson's vertebral venous plexus* is thought to account for the increased frequency of metastases (Fig. 20.S1) to the pelvic bones or the spine from cancers arising in the prostate or the breast[35,56]. Indeed it has been demonstrated that when intra-abdominal pressure is increased in experimental animals undergoing injections of tumour cells into the femoral vein, nearly all develop osseous metastases without lung involvement.

Tumour clusters in the paratrabecular sinusoids are frequently seen in *bone biopsies* of patients with prostatic and breast cancers, and this is compatible with retrograde tumour invasion via the vertebral venous system[26–28]. But not only mechanical and filtration mechanisms determine the distribution of metastases. An interaction is postulated between a clump of circulating cancer cells and the site at which it is arrested – the 'seed and soil' hypothesis of Paget[74]. The manifestations of blood-borne metastasis in bone represent the end-results of a series of *interactions between tumour and host tissue*[27,62]. There is a complex series of interactions between metastases and host[37]. Factors produced and released by the tumour cells themselves stimulate host cells – fibroblasts, endothelial cells, monocytes, macrophages, mast cells, plasma cells and lymphocytes – also to secrete regulatory factors[27]. Despite the complexity involved in these interactions, preliminary pathways regulating tumour growth, invasion and establishment of metastases have now been proposed. Many of the regulatory factors participating in these processes also affect bone cells and thereby bone and its remodelling. The process itself can be tentatively divided into five events (Plate 20.B)[47,62,65,74].

1. invasion, i.e. of lymphatic or blood vessels at site of origin;
2. embolism, single cells or clusters split off into the peripheral blood;
3. extravasation, out of a sinusoid into the interstitium;
4. adherence; and
5. growth, induction of connective tissue and blood vessels (see also Fig. 20.S2).

Within the vascular system, tumour cells tend to form aggregates without or with platelets and lymphocytes, and it is these larger emboli that are trapped in the sinusoidal system of the bone marrow, mostly in the endosteal sinusoids. The tumour cells enter the bone marrow by migrating through the endothelial gaps. Subsequent growth, vascularization and stromal organization of the extravascular tumour cells depend on chemical agents secreted by them which create a suitable environment (the 'seed and soil' hypothesis). Resorption of bone

Distribution of skeletal metastases

Skull 40%

Cervical spine 25%
Scapula/clavicula 10%
Proximal humerus 15%

Ribs 60%
Thoracic spine 70%

Lumbar spine 70%
Pelvis 70%
Proximal femur 45%

Fig. 20.S1 Frequency of skeletal sites involved in metastatic bone disease

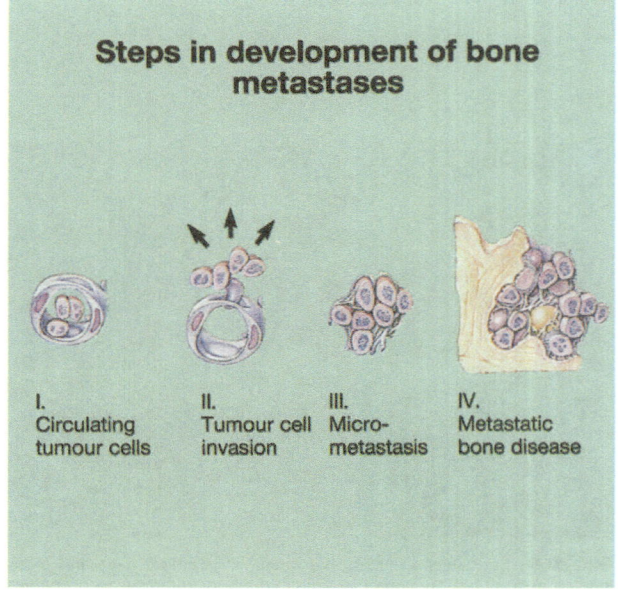

Steps in development of bone metastases

I. Circulating tumour cells

II. Tumour cell invasion

III. Micro-metastasis

IV. Metastatic bone disease

Fig. 20.S2 From circulating tumour cell to metastatic bone disease

Plate 20.B

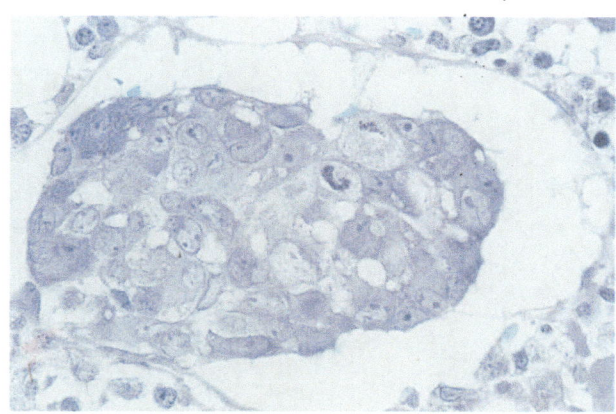

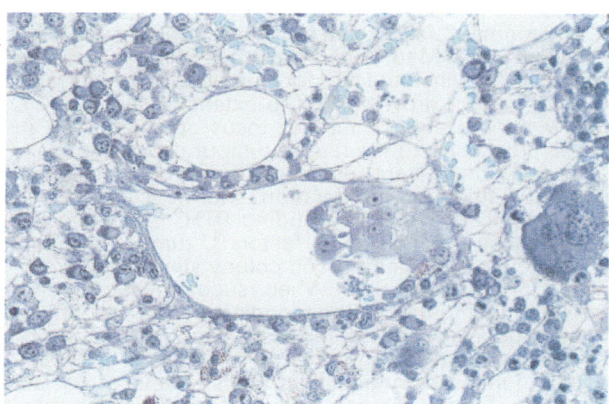

Figs. 20.7–20.21 Steps in establishment of metastasis in bone

Fig. 20.7 Tumour cell embolus in bone marrow showing attachment and penetration of endothelial layer (lower left). Note mitotic figure in tumour cell embolus. Giemsa

Fig. 20.8 Metastatic embolus destroying the sinusoidal wall (right) and invading the interstitial space of the bone marrow. Note mega-karyocyte (right) and inflammatory cells (plasma cells and lymphocytes) surrounding the area of tumour cell invasion. Giemsa

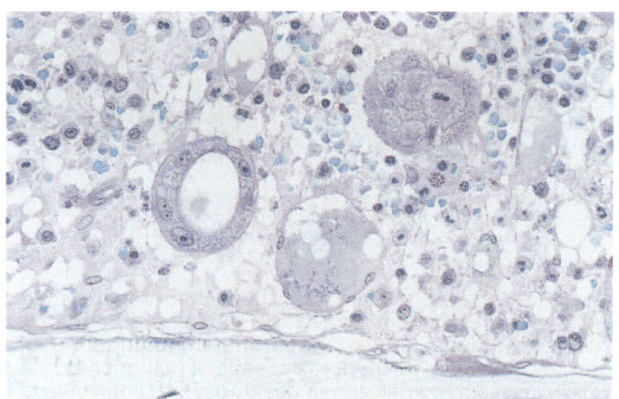

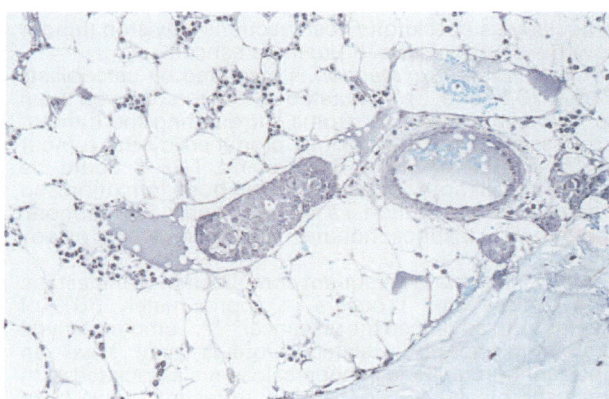

Fig. 20.9 Two metastases, one showing glandular differentiation and the other consisting of a tumour cell cluster including a mitotic figure, together with stromal and osseous reaction (osteoclast lower right). Giemsa

Fig. 20.10 Large intravascular tumour embolus and small interstitial clusters of tumour cells in hypocellular bone marrow. Giemsa

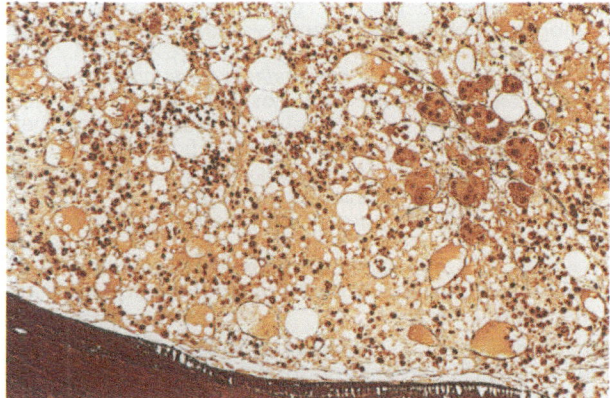

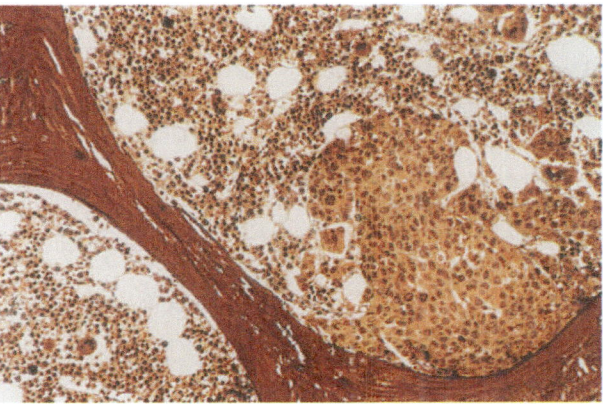

Fig. 20.11 Multiple small tumour cell aggregates in bone marrow exhibiting marked stromal alterations in the surroundings: oedema, vascular hyperplasia, incipient fibrosis and marked reactive lympho- and plasmacytosis. Gomori

Fig. 20.12 Paratrabecular metastasis extending into marrow cavity with minimal stromal and osseous reactions. Gomori

near such a tumour cell aggregate may help to provide an environment favourable for the development of a metastatic focus. Matrix factors released from the resorbed bone can be chemotactic for tumour cells and also promote tumour growth[47,62]. The extent of laying down of new bone around a tumour focus appears to be in inverse proportion to the rate of tumour expansion.

A number of different substances are involved in stimulation of osteoclast proliferation and neoplastic *bone destruction* (Plate 20.C), including PTH[5,38], prostaglandins[30], transforming growth factors[39], tumour necrosis factor[8,41,71], interleukins[63,71] and colony stimulating activities[9,46,62,83] (Fig. 20.S3). When such substances are secreted by tumours into the bloodstream they act on the skeleton generally, when released locally osteolysis of immediately adjacent bone results[29]. Tumours of breast, prostate, lung, kidney and thyroid all secrete osteoclast stimulating factors. Monocytes, often found at the margins of bone metastases, may also stimulate bone resorption via the osteoclast activating cytokines IL-1 and TNF-α[10,60]. Osteoclast-independent mechanisms of bone destruction by cancer are rare and comprise direct tumour-related osteolysis (Fig. 20.EM1) (lytic enzymes secreted by tumour cells), osteocyte-mediated osteolysis, as well as necrosis of bone due to ischaemia or 'pressure atrophy' (Fig. 20.S3)[10,62]. However immunological, fibrotic and particularly osteosclerotic host reactions may stop tumour growth – as often seen in prostatic cancer.

The *osteosclerotic reaction* is mediated by osteoblasts (Plates 20.D and E) stimulated by factors derived from the fibrous and osseous stroma surrounding the tumour; and possibly also by cytokines produced by the tumour cells[62,70,86]. For example, TGF-α and TGF-β could be responsible for both appositional new bone formation and membranous ossification, i.e. woven bone[39]. Furthermore, therapy with bisphosphonates may also evoke osteosclerosis[57,58].

Hypercalcaemia is a frequent complication of metastatic bone disease and it occurs in approximately 30% of patients with advanced breast cancer[59,60]. Tumour-derived parathyroid hormone-related proteins may have an important humoral role in hypercalcaemia associated with metastatic breast cancer[11], and more recently have been

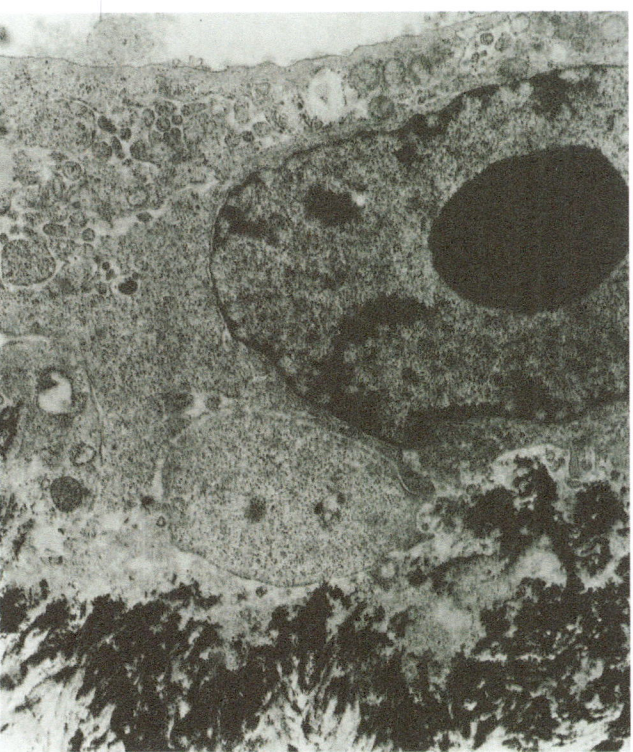

Fig. 20.EM1 Iliac crest biopsy of patient with metastatic carcinoma: tumour cell eroding bone. EM × 33 600

shown to be responsible for the hypercalcaemia associated with other cancers as well[12,77,81]. Some quantitative histomorphometric studies have shown uncoupling of bone cell activity in the hypercalcaemia of malignancy[17,79]. In some cases hypercalcaemia develops in the absence of bone metastases. In this situation the tumour is producing humoral factors that stimulate osteoclastic bone resorption and/or intestinal calcium absorption. Nussbaum *et al.* (1990) described a patient with severe hypercalcaemia and an elevated serum concentration of PTH due to the ectopic synthesis and secretion of the hormone by an ovarian carcinoma[64]. Four histologically normal parathyroid glands were identified. This type of hypercalcaemia is one aspect of the 'paraneoplastic syndrome'; neurological, dermal and haematological manifestations have also been reported[1,34,46].

Hypophosphataemic osteomalacia associated with prostatic carcinoma is not rare. Possible mechanisms are a phosphaturic effect, a humoral substance inhibiting the conversion of 25-(OH) vitamin D_3 to 1,25-(OH)$_2$ vitamin D_3, and treatment with oestrogens. The main symptoms of oncogenic osteomalacia are bone pain and muscle weakness, and these improve with specific treatment for carcinoma of the prostate[44,61,87].

In a *study of 1800 iliac crest biopsies*[27] of patients with carcinomatous disease we investigated the following five points in particular:

1. frequency of bone involvement, that is clinical staging;
2. tumour cell differentiation in metastases, that is biological behaviour;
3. mode of spread in the bone marrow, that is progression of disease;
4. stromal reactions, that is host response to the presence of metastases; and

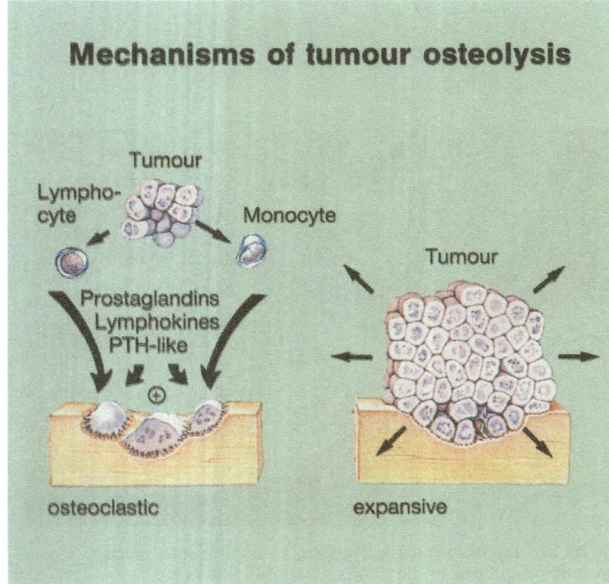

Fig. 20.S3 Cells and factors involved in metastatic osteolysis

Mechanisms of tumour osteolysis

Tumour

Lymphocyte   Monocyte

Prostaglandins
Lymphokines
PTH-like

(+)

osteoclastic

Tumour

expansive

[continued on p. 224]

Plate 20.C

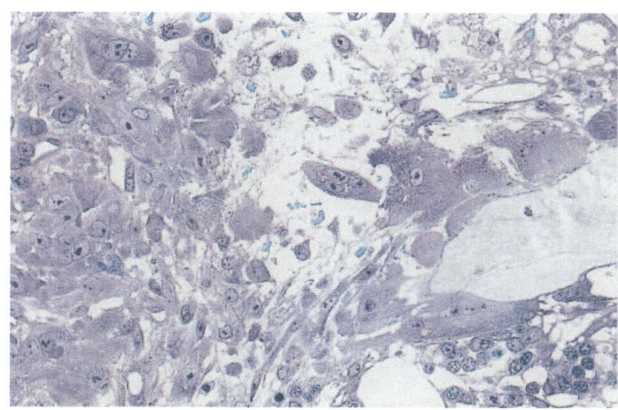

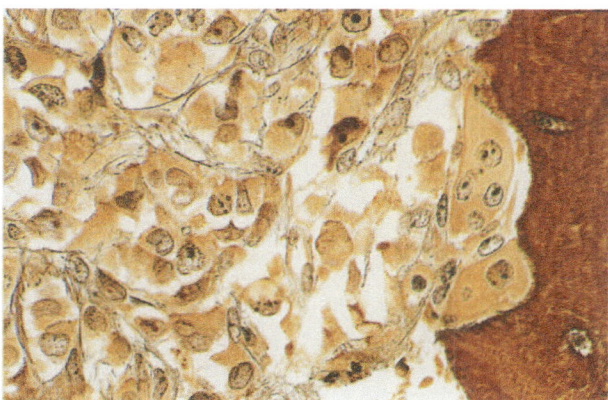

Figs. 20.13–20.18 Iliac crest biopsies illustrating osteoclastic and direct tumour cell osteolyses in metastatic bone disease

Fig. 20.13 Osteoclastic bone resorption at edge of metastatic focus consisting of solid mass of tumour cells. Giemsa

Fig. 20.14 Osteoclasts activated by adjacent tumour cells in resorption cavity. Gomori

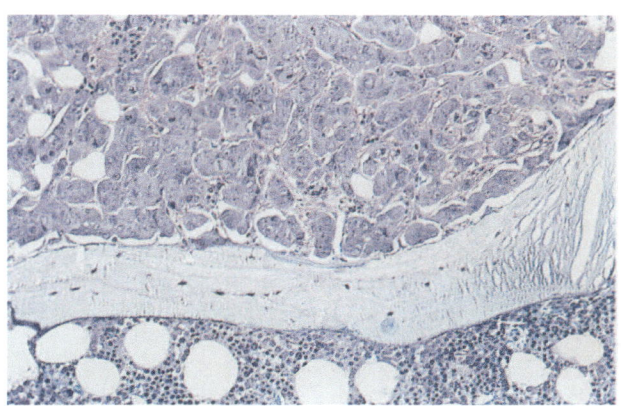

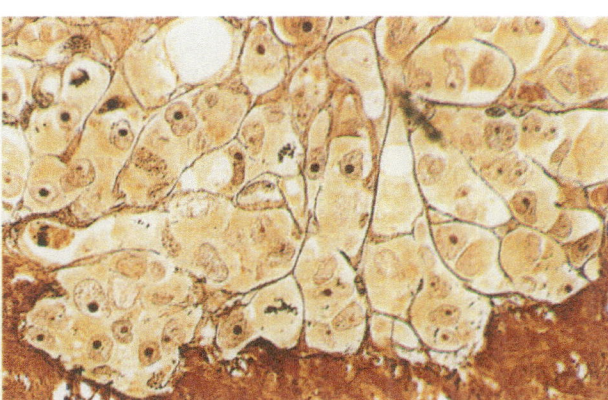

Fig. 20.15 Tumour cells eroding the bone on upper side of a trabecula, with normocellular bone marrow on the opposite side. Giemsa

Fig. 20.16 Excavations on trabecular bone surface indicating direct osteolysis by tumour cells. Gomori

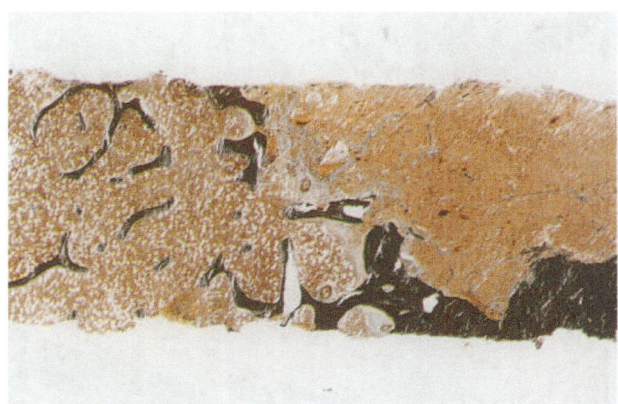

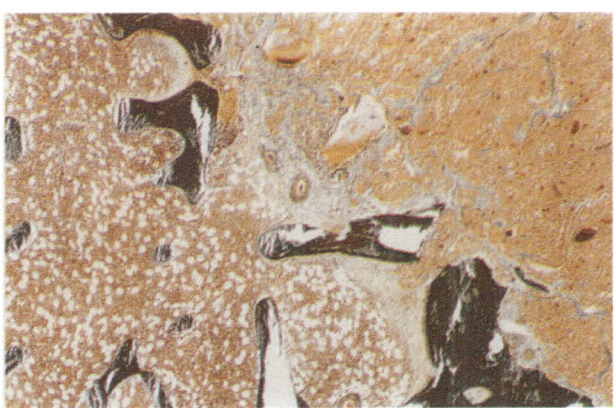

Fig. 20.17 Overview of biopsy showing large osteolytic lesion with marginal reactive osteosclerosis (especially lower right) and normal marrow and trabecular bone (left). Gomori

Fig. 20.18 Higher magnification of biopsy in Fig. 20.17 illustrating marginal fibrosis and sclerosis. Gomori

Plate 20.D

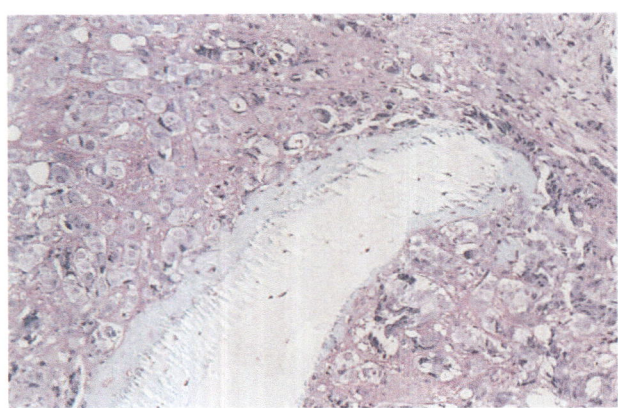

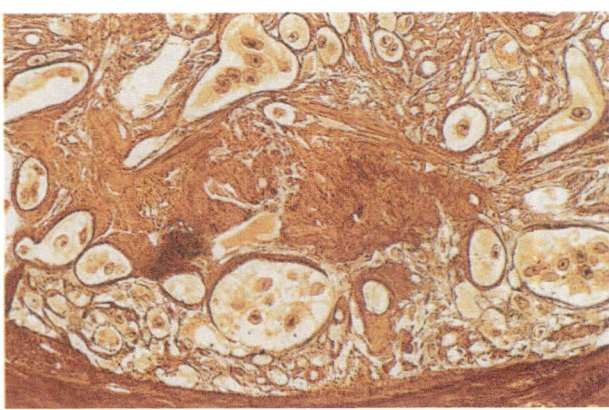

Figs. 20.19–20.24 Iliac crest biopsies illustrating osteoblastic new bone formation in metastatic bone disease

Fig. 20.20 Interstitial deposition of woven bone near trabecular surface. Gomori

Fig. 20.19 Trabecula covered by osteoid seam and surrounded by fibrotic metastasis. Giemsa

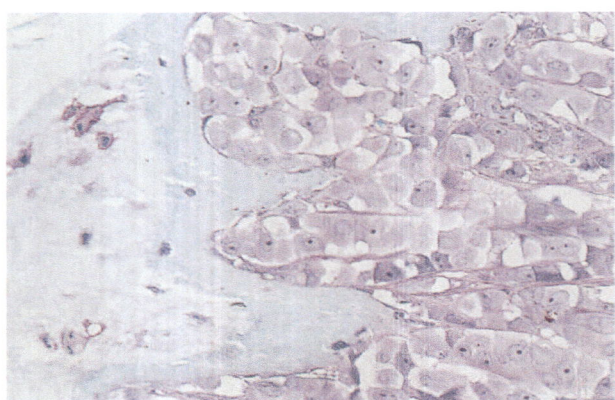

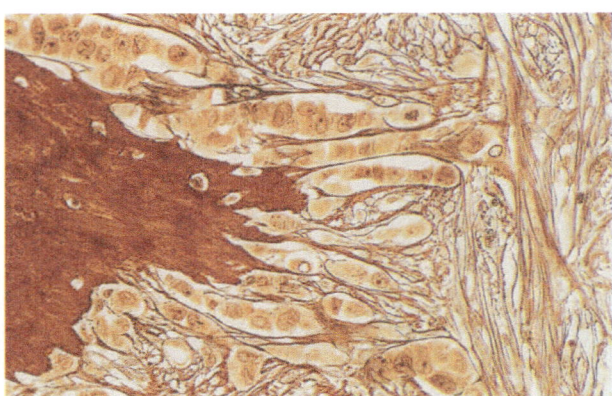

Fig. 20.21 Sprouts of new bone encroaching on marrow cavity. Note broad seam of osteoid and original trabecular surface at upper left-hand corner. Absence of osteoblasts at osteoid surface. Giemsa

Fig. 20.22 Metastasis with pronounced reactive fibrosis. Note coarse collagenous fibres radiating out between the tumour cells from woven bone. Gomori, polar.

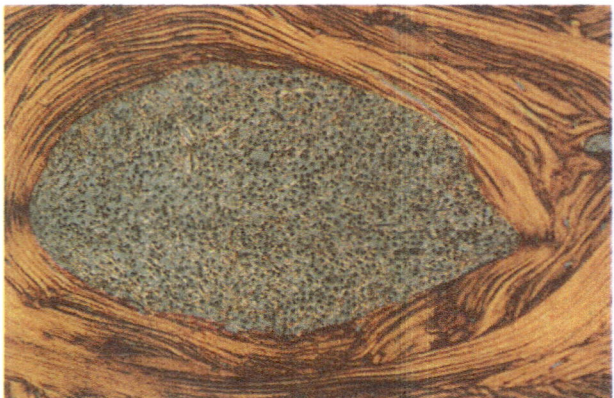

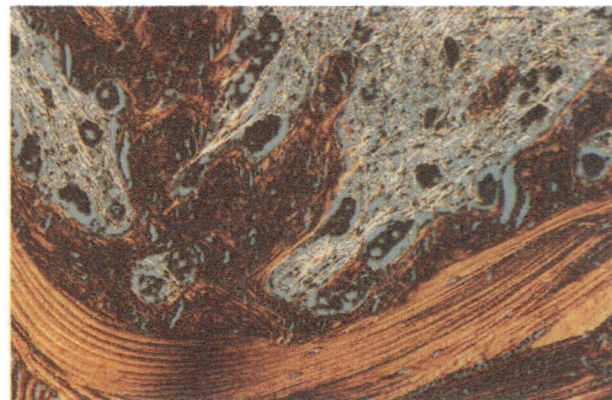

Fig. 20.23 Progressive narrowing of marrow cavity by lamellar bone formation. Gomori

Fig. 20.24 In contrast to Fig. 20.23, diminution of marrow space by woven bone deposited on the trabecula as well as in the marrow cavity. Gomori, polar.

Plate 20.E

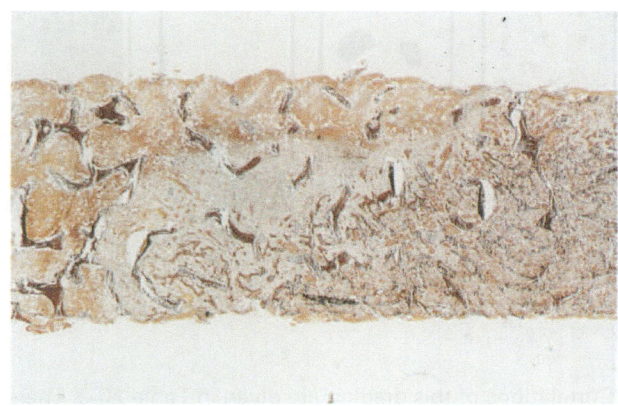

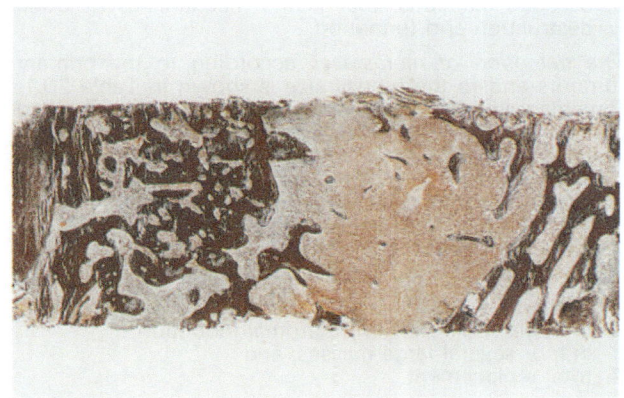

Figs. 20.25–20.30 Aspects of osseous reactions in metastatic bone disease: overviews of iliac crest biopsies. These demonstrate the potential pitfalls of histomorphometry in such cases

Fig. 20.25 Fine sclerosis composed of unmineralized woven bone in metastatic area. Normal trabecular bone volume in the rest of the biopsy. Gomori

Fig. 20.26 Mixed osteolytic/osteosclerotic reaction in involved trabecular region. No metastasis in cortical and subcortical region which contains fibrosis and fatty marrow. Gomori

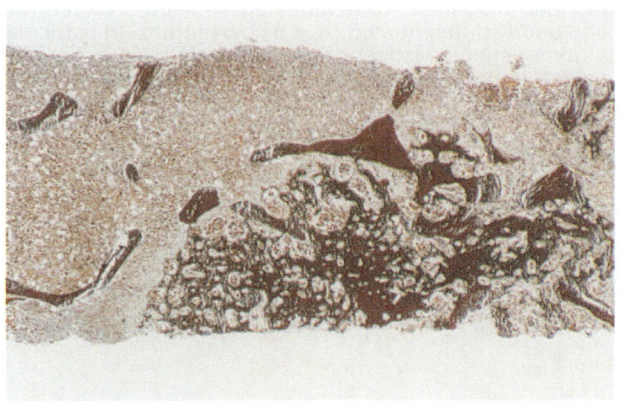

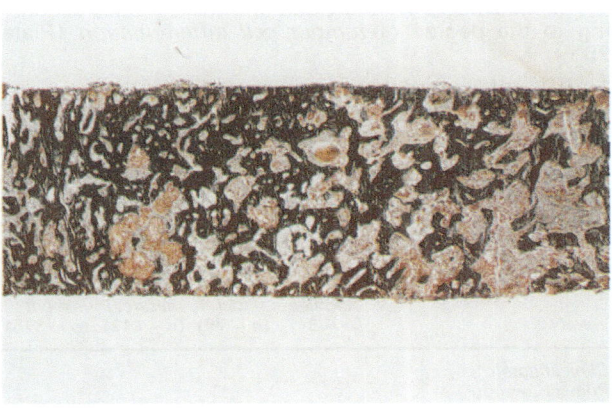

Fig. 20.27 Coarse sclerosis consisting of woven bone in metastatic area. Reduction in trabecular bone volume in non-involved area. Gomori

Fig. 20.28 Complete replacement of trabecular network by dense lattice of woven bone. Gomori

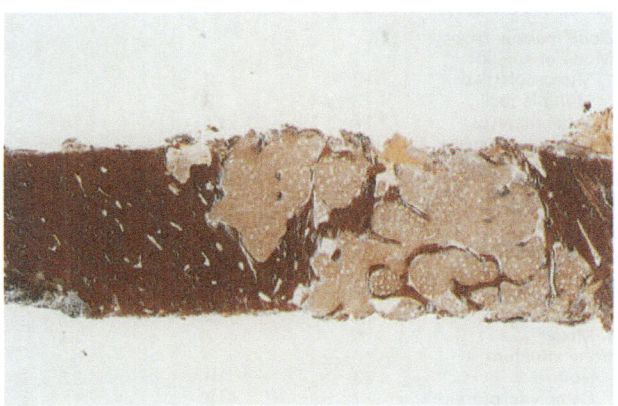

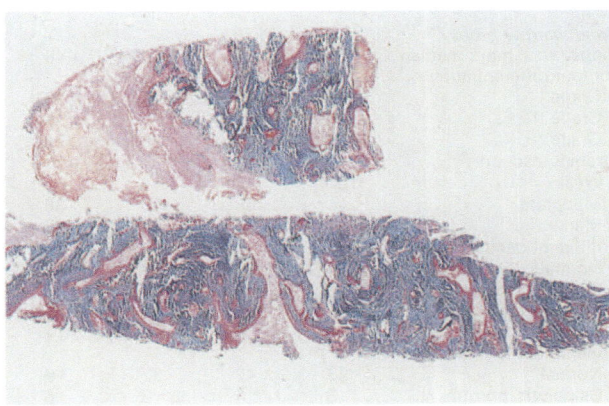

Fig. 20.29 Massive thickening of cortical bone, but some preservation of trabecular structure even in involved area. Gomori

Fig. 20.30 Massive osteosclerosis replacing the whole biopsy simulating osteopetrosis ('marble bone disease'). The red stripes represent osteoid. Ladewig

5. osseous reactions, that is the mechanisms of bone destruction and formation.

The *detection of metastases* according to the primary tumours and to the biopsy size is shown in Table 20.1. Patients with already proven systemic manifestation had a higher incidence of positive biopsies than those without (69% compared with 19%). In breast cancer we found that patients with positive bone biopsies (*n* = 140) had significantly shorter median survivals than those without (*n* = 189) (28 and 18 months respectively)[48,67].

The metastases in the bone biopsy were divided into four groups according to the *mode of spread* (Plate 20.B):

1. micro-colonies, consisting of single cells or clusters;
2. multiple small foci, with stromal induction;
3. one or several large masses; and
4. total replacement.

The distribution of these groups is given in Fig. 20.S4 and in Table 20.2. The micro-clusters were no longer within the sinusoids, but already in the interstitial spaces. Patients with breast cancer and large masses in biopsy (*n* = 118) had a more favourable prognosis than those with multiple small metastases (*n* = 22) (13 compared with 5 months of median survival).

The metastases were divided into three grades according to the degree of *tumour cell differentiation* (Plate 20.F):

1. well differentiated;
2. moderately differentiated, and
3. poorly differentiated.

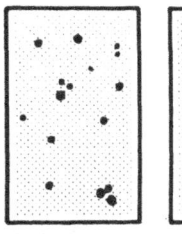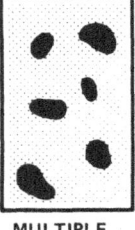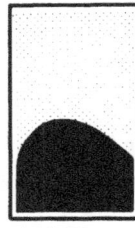

| MICRO-COLONIES 5% | MULTIPLE FOCI 13% | LARGE MASSES 19% | TOTAL REPLACEMENT 63% |

Fig. 20.S4 Metastases and mode of spread in iliac crest biopsy. From Frisch *et al.*[27]

Correlations of this grading are given in Table 20.3. There was also considerable diversity of tumour cells between the metastases of a single primary, usually less differentiated in the osseous metastases than in the initial histology of the primary tumour. Prognostic evaluation of this histological grading of bone biopsies in patients with breast cancer has shown the following median survival times: well-differentiated metastases (*n* = 20), 37 months; moderately differentiated (*n* = 69), 15 months and poorly differentiated (*n* = 57), 5 months. In particular a homogeneous aspect of metastatic cells (*n* = 57) signalled a better prognosis than a heterogeneous one

Table 20.2 Metastatic carcinoma in bone biopsies: grouping is mode of spread[27]

Variables	Micro-colonies (*n* = 34)	Multiple foci (*n* = 79)	Large mass(es) (*n* = 112)	Total replacement (*n* = 375)
Clinical data				
Primary tumour				
Breast	32*	40	30	34
Prostate	19	7	5	17
Lung	16	12	11	8
Others	4	7	9	9
Unknown	29	34	45	32
Peripheral blood				
Haemoglobin < 10 g/dl	19	27	22	38
Leukocytes < 4 × 10⁹/l	8	13	18	27
Platelets < 100 × 10⁹/l	14	23	20	31
Metastatic disease†	41	54	56	57
Bone marrow biopsy				
Biopsy size, mm², median	68	60	60	48
Tumour differentiation				
Grade I	45	20	19	18
Grade II	20	57	5	18
Grade III	35	23	26	24
Stromal reaction				
Weak	100	13	4	–
Moderate	–	58	50	38
Marked	–	29	46	62
Bone remodelling				
Normal	84	36	24	17
Osteoblastic	16	52	56	75
Osteoclastic	–	12	10	1
Mixed	–	–	10	12
Bone structure				
Normal	97	42	32	9
Osteolytic/porotic	3	4	9	6
Osteosclerotic	–	34	37	59
Mixed	–	20	22	26

*Percentage of patients in each histological group
†Indications of systemic metastases present before bone marrow biopsy

Table 20.3 Metastatic carcinoma in bone biopsies: grouping is tumour differentiation[27]

Variables	Grade I well differentiated (*n* = 167)	Grade II moderately differentiated (*n* = 271)	Grade III poorly differentiated (*n* = 162)
Clinical data			
Primary tumour			
Breast	51*	36	42
Prostate	12	18	12
Lung	5	2	9
Others	3	7	11
Unknown	23	37	26
Peripheral blood			
Haemoglobin < 10 g/dl	25	36	29
Leukocytes < 4 × 10⁹/l	12	16	10
Platelets < 100 × 10⁹/l	17	25	34
Metastatic disease†	56	58	45
Bone marrow biopsy			
Mode of spread			
Micro-colonies	12	2	7
Multiple foci	13	13	17
Large mass(es)	17	17	26
Total replacement	58	68	50
Stromal reaction			
Weak	4	2	7
Moderate	44	34	50
Marked	52	64	43
Bone remodelling			
Normal	22	14	32
Osteoblastic	70	73	37
Osteoclastic	2	1	18
Mixed	6	2	13
Bone structure			
Normal	23	16	32
Osteolytic/porotic	7	2	11
Osteosclerotic	48	56	32
Mixed	22	26	25

*Percentage of patients in each histological group
†Indications of systemic metastases present before bone marrow biopsy

Plate 20.F

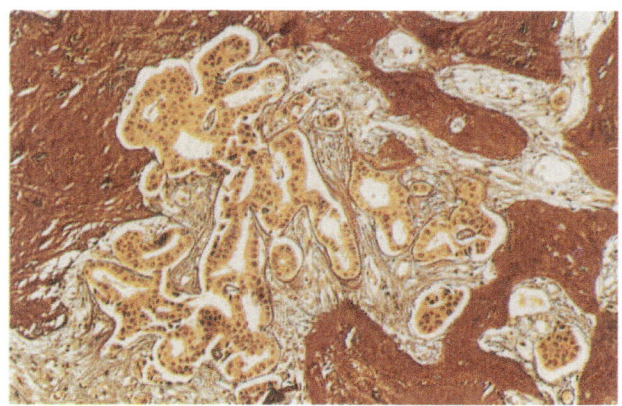

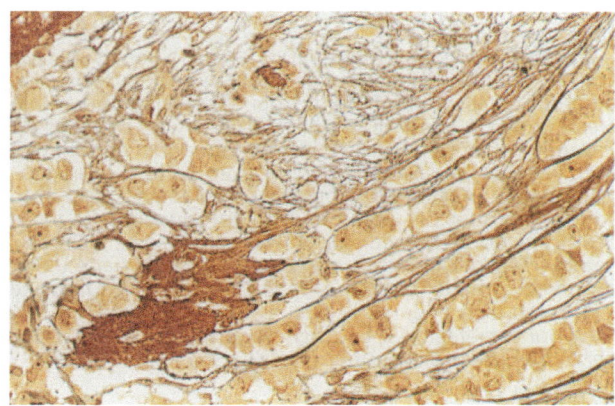

Figs. 20.31–20.36 Cytological aspects of metastatic carcinoma in iliac crest biopsies

Fig. 20.31 Glandular structures of adenocarcinoma in prostatic cancer. Gomori

Fig. 20.32 'Indian file' organization in mammary carcinoma. Gomori

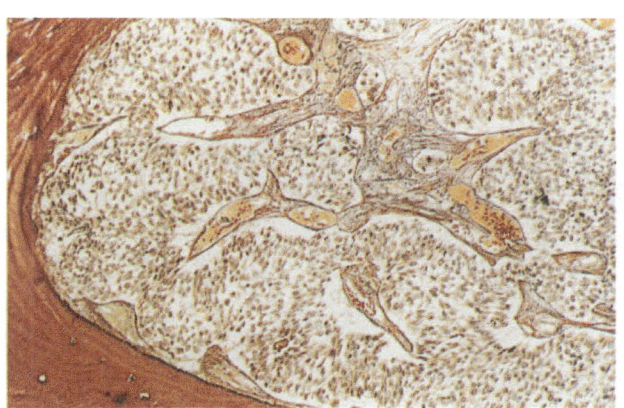

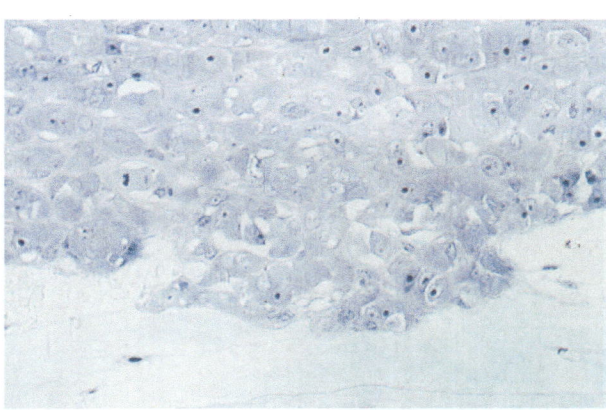

Fig. 20.33 Bronchial carcinoma, small oat cell type. Gomori

Fig. 20.34 Closely packed solid masses of large, nucleolated tumour cells: metastasis of unknown primary tumour. Giemsa

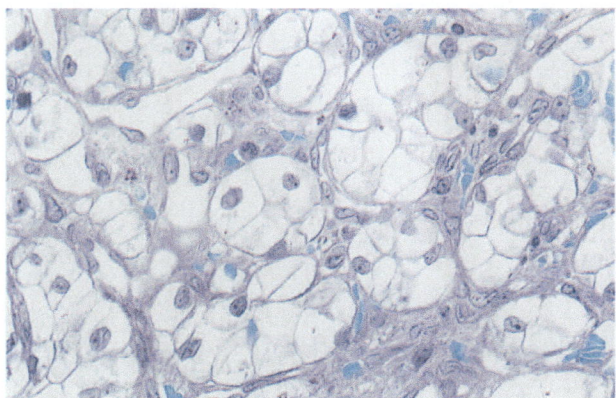

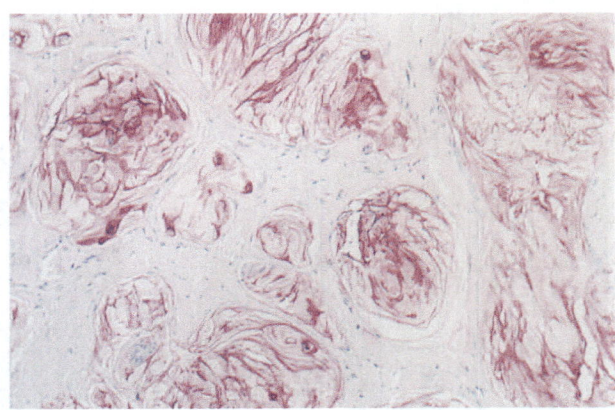

Fig. 20.35 Metastasis composed of 'clear cells' in renal carcinoma. Giemsa

Fig. 20.36 Mucus-secreting adenocarcinoma of gastrointestinal tract. PAS

($n = 57$) (18 compared with 5 months of median survival)[52].

Stromal reactions (Plates 20.G and H) varied in type and in quantity between the metastases, and even in different areas of single large foci. Osseous remodelling was found in over 90% of biopsies with metastases. Though either bone resorption or formation dominated, both were usually present, and destruction of the trabecular architecture resulted. Pronounced osteoclast activation adjacent to sites of tumour invasion produced large areas devoid of bone, sometimes with a patchy osteosclerosis nearby. Marked systemic osteosclerosis was particularly observed in patients with prostatic cancer, though bone resorption also occurs.

In bone metastases five histological patterns of *bone behaviour* were discernible (Fig. 20.S5):

1. normal (7%);
2. lytic (18%);
3. mixed lytic/sclerotic (38%) (Figs 20.R2 and R3);
4. sclerotic/lamellar, with broad lamellar trabeculae and appositional bone formation (10%) (Fig. 20.R4); and
5. sclerotic/woven, with normal trabeculae, but with increase of woven bone in the marrow cavities causing myelophthisis (27%).

The frequencies of these five osseous subgroups in patients with breast, prostate and bronchus cancer are given in Fig. 20.S6. Patients with normal bone structure

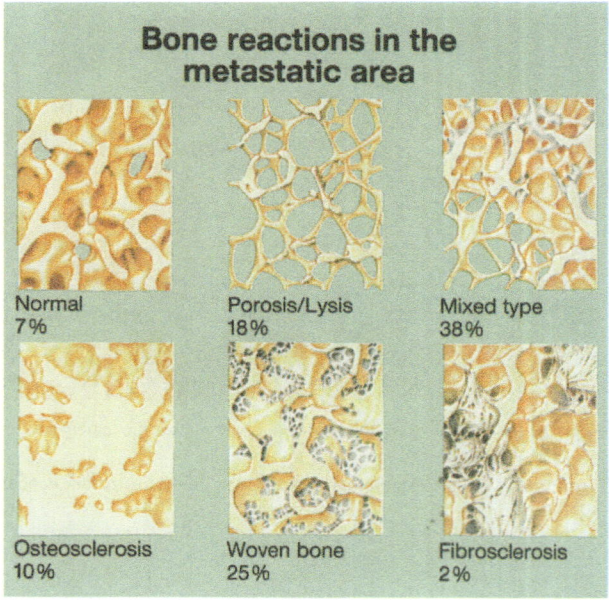

Fig. 20.S5   Range of osseous reactions in metastatic bone disease

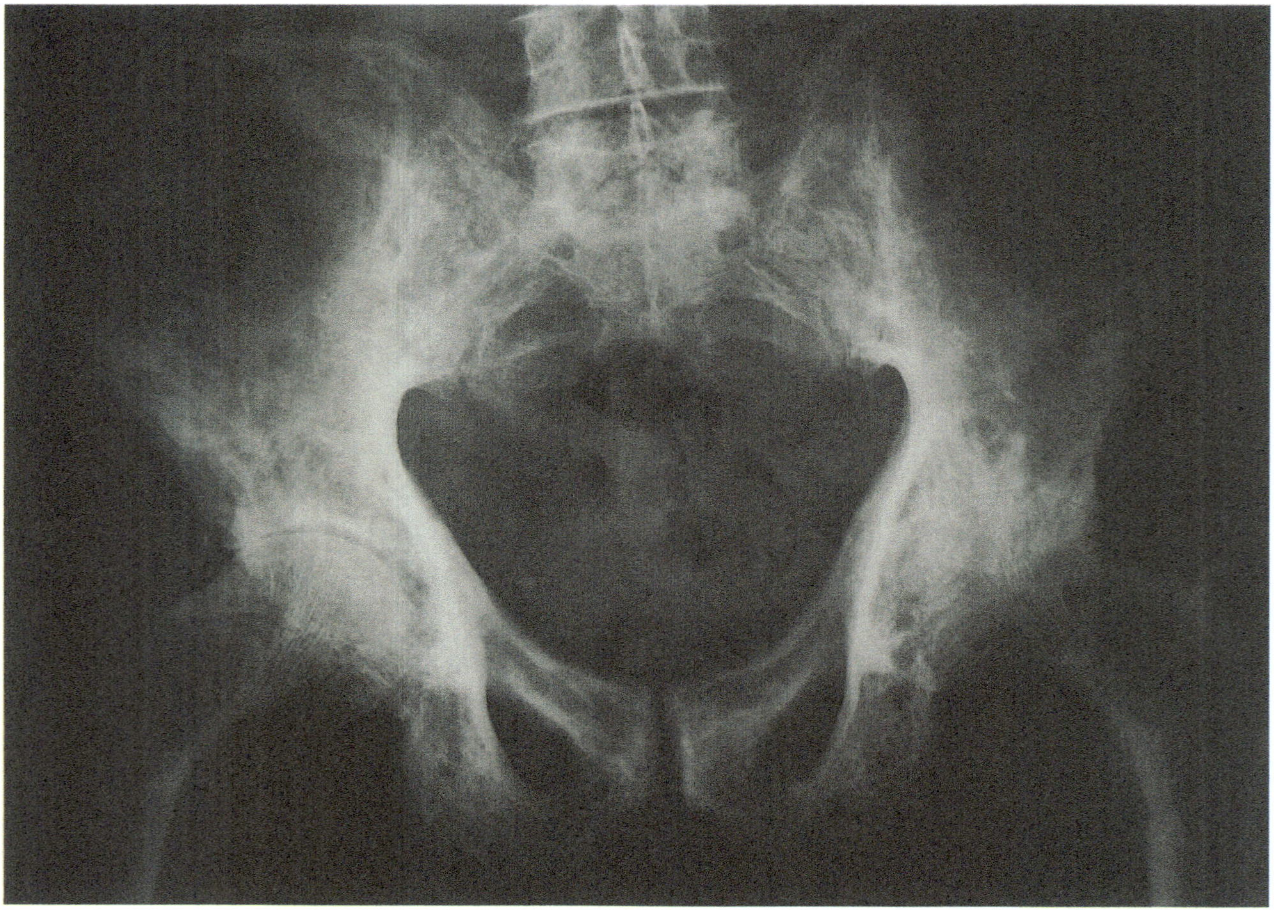

Fig. 20.R2   X-ray of metastatic bone disease of breast cancer, with mixed blastic and lytic lesions in the pelvis

Plate 20.G

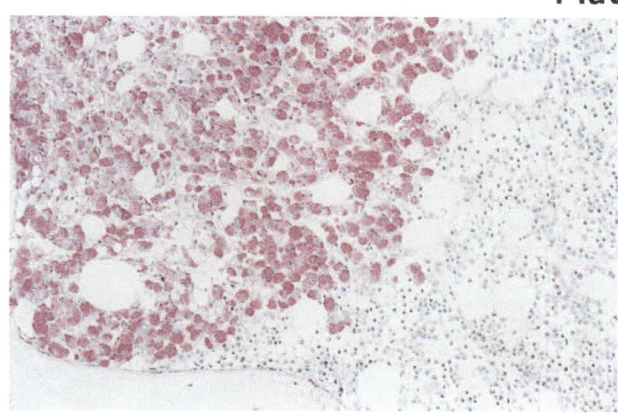

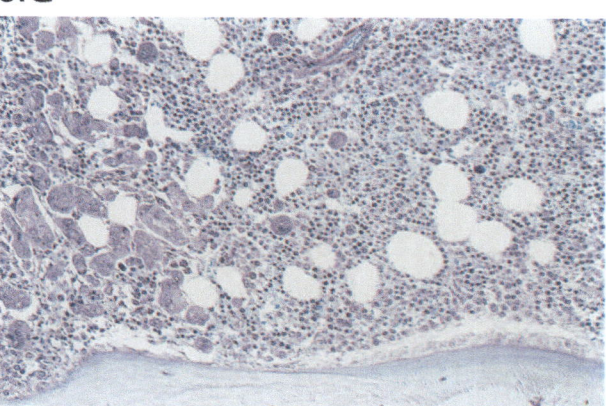

Figs. 20.37–20.42 Aspects of marginal bone and marrow reactions in metastatic carcinoma

Fig. 20.37 No reaction at interface between metastasis, marrow and bone. PAS

Fig. 20.38 Dispersed tumour cell clusters without changes in the bone marrow but an osteoblastic reaction at the trabecular surface. Giemsa

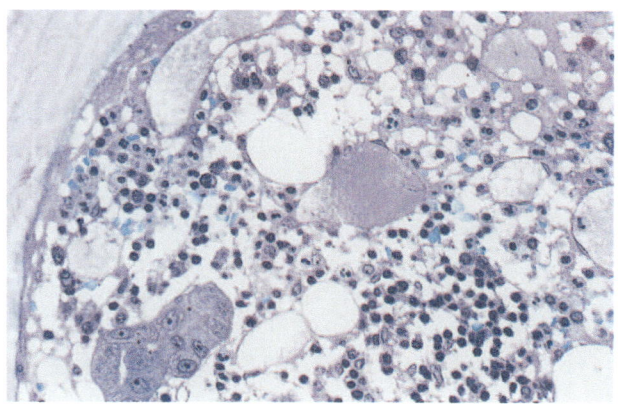

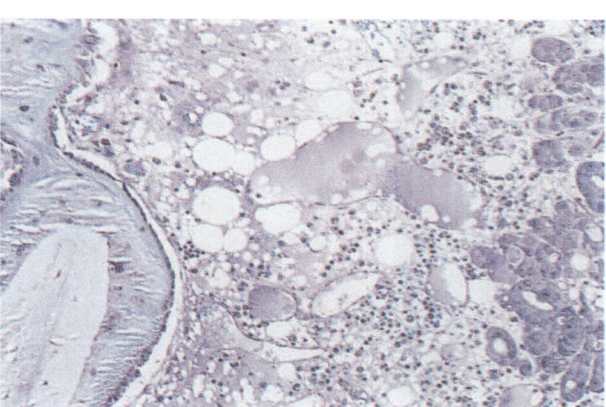

Fig. 20.39 Interstitial tumour cell cluster within oedematous stroma and reactive lymphocytic infiltration. Note ectatic blood vessels. Giemsa

Fig. 20.40 Tumour cell clusters, some showing incipient gland formation, in highly oedematous marginal zone, with hyperplastic ectatic blood vessels (angioneogenesis) with residual haematopoietic cells. Osteoblastic reaction with wide osteoblastic seams. Giemsa

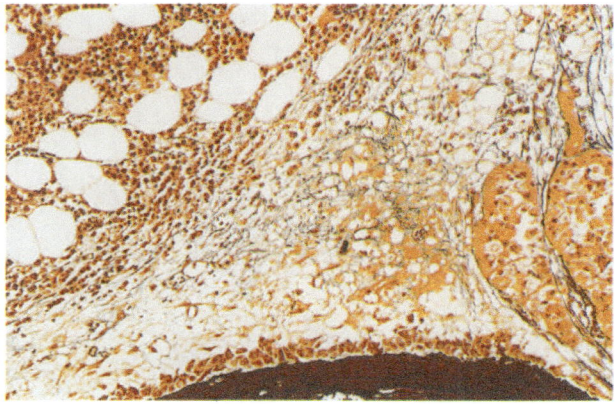

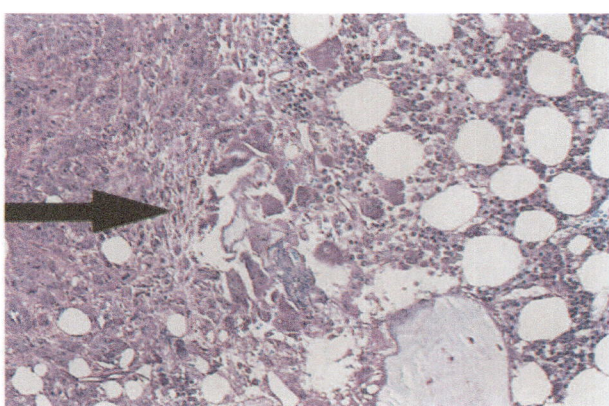

Fig. 20.41 The tumour cells (right) are separated from the normal marrow by a broad marginal zone of hypocellular, oedematous and fibrotic stroma. Note layer of osteoblasts on osteoid seam at trabecular surface. Gomori

Fig. 20.42 Striking destructive osteoclastosis evoked by mass of anaplastic tumour cells with many mitotic figures. No evident bone marrow reaction. Giemsa

Plate 20.H

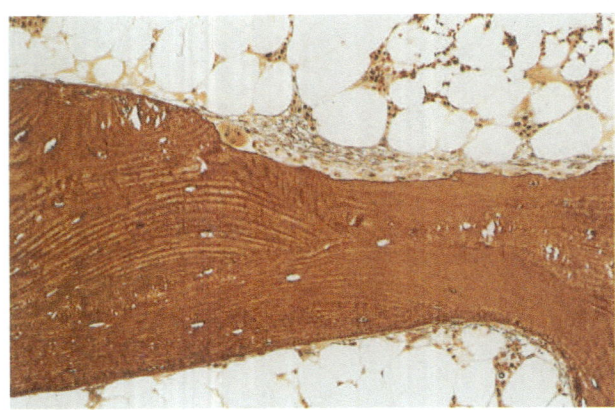

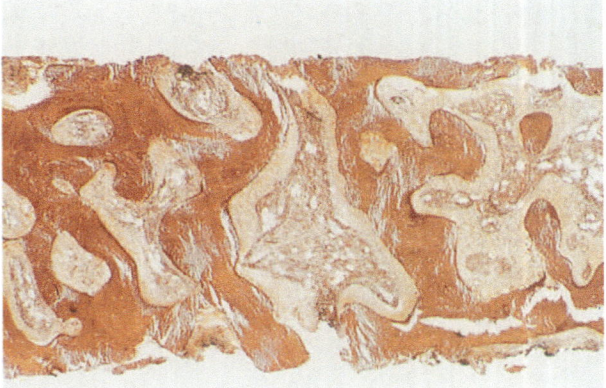

Figs. 20.43–20.45 The extremes of paraneoplastic bone disease in the absence of metastases in iliac crest biopsies

Fig. 20.43 Minimal osteoclastic and osteoblastic bone remodelling, with some paratrabecular fibrosis. Gomori

Fig. 20.44 Pronounced widespread paraneoplastic bone disease accompanied by paratrabecular fibrosis. Gomori

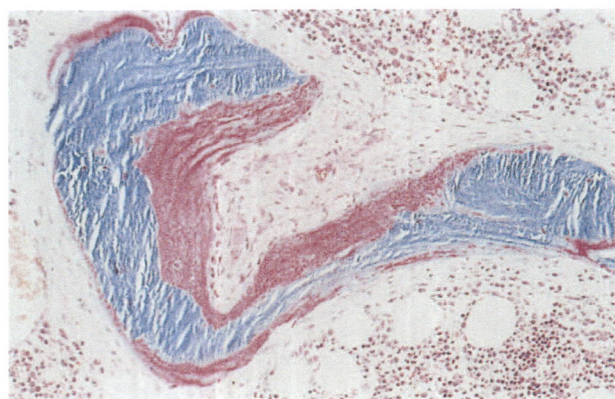

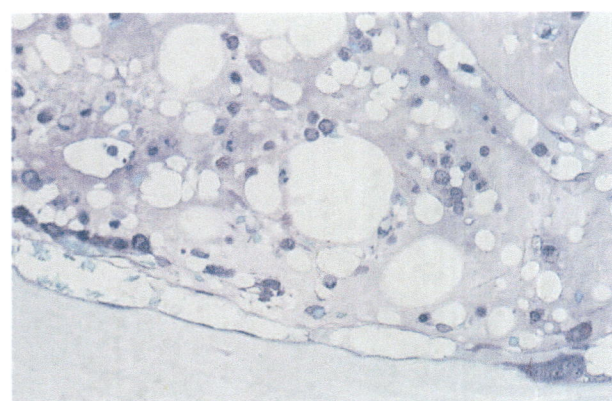

Fig. 20.45 Higher magnification of section of another biopsy of patient with paraneoplastic syndrome: parts of the broad trabecula consist of wide osteoid seams ('oncogenic osteomalacia'). Ladewig

Figs. 20.46–20.48 Post-therapy iliac crest biopsies of patients with metastatic bone disease.

Fig. 20.46 Single tumour cells dispersed in oedematous, almost acellular marrow. Giemsa

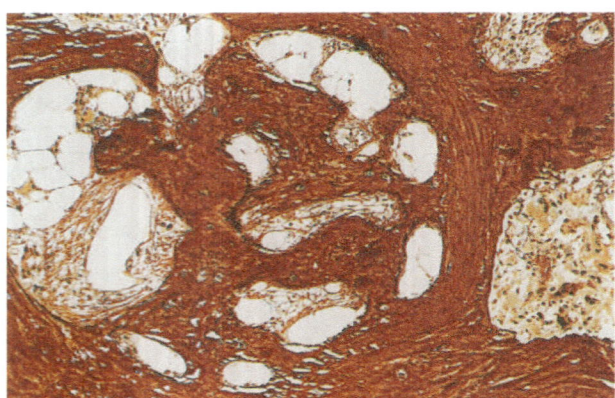

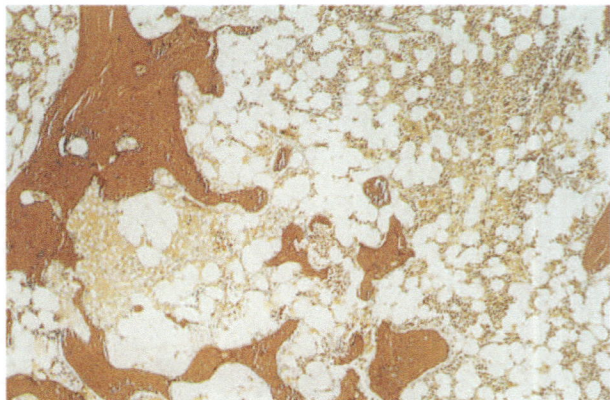

Fig. 20.47 Part of bone biopsy of patient with metastases of prostatic carcinoma showing typical osteosclerotic lesion (woven bone within intertrabecular marrow space). Gomori

Fig. 20.48 Biopsy section showing restitution of haematopoietic bone marrow (upper right); altered trabecular bone structure (lower left) indicating previous presence of metastasis, no residual tumour cells found. Gomori

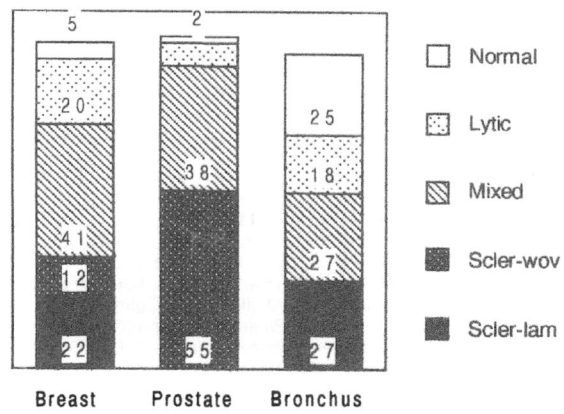

Fig. 20.S6 Bone changes in iliac crest biopsies with metastatic involvement according to primary tumours

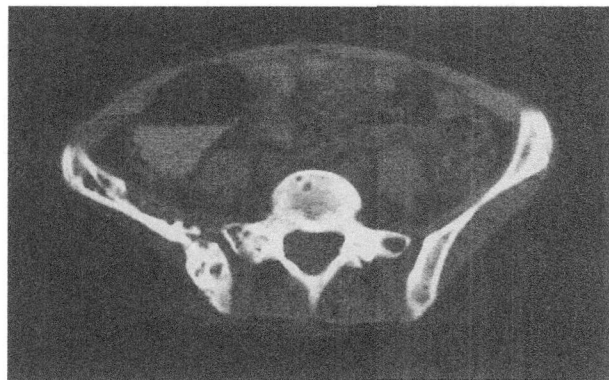

Fig. 20.R3 CT of a patient with metastatic breast cancer. Note unilateral (left) involvement of ilium, showing osteolytic and osteosclerotic lesions with destruction of cortical bone

had a short history of disease, while those with sclerotic bone reaction had the longest history of cancer disease, with the most favourable course. In patients with breast cancer we compared the findings of bone biopsy with radiological methods: 20% of the patients with normal bone scan ($n = 86$) and 30% of the patients with normal skeletal X-rays ($n = 106$) had positive biopsies[52]. Thus

bone biopsy proves to be helpful in the interpretation of equivocal X-rays or bone scans, and may document tumour dissemination even when radiological results are negative[45]. In addition, demonstration of osteoclastic bone resorption now constitutes one of the indications for therapy with osteoclast inhibiting agents[18,51,57,58,75].

A major inadequacy of cancer treatment to date is our

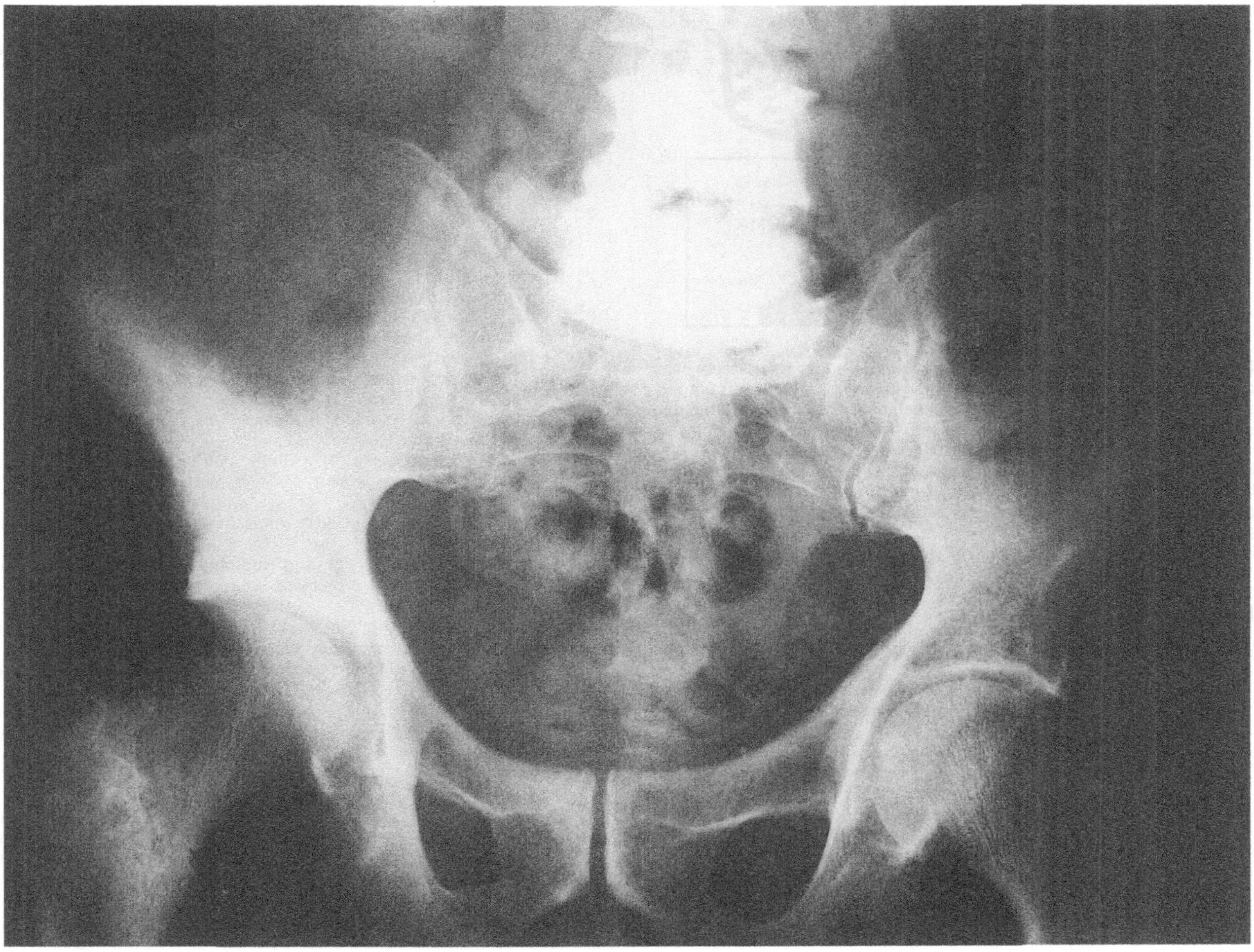

Fig. 20.R4 X-ray of metastatic bone disease in prostatic cancer, with predominantly sclerotic lesions in the ilium and the vertebrae

limited possibility of discovering small occult metastases. There is a need not only to detect circulating tumour cells, for example by culture techniques and immunocytological methods[20,43,72,73,78,84,85], but also to diagnose intrasinusoidal tumour emboli (Fig. 20.S7) and settled bone metastases at an earlier stage ('micro-metastasis'), and bone biopsy may contribute to solving this diagnostic need[6,27].

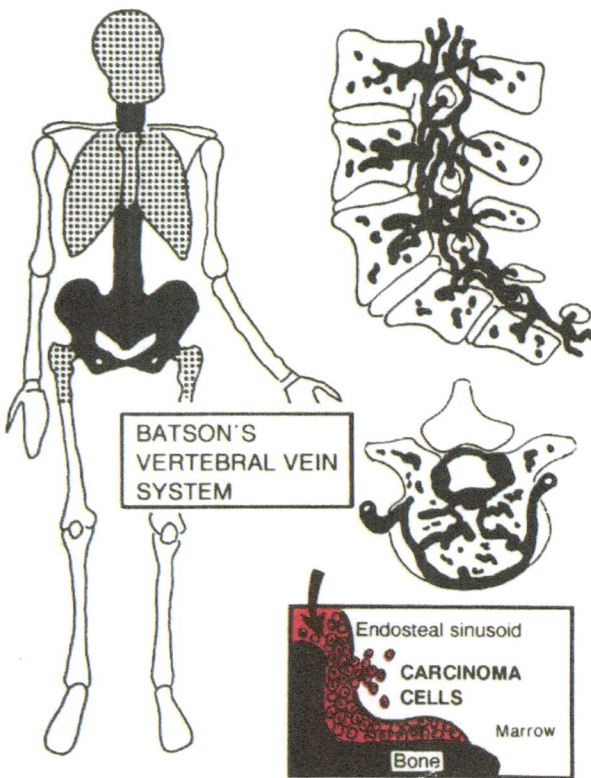

Fig. 20.S7 Illustration of the 'Batson's vertebral vein system'. It consists of a network of thin-walled veins with a low intraluminal pressure communicating with the dural, intercostal and pelvic veins. When intrathoracic or intraabdominal pressures are increased – e.g. in coughing, straining or muscle activity – blood is forced into the low-pressure vertebral vein system, with a retrograde flow into the veins and endosteal sinusoids of the bone marrow. Once carcinoma cells – e.g. from breast, prostate or other pelvic organs – enter this valveless system, they have access to the whole axial skeleton

References

1. Abeloff M. D. (1987). Paraneoplastic syndromes. *N. Engl. J. Med.,* **317**, 1598
2. Abrams H. L., Spiro, R. and Goldstein N. (1950). Metastases in carcinoma. Analysis of 1000 autopsied cases. *Cancer,* **3**, 74
3. Adams J. E. and Isherwood I. (1983). Conventional and new techniques in radiological diagnosis. Stoll B. A. and Parbhoo S., *Bone Metastases: Monitoring and Treatment* (p. 107). New York: Raven Press
4. Anner R. M. and Drewinko B. (1977). Frequency, and significance of bone marrow involvement in metastatic solid tumours. *Cancer,* **39**, 1337
5. Barengolts E., Buschmann R., Shevria D. H., Abramson E. C. and Kukreja S.-C. (1990). Effects of hypercalcemia-producing tumor extract and parathyroid hormone on osteoclast ultrastructure. *Acta Anat.,* **139**, 160
6. Berger U., Bettelheim R., Mansi J. L., Easton D., Coombes R. C. and MunroNeville A. (1988). The relationship between microme-

tastases in the bone marrow, histopathologic features of the primary tumor in breast cancer and prognosis. *Amer. J. Clin. Pathol.,* **90**, 1
7. Berrettoni B. A. and Carter J. R. (1986). Mechanisms of cancer metastasis to bone. *J. Bone Jt Surg.,* **68A**, 308
8. Bertolini D. R., Nedwon G. E., Bringham T. S., Smith D. D. and Mundy G. R. (1986). Stimulation of bone resorption and inhibition of bone formation *in vitro* by human tumor necrosis factor. *Nature,* **319**, 516
9. Bonjour J. P. and Rizzoli R. (1989). Pathophysiological aspects and therapeutic approaches of tumoral osteolysis and hypercalcemia. *Rec. Results Cancer Res.,* **116**, 29
10. Boyce B. F. (1991). Normal bone remodeling and its disruption in metastatic bone disease. Rubens R. D. and Fogelman I., *Bone Metastases: Diagnosis and Treatment* (p. 11). London: Springer
11. Bundred N. J., Ratcliffe W. A., Walker R. A., Coley S., Morrison J. M. and Ratcliffe J. G. (1991). Parathyroid hormone related protein and hypercalcaemia in breast cancer. *Brit. Med. J.,* **303**, 1506
12. Burtis W. J., Brady T. G., Orloff J. J., Ersbak J. B., Warrell R. P., Olson B. R., Wu T. L., Mitnick M. E., Broadus A. E. and Stewart A. F. (1990). Imunochemical characterization of circulating parathyroid hormone-related proteins in patients with humoral hypercalcemia of cancer. *N. Engl. J. Med.,* **322**, 1106
13. Carter R. L. (1985). Patterns and mechanisms of bone metastases. *J. Roy. Soc. Med.,* **78** (Suppl. 9), 2
14. Castello A., Coci A., Magrini U. and Ascari E. (1986). Histopathology of bone marrow metastases. Considerations on 104 cases. *Haematologica,* **71**, 369
15. Ceci G., Franciosi V., Nizzoli R., DeLisi V., Lottici R., Boni C., DiBlaso B., Passalacqua R., Guazzi A. and Cocconi G. (1988). The value of bone marrow biopsy in breast cancer at time of diagnosis. A prospective study. *Cancer,* **61**, 96
16. Clamon G. H., Edwards W. R., Hamous J. E. and Scupham R. K. (1984). Patterns of bone marrow involvement with small cell lung cancer. *Cancer,* **54**, 100
17. Clarke N. W., McChire J. and George N. J. (1991). Morphometric evidence for bone resorption and replacement in prostate cancer. *Brit. J. Urol.,* **68**, 74
18. Coleman R. E. (1987). The pathogenesis, assessment and medical treatment of bone metastases. *Baillière's Clin. Oncol.,* **1**, 651
19. Contreras E., Ellis L. D. and Lee R. E. (1972). Value of the bone marrow biopsy in the diagnosis of metastatic carcinoma. *Cancer,* **29**, 778
20. Cote R. J., Rosen P. P., Old L. J. and Osborne M. P. (1991). Detection of bone marrow micrometastases in patients with early-stage breast cancer. *Diagn. Oncol.,* **1**, 37
21. Edeiken J., Dalinka M. and Karasick D. (1990). *Edeiken's Roentgen Diagnosis of Diseases of Bone.* Baltimore: Williams & Wilkins
22. Evans C. W. (1991). *The Metastatic Cell: Behaviour and Biochemistry.* London: Chapman & Hall
23. Fidler I. J. and Hart I. R. (1982). Biological diversity in metastatic neoplasms: origins and implications. *Science,* **217**, 998
24. Frassica F. J. and Sim F. H. (1988). Pathogenesis and prognosis. Sim F. H., *Diagnosis and Management of Metastatic Bone Disease* (p. 1). New York: Raven Press
25. Frassica F. J. and Sim F. H. (1988). Pathophysiology. Sim F. H., *Diagnosis and Management of Metastatic Bone Disease* (p. 7). New York: Raven Press
26. Frisch B. and Bartl R. (1990). *Atlas of Bone Marrow Pathology.* Dordrecht: Kluwer
27. Frisch B., Bartl R., Mahl G. and Burkhardt R. (1984). Scope and value of bone marrow biopsies in metastatic cancer. *Invasion Metastasis,* **4** (Suppl.), 12
28. Frisch B., Lewis S. M., Burkhardt R. and Bartl R. (1985). *Biopsy Pathology of Bone and Bone Marrow.* London: Chapman & Hall
29. Galasko C. S. B. (1982). Mechanisms of lytic and blastic metastatic disease of bone. *Clin. Orthop.,* **169**, 20
30. Galasko C. S. B. and Bennet A. (1976). Relationship of bone destruction in skeletal metastases to osteoclast activation and prostaglandins. *Nature,* **263**, 508
31. Gittes R. F. (1991). Carcinoma of the prostate. *N. Engl. J. Med.,* **324**, 236
32. Gold R. H. and Bassett L. W. (1986). Radionuclide evaluation of skeletal metastases: practical considerations. *Skelet. Radiol.,* **15**, 1
33. Gowen M., Wood D. D., Ihrie E. J., McGuire M. K. B., Graham R. and Russel G. G. (1983). An interleukin 1-like factor stimulates bone resorption *in vitro. Nature,* **306**, 378
34. Hall T. C. (1974). Paraneoplastic syndromes. *Ann. N.Y. Acad. Sci.,* **230**, 571
35. Harrington K. D. (1988). *Orthopaedic Management of Metastatic Bone Disease.* St. Louis: Mosby

36. Helms C. A., Cann C. E. and Brunelle F. O. (1981). Detection of bone marrow metastasis using computed tomography. *Radiology,* **140**, 745

37. Herlyn M. and Malkowicz S. B. (1991). Biology of disease: regulatory pathways in tumour growth and invasion. *Lab. Invest.,* **65**, 262

38. Hirshon J. E., Vrhovsek E. and Posek S. (1979). Carcinoma of the breast associated with hypercalcemia and the presence of parathyroid hormone-like substances in the tumor. *J. Clin. Endocrinol. Metab.,* **48**, 217

39. Ibbotson K. J., Twardzik D. R., D'Souza S. M., Hargreaves W. R., Todaro G. J. and Mundy G. R. (1985). Stimulation of bone resorption in vitro by synthetic transforming growth factor-alpha. *Science,* **228**, 1007

40. Jaffe H. J. (1958). *Tumours and Tumorous Conditions of the Bones and Joints.* Philadelphia: Lea & Febiger

41. Johnson R. A., Boyce B. F., Mundy G. R. and Roodman G. D. (1989). Tumors producing human tumor necrosis factor induced hypercalcemia and osteoclastic bone resorption in nude mice. *Endocrinology,* **124**, 1424

42. Johnston A. D. (1970). Pathology of metastatic tumors in bone. *Clin. Orthop.,* **73**, 8

43. Joshi S. S., Kessinger A. and Mann S. L. (1987). Detection of malignant cells in histologically normal bone marrow using culture techniques. *Bone Marrow Transplant,* **1**, 303

44. Jowell P. S., Epstein S., Ismail F., Hollis B. and Schwartz I. R. (1988). Alteration in osteoblast activity and nutritional vitamin-D deficiency in non-hypercalcemic malignancy. *Calcif. Tissue,* **42**, 18

45. Kamby C., Guldhamer B., Vejborg I., Rossing N., Dirksen H., Daugaard S. and Mouridsen H. T. (1987). The presence of tumor cells in bone marrow at time of first recurrence of breast cancer. *Cancer.* **60**, 1306

46. Kitamura H., Kodama F., Odagiri S., Nagahara N., Inove T. and Kanisawa M. (1989). Granulocytosis associated with malignant neoplasm: a clinicopathologic study and demonstration of colony-stimulating activity in tumour extracts. *Hum. Pathol.,* **20**, 878

47. Lam W. C., Delikatny E. J. and Orr F. W. (1981). The chemotactic response of tumor cells: a model for cancer metastasis. *Amer. J. Pathol.,* **104**, 69

48. Landys K. (1982). Prognostic value of bone marrow biopsy in breast cancer. *Cancer,* **49**, 513

49. Landys K. E. (1983). Role of bone and marrow biopsy in monitoring metastasis. Stoll B. A. and Parbhoo S., *Bone Metastases: Monitoring and Treatment* (p. 149). New York: Raven Press

50. Lippman M. E., Lichter A. S. and Danforth D. N. (1988). *Diagnosis and Management of Breast Cancer.* Philadelphia: Saunders

51. Lote K., Walloe A. and Bjersand A. (1986). Bone metastasis. Prognosis, diagnosis and treatment. *Acta Radiol. Oncol.,* **25**, 227

52. Mahl G., Burkhardt R., Bartl R., Frisch B., Rieger E., Weybora W., Jäger K. and Kettner G. (1986). The prognostic value of bone marrow biopsy in breast cancer. Bässler R. and Hübner K., *Pathology of Neoplastic and Endocrine Induced Diseases of the Breast* (p. 349). Stuttgart: Fischer

53. Manishen W. J., Sivananthan K. and Orr F. W. (1986). Resorbing bone stimulates tumour cell growth: a role for the host microenvironment in bone metastasis. *Amer. J. Pathol.,* **123**, 39

54. Mareel M. M., DeBaetselier P. and VanRoy F. M. (1991). *Mechanisms of Invasion and Metastasis.* Boca Raton: CRC Press

55. Miller F. and Whitehill R. (1984). Carcinoma of the breast metastatic to the skeleton. *Clin. Orthop.,* **184**, 121

56. Mirra J. M. (1989). Metastases. Mira J. M., Picci P. and Gold R. H., *Bone Tumors: Clinical, Radiologic, and Pathologic Correlations* (p. 1495). Philadelphia: Lea & Febiger

57. Morton A. R., Cantrill J. A., Pilai G. V., McMahon A., Anderson D. C. and Howell A. (1988). Sclerosis of lytic bone metastases after aminohydroxypropylidene bisphosphatase (APD) in patients with breast carcinoma. *Brit. Med. J.,* **297**, 772

58. Morton A. R. and Howell A. (1988). Biphosphonates and bone metastases. *Brit. J. Cancer,* **58**, 556

59. Mosekilde L., Eriksen E. F. and Charles P. (1991). Hypercalcemia of malignancy: pathophysiology, diagnosis and treatment. *Crit. Rev. Oncol. Hemat.,* **11**, 1

60. Mundy G. R. (1990). Hypercalcaemia of malignancy. Avioli L. V. and Krane S. M., *Metabolic Bone Disease* (p. 793). Philadelphia: Saunders

61. Murphy P., Wright G. and Rai G. S. (1985). Hypophosphataemic osteomalacia associated with prostatic carcinoma. *Brit. Med. J.,* **290**, 1945

62. Nielsen O. S., Munro A. J. and Tannock I. F. (1991). Bone metastases: pathophysiology and management policy. *J. Clin.*

Oncol., **9**, 509

63. Nielsen O. S. and Poulsen H. S. (1989). Bone metastases. *J. Danish Med. Assoc.,* **151**, 362

64. Nussbaum S. R., Gaz R. D. and Arnold A. (1990). Hypercalcemia and ectopic secretion of parathyroid hormone by an ovarian carcinoma with rearrangement of the gene for parathyroid hormone. *N. Engl. J. Med.,* **323**, 1324

65. Orr F. W., Buchanan M. R. and Weiss L. (1991). *Microcirculation in Cancer Metastasis.* Boca Raton: CRC Press

66. Parbhoo S. (1985). Usefulness of current technique in detecting and monitoring bone metastases from breast cancer. *J. Roy. Soc. Med.,* Suppl. 9, 7

67. Patanaphan V., Salazar O. M. and Risco R. (1988). Breast cancer: metastatic patterns and their prognosis. *S. Med. J.,* **81**, 1112

68. Paterson A. H. G. (1987). Bone metastases in breast cancer, prostate cancer and myeloma. *Bone,* **8** (Suppl.), 17

69. Perez D. J., Milan J. and Ford H. T. (1983). Detection of breast carcinoma metastases in bone: relative merits of X-ray and skeletal scintigraphy. *Lancet,* **2**, 613

70. Perkel V. S., Mohan S., Herring S. J., Baylink D. J. and Linkhart P. A. (1990). Human prostatic cancer cells (PC3) elaborate mitogenic activity which selectively stimulates human bone cells. *Cancer Res.,* **50**, 6902

71. Pfeilshifter J., Mundy G. R. and Roodman G. D. (1989). Interleukin-1 and tumor necrosis factor stimulate the formation of human osteoclast-like cells *in vitro. J. Bone Miner. Res.,* **4**, 113

72. Porro G., Menard S., Tagliabue E., Orefice S., Salvadori B., Squicciarini P., Amdreola S., Rilke F. and Colnaghi M. I. (1988). Monoclonal antibody detection of carcinoma cells in bone marrow biopsy specimens from breast cancer patients. *Cancer,* **61**, 2407

73. Reske S. N., Gloekner W., Schwarz A., Karstens J. H., Steinstrasser A. and Ammon J. (1989). Radioimmunoimaging for diagnosis of bone marrow involvement in breast cancer and malignant lymphoma. *Lancet,* **1**, 299

74. Rubens R. D. (1991). The nature of metastatic bone disease. Rubens R. D. and Fogelman I., *Bone Metastases: Diagnosis and Treatment* (p. 1). London: Springer

75. Sim F. H., Frassica F. J. and Edmonson J. H. (1988). Clinical and laboratory findings. Sim F. H., *Diagnosis and Management of Metastatic Bone Disease* (p. 25) New York: Raven Press

76. Simon M. A. and Bartucci E. J. (1986). The search for the primary tumor in patients with skeletal metastases of unknown origin. *Cancer,* **58**, 1088

77. Singer F. R. (1991). Pathogenesis of hypercalcemia of malignancy. *Semin. Oncol.,* **18**, 4

78. Stahel R. A., Mabry M., Skarin A. T., Speak J. and Bernal S. D. (1985). Detection of bone marrow metastasis in small-cell lung cancer by monoclonal antibodies. *J. Clin. Oncol.,* **3**, 455

79. Stewart A. F., Vignery A. and Silverglate A. (1982). Quantitative bone histomorphometry in humoral hypercalcema of malignancy: uncoupling of bone cell activity. *J. Clin. Endocrinol. Metab.,* **55**, 219

80. Stoll B. A. (1983). Natural history, prognosis, and staging of bone metastases. Stoll B. A. and Parbhoo S., *Bone Metastases: Monitoring and Treatment* (p. 1). New York: Raven Press

81. Tachimori Y., Watanabe H., Kato H., Yamaguchi H., Nagasaki K., Honda S., Itabashi M. and Yamaguchi K. (1991). Hypercalcemia in patient with esophageal carcinoma: the pathophysiologic role of parathyroid hormone-related protein. *Cancer,* **68**, 2625

82. Tofe A. J., Francis M. D. and Harvey W. J. (1975). Correlation of neoplasms with incidence and localisation of skeletal metastases. *J. Nucl. Med.,* **16**, 986

83. Trump D. L. (1983). Mechanisms of bone destruction by cancer. Stoll B. A. and Parbhoo S., *Bone Metastases: Monitoring and Treatment* (p. 39). New York: Raven Press

84. Untch M., Bartl R. and Eiermann W. (1986). Immunhistochemischer Nachweis von Knochenmarkmetastasen beim primären Mammakarzinom. Wüst G., *Tumormarker* (p 208). Darmstadt: Steinkopff

85. Untch M., Harbeck N. and Eiermann W. (1988). Micrometastases in bone marrow in patients with breast cancer. *Brit. Med. J.,* **296**, 290

86. Vaughan J. (1983). Mechanisms of osteoblastic response to tumor. Stoll B. A. and Parbhoo S., *Bone Metastases: Monitoring and Treatment* (p. 59). New York: Raven Press

87. Weidner H. (1991). Review and update: oncogenic osteomalacia-rickets. *Ultrastruct. Pathol.,* **15**, 317

88. Weiss L. and Gilbert H. A. (1981). *Bone Metastasis.* Boston: Hall

89. Willis R. A. (1973). *The Spread of Tumours in the Human Body.* London: Butterworths

90. Wold L. E. (1988). Pathology. Sim F. H., *Diagnosis and Manage-*

ment of Metastatic Bone Disease (p. 15). New York: Raven Press
91. Zajicek G. (1987). Long survival with micrometastasis. At least 9%
of breast cancer patients carry metastases for more than 10 years.
Cancer J., **1**, 381

The following two references reflect the efforts being made to detect
bone marrow involvement by metastases:

Belske K., Myklebust A. T., Aamdal S., Langholm R., Jakobson E. and
Fodstad O. (1992). Detection of bone marrow metastases in small
lung cancer patients. Comparison of immunologic and morphologic
methods. *Amer. J. Pathol.*, **141**, 531
Lindemann F., Schlimok G., Dirschedl P., Witte J. and Riethmüller G.
(1992). Prognostic significance of micrometastatic tumour cells in
bone marrow of colorectal cancer patients. *Lancet*, **340**, 685

Index

Numbers in *italic* type refer to figures in colour plates

The manufacturer's authorised representative in the EU is Springer
Nature Customer Service Centre GmbH, Europaplatz 3, 69115 Heidelberg,
Germany. If you have any concerns regarding our products, please
contact ProductSafety@springernature.com

Printed and bound by CPI Group (UK) Ltd, Croydon, CR0 4YY

27/04/2026

02097584-0002